RODALE'S
21st CENTURY HERBAL

A PRACTICAL GUIDE
for HEALTHY LIVING USING NATURE'S
MOST POWERFUL PLANTS

MICHAEL J. BALICK, PhD

Foreword by ANDREW WEIL, MD ◆ *Edited by* VICKI MATTERN
and Featuring Top Healing Herbs from TIERAONA LOW DOG, MD

RODALE.

© 2014 by Rodale Inc.

All rights reserved. No part of this publication may be reproduced or transmitted in any
form or by any means, electronic or mechanical, including photocopying, recording, or any other
information storage and retrieval system, without the written permission of the publisher.

Rodale books may be purchased for business or promotional use or for special sales.
For information, please write to:
Special Markets Department, Rodale, Inc., 733 Third Avenue, New York, NY 10017

Printed in the United States of America

Rodale Inc. makes every effort to use acid-free ♾, recycled paper ♻.

Illustrations by Lizzie Harper, www.lizzieharper.co.uk

Photography Credits can be found on page 474.

Book design by Christina Gaugler

Library of Congress Cataloging-in-Publication Data is on file with the publisher.

ISBN 978-1-60961-804-9 hardcover

Distributed to the trade by Macmillan

2 4 6 8 10 9 7 5 3 1   hardcover

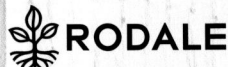

RODALE.

We inspire and enable people to improve their lives and the world around them.

rodalebooks.com

In all that we do, it has been said

that we stand on the shoulders of the

giants who have come before us, building

on their accomplishments. It is in that

spirit that this book honors all of those

people from so many different walks of

life who have helped bring greater clarity

to our understanding of the relationship

between plants and people and the

usefulness of herbs.

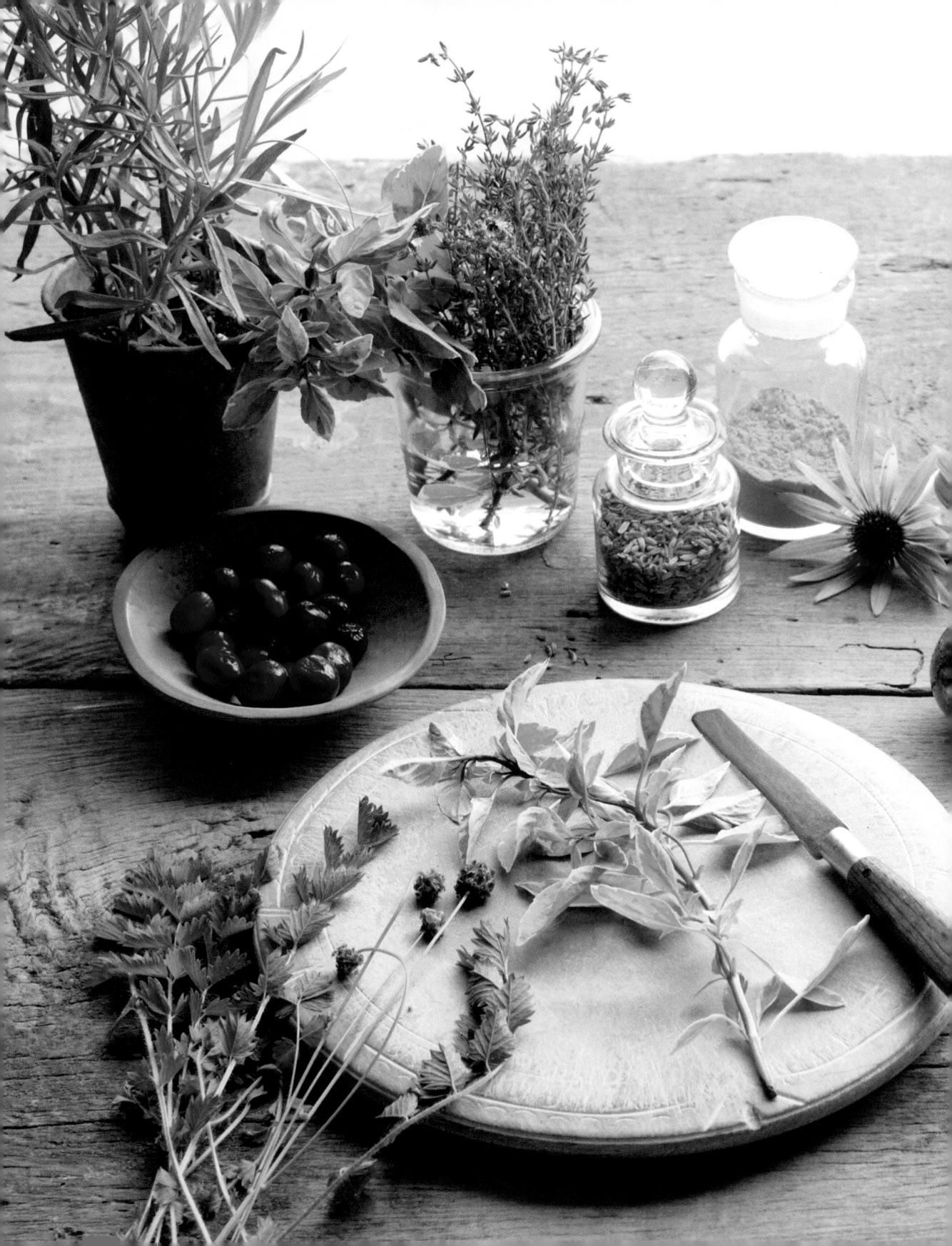

Contents

FOREWORD

Herbs have not only made me a better doctor, but they have also enriched my life in general. I am an avid gardener and home cook, and I enjoy growing and using culinary herbs, both familiar and exotic. Herbs are diverse and fascinating, as are the ways that people interact with them. Whenever I travel, I'm always on the lookout for culturally specific uses of herbs that are new to me, and I'm as likely to find them in developed societies as in more traditional ones.

Dr. Michael Balick loves plants as much as I do. He is one of our foremost ethnobotanical researchers—the best expert I can think of to introduce readers to the world of herbs. Mike and I both had the good fortune to be students of the late Dr. Richard Evans Schultes, director of the Harvard Botanical Museum and the godfather of modern ethnobotany. Dick Schultes inspired in us a passion for understanding the usefulness of plants and teaching their uses to others. I completed my undergraduate studies in ethnobotany under his direction and then attended Harvard Medical School, gaining botanical knowledge and experience that have served me very well in my medical career; they are a foundation of the integrative medicine that I practice and teach.

While still in medical school, I began to travel throughout the world to learn about the medicinal plants used by indigenous peoples. Later, I joined the research faculty of the Harvard Botanical Museum and continued to work with Dick Schultes. I became proficient in botanical medicine and soon was relying more on

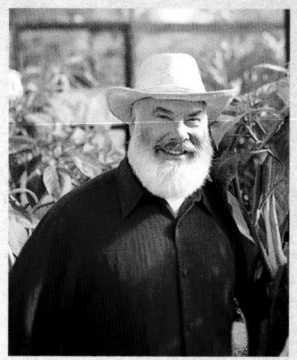

herbal remedies than on pharmaceutical drugs in my practice. Along the way, I also learned as much as I could about culinary and other uses of herbs.

I came to recognize profound differences between whole plants and chemicals isolated from them. The chemistry of plants is wonderfully complex, and the therapeutic actions of herbal remedies are shaped by that complexity, making them safer and often more effective than the highly purified compounds in pharmaceutical drugs. In many areas of contemporary science, theories and models based in complexity have proved very successful in describing and predicting diverse natural phenomena—from weather to the behavior of social insects. Oddly, medicine has made little use of complexity theory, even though doctors deal with the most complex production of nature, the human organism. Integrative medicine is attempting to remedy that by developing research models to evaluate complex treatment protocols, for example, and also by teaching physicians how natural remedies interact with the body in ways different from isolated chemical compounds. It's an exciting—and promising—new approach.

So, delve into the wonderful topics in *Rodale's 21ˢᵗ-Century Herbal*, and see for yourself the rich history and emerging understanding of herbs as ingredients in cuisine, as medicines, and as natural substances for cleaning and adding beauty to the home. I'm right there with you, expanding my knowledge and appreciation for the world's most powerful plants.

Andrew Weil, MD

INTRODUCTION

HISTORICALLY, THE PLANTS WE CALL HERBS have been a keystone of human civilization. They have nurtured, sustained, and healed us and have improved our quality of life in so many ways. The power of that bond between plants and people quickly becomes evident to an ethnobotanist—a scientist who studies the relationship between plants, people, and culture.

As an ethnobotanist, I have been privileged to learn about nature and how people use natural resources. Since the early 1970s, my work has taken me to many fascinating, complex, and distant locations—from deserts that receive less than 2 inches of rain each year to lush tropical rainforests that could receive that same amount of rain on any given day. The focus of my research is on gaining knowledge about botanical diversity and learning about the people who live in these wilderness habitats and depend on plants for their daily survival.

My fascination with the green world started early in life. My youngest memories are of wonderful times spent in my grandparents' garden, watching—with awe—the way seeds responded to a bit of moisture and soil and how vegetables such as cucumbers noticeably grew in size from one day to the next. I am fortunate to be able to continue this childhood interest as a botanist and horticulturist trained first at the University of Delaware and later as a graduate student at Harvard University.

Since 1980, my home has been The New York Botanical Garden (NYBG), acknowledged to be one of the world's premier horticultural, educational, and scientific institutions. Geographically, The New York Botanical Garden's research program spans the world, and through its sophisticated laboratories, collections, and international expeditions, NYBG scientists investigate plants, from the molecular level to whole

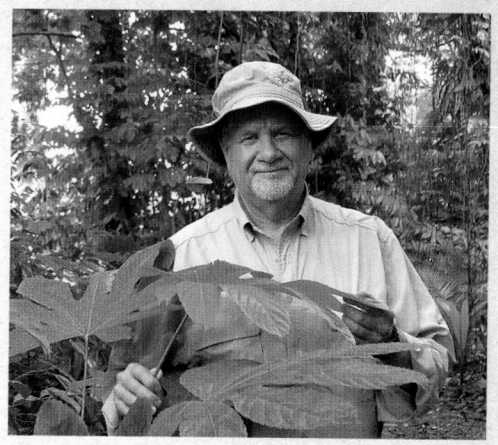

organisms, as well as study and conserve the habitats in which those plants are found. Being an ethnobotanist means living with the people you are working with, and for me this has involved lengthy stays in Central and South America, Oceania, Asia, and the Middle East. But I also believe you can do ethnobotanical research in your own backyard—in most places, including modern cities, you can find people knowledgeable about the historic or contemporary uses of plants. At NYBG we developed a field of study now known as "urban ethnobotany." For 2 decades, we've investigated the ways people use plants in New York City—one of the world's great urban centers (for me, it's an urban laboratory)—where more than 800 different languages are spoken, representing a vast diversity of cultures.

Most of the cultures I've visited recognize hundreds of native and introduced plants used for healing, food, construction, and to improve their quality of life. Just as gardeners eagerly share their horticultural knowledge (and plant cuttings) with other gardeners, the people of the traditional, preindustrial cultures I've lived with have shared their plant knowledge with me. A common language seems to connect those interested in plants, sometimes to the exclusion of other distractions in life.

Many people today suffer a disconnection from nature. Plants offer a life-giving elixir that can sustain us physically, mentally, and spiritually. As an ethnobotanist, I've had many opportunities to learn about plants. Seeing, touching, smelling, harvesting, and discovering how to prepare and use them has resulted in what I would argue is a fuller life. My intention for this book, written with my friends at Rodale, was to produce a guide for healthy living, using nature's most powerful plants: herbs. Getting to know and use these amazing plants—for flavor, health, beauty, and much more—will not only enrich your life in unimaginable ways, but also bring you closer to nature.

Digging into the world of herbs can mean researching the diversity of species you want to grow; planning and planting your garden; nurturing your plants as they grow and mature; and harvesting your herbs and preparing delicious foods, healing teas and salves, fragrant soaps and shampoos, as well as natural products for your home. You'll enjoy the beauty of herbs in your garden and the tranquility you feel as you tend them. You'll value their culinary, aromatic, healing, and cleansing powers. And you'll love sharing your discoveries and accomplishments with a community of like-minded individuals.

Although people have used herbs for health and wellness for tens of thousands of years, the earliest known written instructions for using these powerful plants date back 5,000 years, when they were inscribed on clay tablets by Sumerian healers in the region known today as Iraq. In ancient Egypt, around that same time, medical practitioners wrote of their formulas on papyrus sheets; the most ancient of those documents is known as the Ebers Papyrus, thought to be written around 1500 BCE. In China, more than 4,000 years ago, healers also made careful notes of the plants and plant combinations they used.

Works known as "herbals" were first produced in ancient Greece, ca. 350 BCE. Herbals were medical textbooks of the day, containing descriptions and illustrations of plants, along with recipes and dosages for their use in treating diseases. They also contained information on the culinary uses of plants, as well as their uses as tonics, for cleansing, and in magic, plus information about their toxic qualities. Herbals continued to play an important role in the education of health-care providers and the public well into the 1600s, when the fields of botany and medicine, once allied, began to diverge. The 1800s saw a revival in popular interest in healing with plants and traditional remedies that continues today.

Rodale's 21st-Century Herbal is a celebration of the rich and magnificent history of herbals, providing both ancient wisdom and modern science about herbs and their uses. The book is divided into three sections. The first section discusses how people around the world have utilized herbs—from their uses for healing in prehistory through the development of our earliest medical systems and their use by billions of people today. This section also explores the botany and chemistry of herbs; how plants are classified; and the reasons why herbs can exert a powerful effect on your body, palate, mind, and desires.

The middle section is an encyclopedia of more than 180 of the world's most useful and interesting herbs. It describes their historical importance, healing properties, and culinary and ornamental uses. It also tells how to grow and harvest many of them at home and what cautions to take with certain species.

The final section is a guide for using and enjoying herbs. This section offers dozens of recipes and step-by-step techniques to help you cook and heal with herbs, to make your own beauty-care products, and to make natural products for cleaning, scenting, and decorating your home. It also provides in-depth information on how to grow herbs organically—in gardens, on terraces and patios, and indoors—from planting seeds and cuttings to propagation and harvest. At the end of the book, you'll find a chapter on herb garden design with 12 illustrated sample designs and complete plant lists, followed by a section on herbal resources.

While I can't take you to the places I've seen through my studies or have you at my side as I learn from elders about a plant's use, I try to do just that in a small way by sharing some personal stories in many of the chapters. Far from being a profession filled with excitement, adventure, and life on the edge, as it is sometimes portrayed by the media, ethnobotanists spend a great deal of quiet time listening to the stories we are told, asking questions, and honoring the wisdom of others. Much of my work has been to record that wisdom, as it relates to plants and their uses, before it is lost—particularly among cultures that have never written down this knowledge and people who do not formally teach it to their children. Tragically, in some of our research studies, such as in the remote Pacific Ocean region, we've found that those who stray from a traditional lifestyle and adopt the Western way of life do not live as long as their ancestors and have more illnesses and an overall reduced quality of life.

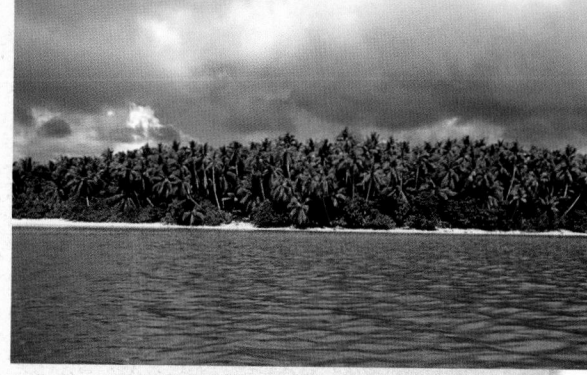

In this book, I've tried to convey the excitement, joy, and purpose that can come from incorporating herbs more prominently into your life and to give you some of the tools and ideas to spark your own explorations. The statement that "education is the kindling of a flame, not the filling of a vessel," attributed to Socrates, has been my approach to university teaching. I encourage students to experience ethnobotany firsthand by developing and implementing their own research projects, rather than by memorizing facts and training to become talented test takers. *Rodale's 21st-Century Herbal* follows that philosophy, and I hope you will use it to explore and learn about plants from around the world, to play in your own personal sandbox as excitedly as perhaps you once did, and to enjoy the plethora of benefits herbs can offer.

Michael J. Balick, PhD

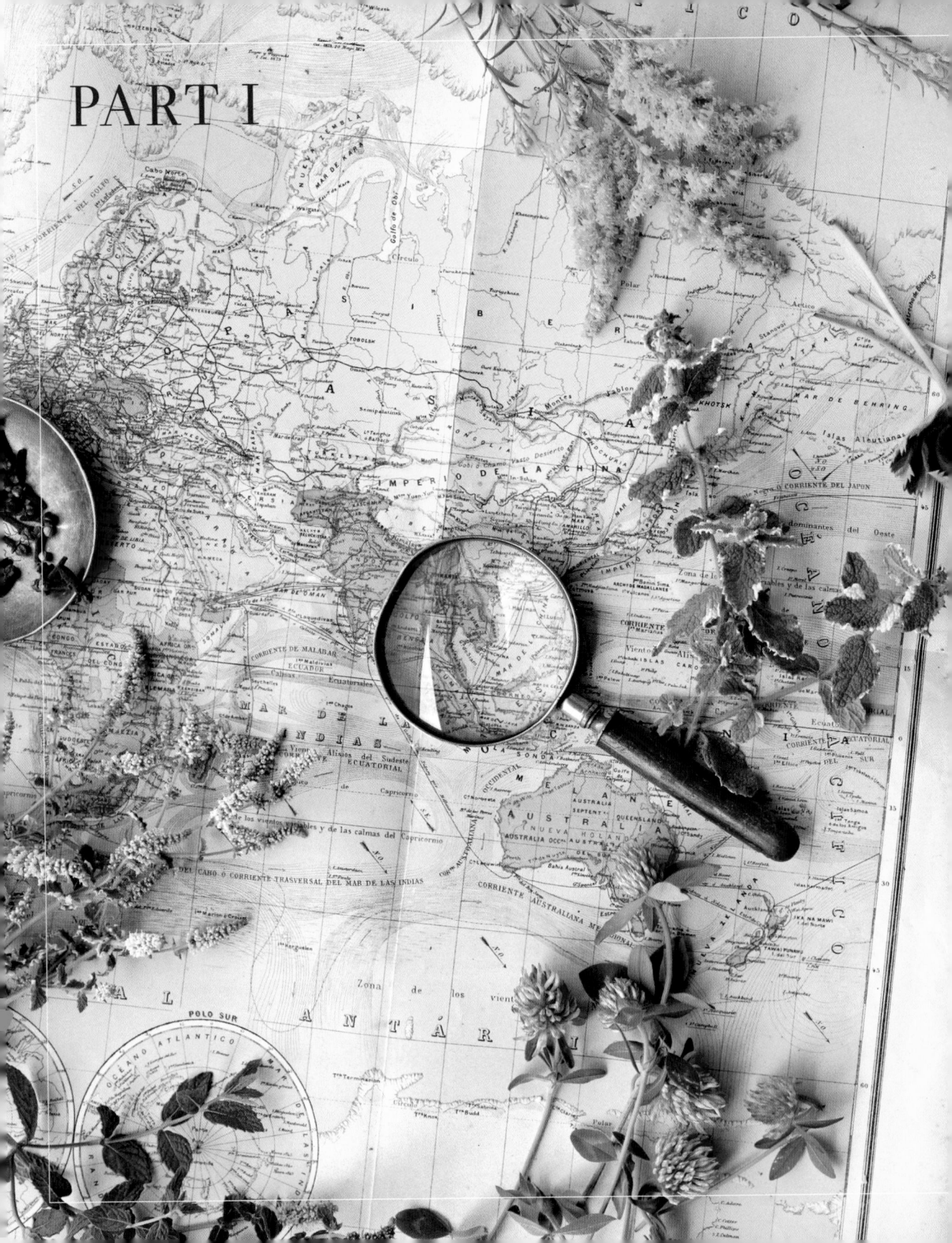

PART I

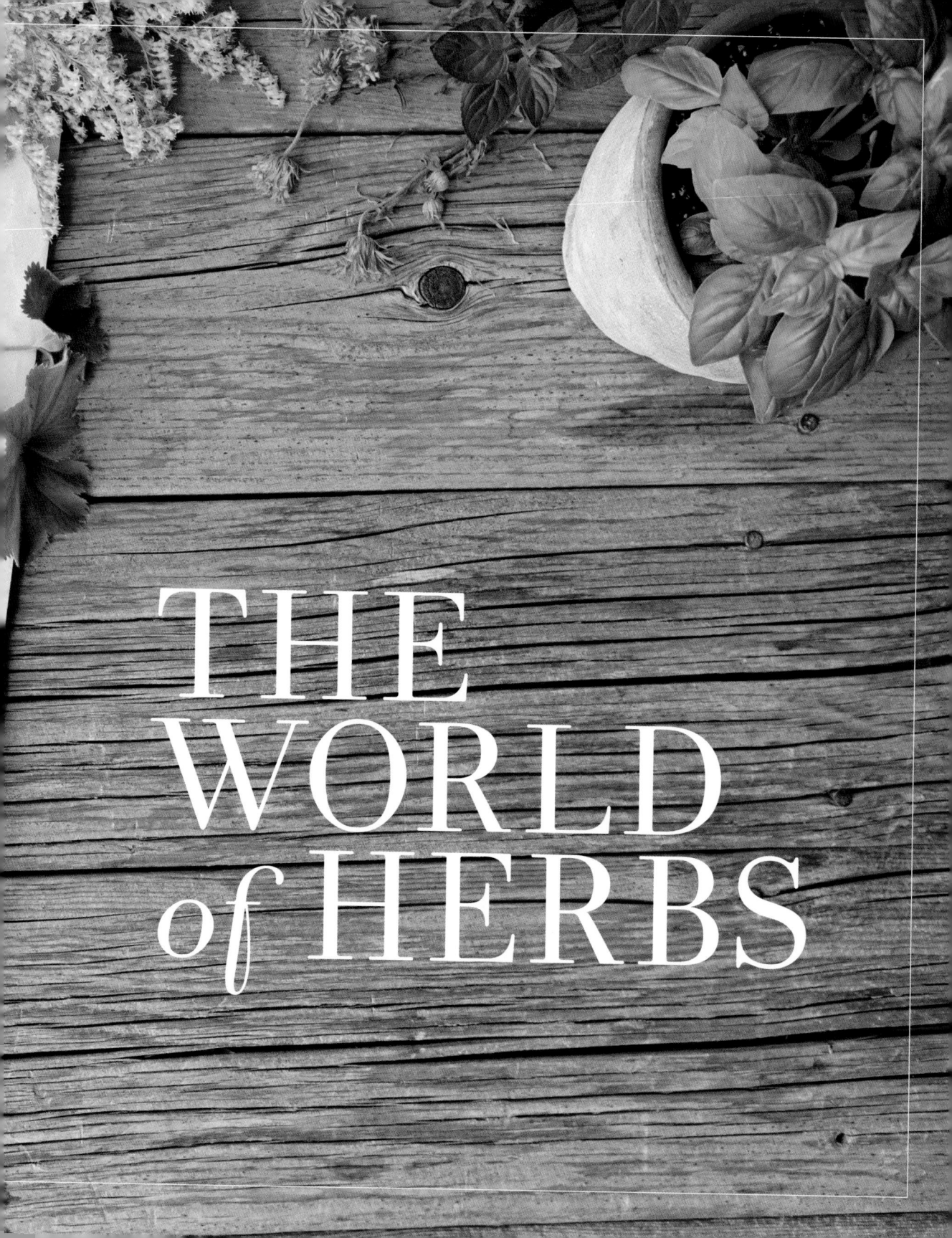

THE
WORLD
of HERBS

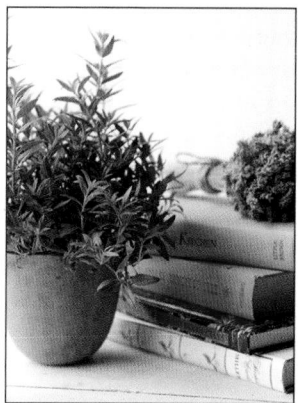

CHAPTER 1

A GLOBAL HISTORY

As an ethnobotanist working to chronicle the relationship between plants, people, and culture, my conversations with traditional healers about the diversity and uses of the plants in their environments—from deserts to temperate regions to rainforests—have been nothing short of extraordinary, even otherworldly. Most of the people I work with are from cultural or ethnic groups that have never codified their healing systems or, as in the case of the Maya, whose great books of learning were destroyed by their conquerors. In most cases, we share common ground—the desire to preserve knowledge, plants, and practices that have sustained people and cultures through millennia and into the present with the hope that, somehow, they will help guide us through the increasingly complex trajectory that is the earth's future.

It is hard not to be affected by an elder's unbridled joy when we present their wisdom back to them and their communities in the form of a published book, video, or scientific paper, the results of a collaborative project and partnership. I feel very fortunate to be one of the relatively few individuals who do this work as their profession, a vocation with a diversity of venues ranging from New York City to some of the planet's most remote regions.

John Gerard (1545–1612) was similarly motivated to capture the essence of herbal medicines traditionally used in England—both native herbs as well as those rare and exotic species brought back from the great explorations of the Elizabethan era. Gerard was a physician, herbalist, and gardener, skills common to those practicing the healing arts of his day. Physicians needed to know the plants they prescribed, so not only did they learn about plant uses, but they also spent a significant amount of their training observing herbs in botanical gardens and other living plant collections associated with medical schools. Gerard's greatest accomplishment was to take the verification process one step further—he codified the herbal knowledge of the time in his famous book *The Herball, or Generall Historie of Plantes*, first published in 1597.

Gerard compiled the work of others and added new knowledge gained through his conversations with healers. *The Herball* contained information on hundreds of herbs, with surprisingly accurate botanical woodcuts providing details of their appearances. This was a way to "publish" a verification of herbs to help physicians grappling with a major problem at the time—how to make certain the plants they prescribed were the ones actually being provided to patients. Mistake the highly toxic digitalis for a plantain species commonly prescribed to treat ulcers, for instance, and the result could be fatal. Gerard's text covered a wide range of culinary and medicinal uses, such as the use of little "flat cakes" of European cyclamen roots as "amorous medicine."

I admit to being a bibliophile, and my sprawling botanical library is the result of decades of travel and obsessive collection. Once confined to a room or two, it now spills out all over my home, into narrow hallways, and throughout my office and laboratory at The New York Botanical Garden. Of these books, my favorite is *The Herball*, a very special original copy obtained for me by a close friend some years ago. I open it, and immediately I am drawn 400 years into the past by the feel of the paper, the smell of the pages, and the extraordinary leather binding—but most of all by the words this priceless book contains. This individual volume also consists of a special sheaf of 18th-century notes made by one of its previous owners. These papers, listing therapeutic family recipes of the time, make it a self-contained and one-of-a-kind reference guide that has survived world wars, pandemics, economic collapse, and the advent of the Internet. It is a remarkable and resilient piece of scholarship.

Health care has made extraordinary and unthinkable advances since 1597, when that book first appeared. Alchemy, famous for its quest to turn lead into gold, also focused on making plant extracts and standardizing remedies, laying the foundation for the eventual development of allopathic (Western or modern) pharmaceutical medicine.

But herbalism persisted as a medical system throughout the world. Today, for example, among indigenous groups that I work with, plant-based traditional medicines are an essential part of healing practices. In fact, scientists estimate that several billion people today use traditional herbal medicines for some aspect of their primary health care. In the West, the field of integrative medicine pioneered by Andrew Weil, MD, partners the use of scientifically validated herbal remedies with conventional allopathic care, optimizing health-care delivery by reuniting the approaches originally rooted in alchemy and herbalism that had been separated for centuries.

Herbs have played a key role in human life since before recorded history. Yarrow, groundsel, and marshmallow, all thought to be ancient medicinal plants, were found in the 60,000-year-old grave of a Neanderthal man unearthed in present-day Iraq. Ancient etchings on cave walls depict people gathering roots, rubbing leaves on their bodies, and arranging plants in ceremonial patterns. Ancestral languages such as Proto-Austronesian had words for herbs, including one for ginger, an herb that may have been carried and traded during the earliest human migrations across Asia. Five thousand years ago, ancient Sumerian healers wrote prescriptions on tablets of clay for treat-ments that used caraway and thyme. As far back as 2700 BCE, Chinese healers produced written records of dozens of plants used to treat the sick. Ancient Egyptian paintings depict some of the earliest herb gardens, including one from 1400 BCE that clearly shows pomegranate trees and grapevines surrounding a fishpond.

The march of progress and the passing of time have not slowed humanity's interest in herbs. Botanical researchers are pursuing a global inventory of plants, discovering more than 2,000 new species each year and cataloging some of their traditional uses. In some ways, we have learned more about certain planets than we have about the earth's biodiversity, and the ongoing age of exploration—aided by modern tools and techniques—continues to yield information that can benefit us all.

EXPLORING THE WORLD OF HERBS

For millennia, people on every continent have incorporated beneficial herbs into their daily lives. Whether used medicinally, in cooking, to enhance beauty, or in gardening and handicrafts, herbs and their lore have been woven into the economic, scientific, and social structures of every culture around the world.

The first organized systems of medicine in China and Mesopotamia centered around herbal treatments. Some of the oldest religions in India and Egypt viewed many herbs as sacred gifts from the gods. For centuries, flavor-enhancing herbs such as pepper and cinnamon, both from the Far East, have been coveted by Western cooks. During eras when regular bathing was rare, perfumes extracted from fragrant herbs made social life in Europe and Africa a little more pleasant. And in the Pacific, royalty bathed themselves daily with coconut oil infused with aromatic and cleansing herbs. Around the world, herbs have long been grown in gardens or collected from the wild, highly valued for their beauty and usefulness.

Much of the knowledge held by early healers was passed down orally from generation to generation, often in sacred teachings. In this way, many medicinal herbs took on an additional, spiritual significance. In traditional Persian weddings, for example, incense made from rue seeds was burned, and bunches of herbs such as mint, parsley, and nigella were spread before the bride and groom to protect them from evil spirits.

One particular ritual, the taking of tea and coffee, has been a part of many cultures on earth. It is said that the tea plant originated when an early Buddhist monk, Bodhidharma, cut off his eyelids and hurled them to the ground in an effort to stay awake while meditating. This produced the first tea plants, which had the power to keep him and his students awake and alert. In England, Japan, and China, the drinking of tea evolved into elaborate rituals that required years of education and practice to perfect. According to legend, coffee originated in Ethiopia when a shepherd named Kaldi noticed that his goats became euphoric after eating the red berries of the wild coffee bush, and he observed that the fruits' seeds had stimulant properties. Ethiopian tribesmen first used coffee as an energizer more than 1,000 years ago; they crushed its red berries with animal fat and molded the mixture into balls, which they then ate as food. By the 1600s, Italian traders had introduced coffee from Arabia to Europe, and it was well on its way to becoming a popular drink.

Over the centuries, people around the world have cooked, steamed, ground, sprinkled, and infused herbs into every conceivable food dish. As early as 3000 BCE, ancient Babylonians included garlic in meals, while in 400 BCE, the Romans created a condiment from mustard by mixing its ground seeds with grape juice. In ancient Europe, parsley, sage, rosemary, and thyme were all widely used to turn cooked meats into palatable meals. Hundreds of years ago, a traveler to East Asia would have been treated to meals saturated in sesame seeds and ginger, and dinner on a Caribbean island would have contained plenty of jerk seasoning made from dried chiles, pepper, and allspice.

Herbs and spices were used not only to enhance flavor, but also to help preserve foods—particularly meats and fish—from spoilage. These properties were validated by Cornell University scientists who published a paper in the late 1990s showing that herbs such as garlic, onions, allspice, and oregano killed most of the potentially harmful bacteria found in foods across a variety of cultures, with other spices such as cinnamon, thyme, cumin, tarragon, and chile peppers substantially reducing the bacterial load, resulting in more healthy consumers.

Many other herbs have been used to beautify human appearances. The ancient Egyptians developed cosmetics made from the oils of herbs and other plants, including olives, almonds, cucumbers, figs, limes, lilies, and generous doses of frankincense and myrrh. Early Arab scientists invented a distillation process for extracting essential oils from flowers, such as roses, which they then used to make soaps, bath oils, and aromatic rose water. In medieval France, both men and women used pomanders—small balls of ambergris with herbs and perfumes added—to mask the stench of unsanitary surroundings.

The world's earliest civilizations also built herb gardens to beautify the land. The legendary Hanging Gardens of Babylon did not actually hang but rather grew on terraced rooftops built to resemble a mountain. The pleasure gardens of Persia, dating from 500 BCE, introduced the concept of arranging plants in regular, straight rows, while the people of ancient Rome grew herbs in the raised beds of their kitchen gardens. In medieval Europe, physic gardens produced a wide variety of culinary and medicinal botanicals.

Culturally and geographically, there are no limits to the uses humans have found for herbs. From the ancient Abyssinians, who stuffed their pillows with fresh celery leaves, to Native Americans who used pennyroyal as an insect repellent, people have always made herbs an essential part of their lives. Today, herbs of all kinds are found in foods and beverages, healing preparations, cosmetics, perfumes, and clothing dyes. They're found growing in gardens and in the pages of medical texts and history books. There is no part of human culture that herbs have not transformed.

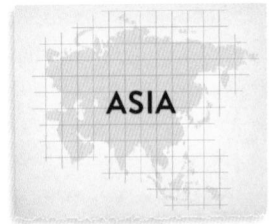

ASIA

A great deal of the world's herb lore, and many of its most highly regarded herbs, can be traced to Asia. The world's largest continent is home to a wide range of plant habitats, from the barren wilderness of Arctic tundra to deserts to lush forests of every type: coniferous, oak, tropical rainforest, and bamboo. With so many people and such a diversity of plants, it's not surprising that Asia has produced some of the oldest known herbal rituals, recipes, gardens, and systems of medicine. The most influential cultures in the region are two of the most populous countries: China and India. Over the millennia, their ancient herbal beliefs and practices spread throughout Asia, adapting to reflect the local flavor of countries such as Korea, Japan, Thailand, and Tibet.

China

According to legend, the first emperor of China, a sage named Fu Hsi (ca. 4000 BCE), single-handedly changed his people from hunter-gatherers to agriculturalists. The plants they grew became integral to the spiritual beliefs of their early society, which included the I Ching, a system of divination.

The stalk of the yarrow plant (*Achillea millefolium*) was particularly significant in the I Ching: Fu Hsi instructed wise men to cast sticks of yarrow on the ground and interpret their arrangement in relation to each other in order to predict future events.

Chinese herbs and philosophy have always gone hand in hand, and they mix particularly well in the history of Chinese cooking. The great philosopher Confucius (551–479 BCE) believed that a good cook must be a skilled herbal matchmaker: Condiments and spices in food must blend harmoniously, or there would be no flavor. He would eat no meal that did not contain a little ginger.

Ancient practitioners of Taoism, another major Chinese philosophy, saw cooking less as the pursuit of beauty and more as the pursuit of health. Leaves, roots, stems, flowers, seeds, bark, and fungi were prepared, tested, and consumed for their health-promoting effects. As a result, most varieties of Chinese cuisine contained plenty of vegetables, grains, and herbs, all cooked in ways that ensured their medicinal value would not be lost.

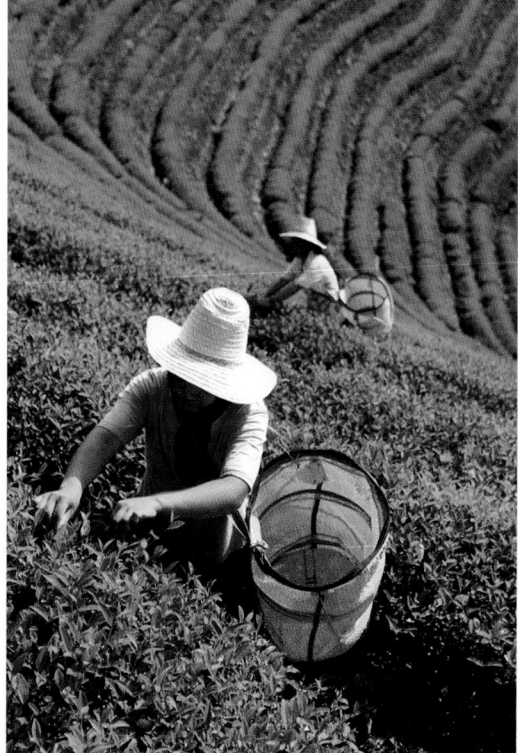

Tea is an important crop throughout Asia. Above, tea leaves are harvested on a plantation in China.

Herbal tea has a long history of use in China, dating back more than 4,000 years. According to legend, one of the first Chinese emperors, Yan Di (2852–2737 BCE), discovered the medicinal powers of tea by accident while he was testing the effects of other herbs on himself. After eating a poisonous plant, he fell to the ground on the verge of death. When a drop of water from the leaf of a tea plant fell into his open mouth, he was cured. During the early Zhou Dynasty (1046–256 BCE), Chinese people used tea as a religious offering and fresh vegetable. Later, during the Tang Dynasty (618–907 CE), the drinking of tea became a cultural event. Tea shops opened throughout China, and a seminal book, *Tea Classics,* by Lu Yu, outlined the rules of growing and processing tea, as well as the etiquette of tea tasting. Tea ceremonies grew successively more refined, elaborate, and lengthy.

The first Chinese gardens were cultivated during the Zhou dynasty. Members of the aristocracy sectioned off particularly beautiful parts of the natural world to use for hunting and strolling. During the Han Dynasty (206 BCE–220 CE), wealthy Chinese developed an interest in constructing more personal gardens where they could display rare plants. By the 4th century, the literati of China became associated with scholar gardens—small, enclosed areas containing unusual rocks, water features, and interesting plants that reflected the personalities and knowledge of their owners. Chinese gardens across all eras were meant to be mirrors of the larger natural world, with the random placement of plants encouraged over geometric shapes and lines, and woody trees and green herbs favored over cultivated blossoms and flowerbeds. Chinese gardens, much like Chinese herbal medicines, were designed to create the perfect balance between the two opposing Taoist life energies, yin and yang.

Chinese Herbal Healing

Traditional Chinese medicine (TCM) has very deep historical roots. Sometime between 2700 and 2600 BCE, the emperor Shen-Nung reputedly created the first Chinese written pharmacopoeia, called the *Pen-ts'ao* (*Herbal*). It was followed by the *Huang-ti Nei ching* (*The Yellow Emperor's Classic of Internal Medicine*), allegedly written by the legendary Emperor Huang Ti (2697–2597 BCE). Near the end of the Han dynasty, a physician named Chang Chung-ching wrote the *Shang Han Lun* (or *Treatise on Colds and Fevers*), which eventually became the theoretical framework for all herbal prescriptions in TCM. It contained more than 100 formulas, many of which are used today.

In 1590, the herbalist Li Shih-Chen (1518–1593) published the *Bencao Gangmu* (*Compendium of Materia Medica*). It contained 11,000 prescriptions and formulas, analyzed 1,094 plant substances, filled 53 volumes, and took nearly 27 years to write. It became the first major Chinese work to be translated into Western languages, and its publication coincided with a dramatic rise in Chinese global exportation of herbs and spices.

In the early 20th century, interest in traditional herbal medicine waned for a time. China's scientists were instructed to examine native plants using Western scientific methods, which resulted in many important discoveries, such as the isolation of the drug ephedrine from the Chinese ephedra (*Ephedra sinica*) plant. Ephedrine quickly became one of the world's most effective decongestants and asthma treatments, and China became its principal supplier. The country also constructed modern hospitals and clinics and began using more advanced instruments and synthetic drugs.

After the People's Republic of China was established in 1949, China's leaders recognized that the most effective health-care system for the populous nation was a combination of Western and traditional methods. Colleges were established to train doctors in both disciplines, and an army of "barefoot doctors" was created to serve the rural population. As the demand for herbs increased, the Chinese government established a program of medicinal plant cultivation, setting aside thousands of acres solely for the production of medicinal herbs. Today, of the 35,000 species of plants

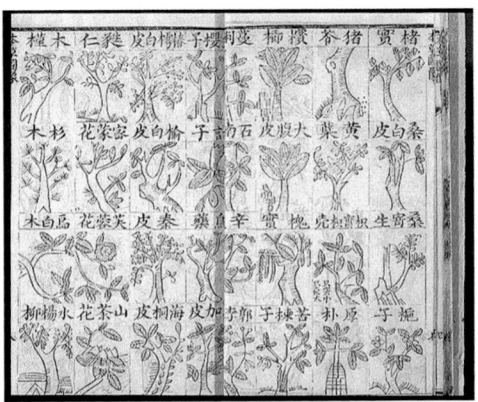

These pages from the 1740 classic text of traditional Chinese medicine, *Hu, Tsung-wen Shen-nung pen ts'ao pei yao i fang ho pien*, or *Herbal and Prescriptions*, illustrate plants used medicinally.

growing in China's various habitats, some 5,000 are used in TCM and provide 40 percent of all China's pharmaceuticals.

Tibet

Now practiced in many countries worldwide, traditional Tibetan medicine traces its history to 300 BCE. According to ancient legend, Tara, the Buddhist god of compassion, commanded two Indian physicians to go to Tibet to teach the ways of Buddhism, including the secrets of herbal healing. For their efforts, the doctors were granted immortality. Current folklore says that they live on today in the sandalwood forests of the region.

The doctors' most famous relative was Yuthog Yonten Gonpo, who reportedly lived to the ripe old age of 125 during the 9th century. Yuthog established the first Tibetan medical school and wrote no fewer than 30 seminal herbal books, each incorporating many aspects of traditional Chinese medicine and Indian Ayurveda. His research led him to reorganize and compile the Four Medical Tantras, the basis of Tibetan medicine. The first three tantras focus mainly on the study of behavior, diet, and the causes of diseases. The fourth is completely devoted to the use of herbs in medical treatment through pills, tonics, ointments, and moxibustion, which utilizes a substance called moxa, made from the herb mugwort (*Artemisia vulgaris*). Heat from burning moxa is applied to specific external points on the body, activating the internal organs, increasing blood circulation, and improving the flow of ki, or life force (similar to the Chinese qi, sometimes spelled chi).

Though many of the medicinal herbs used in Tibet came from India and China, about one-third were unique to the region. The herbs were occasionally used to make powders or tonics, but pills, which were composed of as many as 25 herbal ingredients, were by far the most common form of Tibetan treatment.

In an area as difficult to navigate as mountainous Tibet, pills were the easiest form of medication to transport and administer to patients. They could be prepared in advance at a medical facility with access to a wide variety of herbs, then preserved by rolling them back and forth in cloth to reduce the air inside and prevent the growth of bacteria. Local doctors kept as many as 200 different varieties in stock to treat their patients.

India

Very early in its history, India became a coveted destination for traders eager to profit from the region's bounty of native herbs and spices. In the early Middle Ages, the people of Europe and Mediterranean Africa developed a voracious appetite for the exotic spices of India and the Far East, including cinnamon, cloves, pepper, cardamom, nutmeg, and mace. Arabs, who occupied the middle ground between the two regions, became experts in spice trading, establishing overland east-to-west trade routes. Later, sea routes were added.

By the early 1600s, the Dutch East India Company had established a near-monopoly of the spice trade. The British, seeking a piece of this lucrative market, founded the British East India Company. Soon, British-built factories in India were profitably cultivating herbs such as tea and indigo by the ton. Seeking a permanent foothold in the region, the British negotiated a treaty with India that gave the East India Company exclusive rights to build factories in certain major ports.

By 1690, the British East India Company had become almost a subcountry within India. It minted its own money, acquired its own territories, held criminal jurisdiction, and commanded its own substantial army.

In 1773, lobbyists working on behalf of the East India Company convinced the British Parliament to ratify the Tea Act, which gave the company the right to trade tea tax-free to the American

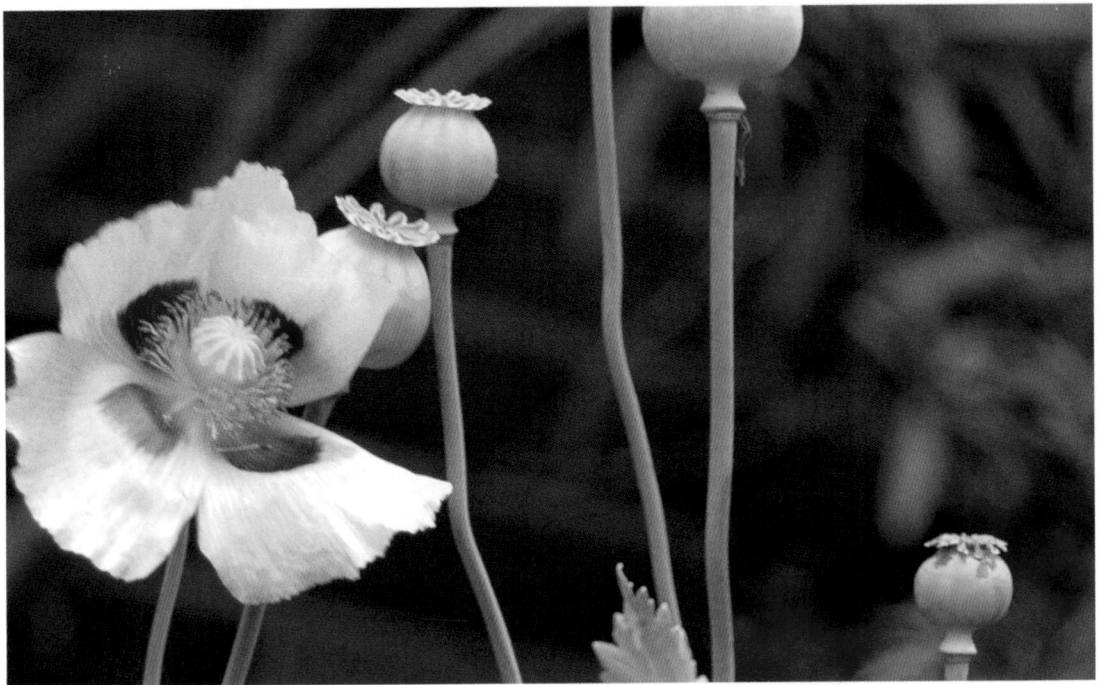

The opium poppy (*Papaver somniferum*), from which morphine and codeine are derived, was first cultivated in lower Mesopotamia more than 5,000 years ago.

OPIUM *and the* EAST

Science has never created a painkiller as effective as opium, a highly addictive natural derivative of the opium poppy. In the early 1800s, most opium poppies came from India, distributed to the world by the British East India Company. The Chinese port of Canton was a key trading hub; tons of opium were exchanged for manufactured goods and tea. As a result, millions of Chinese people became helpless opium addicts, spending their money in squalid urban opium parlors while their families suffered in poverty.

In the late 1830s, the Chinese government made an effort to address the problem. They destroyed opium reserves, prosecuted British traders, and attempted to close the country's borders to opium trade. The British declared war on China, prevailing against them in a series of lopsided battles. In 1842, the Chinese were forced to agree to the Treaty of Nanking, a humiliating agreement that opened new trade ports to the British, exempted British nationals from Chinese law, and more than doubled the trade of opium to China.

The utter defeat of the Chinese in the Opium Wars, however, spurred the modernization of every aspect of Chinese culture. Investing heavily in scientific and technological research, China transformed itself from an undeveloped agricultural society to a world superpower in less than a century. Ironically, the country's newly trained scientists also applied their skills to the study of opium, yielding derivative drugs such as morphine and codeine—important drugs used universally in medical care.

colonies. Outraged American merchants, who could not compete, stormed one of the company's ships and dumped its entire cargo into Boston Harbor. The event, which became known as the Boston Tea Party, was one of the catalysts of the American War of Independence (1775–1783).

Indian Herbal Medicine

The bounty of herbs native to India gave rise to a system of medicinal and spiritual healing known as Ayurveda, meaning "science of life." According to folklore, Ayurvedic herbal remedies were given to the people of India by the gods as early as 10,000 BCE. They were then incorporated into texts called Vedas, upon which the Hindu religion is based. The *Rig Veda,* dating to ca. 2000 BCE, lists more than 1,000 medicinal herbs and tells tales of gifted sages who unlocked the secrets of plants. These trained healers were said to be advanced in their methods: They performed surgery with instruments, cauterized wounds, constructed artificial limbs, and possibly pioneered the use of an anesthetic made from mushrooms.

Between the 4th and 2nd centuries BCE, the *Charaka Samhita* was written. One of the fundamental books on Ayurvedic medicine, the text lists 500 herb- and vegetable-based drugs classified into 50 groups based on their actions on the body. One important drug came from gotu kola (*Centella asiatica*), a key ingredient in a "miracle elixir" purported to extend life and cure leprosy.

Throughout India's history, the influence of Ayurvedic medicine continued to spread, from the expansion of the Roman Empire into the region, to the Islamic invasions of the 16th century, to the period of British control in the 19th century. The Greek physician and botanist Dioscorides (40–90 CE) made many references to Indian herbalism in his *De Materia Medica (The Materials of Medicine). The Book of Simple Drugs,* by 12th-century Arabic pharmacologist Al-Ghafiqi, codified Ayurvedic healing prescriptions for the Islamic world. Today, Ayurvedic medicine is practiced worldwide, using herbal remedies that are much as they were centuries ago.

Other Uses of Herbs in India

India has a long history of vegetarianism, driven mainly by the Buddhist and Hindu religions, which hold many animals as sacred. Evidence suggests that Indian people were eating less meat and more cultivated vegetables, fruits, and cereals as early as 800 BCE. The Muslim invasions of India in the 16th century brought new herbal influences to India's cuisine. The result: an Arabic-influenced Indian cuisine called Mughlai, known for its heavy use of Indian cream, butter, and rice, as well as spices such as cumin, cardamom, coriander, and turmeric. Meat dishes came back into vogue, garnished with pistachios, raisins, almonds, and cashews. Muslims also introduced the idea of ending a meal with dessert, usually a rice cake or wheat bread flavored with sugar, coconut, or rose water.

The cosmetic use of herbs in India coincides with the rise of the Buddhist and Hindu religions.

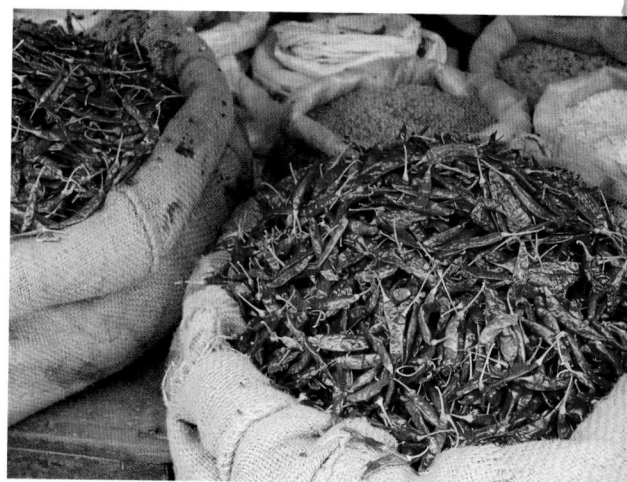

India is the largest consumer, producer, and exporter of chile peppers in the world today. The potency of the peppers is traditionally believed to have supernatural origins.

Paintings found in caves in Ajanta (dating from the 2nd century BCE) and Ellora (dating to the 5th to 7th centuries CE) depict Buddhist men and women applying makeup and perfumes during religious ceremonies. Texts from the period suggest that these cosmetics were made from herbs such as turmeric, saffron, indigo, and nettles. Henna (*Lawsonia inermis*) was widely used as a reddish hair dye and conditioner. Early Hindus used herbal cosmetics as symbols of social class and religious adherence. Applied to the forehead as a sign of auspiciousness, the tilak is a dot of red turmeric powder or sandalwood paste. Perfumes made from agarwood (*Aquilaria malaccensis*) were worn to honor the gods, and incense from the tree was burned in Hindu ceremonies.

Although no archeological evidence remains of the earliest Indian gardens, 3,000-year-old Vedas give accounts of palaces surrounded by gardens of fruit trees and town houses with enclosed outdoor gardens. These cultivated areas were venerated by early Hindus, who saw the trees within gardens as the embodiment of the god Brahma, his roots firmly connected to the primal being of earth.

East and Southeast Asia

Historically, many of China's neighbors borrowed heavily from China's herbal traditions to create their medicinal systems. Over the years, however, Japan, Korea, and Vietnam also developed their own unique uses for herbs.

In Japan, the herbal medicine system of kampo traces its roots to the 7th century, when the empress Suiko sent emissaries to China to study and bring back theories of herbalism. Kampo takes its name from *kan*, meaning "ancient China," and *po*, meaning "medicine." The early practitioners of kampo were Buddhist monks who adhered to a strict vegetarian diet and rejected all Chinese remedies that contained animal products. This—along with the Buddhist ideals of simplicity, safety, and

prevention—led the monks to reduce the tens of thousands of Chinese remedies to several hundred essential herbal treatments that are used in kampo.

In 20th-century Japan, as in China, the use of traditional medicinal methods declined in favor of Western medicine, only to return in recent decades as an integral part of the national health plan. Today, most Japanese physicians use a combination of Western and kampo medicine to treat patients.

Zen Buddhists in the 9th century also carried Chinese tea (*Camellia sinensis*) into Japan, beginning with traditional black tea and evolving into matcha, a powdered green tea. By the 13th century, Japanese samurai warriors had laid the foundations of the formal Japanese tea ceremony, characterized by *wabi*, or quiet, sober refinement.

In Korea and Vietnam, the most important contributions to herbal history were medicinal. Korean healers adapted many of the tenets of Chinese medicine for their own use. Published in 1433, the *Hyangyakjibsongbang* presents more than 10,000 uniquely Korean prescriptions and describes the collection and preparation methods for 700 Korean herbs. The *Uibangryuchi,* a 365-volume medical encyclopedia published a decade later, outlines methods for preventing 95 diseases.

Vietnam's earliest pharmacopoeia is the 14th-century *Thuoc nam,* which describes 650 indigenous herbs and their medicinal uses. The practices described continued even as Western medical techniques and pharmaceuticals were adopted. During World War II, when supplies of antimalarial quinine were cut off, Vietnamese malaria patients were treated using extracts of chang shan (*Dichroa febrifuga*), also referred to in English as Chinese quinine, a shrub found in parts of temperate and tropical Asia.

Western Asia

The civilizations of Mesopotamia, today's Iraq and Syria, were the first to develop irrigated agriculture.

Sometime between 4500 and 3000 BCE, the Sumerians who settled in this fertile area began harvesting crops of barley, growing orchards, and inscribing on stone or clay tablets the medicinal uses of herbs. Their herbal healers were experts at mixing plant resins and animal fat to apply to wounds.

In this same region, from 3000 to 400 BCE, the ancient Babylonians and Assyrians established cities with wondrous gardens. The most famous were the Hanging Gardens of Babylon, said to have been built around 600 BCE by Nebuchadnezzar II as a gift to his favorite wife, Amyitis. He built a mountain of massive stone buildings with terraces so that trees, flowering plants, and herbs could be grown on the rooftops and terraces. Written descriptions of other gardens of the time suggest that the Babylonians grew such herbs as saffron, mandrake, anise, and thyme. One tablet from an Assyrian library, dated ca. 660 BCE, identifies more than 250 plant-based drugs made from opium poppies, myrrh, crocus, cannabis, hellebore, and other herbs.

IMPORTANT HERBS *of* ASIA

HERB	EXAMPLES OF USES
Camphor (*Cinnamomum camphora*)	Muscle and joint pain reliever
Cardamom (*Elettaria cardamomum*)	Flavoring for baked goods and curries
Chinese licorice (*Glycyrrhiza uralensis*)	Treatment for lung conditions and coughs
Cinnamon (*Cinnamomum verum*)	Digestive aid
Ephedra (*Ephedra sinica*)	Bronchial congestion reliever
Forsythia (*Forsythia suspensa*)	Treatment for acute infection
Ginkgo (*Ginkgo biloba*)	Blood circulation stimulant to the brain
Ginseng (*Panax ginseng*)	Chinese culinary ingredient, healthful tonic
Gotu kola (*Centella asiatica*)	Circulatory stimulant
Guggul (*Commiphora wightii*)	Cholesterol reducer
Jasmine (*Jasminum sambac*)	Tea flavoring, used in perfumery
Myrobalan (*Terminalia chebula*)	Considered a cure-all in Ayurvedic medicine
Peony (*Paeonia lactiflora*)	Treatment for gout and osteoarthritis, regulates menses
Pepper (*Piper nigrum*)	Treatment for abdominal pain, vomiting, and diarrhea
Qing hao (*Artemisia annua*)	Treatment for fevers, including those from malaria
Rhubarb (*Rheum* spp.)	Purgative
Sacred lotus (*Nelumbo nucifera*)	Treatment for blood in the urine
Sandalwood (*Santalum album*)	Pain reliever, used in perfumery
Serpentwood (*Rauvolfia serpentina*)	Sedative and tranquilizer, treatment for hypertension
Turmeric (*Curcuma longa*)	Wound healer, antiseptic

After Alexander the Great (356–323 BCE) conquered most of the lands between Greece and Persia, both Greek herbal medicine and the gardening styles of Mesopotamia spread throughout the known world. By late Biblical times (300 BCE–100 CE), cumin, bay, garlic, grapes, marjoram, mustard, pomegranates, and many other herbs were being cultivated in the area. Herbs mentioned in the New Testament include mint and dill (flavorings), spikenard and frankincense (perfumes), and aloe (used to anoint the body of Christ).

Arabic Herbalism

At the height of the Roman Empire, spice traders from the area around present-day Saudi Arabia supplied Roman dinner tables with pepper, cinnamon, and cloves in return for gold. As the power of the empire began to wane, the Arabs began to incorporate the teachings of the great Greek and Roman physicians and herbalists into their culture. From the founding of Islam in the 6th century, the Arabic world became the center of scientific and medical knowledge. By the 9th century, surgical hospitals had been built in Baghdad, as well as pharmacies that dispensed herbal medicines.

Arab physicians used hollow needles to deliver medicines and administered herbal anesthetics. The most important Arabic herbalist and physician was Abu 'Ali al-Husayn ibn 'Abd Allah ibn Sina (980–1037), known to the Western world as Avicenna. His *Canon of Medicine* became the definitive tome on herbal medicine in the Arab world, and its influence spread through Europe as Crusaders carried it back to their home countries from the Middle East; it was widely utilized as a standard medical text until the 18th century.

As early as the 7th century, Arab alchemists had developed a process for distilling rose oil, which was used to purify mosques, infuse prayer

beads with fragrance, sprinkle guests as they entered houses, and flavor everything from sherbet to candy. They isolated the essential oils of other herbs, too, and through this work, aromatherapy developed as a popular medical treatment. During the Middle Ages, much of the Arab world used aromatic baths, powders, and salves to cure a variety of ills. Arabic science and herbal medicine remained highly influential throughout the Western world for hundreds of years.

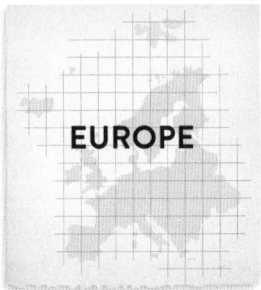

EUROPE

The history of herbs in Europe is a grand collage of plants and traditions from all over the world. Europeans have always imported ideas about herbal medicine, cosmetics, gardening, cooking, and the plants themselves from Asia, Africa, the islands of the Pacific, and the shores of the New World. Today, travelers to Europe are as likely to stumble upon an Ayurvedic bookstore or Japanese garden as they are a French perfumery or Italian spice shop. Europe is also home to some of the world's most famous and sought-after indigenous herbs, including lavender, oregano, rosemary, and bay.

Ancient Greece and Rome

The long culture of herb use in Europe begins with the ancient Greeks and Romans. Greek mythology offers dozens of elaborate legends that explain the origins of important plants and herbs. For instance, as Hera, the queen of the gods, nursed her son Hercules, a few drops of milk are said to have fallen to the ground. In this spot, the first white lily grew. According to another legend, Aphrodite, the goddess of love, is said to have pricked her foot on the thorn of a white rose on the way to meet her lover, Adonis. Her blood turned the rose red, making it the ultimate symbol of love.

One of Greece's most enduring herbal legacies comes from the myth of Apollo and Daphne. Apollo berated the young Cupid one day, saying that a god of love should not play with bows and arrows. In revenge, Cupid fired an arrow into Apollo to ignite love, and another into the beautiful maiden Daphne to repel love. From then on, Apollo pursued Daphne relentlessly until, finally, Daphne begged the river god, Peneus, to help her escape, and he transformed her into a laurel tree. Upon seeing her new form, Apollo declared the laurel (*Laurus nobilis*) sacred and wore a wreath of laurel around his head as a sign of his undying love and honor. This is why athletes in the first Greek Olympic Games were crowned with laurel, and it is the origin of many terms depicting high honors.

Several other herbs gained special, and sometimes superstitious, significance in ancient Greece and Rome. Many Greeks avoided bush basil (*Ocimum minimum*) because they believed that scorpions would breed under pots of it, while the Roman name for basil was *basilescus* because Romans believed that ingesting it protected warriors from the deadly gaze of the basilisk, a mythical serpent. Dittany of Crete (*Origanum dictamnus*) was a symbol of love and peace. The Greeks believed that anointing themselves with this small-leafed herb before they went to sleep would cause them to dream of their future spouses. They also planted it on graves to comfort the dead and provide them eternal peace.

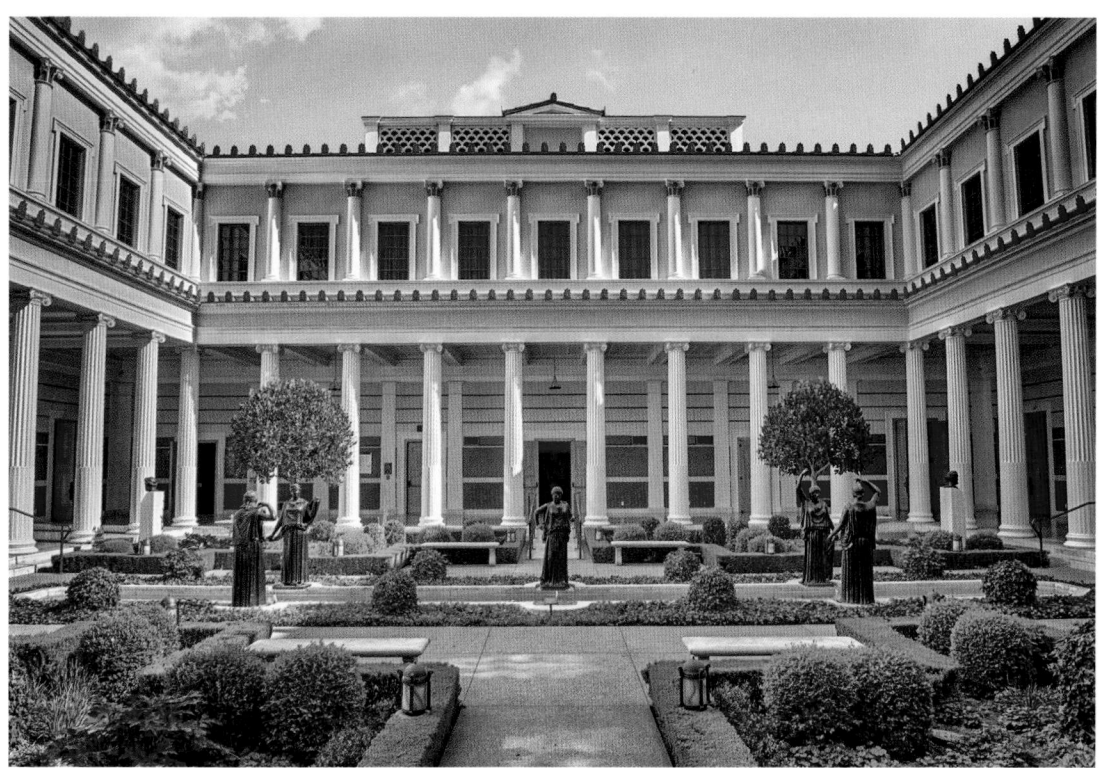

The Getty Villa and garden in Los Angeles, which was inspired by blueprints of an ancient Roman villa, features symmetrical beds of flowers, fruit trees, and herbs, as well as ponds and statues. The herb garden contains wormwood, calamint, lavender, rosemary, and other period herbs.

Greek students wore rosemary braids around their necks or in their hair because they believed it would improve their memory when taking written tests. Romans who were overly fond of food would chew stalks of fennel because they believed it would control obesity. Both the Greeks and Romans used thyme in massage oils, bath oils, perfumes, and incense, and Roman soldiers bathed in thyme-scented water for good luck and honor before going into battle.

According to written records, the Romans ate vegetables and herbs with almost every meal. A light lunch, or *prandium,* often included olives, nuts, and figs. Dinner, or *cena,* was a more elaborate affair, especially for wealthy Romans. The main course typically was meat accompanied by vegetables such as carrots, parsnips, celery, and peas, seasoned with dill, coriander, chervil, and even opium. Wild blackberries, strawberries, and crabapples were served along with cultivated plums, grapes, medlars (*Mespilus* spp.), mulberries, and other fruits.

The Romans grew many of their herbs using gardening techniques developed by the Greeks, Persians, Egyptians, and Mesopotamians, but the enclosed courtyard villa gardens they designed were uniquely Roman. In these villa courtyards, raised flowerbeds were arranged symmetrically alongside herb beds of dill, fennel, bay, rosemary, myrtle, and parsley, all interspersed with topiaries, trees, canals, fountains, and statues collected from Greece. Even in the cities, Roman houses were designed with garden rooms open to the sky. Their orderly rows of herbs and flowers extended to the walls, which were painted with scenes of plant rows extending into the distance to give the impression of a larger villa garden.

Greek and Roman Medicine

Herbs played a prominent role in ancient Greek and Roman medicine. Hippocrates (460–375 BCE), author of the Hippocratic Oath and described by many as the father of modern medicine, was among the first in the Western world to reject the idea that diseases were caused by magic, hexes, or the gods. He offered rational explanations and believed that the body should be treated as a whole, considering all aspects of life to be potential contributors to both sickness and health. Hippocrates assigned health effects to the different herbs used in food, categorizing them as hot, cold, dry, or damp. His natural healing process included a balance of these herb types, along with exercise and fresh air. He rarely prescribed drugs to his patients, instead believing in a gentler approach and that, in many cases, the body would rebalance itself over time.

Like most Europeans throughout history, the Greeks and Romans drew much of their herbal knowledge from other civilizations, such as Egypt, Assyria, Persia, and India. The first of the Greek philosophers and doctors to compile this collected learning was Theophrastus (371–287 BCE). As inheritor of the library of Aristotle and an avid student of the many regions conquered by Alexander the Great, Theophrastus might have known more about the world's botany than any man before him. His two surviving works, *Historia Plantarum* (*The History of Plants*) and *De Causis Plantarum* (*The Growth of Plants*), described the structure, growth, habitat, cultivation, and medicinal uses of hundreds of herbs and became the basis of all botanical understanding for centuries to come.

In 77 CE, the Roman scholar Pliny the Elder (23–79 CE) expanded on Theophrastus's work in his 37-volume *Naturalis Historiae* (*Natural History*). Nearly half of the volumes describe the many uses of plants, from producing olive oil to spinning flax; several explain in detail herbal drugs and treatments for diseases. Pliny was the first to categorize herbal drugs according to the type of plant from which they derived. For example, one volume covered drugs derived from garden plants such as garlic and cabbage, one covered

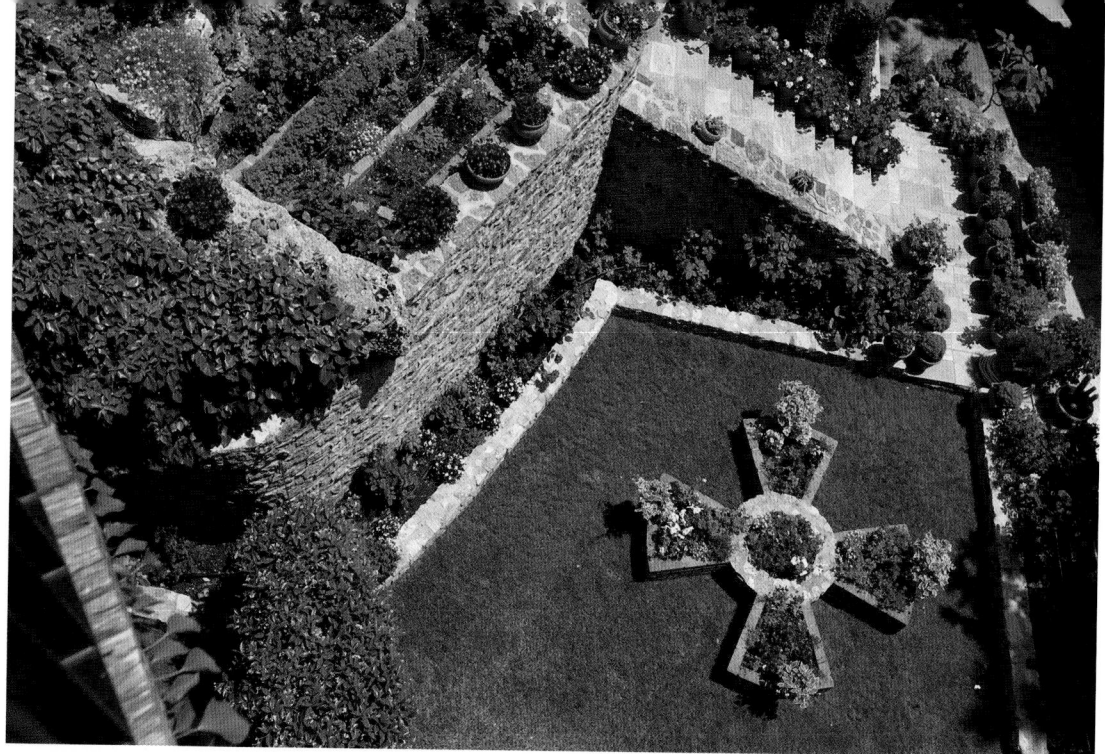

The Great Meteoron monastery in Thessaly, Greece, was founded around 1340 by the scholar monk of Mount Athos, Saint Athanasios Meteorites.

those from wild plants such as aconite and worm-wood, and another covered drugs from forest trees such as cork and juniper.

During the first century, Greek physician, pharmacologist, and botanist Pedanius Dioscorides (ca. 40–90 CE) traveled extensively around the Mediterranean with the Roman legions. Between battles, he studied local herbs and their uses. The result of his research was the first true herbal, *De Materia Medica,* which describes nearly 600 medicinal plants and close to 5,000 cures, including the use of parsley as a diuretic, fennel to promote the flow of mother's milk, and white horehound with honey as an expectorant. The *De Materia Medica* became the chief reference of herbalists from Italy to Scandinavia, and from Britain to Russia. Its influence lasted for more than 1,500 years.

Less than a century after the publication of Dioscorides's pathbreaking work, the great Greek physician Aelius Galenus (130–200 CE)—known as Galen—promoted the idea of a system of four humors—blood, phlegm, black bile, and yellow bile—similar to the Ayurvedic system in India. A higher or lower level of any one of these humors not only affected a person's health, but his personality and mood, as well. Galen wrote more than 500 treatises on medicine, only one of which has survived to this day—a recipe book of 130 herbal antidotes and medicines, each designed to bring one or more of the humors back into balance. Like the writings of Dioscorides, Galen's theories of humors and herbal healing were followed by practitioners throughout Europe for 1,600 years.

The Middle Ages

In Europe, the Middle Ages were a time of few advancements and many superstitions in herbal lore. In an era that witnessed Druid rituals and the practice of witchcraft, herbs played a major role in daily life, even if their uses often were informed by fantasy and imagination rather than scientific experimentation. Nearly every tree, bush, or root in the forest was believed to have some sort of magical power. For instance, the elder tree (*Sambucus nigra*) was considered sacred in Germany and Denmark, particularly among gypsies, who believed that if a cradle was made from its wood, the *Hylde Moer*, or Elder Mother, would strangle the baby in revenge. Pagan fertility rituals in Britain coincided with the annual first bloom of midland hawthorn, or mayflower (*Crataegus laevigata*). On May Day, celebrants would go "a-maying"— they would crown a May Queen with wreaths of hawthorn in the hope that a bountiful harvest would follow.

The folklore surrounding European mistletoe (*Viscum album*) was especially colorful. Druids in Britain and Gaul (France) carried branches of mistletoe to celebrate the New Year, and since mistletoe could only be cut during a certain phase of the moon and with a sacred golden knife, these branches were known as golden boughs. Germans thought that mistletoe gave people the power to see ghosts. The Norse believed the plant was banished to the treetops because a Norse god had been killed by a mistletoe dart, and people meeting beneath a mistletoe branch were required to kiss to compensate for the god's death.

Mandrake (*Mandragora officinarum*) was believed to have even more fantastic powers. European practitioners of witchcraft believed mandrake enabled them to fly. In fact, when the plant is rubbed against the skin or crushed and inhaled, it has an intoxicating effect that could evoke a feeling of flying! This is due to the presence of powerful and potentially toxic tropane alkaloids that produce hallucinations. Because mandrake root resembles a human figure, many believed it would make a shrieking sound when pulled from the ground. They feared that anyone who heard the

shriek would die instantly, so they often harvested the plant by tying a dog to it, then calling to the dog from a safe distance. The 1st-century historian Josephus provided precise directions for harvesting mandrake, noting that the dog pulling it up would die "instead of his master."

For centuries throughout Europe, people continued to believe strongly in the magical power of herbs. They wore them around their necks as amulets to ward off evil spells, mixed them into ointments to prevent baldness and sunburn, hung them from doorways as charms to protect cattle or cure madness, and combined them with ale, milk, vinegar, or honey to create powerful potions.

Medieval Europeans also used herbs liberally in their daily diets, as did the ancient Greeks and Romans. The use of spices was more than a matter of enlivening dull food. With few fresh vegetables and no refrigeration to preserve meat, spices were needed to make such fare palatable, to mask repulsive odors and flavors, and even to reduce contamination by killing organisms that could make a person eating it get sick.

Most people usually gathered herbs such as horseradish, parsley, and fennel locally, from nearby fields and forests, but those with more social status and larger incomes relied on intrepid explorers to import exotic spices from the Far East. The kings and gentry of Europe often ate meals and drank wines seasoned with cinnamon, pepper, and ginger grown and harvested continents away.

Medieval Europeans also had spectacular gardens of their own. While herbal medicine and scientific knowledge advanced little over the course of 1,000 years, the art of gardening went through several phases. After the fall of the Roman Empire, most of the gardening in Europe took place within the walls of monasteries. Gardening was considered a devout duty for monks. By the time the Benedictine order was founded in Italy in the 6th century, the importance of gardening was second only to prayer in the monastic hierarchy. For the

European fiefdoms, monasteries acted as cottage industries that produced fruits and herbs for food, flavoring, medicine, incense, dye, and additives for wine and ale.

The first person to record the monastic theories of gardening was Walahfrid Strabo (ca. 808–849 CE), the abbot of Reichenau, in Switzerland. His book, *Hortulus,* a collection of poems, was an ode to his love of the labor of gardening, as well as an elaborate instruction manual on horticulture and healing herbs. He explained how to grow plants in raised beds just as the Romans had 1,000 years earlier, and he offered planting directions for the dozens of plants he tended.

Saint Hildegard (1098–1179), the abbess of Bingen, followed with four treatises on medicinal herbs. Recognized for her great powers as a healer, Hildegard wrote about the abbey's fragrant herbs and how they were used in perfumes and medicinal concoctions such as lavender water, *aqua mirabilis* (miracle water), Benedictine liqueur, and the highly prized Carmelite water.

By the 13th century, products such as Carmelite water—a fragrance and complexion aid made from lemon balm, nutmeg, coriander, and angelica root—had prompted many wealthy Europeans to seek instruction from monks and nuns on how to grow gardens of their own. These ranged from simple household gardens stocked with herbs for the kitchen and flowers for the table to elaborate pleasure gardens with a center lawn surrounded by sweet-smelling herbs such as sage, rue, and basil,

HORTULUS: THE POETRY *of* HERBS

Walahfrid Strabo was a prolific individual who died tragically in his third decade of life while attempting to cross a river in France. *Hortulus* (*The Little Garden*), a collection of 27 short poems, is his only journey into the world of nature and is thought to be his best and most memorable work. His garden was a kitchen garden—a space protected by the monastery's walls, inside which he grew vegetables, spices, and medicinal herbs, tending his plants with great care. While no original of this work written by Strabo himself still exists, four medieval manuscripts are believed to have been produced by scribes. One of them was translated into English and published by the Hunt Botanical Library in 1966. In the poem "On the Cultivation of Gardens," Strabo noted:

Your labor, if you do not insult with
    misguided efforts
the gardener's multifarious wealth, and
    if you do not
Refuse to harden or dirty your hands in
    the open air
Or to spread whole baskets of dung on
    the sun-parched soil—
Then, you may rest assured, your soil
    will not fail you.

In *Hortulus,* Strabo wrote of 29 plants growing in his garden, most likely his favorites among many more. Of fennel he wrote:

Let us not forget to honor fennel. It
    grows
On a strong stem and spreads its
    branches wide.

Its taste is sweet enough, sweet too its
    smell;
They say it is good for eyes whose sight
    is clouded,
That its seed, taken with milk from a
    pregnant goat,
Eases a swollen stomach and quickly
    loosens
Sluggish bowels. What is more, your
    rasping cough
Will go if you take fennel-root mixed
    with wine.

The plants in his collection of 9th-century garden poems were actually medicines, and the poems were a medical guide for the day, meant to foster health and healing. The poems highlighted food plants, as well as medicinal herbs such as chervil, clary, mint, sage, and tansy.

plus shade trees, benches, and a few resident peacocks for a splash of color.

In 1545, gardening in Europe took an educational turn: The first physic (herbal medicine) garden was commissioned by the University of Padua in Italy for the purpose of teaching botany and herbal medicine. During those days, there was a great deal of confusion about the identity of certain medicinal plants, and it was possible to confuse a healing herb with an ineffective or even toxic species. The Garden of Padua was established to standardize the identification of plants used in medicine and to train botanists and physicians in the plants' proper identification and use.

A century later, universities all over Europe had established physic gardens. How they were used determined much of their design; at the University of Edinburgh, for example, herbs were arranged in rows by alphabetical order. The educational value of physic gardens grew as explorers carried new plant species back to Europe from all over the world and as scientists grew ever hungrier for knowledge about how herbs could be used.

The Global Spice Race

Throughout history, Europeans traveled the world searching for new trade goods and establishing better trade routes. Herbs and spices have been among the most valuable commodities, and the ancient Greeks and Romans were the first Europeans to seek them out. Since the seas were considered treacherous and unpredictable, the majority of trade with the Far East took place over land, until 40 CE, when a Greek merchant named Hippalus made a discovery about the monsoon patterns over the Indian Ocean.

Hippalus realized that a ship leaving Egypt could reach India or the Indonesian Spice Islands faster by traveling with the prevailing southwesterly winds that blow in the summer months, and it could return more easily on the northeasterly winds of winter. Using this knowledge, a major expedition could be completed in just 1 year. The Romans took particular advantage of this insight, importing tons of pepper, cinnamon, cloves, and nutmeg and decreasing their reliance on the overland trade routes through Persia.

Few new trade routes were discovered until the 13th century, when Marco Polo (1254–1324) traveled from Venice through southwestern Asia, across the vast Gobi desert, and into Mongolia and China to be presented at the court of Kublai Khan. When he returned to Europe 24 years later, his travel journal sparked renewed interest in finding quicker, safer trade routes to the Far East. Many explorers followed over the next 200 years. On separate voyages, Bartolomeu Dias (1450–1500) and Vasco da Gama (1469–1524) navigated the Cape of Good Hope in Africa, opening a direct sea route from Europe to the East. Christopher Columbus (1451–1506) set out in search of a westerly route to the East Indies and discovered the herbal riches of the Americas, instead. Ferdinand Magellan (1480–1521) circumnavigated the globe and discovered the Philippine Islands, leading to the establishment of Manila as one of the world's great spice trading capitals.

The Age of Herbals

Advances in gardening and herbal knowledge in 16th-century Europe led to the publication of several new and interesting herbals. In earlier centuries, herbals for the common person were copied by hand from ancient Greek or Roman works, and repeated translations over the years caused many errors. But when printing presses came into use in the 1400s, authors could make more accurate plant descriptions and detailed illustrations available to the public, without the risk of adding errors with each printing. This helped renew interest in botany and the uses of herbs.

New Kreüterbuch (1543) and *De Historia*

CIRCA INSTANS: A 12TH-CENTURY PHARMACOPOEIA

Many botanical gardens and universities have collections of rare books, often kept in a room designated as such. In the fields of botanical and horticultural bibliography, The New York Botanical Garden (NYBG) has one of the world's greatest collections of rare medieval and renaissance herbals, housed in the rare book room of the LuEsther T. Mertz Library. From time to time in the course of my research I've walked through this extraordinary facility, which is filled with shelves and shelves of ancient books and manuscripts.

The oldest item in the collection, a manuscript known as *Circa Instans,* is considered a "fundamental work of Western science." Lacking a title page, the work is known by the first two words of the manuscript, *Circa Instans.* This work of medicinal simples, or basic ingredients used in formulating medicines, is thought to have been written around 1140. Although the original document is believed to be lost, the Mertz Library has the oldest-known existing copy, most likely written around 1190 by Mattheus Platearius, a physician from the medical school at Salerno.

The book's original purpose was to help standardize information about the ingredients used to produce early medical prescriptions, replacing chaos with order—with the goal of improving a patient's chances of recovering from his or her specific health condition. It describes, for instance, three types of aloe recognized at the time—*citrinum* (lemon yellow), *epaticum* (liver colored), and *caballinum* (horse aloe).

Recently, I went through the notes on this book made by my late colleague Frank J. Anderson, an internationally recognized scholar on herbals who translated the manuscript in the 1970s. Regarding the beneficial properties of aloe, his translation noted:

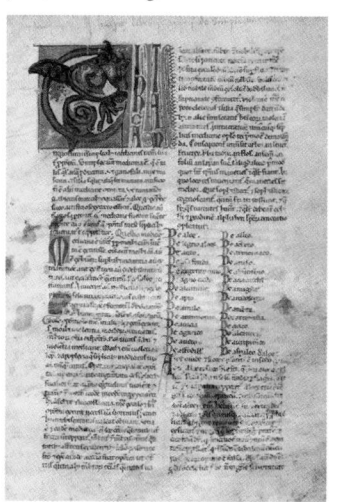

> It [aloe] clears the vision, opens stoppages of the spleen and liver, brings on menstruation . . . and purifies scabies. It will also restore color to the body if the pallor resulted from a preceding ailment, and is curative of alopecia and falling hair. . . . Although aloe is bitter in the mouth, still the stomach is sweetened by it. From which words rises the saying, "cure the pain of the stomach by way of the stomach's mouth," which is to say, "a bitter mouth makes a sweet stomach."

Anderson called *Circa Instans* the "prototype of the modern pharmacopoeia," and it was an influential reference in medicine until the beginning of the 15th century. "Of course modern science has long since outgrown the *Circa,* just as Newton surpassed Euclid, and Einstein overshadowed Newton, but each built on work that had gone before and gladly acknowledged their debt," wrote Anderson in his classic 1977 work, *An Illustrated History of the Herbals.* "The *Circa* may not be consulted nowadays in the prescription room of your corner drugstore, nor in pharmaceutical laboratories, but it was a major instrument in making those places possible."

Described by Marie Long, NYBG's reference librarian, as ". . . some of the first real scientific work in medicine that we know of," *Circa Instans* documented firsthand experiences and observations of the physicians at the School of Salerno and guided healers of the day in identifying the exotic plant material arriving from around the world to the Mediterranean region. Carefully preserved, protected, and translated, this wonderful volume is the "rarest of the rare" in this great bibliographic collection.—M. J. B.

Stirpium (1545) by Leonhard Fuchs (1501–1566) of Germany were pioneering works in herbal publishing. The books contained more than 500 large, clear, woodcut prints of plant specimens with little or no text. As a doctor and professor of medicine, Fuchs felt compelled to create accurate depictions of medicinal herbs, having witnessed ignorance among the general public and even among his fellow physicians. Although his illustrations became extremely popular and were widely copied throughout Europe, Fuchs's writing didn't include anything new. Like most European authors before him, he simply rehashed the herbal remedies of Theophrastus and Dioscorides.

While Fuchs borrowed from the works of the ancient Romans, a charismatic Swiss physician and alchemist who called himself Philippus Aureolus Paracelsus (1493–1541) built on them. He traveled throughout Europe, Egypt, and the Middle East researching folk remedies and considered himself a practical man who spoke for the common people. He rejected Latin and wrote most of his books in German. He also rejected Galen's theory of four humors, which had been practiced and mandated by the medical establishment for nearly 1,500 years.

Paracelsus was the first European to promote the idea of evidence-based medicine. He believed the active ingredient in each substance (animal, vegetable, or mineral) could be identified, extracted, and purified, and then prescribed in the

LIKE CURES LIKE?

The Doctrine of Signatures maintains that a plant's therapeutic value can be determined from its unique shape, color, aroma, and other characteristics. For instance, a plant with a thick, curled root would be useful for curing snakebite. *Rauvolfia serpentina*, also known as Indian snakeroot, was used in Ayurvedic medicine to treat snakebites (as well as other conditions) and eventually found its way into Western medicine as an early antihypertensive drug. According to the Doctrine, a plant with a yellow root or leaf might be useful to treat jaundice, associated with yellowing of the eyes and skin.

Exploring the Doctrine of Signatures in a 2008 article in *HerbalGram*, ethnobotanist Dr. Bradley Bennett wrote, "Some believe that the Creator gave physical clues about the value he imbued to plants. In 1669 Oswaldus Crollius wrote: 'All herbs, flowers, trees and other things which proceed out of the Earth, are books, and magick signs, communicated to us, by the immense mercy of God, which signs are our medicine. . . . for every thing that is intrinsic, bears the external figure of its occult property . . . '"

So many of the traditional cultures I have worked with—in habitats ranging from deserts to rainforests to high mountains—believe that many plants *indicate* their uses in this way. An inflorescence shaped like the stinger of a venomous insect can be used to treat the injury from that insect; plants with red leaves are good for treating the blood; and so forth. It really is impressive how ubiquitous this belief is and how well it was embedded in the most ancient of medical theories on the initial identification of plants with therapeutic properties.

But Dr. Bennett offers a more likely interpretation: This theory was not used to *discover* plants, but to *explain* and *teach* their therapeutic uses, as a mnemonic device to help retain and communicate this information to the vast audience of people interested in healing techniques and tools.

As any contemporary student knows, mnemonics are effective for memorizing and retaining information about complicated processes and phenomena. In this case, could there be any better way to learn about the therapeutic properties and preparation of so many medicinal plants?—M. J. B.

correct dose to heal the sick. This approach led to the development of new herbal treatments—he dissolved opium in alcohol to produce laudanum, a highly effective painkiller—and to the debunking of current ones—he demonstrated that guaiac (*Guaiacum officinale*) imported from the West Indies was not an effective treatment for syphilis, as most Europeans believed, but that small doses of toxic mercury were very effective.

The Doctrine of Signatures

Paracelsus also believed that each and every plant was marked by God with a distinctive sign. This sign was both the key to unlocking the plant's active ingredient and a clear indicator of God's purpose for the plant. This theory was not entirely new, but it did take on new prominence in the world of herbalists when Jakob Böhme (1575–1624) codified it in *Signatura Rerum* (*The Signature of All Things*). This Doctrine of Signatures was extremely popular with the public because it made herbal remedies more identifiable and accessible. The spotted leaves of lungwort (*Mertensia* spp.), for example, were shaped vaguely like lungs, so

clearly, the plant could be used to treat lung ailments. Goldenrod was yellow, so it must be an effective treatment for jaundice. Unfortunately, these simplistic "signatures" rarely corresponded with the actual medicinal values of their plants, and hundreds of new herbal myths grew without thorough scientific testing.

Gerard, Parkinson, and Culpeper

In the late 16th century, English herbalists began to make their mark with books that added to both the fact and fiction of herbal knowledge. John Gerard's classic *Generall Historie of Plantes* relied very heavily on an earlier Belgian herbalist's work. It was supplemented by Gerard's personal observations, some quite accurate and others based more on popular beliefs of the time. Gerard's book painstakingly described the proper care and use of thousands of herbs, including many exotics given to him by traveling friends.

Besides advocating aromatherapy and the absorption of herbal oils through the skin, Gerard believed herbal tonics could soothe the mind and

IMPORTANT HERBS *of* EUROPE

HERB	EXAMPLES OF USES
Calendula (*Calendula officinalis*)	Treatment for skin irritations and wounds
Dandelion (*Taraxacum offinale*)	Strong diuretic
Deadly nightshade (*Atropa belladonna*)	Poison, sedative
Hops (*Humulus lupulus*)	Sedative
Horse chestnut (*Aesculus hippocastanum*)	Shampoo ingredient
Lavender (*Lavandula* spp.)	Perfumery, aromatherapy
Oregano (*Origanum* spp.)	Culinary herb
Saffron (*Crocus sativus*)	Dye and culinary herb
Sage (*Salvia officinalis*)	Culinary herb, digestive aid
Yellow gentian (*Gentiana lutea*)	Treatment for gastrointestinal disorders

spirit. Among his recommended herbal treatments were peony seeds in wine, taken to ward off nightmares, and concoctions made from rosemary, taken to comfort the brain.

In 1640, another English herbalist, John Parkinson (1567–1650) published a far more ambitious work. The *Theatrum Botanicum* consisted of 1,700 pages covering more than 3,800 plants from throughout the world. Unlike his predecessors, Parkinson combined horticulture, botany, pharmacy, and history in one volume. He made the first serious attempt to classify plants into similar groups, which he called "tribes." Among his fascinating tribe descriptions are "hot and sharpe biting plants," "strange and outlandish plants," and "venomous sleepy and hurtfull plants and their counter poisons."

The most successful English herbalist was Nicholas Culpeper (1616–1654). First, he translated the London Pharmacopoeia from Latin to English and published it for the masses as *A Physical Directory*. In effect, this put herbal medical knowledge, previously accessible only to doctors, into the hands of the apothecaries who, at the time, did most of the prescribing. This made Culpeper popular with members of the general public, but decidedly less so with the medical establishment.

In another book, *The English Physician,* published in 1652, Culpeper, a devoted astrologer, ascribed a celestial cause to every illness, with a corresponding treatment based on the planetary aspect of every plant. He believed the planet Venus, for example, governed the sexual organs and that emollients made from heavily scented Venusian plants, such as the Damascus rose or apple blossom, could be used to create a desired sexual effect. Jupiter, decreed Culpeper, ruled the liver, spleen, and kidney, so plants that astrologers associated with Jupiter, such as chestnut and apricot, could be used to treat problems with these organs.

Culpeper's books and theories soon were eclipsed by the more rigorous science of his contemporaries. In 1646, Sir Thomas Browne published *Pseudodoxia Epidemica* (or *Vulgar Errors*), which challenged some of the superstitions and beliefs of his day. This book went through five editions, the final one appearing in 1672. As explorers brought home new plants from newly discovered continents and physic gardens appeared in more and more universities, European physicians, scientists, and pharmacologists made concerted efforts to unlock the true medicinal values of all herbs, familiar and new.

Science and Cross-Pollination

In the 18th century, colonists traveling to the New World carried with them European plants, herbal books, and gardening styles. In return, traders carried back New World herbs such as tobacco,

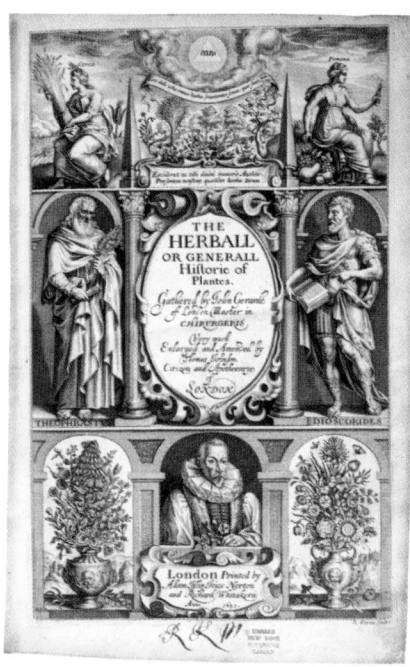

The Herball or Generall Historie of Plantes by botanist and herbalist John Gerard, first published in 1597, was one of the most well known of the English herbals. It discussed the therapeutic application and folklore of healing plants.

tomatoes, and corn. The European public quickly found domestic uses for these plants, while the scientific community explored the medicinal possibilities of herbs such as Jesuits' bark (several species in the genus *Cinchona*), the source of antimalarial quinine, and sassafras (*Sassafras albidum*), which was believed at the time to cure venereal diseases.

In Europe, as the Age of Reason led to the Industrial Revolution, scientists became ever more disciplined in their approach to herbal medicine. They learned how to distill the active ingredients in plants and, eventually, were able to chemically synthesize beneficial molecules and oils. The science of botany continued to develop, with writers and artists creating highly accurate textbooks on the plant world that supplanted the sometimes highly subjective herbals.

In gardening, the formal gardens of the French chateaux gave way to a deliberately informal approach. Symmetry was discarded in favor of the creation of natural landscapes. Yet simple cottage and kitchen gardens never went out of style. In urban centers, the limitations of space led to the invention of the window box, and more and more people moved their plants indoors to grow in pots. Even as scientific advances moved Europeans further from nature, they still found ways to connect with the textures, scents, and flavors of their favorite herbs.

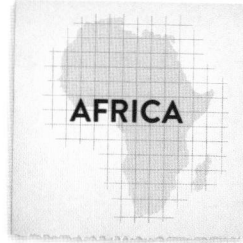

Africa hosts a large variety of herbs that are the result of its many climatic regions. The range spans from the culinary herbs of the fertile Mediterranean coast to the cosmetic herbs of the northeastern regions to the medicinal plants found in the desert oases, dry savannas, mountainous woodlands, and lush rainforests of the central and southern parts of the continent.

Ancient Egypt

The history of herb use in Africa begins in ancient Egypt, where pharaohs and commoners alike used herbal medicines extensively. Some of the world's earliest known herb gardens were planted nearly 4,000 years ago in Egypt, often near temples where certain herbs and flowers were needed on a daily basis for worship. One such flower, the water lily or lotus (*Nymphaea lotus*), was considered sacred, and every part of the lotus plant was used in Egyptian art, food, and medicine.

Another very important herb, garlic, was found in the tomb of Tutankhamen (1341–1323 BCE) and was thought to possess magical powers. If Egyptians took a solemn oath, they swore on a clove of garlic, and garlic was eaten by slaves as they built the great pyramids at Giza because it was believed that it would endow the workers with strength and endurance. Frankincense and myrrh were important in Egyptian rituals, as well. Reliefs in the tomb of Queen Hatshepsut (ca. 1512–1457 BCE) in Luxor show frankincense trees growing in pots. Myrrh was believed to cure cancer, leprosy, and syphilis and was used in embalming.

Believing they could keep alive the souls of the departed by preserving their bodies, the Egyptians developed embalming and mummification. They first removed the brain and all internal organs except for the heart, which was believed essential to the survival of the soul. The body cavities were then cleansed with frankincense, myrrh, and palm wine. Moisture was removed with natron (a mix of sodium compounds), and the cavities were packed with linens, salt, muslin packets of wood shavings, and spices such as cinnamon, chamomile, cassia, anise, marjoram, and cumin. The eyes were replaced with glass or gems, the skin was painted to give it a lifelike hue, and the body was rubbed with a mixture of five oils: frankincense, myrrh, lotus, palm, and cedar. Finally, the body was wrapped in linen and sealed with natural resin. The process took about 70 days.

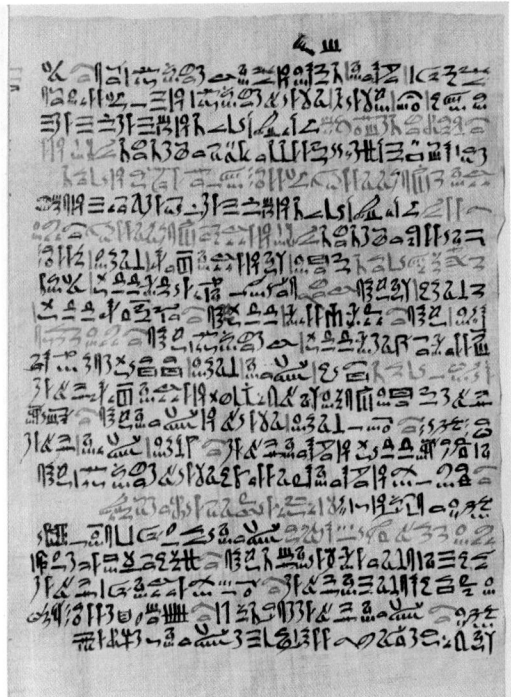

The Ebers papyrus records Egyptian herbal drugs and treatments, some of which date to the first Egyptian dynasty.

The earliest surviving scrolls date to 2000 BCE, but the Egyptians were administering herbal treatments long before that. The most valuable source of herbal information is a remarkable papyrus dated to ca. 1550 BCE and looted from a tomb of the 18th dynasty. Bought by the German Egyptologist Georg Ebers (1837–1898), the Ebers papyrus is a complete, undamaged scroll about 65 feet long and containing 3,000 lines of hieratic text (an ancient Egyptian writing system). It compiles treatments, diagnoses, prescriptions, and even surgical techniques dating back to the first Egyptian dynasty, or around 3400 BCE. It lists 811 medicinal drugs and their presumed effects, including poppies to induce sleep, aloe to treat excess mucus, and crocus to be used as a diuretic. It also describes the healing effects of anise, mustard, linseed, peppermint, watermelon, fenugreek, caraway, worm-

wood, elderberry, fig, nasturtium, flax, and—of course—garlic. These herbs are prescribed in complex and carefully measured recipes and are recommended for administration as ointments, infusions, pills, gargles, snuffs, poultices, suppositories, and enemas.

Perfumes and Cosmetics in Ancient Egypt

Wall paintings show that most Egyptians, from childhood on, wore a heavy black makeup called kohl. Kohl was a fairly toxic mixture of galena (lead sulfate), powdered malachite, frankincense gum, and goose fat placed in cow dung and burned, then pounded in a mortar with milk and rainwater, decanted, and finally dried and formed into tablets or eye pencils. These valuable beauty products were kept in ceremonial jars, many of which have been found buried in tombs with the kohl still inside.

The Egyptians used the dried powdered leaves of henna (*Lawsonia inermis*) to dye their nails, palms, soles, fingertips, and moustaches a rich orange-red color. Mixed with indigo, henna was used as early as 3200 BCE to dye hair, as well as the manes and tails of horses. Henna tattoos were applied to the chests, shoulders, arms, and thighs of exotic dancers, musicians, and servants.

Beauty creams were commonly used by ancient Egyptians. These included depilatories made of gum, cucumber, and fig juice; cleansing lotions of oil and lime; and hair tonics of lettuce, fir oil, and juniper berries. Daily applications of wrinkle creams were made from frankincense gum, the oil of the moringa tree, and fermented cyperus grass. Papyrus scrolls dating from 2700 BCE describe fragrant herbs, oils, perfumes, and incense being used in ceremonies and as protective skin salves.

Perfumes were commonly made from frankincense and myrrh, combined with animal fats and oils, mixed into gum resins, and burned as incense or applied liberally as ointments. Other popular scents included almond, sesame, olive, and balanos oil as well as lily oil, which was made from the petals of 2,000 lilies mixed with cardamom, cinnamon, and sweet flag. One powerful fragrance, called *kyphi*, was made from pistachio resin, cinnamon, frankincense, myrrh, spikenard, henna, and calamus. Kyphi was burned at sunset to honor the sun god Ra and was used as an aromatic oil to eliminate sorrow and anxiety and to increase the vividness of dreams. Ancient Egyptians rubbed fragrant gums and creams under their arms and between their legs. Some made pomades of herbal extracts mixed with animal fats, shaped them into mounds, and wore them on their heads, where they gradually melted down over their hair and bodies as the day progressed, spreading a pleasing fragrance and oil.

North Africa

The history of North Africa is one of conquest, survival, and lucrative trade. The indigenous people of the areas now called Libya, Tunisia, Algeria, and Morocco were the Berbers. The first invaders of this region were the Phoenicians, who established the city of Carthage in present-day Tunisia. Though the Berbers eventually gained control of Carthage, it finally succumbed to Roman rule. The Berbers then moved southward and westward, establishing important trading posts throughout most of North Africa, particularly in today's Morocco, which became an important stop for spice-trading ships traveling to and from Europe.

Many of the foods and spices now associated with Moroccan cuisine came from the influence

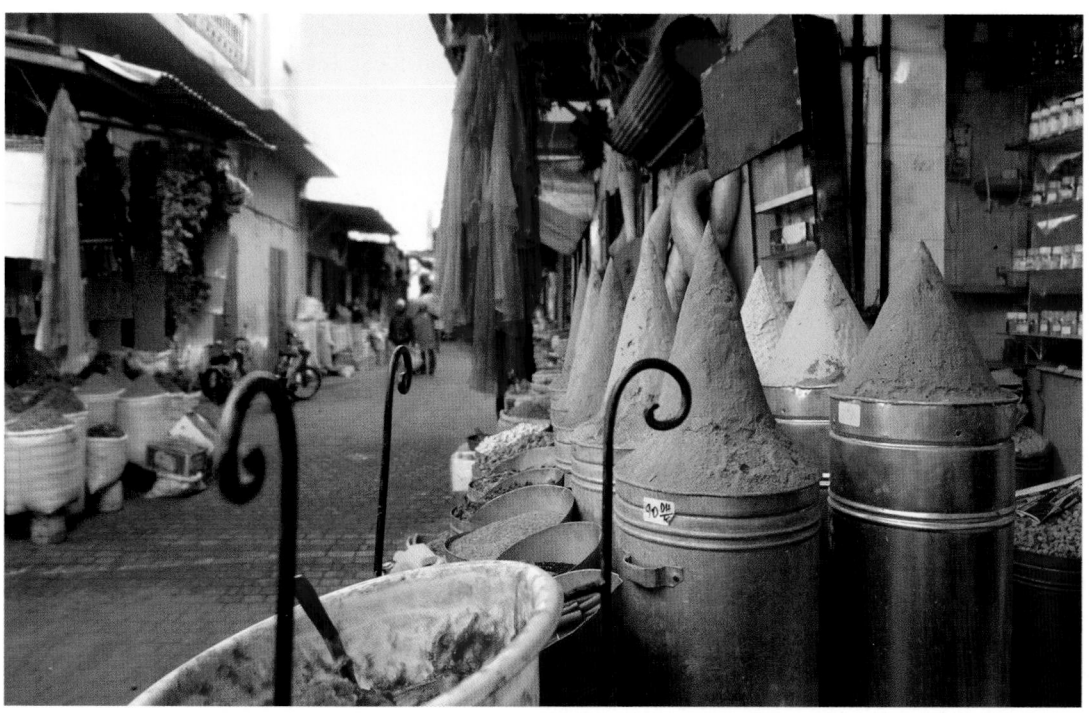

Spice shops add color to the streets of Morocco, which was once an important stop on the spice trade route. Paprika, turmeric, ginger, and cinnamon are often used in the regional cuisine.

of Islamic Arabs, who conquered the region in the 7th century. In the centuries that followed, most of the countries of Europe battled for control of Morocco, a fight finally won by France in 1912. Morocco gained its independence in 1956, inheriting a population that was 80 percent Berber, with heavy Arabic, Spanish, and French influences.

Over the centuries, Morocco has grown almonds, dates, walnuts, chestnuts, prickly pears, cherries, oranges, lemons, apricots, olives, and mints. Spices imported and incorporated into the region's foods include paprika, black pepper, nutmeg, turmeric, ginger, cinnamon, cumin, cloves, and saffron. Proprietors of spice shops developed secret mixtures known as *ras el hanout* ("head of the shop"), which contained as many as 100 carefully blended spices. While there are subtle variations in cuisine across North Africa today—Tunisian foods contain more fiery spices than Moroccan foods do—the blended influence of indigenous Middle Eastern and European people has created a cohesive herbal tradition that stands on its own.

West, Central, and East Africa

In many areas of Africa, local systems of herbal medicine began as religious rituals, such as holy men drinking herbal tonics to better commune with a god or gods. Over time, religious leaders also became tribal healers, harvesting herbs, tree barks, roots, and berries to cure common ills and combat diseases such as malaria and yellow fever.

In the Yoruba religion, which dates back thousands of years, medicinal plants and herbs, called *ewe,* were believed to possess strong spiritual powers. Cemeteries, for example, were the territory of Oya Orisha, the goddess of change, so ewe harvested there was thought to possess her ability to bring about violent but necessary transformations. Many herbs used in Yorubic medicine, including cola, buchu, and ginger, were steeped and prepared as teas, and some were administered as enemas. One medicinal soup, or *ose,* recipe includes water, oil, salt, pepper, cooked melon, and locust seeds.

In much of Central Africa, the history of herb use varied depending on the local flora and the traditions of individual tribes. Natives of Cameroon,

IMPORTANT HERBS *of* AFRICA

HERB	EXAMPLES OF USES
Aloe (*Aloe vera*)	Treatment for skin irritations and burns
Buchu (*Agathosma betulina* and *A. crenulata*)	Treatment for gastrointestinal ailments
Castor bean (*Ricinus communis*)	Oil used as laxative and motor lubricant
Devil's claw (*Harpagophytum procumbens*)	Treatment for arthritis
Iboza (*Tetradenia riparia*)	Fever reducer
Lotus (*Nymphaea lotus*)	Sacred flower
Milk bush (*Euphorbia tirucalli*)	Treatment for warts
Rooibos (*Aspalathus linearis*)	Caffeine-free tea substitute
Wormwood (*Artemisia afra*)	Treatment for bronchitis
Yohimbe (*Pausinystalia yohimbe*)	Aphrodisiac, treatment for fevers and coughs

Gabon, and the Congo have long believed that the bark of the tall evergreen yohimbe could cure coughs, fevers, and leprosy. The long-standing trade of cola nuts (*Cola nitida*) began with the tradition of chewing cola before each meal to aid digestion and sustain strength.

In Ethiopia and Somalia, traditional herbal medicine has been practiced for nearly 2,000 years, with recipes being passed down from healer to healer by word of mouth because people believed the herb would lose its medicinal power if a patient knew its name. For centuries, Ethiopian healers have prescribed ground twigs and buds of African pencil cedar (*Juniperus procera*) to treat stomach worms, flaxseed as a laxative and to speed the healing of deep wounds, and bosoke (*Kalanchoe* spp.) to treat boils and wounds.

Other tribes had traditional uses for herbs. Slukari hunters in the Congo rubbed the gel of aloe over their bodies to mask their scent from prey. The algum tree of Somalia, probably a type of sandalwood, was prized for its ability to produce fragrant incense. The Masai people of eastern Africa have always supplemented their staple foods of beef, milk, and yogurt with wild weeds, tree bark,

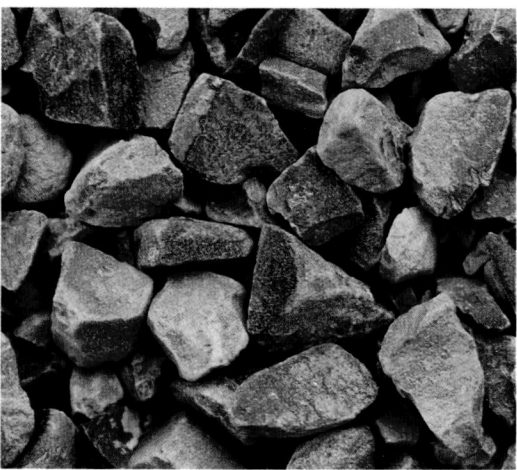

Cola nuts, native to the rainforests of Africa, are valued for their stimulatory properties.

and tree gums that might help counterbalance their cholesterol-rich diet. Traditionally, cassava tubers have been the primary food of millions of people in Uganda. In times of famine, when grain crops failed, Ethiopians routinely gathered and ate the roots and stems of the wild treelike herb *Ensete ventricosum*, known as the Ethiopian banana, to survive. This plant, also known as ensete, is cultivated as an important food source, mixed with other crops such as sorghum or coffee, depending on the region.

South Africa

In 1652, an outpost of the Dutch East India Company was established at the Cape of Good Hope. Initially, the purpose was to resupply company ships traveling between Europe and the East Asian spice ports. But soon, a full Dutch colony was established. As colonists planted kitchen gardens for their own use in the early 1700s, they began to learn more about the local herbs. Probably by observing local tribes such as the Khoisan, the Dutch learned that honeybush (*Cyclopia genistoides*) was a pleasant substitute for tea. Honeybush tea also proved to be an effective treatment for coughs and other respiratory conditions, so before long, it became another profitable export for the Dutch East India Company. The popular herb rooibos (*Aspalathus linearis*), long used by tribes as a mild sedative and to relieve colic in babies, gained worldwide acceptance as another tea substitute. Blended with cinnamon, cardamom, and nutmeg, rooibos creates a full-bodied, caffeine-free red tea filled with antioxidants.

Through the centuries, practitioners have gone by a variety of names: *inyanga*, or herbalist; *sangoma*, or diviner; and, after the arrival of the Dutch, *bossiedokter*, or bush doctor. These healers all collected herbs from the wild, or "bush." Some of the more popular herbs in traditional South

African medicine were devil's claw (*Harpagophytum procumbens*), used for arthritis and gastrointestinal disorders; pepper-bark (*Warburgia salutaris*), used for sinusitis and disorders of the lungs; African wormwood (*Artemisia afra*), used for measles and malaria; and wild willow (*Salix mucronata*), used for arthritis and fevers.

Herbal healing remains popular in South Africa, and large quantities of herbs collected from the wild are still prescribed and sold. Even newly introduced diseases are treated herbally. African potato (*Hypoxis hemerocallidea*)—used for centuries by Zulu healers to treat urinary tract infections, cardiac disorders, tumors, and nervous disorders—is used today as an immunostimulant for HIV/AIDS patients.

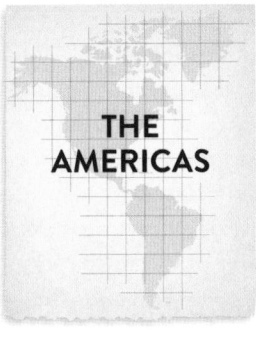

THE AMERICAS

Isolated from the rest of the world's landmass for millions of years, the Americas developed a fascinating flora and fauna, with many unique species. The people who migrated to the western hemisphere over the Bering land bridge many thousands of years ago learned numerous uses for the plants that grew around them. The Navajo Indians used desert plants of present-day Arizona in religious ceremonies. Maya Indians incorporated Mexican rainforest plants into daily spiritual rituals. And Incas created medicines from the high-altitude herbs of the Peruvian mountains. Over time, each culture developed its own uses and recipes for therapeutic herbs.

North America

Many of the first North American inhabitants became expert botanists and developed sophisticated systems of herbal medicine and healing, represented most clearly by the medicine wheel. On the wheel, the four cardinal directions—north, south, east, and west—represent the proper balance of bodily energies, an idea remarkably similar to Chinese, Indian, and Greek herbalism. On a Native American herb wheel, the directions are represented by different animal totems, personality types, colors, and herbal medicines. Shamans used these symbols to travel spiritually through the cosmos, searching for the souls of the sick and seeking spirit guides to assist in their healing.

To become a shaman, individuals were required to learn plant identification, preparation, and medicinal use, as well as patient diagnosis and tribal rituals and songs. Sometimes they underwent a spiritual awakening, called a vision quest, which required them to spend time alone in the wilderness. Initiated shamans were expert healers who were well versed in the medicinal powers of their region's native herbs.

Navajo shamans used a tea prepared from Fendler's bladderpod (*Lesquerella fendleri*). The Meskwaki tribe ground the flowers of goldenrod into a lotion and applied it to bee stings. Plains Indian tribes applied purple coneflower to insect or animal bites. Cherokees covered their bodies with an insect repellent made of a mixture of pounded goldenseal roots (*Hydrastis canadensis*) and bear fat. Many tribes had natural treatments for more serious ailments, as well. The Winnebago and Dakota peoples ate or smoked the roots of skunk cabbage (*Symplocarpus foetidus*) to remove excess phlegm produced by asthma, whooping cough, bronchitis, and hay fever. Many Native Americans used dandelion as a tonic for problems ranging from liver spots and kidney pain to sore throats and indigestion.

The process of childbirth was aided by many natural remedies, too. Healers used the tubers of the wild yam (*Dioscorea villosa*) to relieve pain during childbirth. Cherokee and Iroquois women used partridgeberry (*Mitchella repens*) to speed labor, while other tribes used warm infusions of blue cohosh (*Caulophyllum thalictroides*) to produce the same effect. The Navajos made a tea from the broom snakeweed plant (*Gutierrezia sarothrae*) to promote the expulsion of the placenta, and the Omahas boiled smooth upland sumac (*Rhus glabra*) and applied the liquid as an external wash to stop bleeding after birth. To ease labor pain, the Alabama and Koasati tribes made a tea of cotton roots (*Gossypium herbaceum*).

To prevent pregnancy, the women of many tribes consumed a tea made of ragged leaf bahia (*Bahia dissecta*) or dogbane (*Apocynum cannabinum*). Hopi women drank Indian paintbrush (*Castilleja mutis*) tea to stop their menstrual flow. Mendocino tribes drank an American mistletoe tea (*Phoradendron leucarpum*) to induce abortion, and in the Shoshoni tribe of present-day Nevada, women drank cold-water infusions of stoneseed roots (*Lithospermum ruderale*) in a quest for permanent sterility.

Native Americans also used herbs in spiritual ceremonies. Many of these occurred in sweat lodges—special huts or teepees where tribesmen and women would heighten their spiritual consciousness, mentally prepare for important events like war or a hunt, and physically "sweat out" toxins or illness. To create a saunalike atmosphere inside, rocks were heated over fires and then placed in a depression in the middle of the lodge floor. Water—often mixed with healing herbs such as cedar (*Thuja* spp.), sage (*Salvia* and *Artemisia* spp.), and sweetgrass (*Hierochloe odorata*)—was poured onto the rocks to create steam. Participants would sit inside for hours on freshly cut flat cedar boughs, smoking a ceremonial pipe filled with exactly four pinches of tobacco.

Another herb-based ritual was the peyote ceremony, first documented in 1560 but practiced by Plains Indians such as the Osage, Ute, Navajo, and Mescalero Apache tribes for centuries before that. Participants sat around a fire and an altar inside a teepee, smoking pipes, as everyone was invited to speak about an illness or problem. After purifying their bodies with sprigs of sagebrush, each person chewed four buttons of hallucinatory peyote (*Lophophora williamsii*), then sat silently in prayer as they experienced plant-induced visions.

Tribes who settled in the far northern regions of present-day Canada and Alaska used herbal teas to provide essential vitamins during long winters when no crops could be grown. The Anishinabeg people of Ontario drank tea made from dried leaves, flowers, and twigs of chokeberry, wintergreen, pine, slippery elm, mint, clover, and goldenrod. Many natives of the North drank swamp tea, also known as Labrador tea (*Ledum glandulosum*). This plant grew year-round, even in cold, wet conditions. Rich in caffeine and tannins, it provided them with a coffeelike drink to help ward off the cold. Interestingly, it contains a toxic compound and must be prepared and consumed in a specific way to avoid poisoning.

The Arrival of Europeans

European settlers exchanged herbs and knowledge of their uses with Native Americans. They introduced native people to thyme, caraway, basil, rosemary, chamomile, licorice, and plantain, the latter also known as "white man's foot" to the natives because it seemed to appear wherever the settlers lived. In return, Native Americans offered crop plants such as corn, beans, squash, and tobacco, as well as medicinal plants such as American ginseng, goldenseal, sassafras, purple coneflower, pleurisy root, and witch hazel.

Early French explorers noted the prominence of tribal shamans and called them "medicine men." The medicine men taught colonists how to heal wounds and diseases, and they were often better educated than the settlers themselves in safe childbirth practices, surgical procedures, and the herbal treatment of infections.

Soon, the bounty of botanicals led to the publication of New World herbal texts. In 1565, a Spanish physician and botanist, Nicolas Monardes (1493–1588), published the first-ever illustrations of tobacco, coca, sunflowers, and sarsaparilla in an herbal translated by the English merchant John Frampton as *Joyfull Newes Out of the Newe Founde Worlde*. More than a century later, Englishman John Josselyn (1610–1675) published *New England's Rarities, Discovered in Birds, Beasts, Fishes, Serpents, and Plants of that Country* in 1671. Following Josselyn's guidelines, the colonists were able to grow a wide variety of herbs. For preparing sallets (salads of greens sometimes mixed with bacon fat) and potages (hearty stews made of meat, poultry, game, and fruit), they grew sorrel, burnet, and purslane; for general flavoring, they grew chervil, mint, fennel, dill, and savory; and for dyeing clothes, they grew saffron, woad, alkanet, and calendula.

Exploration and Industrialization

In the early 1700s, cash crops of tobacco, cotton, sassafras, and ginseng were grown on the abundant farmlands of North America and Canada and then exported to Europe. A Pennsylvania Quaker farmer, John Bartram (1699–1777), sent hundreds of drawings, seeds, and specimens to England for cultivation and study. Swedish scientist Carolus Linnaeus (see page 44) described Bartram as the "greatest natural botanist in the world" and relied heavily on the specimens for his classifications of American plants. In 1728, Bartram founded North America's first botanical garden near Philadelphia. He also treated the sick with herbal medicines, called simples, made from licorice, green figs, spearmint, pennyroyal, or marshmallow.

Samuel Thomson (1769–1843) transformed Native American herbalism and simple colonial remedies into a national movement known as physiomedicalism. He used natural healing practices such as herbal treatments, mineral baths, and body heating to create "Thomson's Improved System of Botanic Practice of Medicine," a kit for self-diagnosis and treatment. Thomson classified herbs as stimulating, sedating, relaxing, or astringent, and he prescribed a balanced regimen of these four types for each illness. Many of the herbs he promoted, such as black root, black and blue cohosh, agrimony, cayenne, and true unicorn root, were already familiar to Native Americans. By the mid-1830s, three million Americans owned one of his kits.

Around the same time, the Shakers, an offshoot of the Quaker religious sect, created large "physick" gardens stocked with as many as 200 herbs, such as bayberry, feverfew, sage, calendula, and rue. They harvested the herbs and either pressed the dried, chopped plant materials into bricks or mixed them into tonics, which they labeled and sold. In the mid-1800s, the Shakers even established a mail-order business, offering several hundred medicinal herbs and extracts.

By the 1840s, a more scientific approach to herbal healing emerged, called Eclecticism. The Eclectics established a medical school in Cincinnati, Ohio, where they analyzed the chemical composition of herbs, isolated many active ingredients, and created liquid extractions for medical use. Though the American pharmaceutical industry can trace its roots directly to the Eclectic movement, its influence waned early in the 1900s, when philanthropists such as John D. Rockefeller and Andrew Carnegie began to support "orthodox" medical schools.

In the first half of the 20th century, America's reliance on scientific medicine and synthesized drugs grew, and popular interest in herbs declined. In the United States, a rebirth of interest in herbal remedies began around the 1960s, when groups of Americans—motivated by political, philosophical, or spiritual beliefs—began to feel distrust for clinical medicine and started to explore herbal therapies. Shops selling herbs opened all across the nation, people began to visit herbal practitioners in record numbers, and popular interest in this topic began to grow exponentially.

Along with his colleagues, Dr. Andrew Weil, a medical doctor who championed the concept of incorporating evidence-based so-called "alternative" medical practices into conventional medical care, developed the concept of integrative medicine, a holistic approach to health care and wellness now widely practiced in the United States and internationally. Today, the herbal, vitamin, and supplement industry is flourishing—these products fill the shelves of our supermarkets, drug stores, and health food shops—as people seek ways to optimize wellness and improve their quality of life. This has led to a renewed interest in herbal cuisine and organic foods, which today has driven unprecedented growth in the demand for a wide variety of herbs all over North America.

THE MORAVIANS: PIONEERS *of* AMERICAN HERBALISM

In 1735, members of a Protestant sect known as the Unity of the Brethren, or Moravians, began arriving in North America from central Europe to evangelize to Native Americans and fellow European immigrants. Because they were expected to sustain themselves and build strong, self-sufficient settlements, the Moravian missionaries were well versed in healing practices and in the identification, cultivation, and use of local flora and fauna.

In 1741, Moravians purchased land that would become the community of Bethlehem, Pennsylvania, and by 1742, the village's first physician had arrived. Dr. Johann Adolph Meyer, trained in Germany, deputized a group of 15 men and women as assistants and caretakers. They had brought some plants with them from Europe, but now they scoured forest and field for indigenous specimens for use in medicines. The resulting botanical preparations were dispensed from one of the earliest apothecaries in the country, located in the communal dwelling house, or *Gemeinhaus*. By fall of 1742, they established separate hospitals for men and women—among the first, if not *the* first, hospitals in America. They recognized the contributions of women to treating the sick by compiling a collection of their most valuable household remedies. And by 1747, they laid out an extensive garden that included medicinal plants.

Moravian evangelists traversed the Eastern seaboard on foot and on horseback; one missionary alone covered more than 30,000 miles. En route, they recorded the habits and customs of Native Americans, including their curative practices, and they often returned to base villages like Bethlehem carrying botanical specimens for further study and propagation. They maintained meticulous notes both for themselves and for the home church in Germany.

Thanks to this attention to detail, we know that Moravians at what is now Winston-Salem, North Carolina, also established early physic gardens. Detailed garden plans show the plants cultivated, and other community records document their medicinal applications. The records demonstrate a sophisticated understanding of herbal cures employing a broad range of plants—including tropical species such as those in the genus *Citrus*; naturalized European herbs such as borage, caraway, and catnip; angelica, native to Scandinavia but naturalized in Europe; and marshmallow, originally from Africa.

Today, the medicinal garden of the defunct Moravian settlement of Bethabara, known as the Hortus Medicus, has been carefully restored on its original 1761 site in Historic Bethabara Park in Winston-Salem, North Carolina. The Gemeinhaus and the Old Apothecary in Bethlehem, Pennsylvania, are available for tours through Historic Bethlehem, an affiliate of the Smithsonian Institution.—Nancy Rutman

Central America and the Caribbean

The warm, tropical climate of vast areas of Central America and the Caribbean, along with its great diversity of plant and animal life, promoted human settlement beginning at least 15,000 years ago, and perhaps even earlier in some areas. In the millennia that followed, a number of major civilizations arose, each developing a multitude of uses for the herbs that grew around them or were obtained through travel and trade.

The first of Central America's ancient civilizations was the Olmecs who, from 1500 BCE, grew to prominence in present-day Veracruz. Little is known of how they used the richness of the Mexican rainforest in their daily lives, but it is clear that cacao, or chocolate (*Theobroma cacao*), was valued as a food, flavoring, and diuretic, as well as for use as a skin balm.

By the 3rd century CE, the Maya people had established a civilization that spanned most of Central America. They built underground reservoirs to store rainwater for irrigation and cleared large sections of rainforest to grow corn, manioc, sunflowers, cacao, chile peppers, and squash, sometimes in raised gardens or on terraced mountainsides. They also gathered wild avocado, coconut, mamey (*Pouteria sapota*), and breadnut (*Brosimum alicastrum*). Their spiritual healers, both men and women, were highly trained, and some of their remedies were innovative, such as the practice of blistering the leaves of hierba santa (*Piper umbellatum*) over an open flame before wrapping them around a wrist or ankle to reduce inflammation. Yucca was given to patients who suffered from joint pain. The boiled stems of cliffrose (*Purshia mexicana*) were used to cleanse wounds and suppress coughs. The Mayas also developed a variety of aromatic facial astringents and antibacterial topical tonics that incorporated local herbs such as creosote bush (*Larrea tridentata*) and cat-claw acacia (*Acacia greggii*).

By the 12th and 13th centuries, the Aztec civilization had become established in the area now known as the Valley of Mexico. The Aztecs instituted a remarkable system of landfilling the swampy area. They covered floating rectangular log rafts with mud and planted certain trees at the corners to help secure the rafts and create root systems and soil. Before long, a network of artificial islands, or *chinampas*, had been formed. On top of

IMPORTANT HERBS *of* NORTH AMERICA

HERB	EXAMPLES OF USES
American ginseng (*Panax quinquefolius*)	All-purpose medicine and tea
Bloodroot (*Sanguinaria canadensis*)	Insect repellent, treatment for ulcers and sores, emetic
Cranberry (*Vaccinium macrocarpon*)	Beverage, treatment for urinary tract infections
Echinacea (*Echinacea* spp.)	Treatment for colds and flu
Goldenseal (*Hydrastis canadensis*)	Treatment for infection, dye
Mayapple (*Podophyllum peltatum*)	Topical treatment for warts, chemotherapy
Pokeberry (*Phytolacca americana*)	Antiviral and pesticide
Sassafras (*Sassafras albidum*)	Tea and cure-all
Saw palmetto (*Serenoa repens*)	Prostate treatment
Witch hazel (*Hamamelis virginiana*)	Astringent

these they cultivated food crops: beans, squash, cacao, chiles, vanilla, a wide variety of corn (maize), amaranth (for its protein-rich seeds), and maguey, or century plant. They developed a unique system of traditional medicine using nearly 3,000 herbs gathered from the wild and grown on extensive medicinal *chinampas*. The rest of the world knew nothing of their herbal cures until the mid-16th century, when Spanish scholars and priests began to translate written Aztec works.

Invasion and Slavery

The Arawak tribe, also known as the Tainos, dominated the islands of the Caribbean when Christopher Columbus arrived in 1492. Arawak herbal healers, known as *butuous*, gathered herbs from the lush island forests and grew healing plants and fruits in raised-bed gardens known as *conucos*. These healers prescribed treatments for a variety of illnesses, including teas made from large-leaf thoroughwort (*Hebeclinium macrophyllum*) and aloe for the common chest cold; sucking on the bark of *Unonopsis glaucopetala*, a tree in the custard apple family, to treat snakebite; and burning the foul-smelling leaves of huamansamana (*Jacaranda copaia*) under the hammock of a person with an "illness caused by spirit attack."

The era of two-way commerce between the Eastern and Western hemispheres began with the arrival of Columbus on the islands of the Bahamas, Cuba, Hispaniola, and Dominica. A system of agriculture called *encomienda*, established by the Spanish, subjected the indigenous people to a form of slavery that required them to labor in fields to produce cotton, sugar, and tobacco for export. The conditions of slave labor—compounded by malnutrition and introduced diseases such as smallpox—nearly wiped out the Arawaks within 30 years.

One New World plant quickly exported to Europe was the chile pepper (*Capsicum* spp.). Rum—fermented molasses syrup mixed with cinnamon, rosemary, or caramel—also became a popular export, which spurred the establishment of sugarcane plantations and importing of slaves. Although slavery was finally abolished in the 19th century, the religious beliefs of Santeria (a New World hybrid of Yoruba and Christianity) had become rooted within the former slave populations of many islands, as well as in parts of Central America and the United States. Practitioners used hundreds of different plants and flowers in magic rituals to obtain the power, or *ashe*, of the saints to live their arduous lives. Even today, it is not uncommon for practitioners to use basil to drive away the evil eye, marigold to produce lucky number dreams, juniper berries to increase virility in men, and oregano to keep away annoying in-laws.

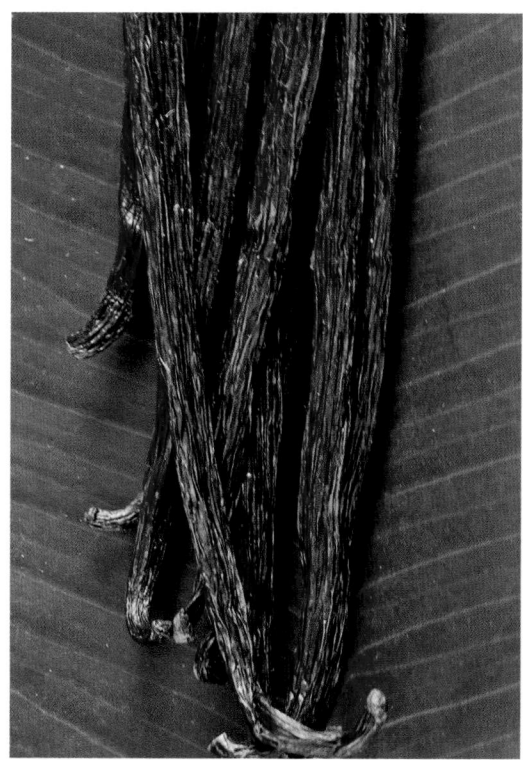

Vanilla pods, which produce the popular flavoring, are the fruit of a South American vine.

South America

The continent of South America is unparalleled for the richness of its flora; Brazil alone is home to 55,000 species of flowering plants. But much of the indigenous peoples' traditional uses for these plants remained largely unknown to the outside world until recent centuries, when ethnological and ethnobotanical studies were begun of these sophisticated peoples and their plants. The Yanomami people of Brazil and Venezuela, for example, are believed to have moved to the region nearly 8,000 years ago and have lived very much the same way ever since (although this is rapidly changing). The Amazon forest has provided them (and many other tribes) with berries of urucú, also known as annatto (*Bixa orellana*), for red dye to decorate their bodies and loincloths, and with fibers of the kapok tree (*Ceiba pentandra*) to make deadly poison-tipped blowgun darts for hunting.

In the Siona tribe of Colombia, shamans collected stems of yage (*Banisteriopsis caapi*) and leaves of chagropanga (*Diplopterys cabrerana*) to make a ritual drink that produced hallucinatory visions of the spirit world, through which they could offer healing to their patients. In the western Amazon region, shamans made a medicine by combining the same vine, there called ayahuasca (*B. caapi*), or "vine of the soul," with the leaves of chacruna (*Psychotria viridis*) to cure a wide range of physical, psychological, and spiritual illnesses.

Interestingly, the psychoactive effect results from the potent chemicals released by the combination of the two plants used together—either plant used alone will not produce the same results. The discovery of the synergistic effects of different plant species from two different plant families, first reported more than 150 years ago by the botanist Richard Spruce, is a most remarkable feat of indigenous technology. This level of sophistication, also seen in the preparation of food plants to remove toxic compounds and make them palatable, can be found repeatedly among indigenous cultures.

The Andean highlands of Peru are home to several plants with a long history of use—potato, maca root (*Lepidium meyenii*), and coca (*Erythroxylum coca* and *E. novogranatense*). Maca is said to enhance physical strength and endurance, as well as sexual prowess. In its leaf form, the coca plant was used to energize the body and stave off the fatigue and hunger associated with living in the rugged mountains or remote rainforest. Andean and Amazon civilizations chewed coca leaves (the source of the purified drug cocaine) as early as 2,000 BCE—some references even suggest that its use began 8,000 years ago. Known as *soroche* in the Andean region, coca leaf tea has long been recognized as an effective cure for altitude sickness. Because of its importance in sacred rituals, coca was highly valued in early societies, and today this plant remains a revered species within its native region.

Around 1450 BCE, the Incas rose to power in the Andean mountain region, and in less than a century, they developed a civilization nearly as sophisticated as that of the ancient Romans. The Incas built reliable irrigation systems by diverting rivers, building aqueducts, and digging canals along terraces on which they produced maize, cotton, quinoa, peanuts, coca, potatoes, and tomatoes. They also produced medicinal herbs such as *vilcacora* or cat's claw (*Uncaria tomentosa*), an anti-inflammatory; manayupa (*Desmodium adscendens*), a detoxicant and blood purifier; and sangre de drago, or dragon's blood (*Croton lechleri*), a treatment for wounds.

From the time of the Spanish conquest to the present day, thousands of important herbal medicines have been "discovered" by Europeans in South America—of course, the true discoverers were the local people in the region who taught the early explorers. Legend has it that an Andean Indian with a terrible fever drank bitter-tasting water from a pond that was contaminated by the stems and leaves of the quinine trees that grew around it. Miraculously, his fever disappeared and word about the power of this tree spread. The bark was later found to contain the alkaloid quinine, a drug that reduces fevers and helps prevent malaria. Quinine remained the world's most effective antimalarial agent until the invention of a synthetic equivalent several hundred years later.

Curare, extracted from the stem of *Chondrodendron tomentosum,* was the basis for a deadly poison used to coat the tips of arrows and blowgun darts. Hunters could use this poison to kill large or distant animals simply by shooting an arrow or dart at their quarry and penetrating the skin. Curare would paralyze the skeletal muscles and cause asphyxiation, leading to death. Curare later became useful as a surgical anesthetic and treatment for chronic muscle spasms.

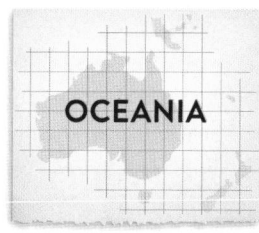

Oceania is a 3.5 million-square-mile region, mostly ocean, containing within it thousands of tropical Pacific islands. This includes the island groups of Melanesia, Micronesia, and Polynesia, as well as Australia, New Zealand, Indonesia, and other areas. In this part of the world, the use of herbs for food, medicine, and spiritual practices originated with indigenous peoples whose cultures date back thousands of years. Antiseptic tea tree oil, for example, was first prepared by Australian Aboriginals from the leaves of the melaleuca tree (*Melaleuca* spp.). Australian forests also hold the promise of new medicines, such as from the black bean (*Castanospermum australe*), which produces the powerful antiviral compound castanospermine, a substance of interest to medical researchers.

Indonesia's dense tropical rainforests have been home to some of the world's most important spice plants, such as nutmeg, cloves, and mace, as well

IMPORTANT HERBS *of* CENTRAL *and* SOUTH AMERICA

HERB	EXAMPLES OF USES
Allspice (*Pimenta dioica*)	Pungent culinary flavoring
Annatto (*Bixa orellana*)	Cosmetic colorant, culinary flavoring
Epazote (*Dysphania ambrosioides*)	Mexican cooking herb
Ipecac (*Carapichea ipecacuanha*)	Potent emetic, expectorant
Lignum vitae (*Guaiacum officinale*)	Mild laxative, diuretic
Mexican yam (*Dioscorea macrostachya*)	Source of raw material for steroids
Papaya (*Carica papaya*)	Insect sting remedy, digestive aid, culinary uses
Vanilla (*Vanilla planifolia*)	Popular flavoring, perfume
Yerba mate (*Ilex paraguariensis*)	Stimulating tea

as important plant families, such as Apocynaceae, a source of cardiac and tranquilizing alkaloids. From the Pacific islands come the noni plant (*Morinda citrifolia*), which some consider a panacea, and the starchy taro (*Colocasia esculenta*), a food plant that's also used to treat complaints from boils to heart conditions.

Australia

Northern Australia has a tropical climate, while the southern coast is relatively cool and moist. A vast, arid desert covers the interior. Much of the continent is subject to brush fires, and many native plants, such as eucalyptus, have oils and resins in their aerial parts that encourage a rapid burning that leaves woody tissues and underground parts unharmed.

The early Aboriginal people of Australia were hunters and gatherers who traveled vast distances on foot. They are believed to have used more than 150 different herb species just for the treatment of inflamed wounds and eyes. To alleviate the hunger and fatigue of long journeys, they commonly chewed *pituri,* a substance made from nicotine-containing plants of the nightshade family (Solanaceae). Gum from *Eucalyptus* species, produced by wounding the tree, was used to control infections, bleeding, and diarrhea. The native people also mixed herbal medicines to treat burns, headaches, digestive upsets, jellyfish and insect stings, and snakebites.

According to the Aboriginal belief system, many ailments and accidents were caused by spirits. Spiritual healers, both men and women, performed sacred rites using herbs to counteract the sorcery. Treatments included steam inhalation, sleeping pillows, and infusions. Many remedies were applied topically: A patient could be rubbed with crushed seed paste, fruit pulp, or sap. Newborn babies and new mothers were exposed to steam or rubbed with oils to give them strength.

Bush medicine focused on commonly found plants, such as the fuchsia bush (*Eremophila* spp.), the bloodwood tree (*Corymbia terminalis*), and lemongrass (*Cymbopogon* spp.). Some medicines varied in strength with the seasons—for a toothache, the wet season growth of green plum leaves (*Buchanania obovata*) was considered a stronger remedy than the plant's dry season growth.

In 1770, Captain James Cook (1728–1779) arrived and claimed Australia for the British crown. The land was established as a British penal colony, and for the next 80 years nearly 160,000 men and women were transported from England to Australia as convicts. The new arrivals brought with them a host of nonnative crops, from cereal grains to potatoes, onions, sugarcane, tobacco, and grapevines. The Europeans also named native plants after species the plants resembled in their homeland. Today, native or "bush" potatoes, bananas, cherries, pears, and plums unrelated to their European namesakes are found throughout Australia. These plants—intertwined with exotic imports and edible and medicinal plants cultivated by settlers—spread into the wild.

In all, at least 2,700 new plants were introduced in Australia, where they have now established populations. Some, such as arum lily (*Zantedeschia aethiopica*), fleabane (*Conyza* spp.), and the ubiquitous lantana (*Lantana camara*), have become invasive weeds, spreading throughout the country and edging out indigenous species. Others, such as wild tobacco (*Nicotiana glauca*), were simply integrated by Aboriginal people into traditional medical practices.

New Zealand

The plant life of northern New Zealand resembles that of tropical southeastern Asia, while the country's central regions have a temperate climate, and the southern zone is cool and wet. New

Zealand's first inhabitants were the Maori people, who are believed to have arrived from southeastern Asia around 1000 CE. They had an intricate healing system that centered on the *tohunga*, who was both doctor and spiritual leader. The tohunga administered herbal remedies, known as *rongoa*, that prevented and cured illnesses as well as spiritual rituals and vapor baths. Native species such as New Zealand flax (*Phormium tenax*) and manuka (*Leptospermum scoparium*), now familiar as ornamental plants, were used to treat a wide range of ailments, including topical wounds.

The Pacific Islands

The islands in the Pacific are home to hundreds of interesting herbs: Fiji has 2,000 native plant species, Papua New Guinea has 15,000, and Samoa has 550. Much of the collective history of the Pacific Islands is fundamentally linked to the use of these plants, which include kava (*Piper methysticum*) and noni (*Morinda citrifolia*).

Kava contains compounds known as kavalactones, which have analgesic, anesthetic, and tranquilizing effects. The herb has gained worldwide popularity as a stress and anxiety reliever. Noni, or Indian mulberry, is the fruit of a shrubby, evergreen tree. Fermented noni juice is consumed throughout the Pacific as a traditional prophylactic against illness, and the fruit is traditionally believed to cure sore throats and the sting of the poisonous stonefish. Noni fruit and juice contain compounds that are locally believed to help treat a variety of ailments, including high blood pressure, arthritis, and cancer. The vanilla bean is also grown and exported from some Pacific islands. A climbing vine of the orchid family, vanilla produces seedpods—known in commerce as beans—used for manufacturing extracts, oleoresins, and alcoholic tinctures, as well as flavorings for ice creams, baked goods, chocolates,

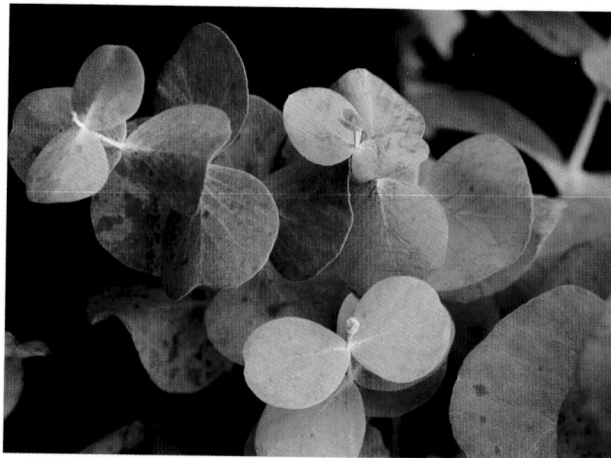

The leaves of the Australian *Eucalyptus globulus* contain eucalyptol, the active ingredient in many over-the-counter chest rubs.

liquors, soft drinks, tobaccos, and perfumes.

The screwpine, or pandanus (*Pandanus tectorius*), is one of the South Pacific's most useful plants. In Samoa, fragrant pandanus flowers are used to make wreaths called *lei*, which are worn by chiefs. In Tahiti, juice from pandanus root tips is used to treat skin inflammation. In Tonga, the juice is mixed with turmeric (*Curcuma longa*) and grated coconut and is applied to topical sores. The skin of ripe pandanus fruit is used to treat urinary tract problems, and in Fiji, a tea made from pandanus leaves is consumed as a remedy for diarrhea. Numerous other medicinal uses for the herb include the treatment of asthma, back pain, heart conditions, and internal fractures.

These few examples, from among the tens of thousands of plants recorded to date with medicinal or related uses around the world, show just how strongly plants have influenced the trajectory of human civilization. Despite the advent of virtual living through the extraordinarily sophisticated array of technology available today, it's clear that plants will continue to play a central role in our lives and remain key to our survival as a species.

Quite often in the Pacific, as well as elsewhere, common foods are also used as medicines. *Colocasia esculenta,* known as taro and by other names in the Pacific region, is a staple food crop, providing starch, essential minerals, vitamins, and fiber to the people who prepare and eat the root. The leaves, after being properly prepared to eliminate the irritating calcium oxalate crystals they contain, are cooked, mashed, often mixed with coconut milk, and eaten as a delicious green vegetable. People on each island can recognize a dozen or more cultivars of taro, each with a distinctive appearance, taste, or other trait. Taro leaves are often rolled into cups for drinking beverages and medicinal teas, and on Fiji a boiled extract of the macerated leaves is used to promote menstruation. The leaves, mixed with other herbs, are used to treat conditions ranging from stomach disorders and cysts to wounds and boils. A multiherb mix containing the scraped stem of taro is administered to children to build their appetites. However, no matter what the use, all parts of this plant must be thoroughly cooked to eliminate the chance of oxalate toxicity.

IMPORTANT HERBS *of* OCEANIA

HERB	EXAMPLES OF USES
Corkwood (*Duboisia* spp.)	Stimulant
Gum tree (*Eucalyptus* spp.)	Astringent, cough medicine
Jequirity (*Abrus precatorius*)	Aboriginal body ornament
Kava (*Piper methysticum*)	Anxiety reliever
Mint bush (*Prostanthera* spp.)	Antibiotic, fungicide
Mountain pepperberry (*Tasmannia lanceolata*)	Hot, pepperlike spice
Myrtle (*Backhousia* spp.)	Fragrance
Old man saltbush (*Atriplex nummularia*)	Treatment for scurvy
Sticky hop bush (*Dodonaea viscosa*)	Toothache and insect sting remedy
Taro (*Colocasia esculenta*)	Staple food, all-purpose medicine

ETHNOBOTANICAL RESEARCH *in* MICRONESIA

I first visited Micronesia in 1997, traveling to Pohnpei and Kosrae in the Federated States of Micronesia, and then on to the Republic of Palau. The goal of my monthlong trip was to find the setting for the next chapter of my career as an ethnobotanist at The New York Botanical Garden: an island whose people, faced with the pressures of globalization, wanted to inventory their natural resources and record their plant-based traditions before Westernization replaced them with a modern perspective and lifestyle. For a variety of reasons detailed in our 2009 book, *Ethnobotany of Pohnpei: Plants, People, and Island Culture*, the 138-square-mile

volcanic island of Pohnpei, situated in the Western Caroline Islands, was to be the next stop on my ethnobotanical journey.

I was fascinated from the moment I landed on the island, as I noted in the introduction to our book: "Pohnpei is a special part of the world. It is a small island where people are openly friendly, extremely helpful, and genuinely interested in the welfare of others. . . . What is most lacking in many Westerner's lives—a sense of community—is omnipresent in Pohnpei."

From my earliest visits, and continuing through dozens of intensive collecting trips to explore the most

remote areas of the island, people were eager to discuss and record the uses of plants. Their traditional leaders were particularly devoted to preserving knowledge of their traditional uses of plants and the sustainable management of their natural resources.

We recruited teams of local people to survey and record how plants provide food, medicine, and construction materials, as well as how they are used for fishing, canoe building, and in the spiritual beliefs of this culture. The people I was so privileged to work with prioritized their most important and endangered traditional skills, and they worked hard to gather information about ancient plant-based practices such as making houses, clothing, fishing nets, and baskets; preparing local medicines; and cultivating crops as their ancestors had done for generations.

More than 150 local experts on the traditional uses of plants participated in this 10-year program. They recorded information on the local names and uses of more than 350 different species—on an island with fewer than 1,000 species of plants. Currently, a group of Micronesians have expanded this effort to record plant diversity, distribution, use, sustainable management, and conservation to islands such as Kosrae and Palau. This information can help the people of these remote parts of the world become more self-sufficient and promote the sustainable use of their natural resources.

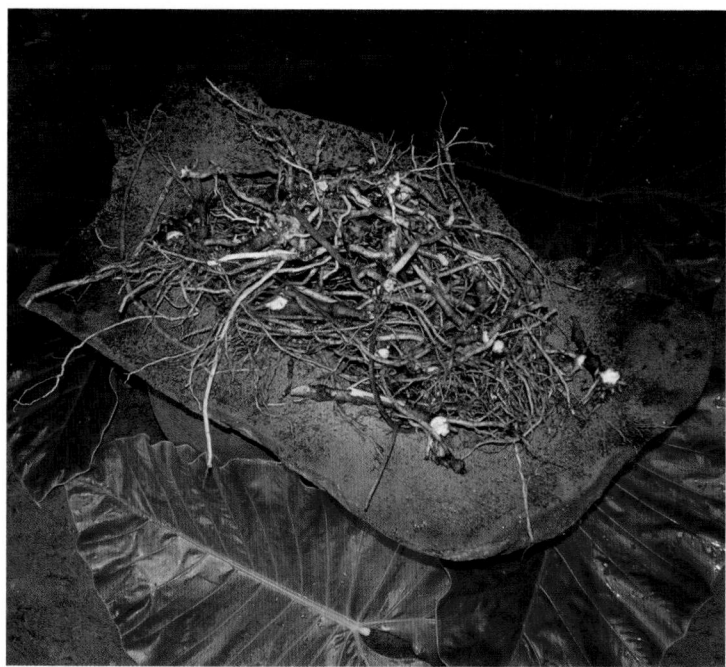

The most important plant on Pohnpei is *Piper methysticum*, locally known as *sakau* and elsewhere in the Pacific called kava. Here the roots of sakau are placed on a stone ready for pounding that will allow their processing into a beverage. Leaves of a local taro species, *Alocasia macrorrhizos*, surround the base of the stone to keep the roots clean and pure should they fall.

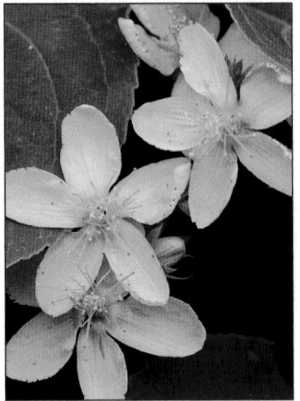

CHAPTER 2

THE BASICS *of* HERBAL BOTANY

W hat are herbs? To a botanist living in the temperate region, an herb is simply an herbaceous plant—that is, a plant that does not produce persistent woody tissue and usually dies back in winter. Height isn't a factor. One of the largest herbaceous plants, the banana—which does not produce a woody stem, but rather a fleshy "pseudostem"—can grow to 20 feet tall or more.

To a chef, the definition is completely different: An herb is any of a vast number of aromatic or savory plants used to add flavor and character to foods. To a gardener, an herb is a delightful, easy-to-grow addition to the landscape, perennial border, or terrace urn. And to anyone who uses plants medicinally, an herb is a plant or plant part that helps promote health and healing when it's either taken internally or applied externally.

Yet none of these definitions wholly describes the many attributes of an "herb." The botanist's definition of an herb—any "nonwoody" plant—does not encompass many plants known today as "medicinal herbs" or "botanicals." Medicinal herbs come from all kinds of plants: trees, shrubs, vines, grasses, and ferns—as well as mushrooms, lichens, mosses, and seaweeds. The chef's emphasis on flavor does not address the powerful medicinal properties of many common culinary herbs, such as garlic, ginger, turmeric, and cayenne. And the ornamental gardener does not consider the value of dandelion for cooking, healing, or making dyes—she's far more likely to dig out this herb as a "weed" than to plant it.

So just what is an herb—a nonwoody plant, culinary staple, garden ornamental, health-promoting remedy, or a weed? The answer is all of the above, depending on the plant and how it is used. Indeed, usefulness could be the most defining characteristic of an herb: An herb is a plant that humans use, or have used, to enhance their lives.

NAMING PLANTS

A rose is a rose is a rose? If only it were that simple! The truth is, most well-known plants go by several names: a scientific name and one or more common (or vernacular) names, depending on where the plant is found or grown. Making matters more confusing, a single common name can often refer to plants of several different botanical species. For instance, in the United States, "corn" is the common name for *Zea mays,* the vegetable enjoyed "on the cob." Say the word "corn" to a farmer or baker in England, and they will think you are speaking about wheat (*Triticum* spp.). In Scotland, "corn" might refer to oats (*Avena sativa*).

The common name, as the term implies, is a name people coin to identify a local plant—for example, sweet violet, catnip, and dandelion are common names. Often, common names are colorfully descriptive, and they can provide valuable information about a plant's traditional uses, characteristics, or growth habits. The name dandelion, for example, comes from the French *dente de lion,* which means "tooth of the lion" and describes the serrated edge of the leaf. Another common French name for dandelion, *pis en lit,* translates as "wet the bed," a reference to the powerful diuretic properties of the dandelion leaf.

Botanically speaking, sweet violet, catnip, and dandelion are known as *Viola odorata, Nepeta cataria,* and *Taraxacum officinale,* respectively. Just like common names, botanical names offer fascinating clues about what plants look like, what they smell like, where they come from, and even how they are used medicinally. Using the same three plants as examples, it is possible to infer from the species name *odorata* that this violet has a distinctive fragrance. The name *cataria* indicates that

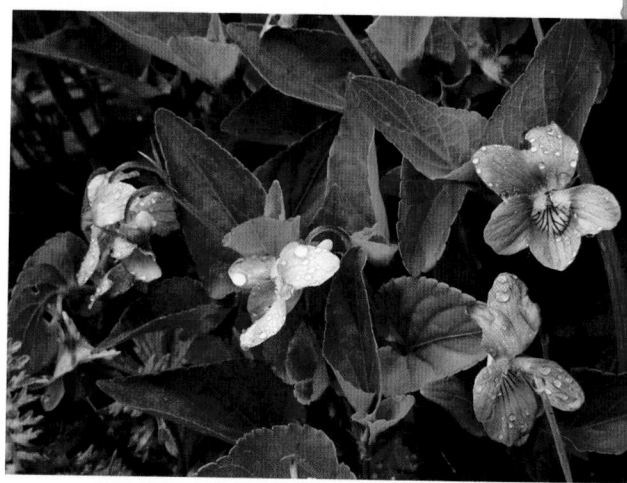

Sweet violet has several common names, including wood violet or English violet. But it has only one correct scientific name: *Viola odorata.*

this member of the genus *Nepeta* is linked in some way to felines. And the name *officinale* (or *officinalis*), which originally referred to a monastic storeroom or pharmacy, is an indication that a plant was utilized as a medicine based on its healing properties.

SCIENTIFIC NAMES: LINNAEUS AND THE BINOMIAL SYSTEM

Although a plant might have several common names, it will have only one officially recognized botanical or scientific name. The advantage of using botanical names, or scientific nomenclature, is that it allows one—no matter what his or her native tongue—to understand exactly which herb is being discussed. For example, the spiny shrub *Eleutherococcus senticosus*—commonly called Siberian ginseng or eleuthero in the United States and devil's shrub or thorny pepper bush in Russia—is understood to be *Eleutherococcus senticosus* whether one is a citizen of the United States or Russia. This is an important and basic standard, not only to botanists and other scientists, but also to herbalists, practitioners, and members of the botanical trade, who need to be absolutely certain about the identities of the plants they use.

Early plant scientists recognized the need for a system of terms that could be used to distinguish one particular plant species from all others in the world. This task was successfully accomplished by the Swedish botanist Carolus Linnaeus (1707–1778), who in 1753 established what's known as the binomial system of plant nomenclature. Linnaeus's goal was to name and describe all known types of plants, as well as animals and even minerals. He believed that in so doing, he would reveal the grand pattern of creation. In a two-volume work called *Species Plantarum*, Linnaeus introduced a workable botanical classification system that would eventually bear his name.

Scientists quickly adopted Linnaeus's system as

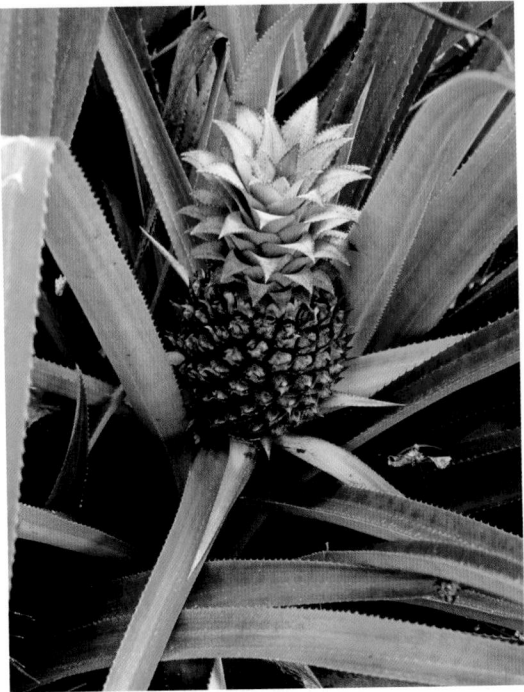

Originally named *Bromelia comosa* by the Swedish botanist Linnaeus, the pineapple plant was renamed *Ananas comosus* by Elmer Drew Merrill in 1917.

a means of sorting out the vast numbers of new species being discovered at the time. Nearly 20 years before publishing *Species Plantarum*, Linnaeus proposed a polynomial (multiple-word) naming system to describe species, but in later editions of his works, this evolved into the basic binomial (two-word: genus and specific epithet) naming system used today. The Linnaean system of classification is based on relationships among living organisms, from the most general (kingdom) to the most specific (species). A species, the most basic unit of organization in the system, is composed of individuals that resemble one another more nearly than they resemble individuals of any other species.

Using the plant *Ginkgo biloba* as an example, *Ginkgo* is the genus name and *biloba* is the specific epithet. In more formal use, such as in a scientific paper, the name of the botanist who first described the plant is also included. For example, *Ginkgo biloba* was described by Linnaeus, which is noted as part of the scientific name following the species: *Ginkgo biloba* L. And over time, if a different botanist decides that the plant belongs to another genus, then the original author's name is put in parentheses, with the later author's name following. For example, the scientific name of the pineapple is *Ananas comosus* (L.) Merr. While this wonderful fruit was first described by Linnaeus as *Bromelia comosa* L., in 1754, the species was moved to the genus *Ananas* by the renowned Pacific botanist Elmer Drew Merrill in a 1917 publication. Nearly 100 years later, the term *Ananas comosus* is still used to describe the pineapple plant.

But that's not the case with all species. As our understanding of relationships among plant species and among plant families becomes more sophisticated, plants are moved into more precise alignments based on their evolutionary position in the "tree of life." In this book, to simplify the binomials, we will not include the botanist's names. If you are interested in this element of botanical history, the names and stories of the scientists who first applied them can be found in many other books and on the Web.

Far from static, these classifications change as new information alters scientists' understanding of the relationships among organisms. Originally, all organisms were classified into two kingdoms: animal and plant. Now, based on information such as data obtained by molecular studies unavailable when the Linnaean system was introduced, most scientists use a six-kingdom classification scheme that separates fungi and certain other kinds of creatures into kingdoms of their own. Increasingly, biologists are recognizing a new rank—domain—above the grouping of kingdom. There are three domains: Bacteria, Archaea, and Eukarya. Herbs belong to the domain Eukarya, which contains animals, plants, fungi, and protists.

Kingdoms

The kingdom is the largest, most inclusive classification in the Linnaean system. Most scientists recognize these six kingdoms: Animalia (animals), Plantae (plants), Fungi (fungal organisms, including mushrooms), Protista (simple organisms, such as protozoans and algae, whose cells have nuclei and organelles), Archaea (single-celled microorganisms with cells that do not have nuclei or organelles and that do not carry out chlorophyll-based photosynthesis), and Bacteria (single-celled organisms with cells that do not have nuclei or organelles; some species carry out chlorophyll-based photosynthesis).

Within the plant kingdom, organisms are sorted into angiosperms (plants with seeds enclosed in an ovary), gymnosperms ("naked seed" plants), ferns, fern allies, mosses, liverworts, and hornworts. Recent classification systems based on a more precise understanding of plant relationships and evolution refer to groupings as clades (see "A Modern Understanding of the Plant Kingdom" on page 47), signifying branches on the tree of life and, to a degree, they dispense with certain elements of the Linnaean system.

Families

Groups of related genera make up plant families. Some plant families are quite large—the orchid, aster, and pea families are the three biggest—while others, such as the ginkgo family, contain only one species.

In an ongoing effort to standardize the classification and naming of plants, botanists in recent decades have modernized the naming of plant families. According to the current system, family names end with the suffix "-aceae" and are taken from the name of an included genus that typifies the family. (Genus and species names are italicized in print, but family names are not.) For example, *Acorus calamus,* sweet flag, is a member of the plant family Acoraceae. Plant families also are sometimes referred to by the common name of a genus associated with that family, such as "rose family" (for Rosaceae). So, while the English hawthorn (*Crataegus laevigata*) is not of the same genus as garden roses (*Rosa* spp.), as a member of the Rosaceae, it shares "rose family" traits, along with species of the genus *Prunus,* where plums, peaches, and apricots are found. However, there is no standardized list of common names for plant families, and some families are referred to using various names. For example, common names for the Marantaceae, a group of tropical species, include the prayer plant family and arrowroot family. And the Asteraceae is known variously as the daisy, sunflower, or aster family.

Botanists have agreed upon protocols for naming plants, known as the rules of nomenclature. For eight plant families, alternative family names are permitted under the current rules: These alternatives are (with modern equivalents in parentheses) Compositae (Asteraceae), Cruciferae (Brassicaceae), Gramineae (Poaceae), Guttiferae (Clusiaceae), Labiatae (Lamiaceae), Leguminosae (Fabaceae), Palmae (Arecaceae), and Umbelliferae (Apiaceae).

Some plant families are so large and complex that they are further divided into subfamilies and what botanists call "tribes." The sunflower family (Asteraceae), one of the largest of all plant families, at one time was subdivided into two subfamilies. But now, after much more sophisticated analysis of the evolutionary relationships of this group, it is considered to have 12 subfamilies. Such distinctions are not always clear-cut, and botanists continue to study and refine our understanding of plant relationships and how species should be classified.

Genus

A genus consists of a group of species closely related to one another, determined primarily by the reproductive parts of their flowers. Some of the many genera in the mint family (Lamiaceae) are *Lavandula* (lavender), *Mentha* (mint), *Thymus* (thyme), *Salvia* (sage), *Rosmarinus* (rosemary), *Monarda* (bee balm), and *Melissa* (lemon balm). The rose family (Rosaceae) includes the genera *Rosa* (rose), *Prunus* (plum, almond, and cherry), *Crataegus* (hawthorn), *Malus* (apple), *Rubus* (raspberry and blackberry), *Fragaria* (strawberry), and many others.

Species

The species is the most basic of all classifications. For example, *Salvia officinalis* (common garden sage) and *S. sclarea* (clary sage) are both highly aromatic plants, yet each has unique characteristics. In a publication, once the genus name has been established, it may be abbreviated thereafter in that same paragraph. When a species or species name is unspecified, it may be indicated with the abbreviation "sp." For example, *Salvia* sp. indicates an unspecified species of sage. More than one species is indicated by the abbreviation "spp."—for example, *Salvia* spp. refers to a group of *Salvia* species. These two abbreviations are not italicized.

Plant Subspecies and Varieties

A plant that differs genetically from some members of its species, but not enough to be classified as a species of its own, may be designated as a subspecies. Subspecies often result from interbreeding in geographically isolated populations. A subspecies is indicated by the abbreviation "ssp." or "subsp."

Plant subspecies can be further categorized into varieties. A variety, or variation in a species, is designated by the abbreviation "var." followed by an italicized variety name, as in *Achillea millefolium* var. *rubrum*. This name indicates that the plant is a variety of common yarrow (*Achillea millefolium*) that has red (*rubrum*) flowers rather than white

A MODERN UNDERSTANDING *of the* PLANT KINGDOM
The Work of the Angiosperm Phylogeny Group

Botanists now have advanced tools to help them understand the evolution of, and relationships among, plants. In the past, systematic botanists—those who study classification and evolutionary relationships between plants—depended mostly on characteristics from morphological studies (analyses of the form and external structure of a plant) as well as analysis of their different chemical compounds to produce classification systems. Today, modern molecular tools for studying the composition of DNA—deoxyribonucleic acid, which contains the genetic code essential to the development and functioning of all living organisms (except viruses)—have revolutionized botanists' ability to classify plants. Now a botanist can classify a plant by the DNA sequence found in an individual species.

The process is similar to what's used to help solve a crime or absolve the accused. This technology, along with new analytical approaches, has provided a wealth of information that can be analyzed using phylogenetics—the study of evolutionary relationships among organisms (in this case, plants). Perspectives obtained from phylogenetic analysis can be used to clarify and test plant classification systems and to further understand the plant kingdom and the groupings of its components.

Beginning in the late 1990s, a group of systematic botanists created the Angiosperm Phylogeny Group

(APG) to produce a more precise classification system for flowering plants (angiosperms). APG retains some parts of the Linnaean system, plant orders and families, and requires that plants be grouped by their descendants from a common ancestor; this is known as the monophyletic approach. As a result, the placement of many families has changed. The term *clade*—a lineage—is used to group naturally related orders, families, genera, and species.

This work has led to the placement of some plant families within others, resulting in species that were formerly in one family now being recognized as part of another. Information on these new concepts can be found through an online search of "Angiosperm Phylogeny Group."

Studying plants this way, at the molecular level, has truly revolutionized our ability to determine the relationships between and among species, genera, families, orders, and other groupings used to categorize plants—giving us a much greater understanding of plant classification. The closer scientists get to understanding how plants evolved and are related, the greater the ability of those who work on applied aspects of plant biology—including plant breeders, medicinal chemists, biofuel scientists, conservationists, and others who apply plant biology—to help feed, clothe, heal, fuel, and protect a growing world popula-

tion and its environment.

For example, consider Taxol (paclitaxel), an extremely valuable plant-based medicine originally isolated from the endangered tree *Taxus brevifolia*. The quantity of bark needed for the production of a single therapeutic dose meant that there weren't adequate supplies for patients' needs; scientists eventually found compounds in a related, widely available *Taxus* species, allowing this vital medicine to be produced in the quantities needed. Having a precise understanding of plant relationships provided new insights into the search for biologically active molecules needed to make a drug in short supply. Far from an ivory tower exercise, obtaining an understanding of the evolution and relationships of plants, combined with an accurate classification system, greatly benefits us all.

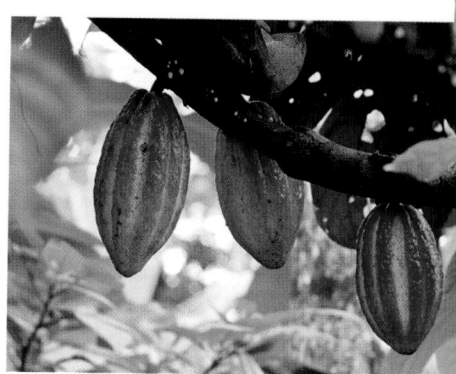

Through DNA analysis, plant scientists have determined that chocolate (*Theobroma cacao*) belongs to the mallow family (Malvaceae), which also includes cola, cotton, and okra.

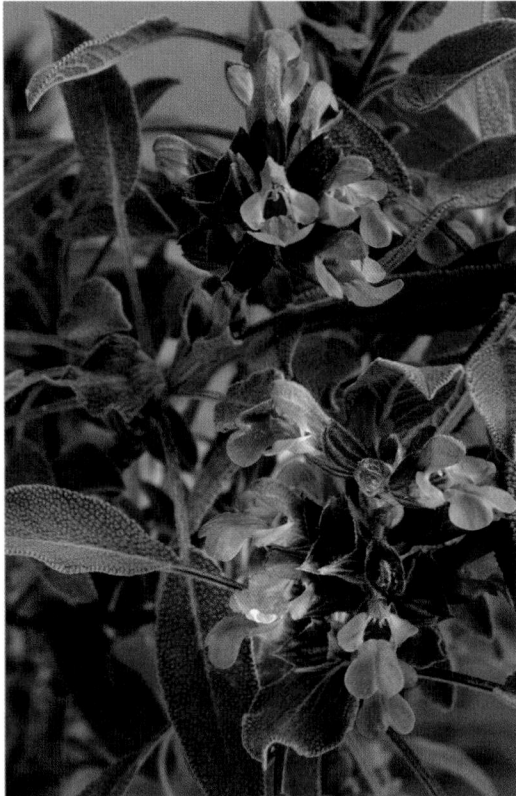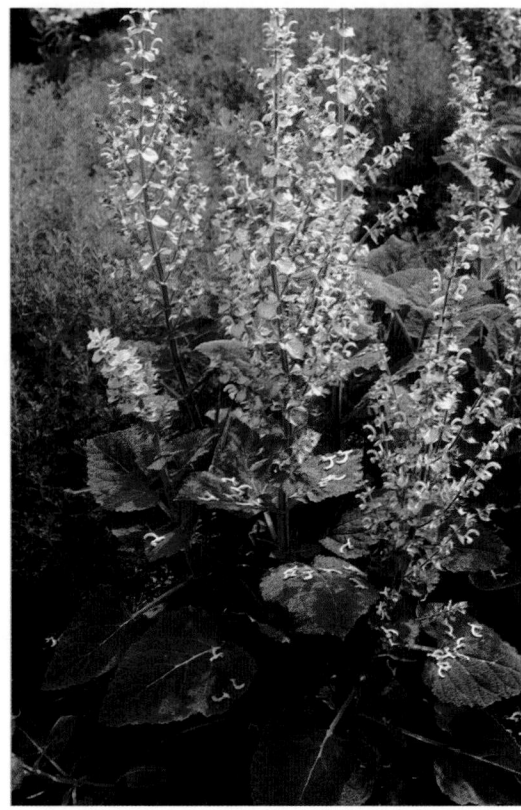

Although both of these plants are from the genus *Salvia*, *Salvia officinalis* (garden sage, left)
and *Salvia sclarea* (clary sage, right) each have distinctive characteristics distinguishing them as separate species.

ones. Variety names are italicized; cultivar names
are not.

Cultivars and Hybrids

Unlike subspecies and varieties, cultivars do not
occur naturally, but rather have been developed
and perpetuated by cultivation. The term "cultivar" was coined from the words "cultivated" and
"variety." Cultivars can be hybrids created by
breeding members of different species, or they may
simply be desirable selections made from one species, chosen for a specific shape, flower color,
aroma, or tolerance to certain environmental conditions. Cultivar names can be trademarked and

registered with an International Cultivar Registra-
tion Authority according to specific nomenclature
rules. Names of cultivars appear in single quota-
tion marks after species names. Wandering
through your local nursery, you might see a tree
labeled *Ginkgo biloba* cv. 'Autumn Gold', indicating that this is a cultivated variety that someone
has selected, named, and registered. Compared to
the usual variant of the species, the cultivar
'Autumn Gold' has particularly beautiful golden
leaves in fall and a more compact shape.

Hybrids occur when two different species cross
(either in nature or by the hand of humans) to produce a new plant, usually with traits from both of the
parents. They are denoted with an "×" between the

genus and species names, as in *Mentha × piperita,* a cross between watermint (*Mentha aquatica*) and spearmint (*Mentha spicata*) that produces a plant known to all gardeners as peppermint.

MORPHOLOGY: PLANT FORM AND STRUCTURE

Learning to identify herbs, understand their structure, and recognize them in their native habitats can open a new dimension of appreciation for plants and the natural world. In fact, many herbalists believe that developing a bond with a healing plant by admiring its beauty, learning to recognize it in the wild, or growing it in a garden is part of the benefit that plant has to offer.

On a basic level, flowering plants are classified by the number and arrangement of their flower parts, so understanding flowers is extremely important in plant identification. Biologically speaking, flower parts are the plant's reproductive organs, so they're essential to plant survival. The colors, fragrances, and shapes that make flowers irresistible to humans also, in many cases, function to lure pollinators to visit and pollinate the plant, thereby producing the seed that becomes the next generation of the species.

Leaves, too, are vital to a plant's survival. One of the main functions of leaves is photosynthesis, the process that causes plants to transform sunlight, water, and carbon dioxide into food (sugars) and oxygen. Leaves also produce a vast variety of chemicals in highly specialized cells and glands. These chemicals perform functions vital for plant survival (not all of which are completely understood) and give plants their characteristic tastes, colors, aromas, and medicinal properties.

IDENTIFYING PLANTS

One of the best ways to learn to identify plants is to become familiar with the characteristics of whole plant families, not just individual plants. This is easier to do than it might sound and can streamline the entire process of plant identification.

The reason is simple: Plant families display patterns that remain consistent from species to species. For example, flowers in the mustard family have four petals in a crosslike pattern and six stamens. Pea family flowers have five petals: two wing petals, one banner petal, and two petals fused into what botanists call a keel. And lily family flowers have three petals, three sepals, and six stamens.

Developing the ability to recognize family characteristics and identify plants takes a bit of practice and perseverance. Begin by looking closely at plants to become adept at recognizing subtle similarities and differences among them. How many petals does each flower have? Do the flowers grow singly or in clumps on the stem? Are the leaves shiny or fuzzy? Are they oval or pointed, round or heart-shaped? Are their edges smooth or serrated? How are the leaves arranged on the stems? Does the plant live in a shady habitat near water, or is it found growing only in dry, sunny locations?

Choose a particular plant and observe its life cycle as it grows throughout the seasons. Learn what it looks like as a seedling and when it is flowering. Watch as the flowers mature and produce fruits and seeds, and examine the seeds. Finally, see what happens as winter approaches and the plant dies back or enters dormancy. By becoming intimately acquainted with a plant in this manner, it will always be recognizable, like the familiar face of a friend in a crowd. The following 10 plant families, each of which contains numerous herbs, are a good place to start.

BASIC PLANT STRUCTURES

*Plant morphology includes vegetative structures
(stem, leaf, and root) and reproductive structures
(such as flowers and fruits).*

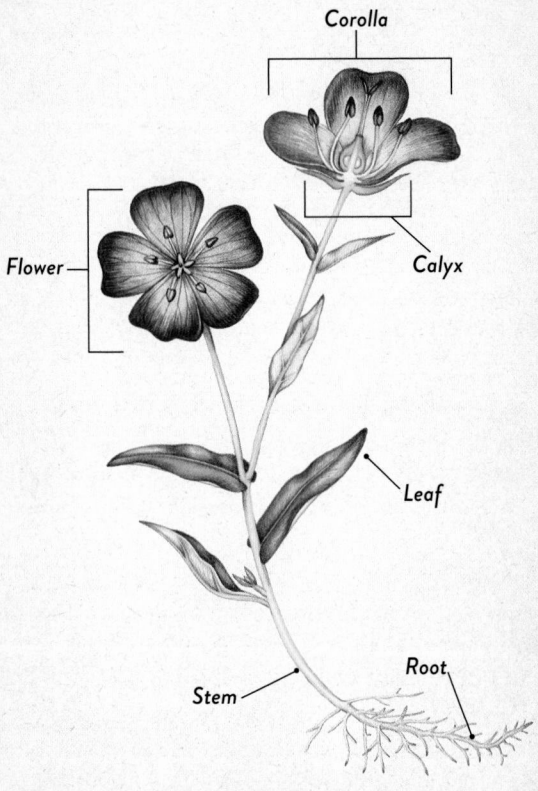

Corolla

Flower

Calyx

Leaf

Root

Stem

Plant Families

These 10 plant families offer an opportunity to explore a variety of plant characteristics.

Apiaceae (carrot and parsley family)

Asteraceae (aster and sunflower family)

Boraginaceae (borage family)

Brassicaceae (mustard family)

Fabaceae (pea family)

Lamiaceae (mint family)

Liliaceae (lily family)

Ranunculaceae (buttercup family)

Rosaceae (rose family)

Scrophulariaceae (snapdragon family)

While learning to identify herbs, a local field guide is an invaluable resource. Another good tool is a magnifying glass, which is helpful for examining small flower parts. The best kind of magnifying glass for plant identification is a jeweler's loupe with a magnification of at least 10x.

Nontechnical field guides are often organized according to flower color, which can be helpful for beginners. Technical field guides, or floras, are more challenging because they utilize what is known as a dichotomous key. It functions as a sort of flowchart that requires you to choose between two options at each point in the identification process, necessitating a working knowledge of botanical terms.

WHAT DO I NEED *to* KNOW?

For herb enthusiasts and gardeners, the most important categories of classifications to learn and understand are family, genus, species, and—when applicable—variety, cultivar, and hybrid. A good understanding of these will allow you to select, acquire, grow, and utilize the plants with the specific qualities you are seeking. Many people feel more comfortable using common names for plants simply because they are more familiar and easier to pronounce, and because plants can be purchased under those names from local nurseries and plant catalogs. If you feel intimidated by the thought of learning botanical names, consider that many common plant names—such as iris, crocus, chrysanthemum, and gladiolus, to name just a few—are actually scientific names that have been so widely used that they have become household words.

Botanists use a rich variety of highly specialized words to describe plant characteristics. Don't feel overwhelmed by the prospect of learning all of these terms. Become familiar with some of the most common ones, and look up unfamiliar words. Nearly all plant identification books provide a glossary of essential terms.

FOCUS ON FLOWERS

Biologically speaking, flower parts are all about reproduction. A flower's showy, colorful petals are designed to attract pollinators such as insects, birds, and even bats. The grouping of petals together is called the corolla. Around the outside of the corolla are sepals, leaflike structures that enclose the flower before it opens. Sepals are often green, but they can also be so colorful that they are mistaken for petals. The grouping of sepals together is called the calyx.

Most flowers include both "male" (staminate) and "female" (pistillate) parts. The stamen, or male flower part, consists of a thin stalk called a filament, topped by an anther, the pollen-bearing structure of the flower. The pistil, or female flower part, is an upright structure in the center of the flower that consists of one or more styles, which are tubelike stalks. The style supports the stigma, the part of the pistil that receives the pollen. Once pollen is deposited on the stigma, it travels down

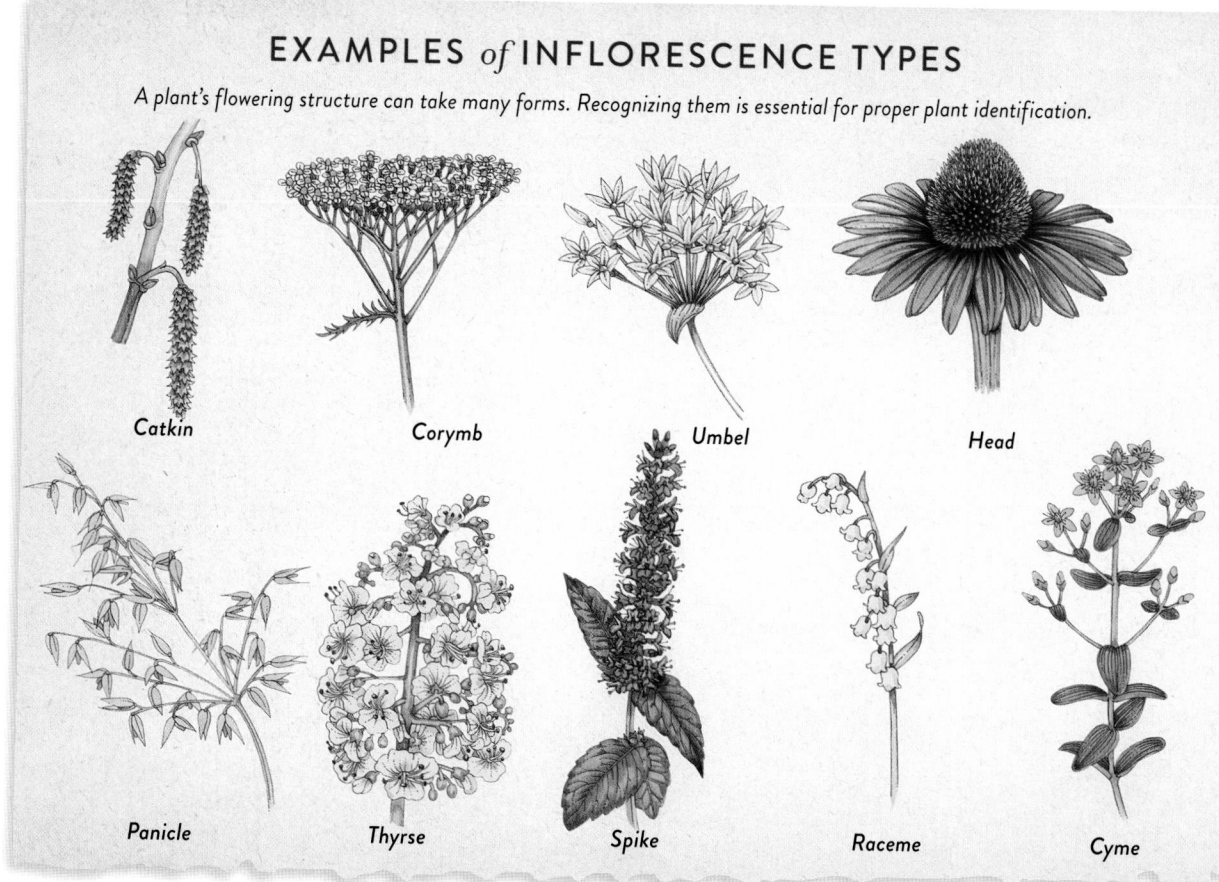

EXAMPLES *of* INFLORESCENCE TYPES

A plant's flowering structure can take many forms. Recognizing them is essential for proper plant identification.

Catkin Corymb Umbel Head

Panicle Thyrse Spike Raceme Cyme

the style to the ovary at the bottom of the pistil. The ovary contains a number of ovules that, when fertilized by pollen, develop into seeds.

Although most flowers have both male and female parts, single-sex plants are not uncommon. Technically known as dioecious plants, these bear male and female flower parts on separate plants, which means that both male and female plants must be present for pollination to occur. Dioecious herbs include ginkgo (*Ginkgo biloba*) and nettle (*Urtica dioica*). Single-sex flowers are called imperfect flowers; flowers that have both male and female parts are called perfect flowers.

In terms of plant identification, flowers are the most important part of a plant. When identifying a plant, begin by determining how many petals and sepals the flower has. Depending on the flower, this can be straightforward or tricky. Petals can be fused (joined together) or free. Flowers can be regular (symmetrical, with all petals the same

INSIDE a COMPOSITE FLOWER

Plants in the daisy family (Asteraceae), including purple coneflower, have composite flowers; each is composed of hundreds of tiny flowers.

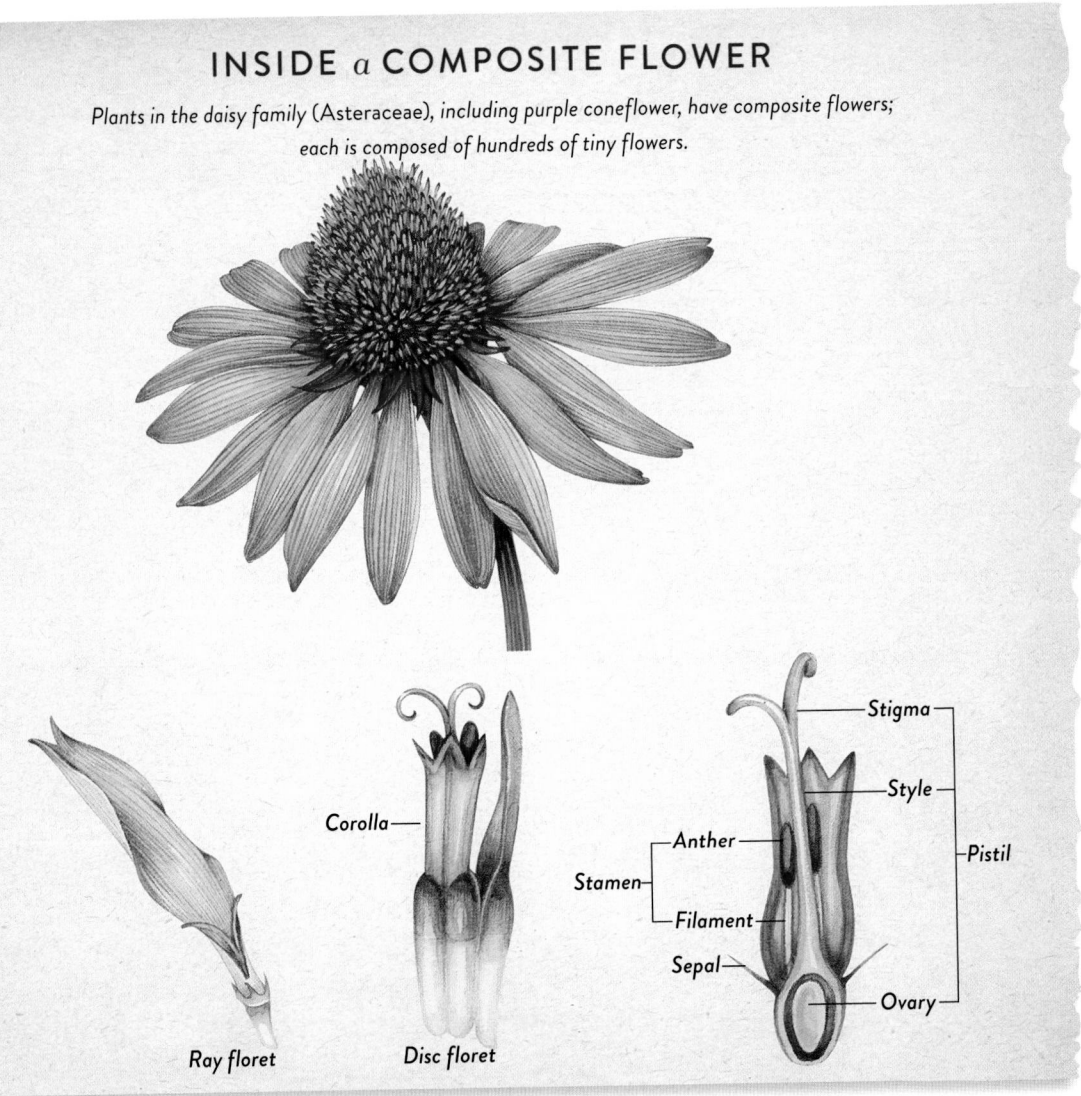

Ray floret

Corolla

Disc floret

Stigma

Style

Anther

Stamen

Filament

Sepal

Pistil

Ovary

THE LANGUAGE *of* FLOWERS

Flowers play an essential role in reproduction. The color and fragrance of a flower attract pollinators, which play a vital part in a plant's reproductive process. The color and fragrance also attract people, who in turn widen the plant's distribution by planting it in other localities and even on other continents. Here are some useful terms to know about flower parts and related structures.

Axis	An elongated, central, supporting structure running through the leaf or stem
Calyx	A collective term for the group of sepals (leaflike structures) that enclose a flower bud and encircle the petals when the flower is open
Corolla	A collective term for petals
Corymb	A short, broad, flat-topped flower cluster with individual flower stalks emerging at different points along an axis; the outermost flowers in a corymb open first
Cyme	A short, broad flower cluster that always has a flower on the tip of the axis; in a cyme, the central flowers open first
Inflorescence	The flowering part of a plant, usually used to denote a flower cluster or arrangement of flowers on an axis
Panicle	An open flower cluster, sometimes pyramid shaped, with no terminal flower on the tip of the axis; a branched raceme
Pedicel	A stalk of one flower in a multiflowered inflorescence
Peduncle	A stalk of a solitary flower or inflorescence
Perianth	The collective term for the corolla (petals) and calyx (sepals) together
Petal	A set of modified floral leaves, usually white or colored, that surround the stamens and pistils
Pistil	The "female" organ of a flower, composed of three parts—ovary, style, and stigma
Raceme	A simple, elongated stem with flowers on short stalks; flowers on the lowest part of the stem bloom first
Sepal	A leaflike flower structure that encloses a flower bud and encircles the petals when a flower is open
Spike	A simple, elongated stem with stalkless flowers or flower heads; flowers on the lowest part of the stem bloom first
Stamen	The "male" organ of the flower, composed of an anther containing pollen, most often on a filament
Umbel	A cluster of flowers with stalks of almost equal length attached to a common point; individual flowers form a flat or nearly flat top

size and shape, such as a mustard or rose family flower) or irregular (with some petals different from the others, as in a mint or pea flower). The color of the flower can provide some help, but flower color can be highly variable within a single species, making it an undependable characteristic for identification.

The aster family (Asteraceae) is one of the two largest flowering plant families. (The other is the orchid family, Orchidaceae.) The aster family's daisylike flowers—called composite flowers—are unique in the plant world. Learning to recognize the basic characteristics of this kind of flower makes it easy to quickly rule out other possibilities when trying to identify a plant.

The sunflower, which is a typical composite flower, is not a single big flower but instead is made up of hundreds of tiny flowers; this is called a composite flower head. A typical composite flower head is composed of numerous ray and disk flowers. Ray flowers are longer, strap-shaped flow-ers that circle the edge of a flower head. Disk flow-ers are short, bristly flowers in the center of a flower head.

Sunflower plants have both ray and disk flow-ers, as do feverfew and echinacea plants. Some composite flower heads, however, are composed solely of either ray or disk flowers. For example, dandelion and chicory flower heads are made up of ray flowers only. Pineapple weed (*Matricaria matricarioides*), a close relative of German chamomile (*M. recutita*), has only disk flowers. The arrangement of flowers on a plant's stem determines its type of inflorescence (flower clus-ter). This is another important identification fea-ture. (See "Examples of Inflorescence Types" on page 51.)

A CLOSER LOOK AT LEAVES

Leaves, although not as important as flowers in terms of classification, nonetheless provide essen-tial clues for plant identification. When examin-ing a plant, look at the way its leaves are arranged. The leaves can be opposite (arranged in pairs along the stem, as in plants of the mint family) or alternate (unpaired, occurring in an alternating pattern along the stem, as in plants of the borage family). Whorled leaves encircle a plant's stem, a pattern that can be seen in many plants of the lily family. The leaves of some plants, such as mullein and plantain, form what is called a basal rosette—a cluster of leaves arranged in a circular pattern on the ground at the base of the flower stalk.

The structure of a leaf is an important ele-ment of plant identification. Leaves can be simple (consisting of only one part) or compound (com-posed of multiple parts, or leaflets). In the rose family, for example, five rounded leaflets attached to a stalk make up a single compound leaf. Plants in the carrot and ginseng families also have compound leaves.

LEAF COMPLEXITY

Learning the kinds of leaf complexity can help you identify the plant.

Simple

Trifoliolate

Palmately Compound

Pinnately Compound (even pinnate)

Pinnately Compound (odd pinnate)

THE LANGUAGE *of* LEAVES

Along with roots and stems, leaves are a basic organ of plants. Their primary function is photosynthesis: the process by which a leaf uses energy from sunlight to process water and carbon dioxide into carbohydrates, such as sugars, which the plant uses as food. The following terms are used to describe leaves, leaf shapes, and leaf structures.

Apex	Tip
Basal	At the base (as in a basal rosette of leaves); arising at the base of the stem
Bract	A reduced or modified leaf located close to the base of a flower or inflorescence
Compound leaf	A leaf having two or more distinct leaflets
Cordate	Heart-shaped
Dentate	Toothed
Dissected	Divided deeply into many narrow segments
Elliptic	Having the approximate shape of an ellipse
Entire	Leaf margins with no teeth or lobes
Lanceolate	Lance-shaped, several times longer than wide; widest at the base and tapering toward the tip
Linear	Narrow and flat with parallel sides, like a blade of grass
Lobe	A segment of a leaf, especially when rounded
Node	The place on a stem from which leaves or branches originate
Oblong	Somewhat rectangular; having greater length than width and a rounded, not squared, base and tip
Obovate	Shaped like a hen's egg, but having the wider end toward the tip
Ovate	Similar to obovate, but with the wider section at the base of the leaf, where it is attached to the stem
Palmate	With numerous leaf divisions radiating from one point at the base of the leaf
Petiole	The stalk of a leaf blade or a compound leaf
Pinnate	Leaf divisions (leaflets) arranged along the axis or stalk
Serrate	With sharp teeth, pointed forward
Sessile	Having no stalk
Simple	A leaf with a blade in one piece, not compound; sometimes lobed
Stipule	A modified leaf part, usually paired, found at the base of the petiole in certain plant families, such as the rose family
Trifoliolate	Leaves having three leaflets

LEAF SHAPES *and* MARGINS

An herb leaf's shape and margins are defining characteristics associated with the plant's genus and species.

Leaf Shapes

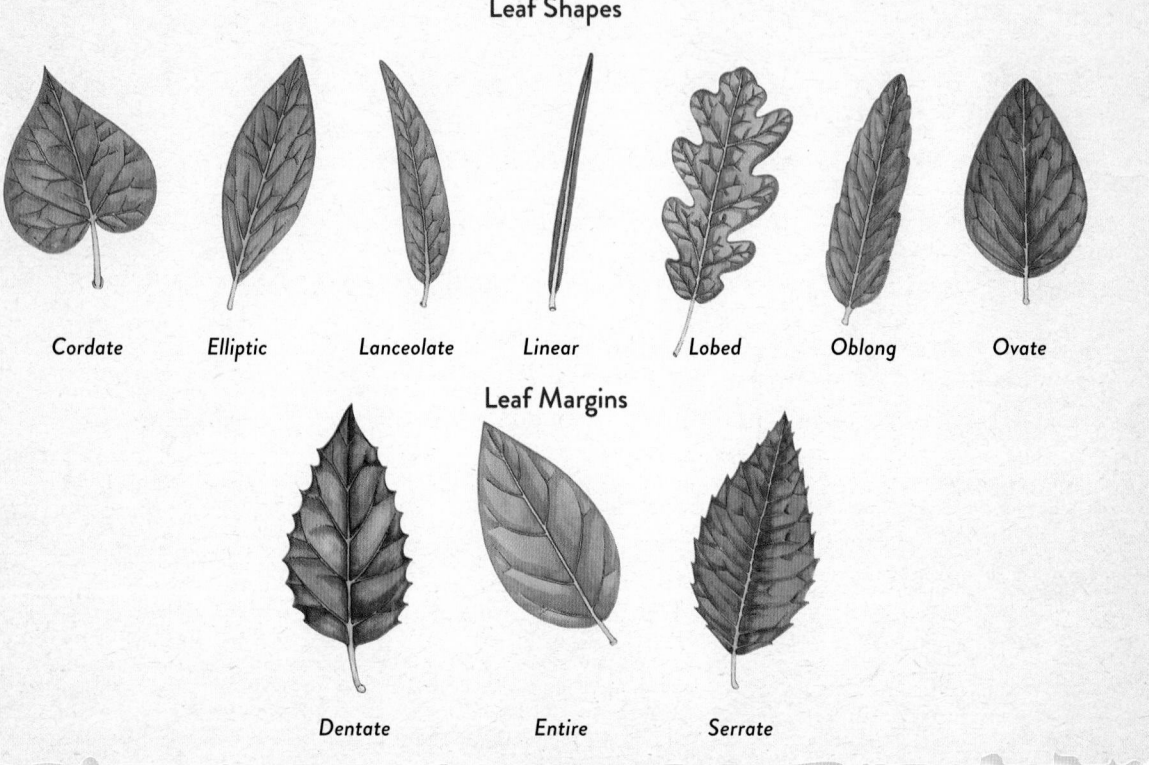

| Cordate | Elliptic | Lanceolate | Linear | Lobed | Oblong | Ovate |

Leaf Margins

| Dentate | Entire | Serrate |

The leaflets of palmately compound leaves are all attached to the leaf's petiole at one point. A pinnately compound leaf is composed of leaflets arranged on opposite sides of an axis. Even pinnate leaves have an even number of leaflets, odd pinnate leaves have an odd number.

After determining whether a plant's leaves are compound or simple and how they are arranged on the plant's stem, note the shape and texture of the leaves. Leaves can be glabrous (hairless) or pubescent (hairy); the edges (or margins) can be serrate (toothed) or entire (untoothed). And the leaves can be round, oval, heart-shaped, lancelike, or one of many other shapes.

EXAMINING FRUITS AND SEEDS

A fruit is the fertilized, ripened ovary of a flower. It contains the plant's seeds, fertilized ovules that hold the genetic material for a new plant. While some fruits are juicy, tasty structures such as apples, tomatoes, and plums, others are merely hard, dry seedpods.

Simple fruits ripen from an ovary with one pistil and can take many forms. Examples of dry simple fruits include an achene (buckwheat), a capsule (poppy), a caryopsis (grass), a cypsela (daisy), a follicle (milkweed), a legume (pea), a nut (acorn), a samara (elm), a schizocarp (parsley), and a silique (mustard plant). Examples of fleshy simple

FRUITS and SEEDS

A fruit and its seeds contain the genetic material for a new plant. These are a few of their many possible forms.

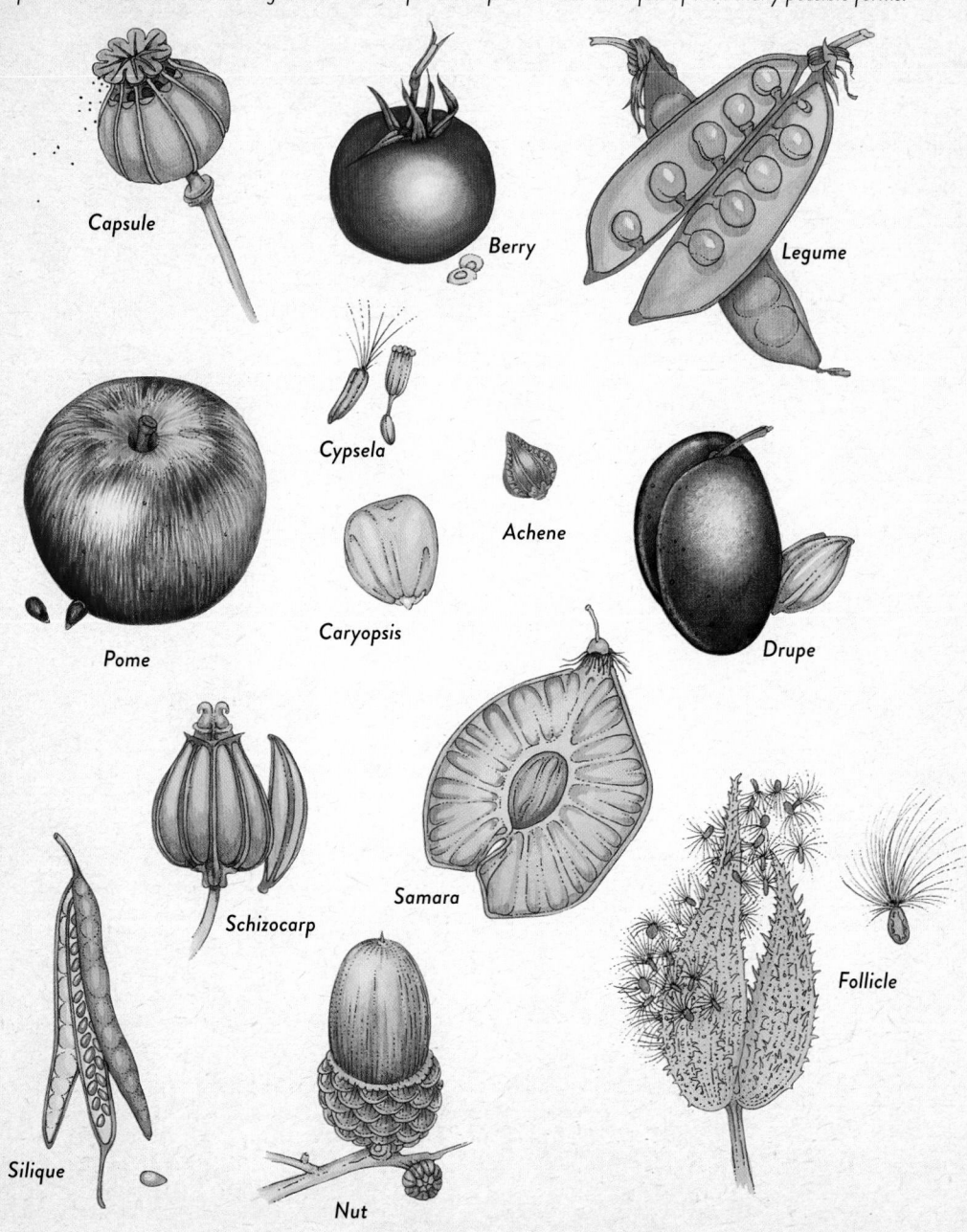

Capsule

Berry

Legume

Cypsela

Achene

Pome

Caryopsis

Drupe

Schizocarp

Samara

Follicle

Silique

Nut

fruits include a berry (tomato), a drupe (plum), and a pome (apple).

Other classifications of fruits include multiple fruits (formed from a cluster of flowers, as in a pineapple), aggregate fruits (formed from single flowers with multiple pistils that are not fused together, as in a raspberry), and accessory fruits (not originating from an ovary but from tissue outside of the carpel, as in a strawberry). Fruits and seeds provide important foods and medicines and can be vital for plant identification.

THE ANATOMY OF STEMS AND ROOTS

A plant's stem offers structural support and serves as a transport and storage system for nutrients and water. Along the stem, nodes or swellings indicate where leaves, buds, or branches will arise. A stolon sprouts from the main stem and grows horizontally along the surface of the soil or just below the ground, referred to by gardeners as a runner. Stems can take many forms, both above and below the soil. A tuber such as a potato, for example, is actually a thickened underground stem, usually with numerous buds (eyes). Similarly, a rhizome, although often mistaken for a root, is actually an underground part of the main stem with roots attached. A bulb is a shortened stem covered by leaf bases or scales that enclose fleshy leaves.

Roots are underground structures that anchor and support a plant, absorb nutrients and water, and store food for the plant. Some plant roots are composed of a main axis with smaller roots coming off the primary root, known as secondary roots. Other plants, such as corn, have a fibrous root system that consists of many fine, threadlike roots. A taproot is a fleshy root that grows downward, sometimes swelling into a storage organ that is eaten, such as a beet or carrot. Roots of an individual plant can grow out several feet beyond the stem, thus competing for resources such as water and fertilizer. That's why plant spacing, depending on the species grown, is important in the garden or farm field.

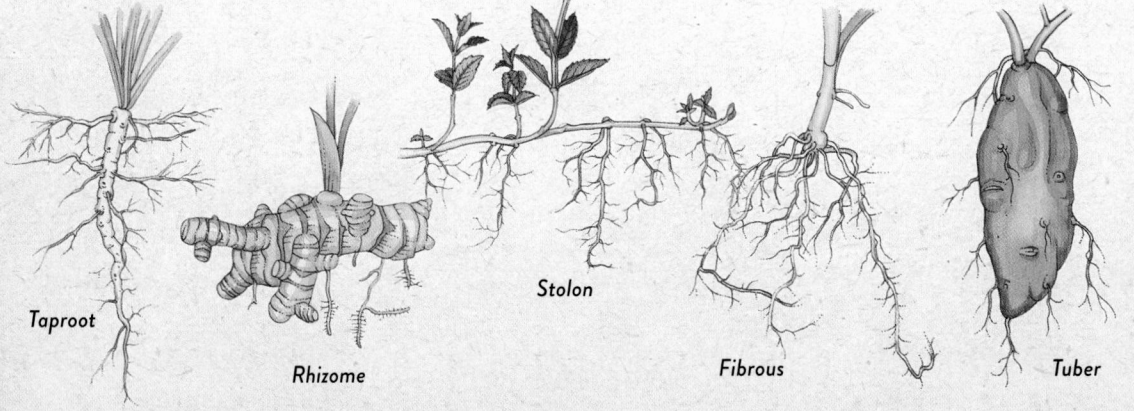

ROOTS *and* UNDERGROUND STEMS

Roots provide structural support and absorb nutrients and water. Some also serve as a storage organ for the plant.

Taproot

Rhizome

Stolon

Fibrous

Tuber

COLLECTING PLANTS FROM THE WILD

If you plan to collect plants from the wild, strong plant identification skills are essential. First, it is a matter of safety: You must be absolutely certain of the identity of the plants you gather, especially if you plan to use them for culinary or medicinal purposes. In the book *Identifying and Harvesting Edible and Medicinal Plants in Wild (and Not So Wild) Places,* noted forager "Wildman" Steve Brill cautions that if you are not 100 percent certain of the identity of a plant, do not eat it: "Look up *all* of a plant's identifying characteristics, and make sure they match *all* your observations." He also recommends looking up any descriptions of poisonous look-alikes and cross-checking multiple sources to be absolutely certain of the identification, palatability, and properties of a plant.

At The New York Botanical Garden, we often receive calls from local physicians, referred through a poison control center, about identifying plants that have been ingested or touched, in cases of possible poisoning or injury. Keep this number handy: 800-222-1222. It is the Poison Help Line number for the American Association of Poison Control Centers. These highly trained professionals can assist you in the case of a suspected poisoning—plant or otherwise. While most of the plant-related calls do not turn out to be life-threatening cases, others *are*—particularly those involving inexperienced mushroom foragers who mistake deadly species for those that are edible. There have also been cases of people poisoning themselves and their families after mistaking foxglove—a deadly poisonous plant—for comfrey. Others have died after harvesting the wrong member of the carrot family, which includes extremely poisonous plants, such as poison hemlock (*Conium maculatum*), in addition to wild medicinal herbs and edible varieties. Plants in the carrot family can be notoriously difficult to identify, even for experienced field botanists. While relatively few plants are as toxic as foxglove or water hemlock (*Cicuta maculata*), the wisest policy is not to taste or sample unknown plants.

Another important issue to consider when harvesting plants from the wild is conservation. As

DANGEROUS LOOK-ALIKES

In the wild, plant identification can be a matter of life and death. Purple-stem angelica (*Angelica atropurpurea;* below left), which has been used for healing, could be confused with highly toxic water hemlock (*Cicuta maculata;* below right). Both have white flower umbels and hollow purple-tinged stems, and both grow in moist woodlands.

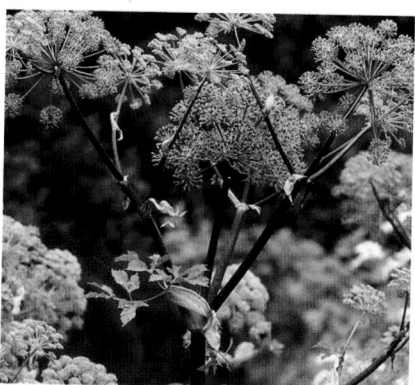 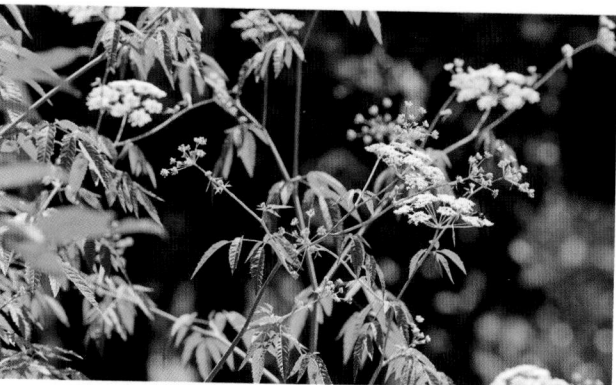

habitats dwindle, wild plant communities increasingly face pressure from the encroachment of human activities, such as development, deforestation, recreation, and, in some regions, commercial harvesting. As more people work to improve their health and well-being with herbal medicines, it's also essential to protect the well-being of the planet and its life-sustaining plants. Before collecting any plants, learn which ones are rare or endangered in that area.

When gathering plants from the wild for any reason, be aware of good wild-harvesting practices, and obtain permission in advance if you wish to collect on any land, private or public, that is not your own. Knowing how to harvest plants sustainably and in ways that minimize damage to their habitats will ensure the survival of the individual plant community. Here are a few general rules.

- *Never harvest rare herbs or plants of any kind.* Some species are protected by law, and the penalties for harvesting them can be severe. Even if the plant being collected is not rare, never harvest when there are only a few specimens growing in one place.

- *Do not harvest more plant material than needed.* When a collector takes the root of a plant, the plant itself is destroyed. Harvesting bark harms trees, and removing a ring of bark from around a trunk can be fatal to a tree.

- *Be sensitive to the surrounding vegetation.* Don't trample nearby plants in a burst of enthusiasm to collect a plant.

- *Be cautious about potential pollutants that can contaminate the plants being gathered.* Those collected near roadsides, for example, could contain unacceptably high levels of toxins, both from automobiles (lead and other heavy metals) and from chemical spraying. Plants gathered from streams could contain the same contaminants and microorganisms as do the waters, including bacteria such as *E. coli.*

In the end, the best course of action might simply be to grow medicinal plants or purchase herbs from a reputable supplier.

Whether you have taken a botany class at some point in your life or these concepts of plant identification are new to you, getting your arms around them will pave the way for greater enjoyment of the herbs you grow, collect, and purchase. When working in your garden, take the time to observe each plant. How does it differ from the ones alongside it? What are the shapes of its leaves? What type of inflorescence does it have? What does its root system look like?

If you are weeding, think about the difference between a weed and a useful plant. Certainly, plants considered weeds are not only in the "wrong" place, but they're also aggressive. I can recall spending part of one beautiful spring weekend "weeding" a collection of mints I had purchased and planted the prior year—their stolons had spread throughout the garden like lava from a spewing volcano, and if not removed, they would have crowded out the other useful and ornamental plants struggling to grow there. The morphology and aggressive growth characteristics of certain mints make these species a weed in some cases and in other cases a most valued herb that can be harvested throughout the growing season.

Part of the great joy of spending time in the garden is observing its natural history—the interactions with pollinators, predators, soil, rain, and people—as well as the growth of each individual plant in your collection. Growing and using herbs in your daily life—strengthening that connection with your natural environment—can certainly help address the health condition that Richard Louv refers to as "nature-deficit disorder" in his wonderful book *Last Child in the Woods.*

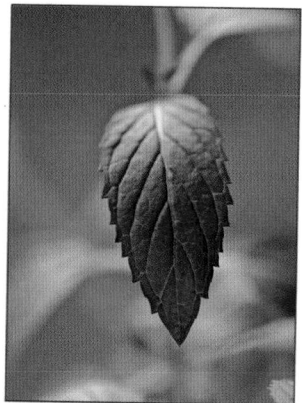

CHAPTER 3

HOW HERBS WORK

Modern research has shed much light on the chemical composition of herbs and how they work. For certain very powerful herbs, scientists have been able to identify a single constituent that stands out as the herb's primary "active ingredient." The anthraquinone compounds in purging buckthorn (*Rhamnus cathartica*), for instance, clearly are responsible for the herb's strong laxative effect. Scientists have also identified many of the compounds that give culinary and aromatic herbs their familiar flavors and scents. For other herbs, especially those used medicinally, explanations are less clear-cut. Scientists try to isolate active ingredients to better understand how herbs work, and some herbal products are "standardized" to a specific chemical—with the implication that the chemical is the single active component. But clinically oriented herbalists and others who study herbal therapies believe that the medicinal properties of most herbs derive from the whole plant—a synergy created by its constituents working *together* to produce a desired effect in our bodies. In this chapter, we explore phytochemistry—the study of chemical compounds made by plants—as it relates to our use of herbs for the treatment of health conditions and for the promotion of wellness.

PLANT CHEMISTRY: AN INTRODUCTION

Plant chemistry, also known as phytochemistry, is the study of the chemical compounds in plants. All living things on earth are made of chemicals. In fact, the chemical composition of plants and people is very similar. Both consist of common elements, including carbon, hydrogen, oxygen, and nitrogen. Chlorophyll—the green pigment essential to photosynthesis, the process plants use to transform water and sunlight into food—has been called "green blood" because its chemical makeup is similar to the hemoglobin in human blood. A molecule of chlorophyll and a molecule of hemoglobin each consist of carbon, nitrogen, and oxygen atoms, but in different proportions. There are other important chemical differences between hemoglobin and chlorophyll, but the basic similarities are striking.

PLANT METABOLITES

Plants produce a variety of chemical compounds, called metabolites, as part of their normal life processes. Some of these compounds allow plants to store energy in the form of sugar, for example, while others, such as toxic compounds, help plants defend against diseases or predators. After all, plants cannot run away from insects and other animals trying to eat them! Some compounds might offer the plant a sort of evolutionary "fitness," allowing it to survive and even thrive under conditions such as drought or an increase in average temperature that could wipe out other plant species.

There are two types of plant metabolites: primary and secondary. Primary plant metabolites include carbohydrates, lipids, proteins, and nucleic acids. These are compounds essential not only to the life of the plant but also to human health and nutrition. Plants use pieces of primary metabolites as building blocks to produce secondary metabolites. Secondary metabolites include terpenes, phenols, alkaloids, and their glycoside derivatives. These are largely responsible for the characteristic aromas, flavors, colors, nutritional values, and medicinal actions of the herbs and spices we use as foods, medicines, dyes, perfumes, and other products, from disinfectants to poisons. These properties also serve a vital purpose for plant life. For example, secondary metabolites give a flower its fragrance and color, both of which attract the pollinators the plant needs in order to set seed and produce the next generation of the species. The dividing line between primary and secondary metabolites is not always clear, and the two are integrally linked. Learning basic information about both primary and secondary metabolites will help you understand how they impact the properties and effects of herbs.

Primary Metabolites: Carbohydrates

Carbohydrates are essential to life and are part of the makeup of all living creatures. They provide animals, including humans, with energy and fiber and are the basic building blocks for all other plant chemicals.

Carbohydrates are composed primarily of sugars (saccharides) whose molecules are arranged in particular ways. Monosaccharides, for example, contain 1 sugar unit (mono means "one"), while polysaccharides contain 10 or more sugar units linked together (poly means "many"). Oligosaccharides contain between 2 and 10 sugar units (oligo means "few"). Glucose and fructose are two of the most common monosaccharides found in plants. Sucrose, found in sugarcane, is a disaccharide (di means "two") formed by a link between the glucose and fructose.

Cellulose, the main component of plant cell walls and the most abundant organic compound on earth, is a homopolysaccharide—a compound made of chains of a single type of monosaccharide. Other important homopolysaccharides include starch, fructans, and inulins. These important dietary substances are commonly called complex carbohydrates.

Many other categories and subcategories of carbohydrates are found in plants and fungi. For example, myco-polysaccharides form the cell walls of mushrooms and are rich in fibrous carbohydrate substances called ß-D-glucans (pronounced beta-D-glucans), which have been studied for their immune-stimulating effects. Other ß-glucans are found in grains, including oats. They are an important source of soluble fiber.

Gums and mucilages—two other types of carbohydrates with various uses as food and herbal medicines—also consist largely of monosaccharides. The term *gum* generally is understood to mean a sticky plant substance, such as gum arabic, made from black catechu (*Acacia catechu*). Mucilages are slippery substances used in herbal medicine to coat and soothe irritated or inflamed tissues (such as a sore throat). Marshmallow (*Althaea officinalis*), psyllium (*Plantago ovata*), and comfrey (*Symphytum officinale*) are all rich in slippery mucilage. Another important mucilage is carrageenan, derived from the Irish moss (*Chondrus crispus*), a seaweed, and from other species. Carrageenan is commonly used as a thickening agent in commercial food products.

Primary Metabolites: Lipids

Lipids—more commonly known as fats—are a major component of membranes in both plants and animals; they're also found in various hormones, as well as in vitamins E and A. They serve as reservoirs

EACH PLANT IS UNIQUE

Plants of the same species or even cultivar can vary in their plant chemistry, depending on their growing conditions and time of harvest. The compounds in St. John's wort (*Hypericum perforatum*) thought to be responsible for its therapeutic activity can vary by as much as 50-fold in concentration, depending upon the season of harvest. Plant compounds can even vary on a daily basis. The chemical compound eugenol, when measured as a total concentration in the essential oil produced from a species of wild basil (*Ocimum gratissimum*), varied from 98 percent for a plant harvested at 12 a.m. to 11 percent for a plant harvested at 5 p.m. Researchers must consider these variations in concentration levels when testing an herb or herbal product in the lab.

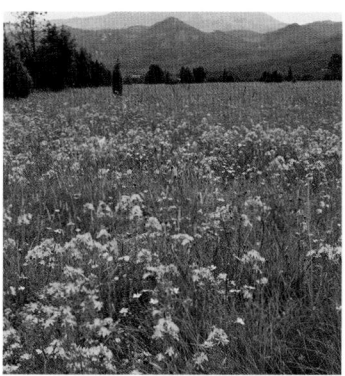

of energy to fuel essential cell functions and, like carbohydrates, are building blocks for a range of secondary plant metabolites.

Among the most important plant lipids for human health and nutrition are fatty acids. Unlike the fats found in animal products, plant fats are rich in unsaturated fatty acids, which research shows are critical for heart health. The human body is capable of producing almost all fatty acid structures; however, some fatty acids cannot be manufactured by your body and therefore must be supplied through your diet. These fatty acids are of critical importance to human health and are called essential fatty acids.

The two essential fatty acids most closely linked to human health are omega-3 and omega-6. Although fish oils from tuna, mackerel, herring, and sardines may be the best sources of omega-3s,

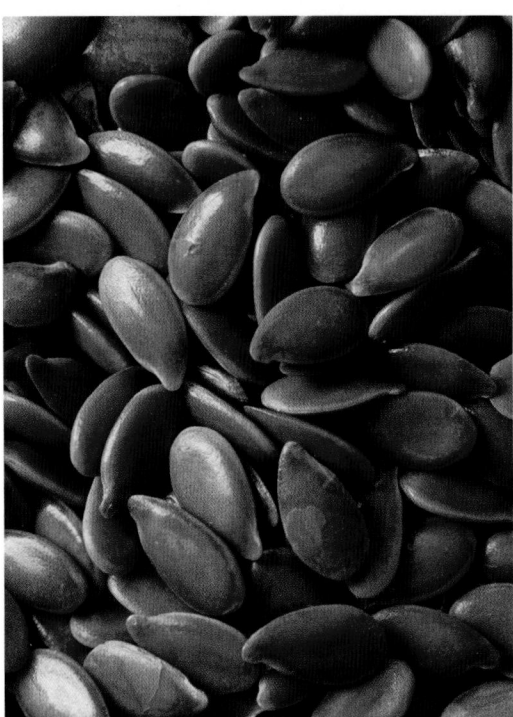

The seeds of flax (*Linum usitatissimum*) contain omega-3 fatty acids, as well as fiber and lignans—all important for health.

flaxseed (*Linum usitatissimum*) and the seeds of hemp (*Cannabis sativa*) contain omega-3 alpha-linolenic acid, providing valuable nonanimal sources of essential fatty acids.

Primary Metabolites: Proteins

Proteins are large molecules with different but very important functions. Besides serving as structural components of cells and tissues, they also regulate biochemical processes in both plants and animals. In fact, every chemical reaction that occurs in living cells is controlled by a special type of protein called an enzyme.

Proteins are composed of hundreds of units called amino acids. There are about 20 different types of amino acids, and most plants can synthesize those necessary for survival. This isn't the case for animals, which can synthesize only a few amino acids. For this reason, all animals—including humans—must obtain the missing, essential amino acids through their diets.

Vegetable proteins can be found in beans, nuts, and seeds, including peanuts (*Arachis hypogaea*), cashews (*Anacardium occidentale*), almonds (*Prunus dulcis*), walnuts (*Juglans regia*), sesame seeds (*Sesamum indicum*), sunflower seeds (*Helianthus annuus*), and soy beans (*Glycine max*).

Secondary Metabolites: Terpenes

Terpenes comprise the largest group of secondary plant metabolites. Thousands of different terpene compounds are found in a wide variety of plant species, and many appear to have important functions for the plants that produce them. For example, some give off aromas that lure pollinators or deter predators.

Terpene-rich volatile (essential) oils have great importance in herbal medicine and cooking. These aromatic compounds are responsible for the fragrances and flavors of kitchen favorites such as thyme (*Thymus* spp.), ginger (*Zingiber officinale*), peppermint (*Mentha × piperita*), and peel from citrus (*Citrus* spp.). These plants are not only tasty and aromatic, but they also have valuable antispasmodic, antimicrobial, and carminative (digestion-enhancing) effects.

Terpenes give us many other valuable medicinal compounds as well, including bitters, anti-inflammatory agents, expectorants, and sedatives. Limonene, a monoterpene found in citrus peel as well as mint, dill, and caraway, has been studied for potential cancer-preventive effects. Another important group of terpenes are the carotenoids—orange plant pigments found in oranges, peppers, and carrots—that the body converts into vitamin A.

Secondary Metabolites: Phenols

This group of plant chemicals includes thousands of different compounds that share one common chemical characteristic: All contain at least one phenol group. This is probably the largest group of plant secondary metabolites, and its compounds are widespread in nature. Plant phenols range from very simple structures to highly complex ones, such as tannins and lignins.

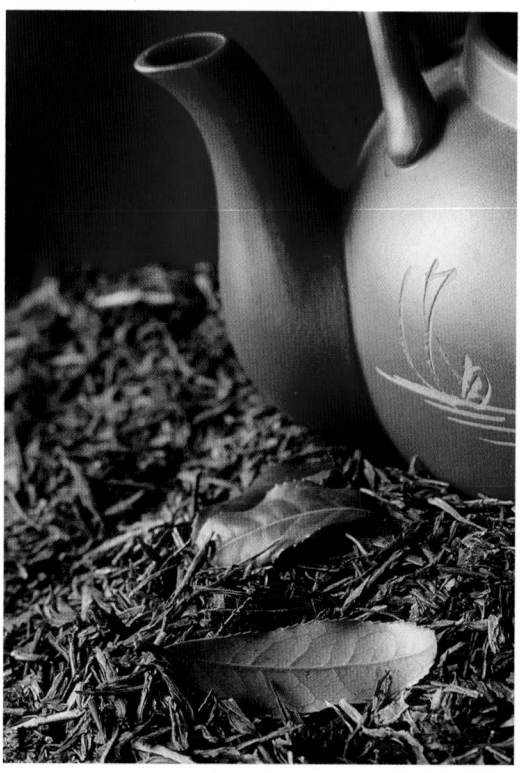

Green teas are rich in antioxidant polyphenols, powerful plant chemical compounds that are thought to protect your body against cell damage that can lead to cancer and heart disease.

THE A-TEAM: ANTIOXIDANTS

The term antioxidant seems to show up in nearly every health food claim and on every label—but just what does it mean? Antioxidant compounds defend your body against the effects of harmful chemicals called free radicals. Free radicals are unstable compounds that are products of oxidation in your body. Plant antioxidants are composed of a broad variety of substances that include phenols and some terpenes.

The human body produces free radicals in response to airborne pollutants such as cigarette smoke, stress, recreational drugs, food additives, and many other things. Free radicals can wreak havoc in your body, damaging cells and contributing to accelerated aging and a host of health problems, including serious conditions such as heart disease.

Antioxidants "scavenge" or "quench" free radicals to protect the human body against these harmful effects. Antioxidants are found in plants, especially fruits, vegetables, and herbs. Herbs that have particularly potent antioxidant actions include green tea (*Camellia sinensis*), milk thistle (*Silybum marianum*), turmeric (*Curcuma longa*), ginkgo (*Ginkgo biloba*), ginger (*Zingiber officinale*), garlic (*Allium sativum*), and horse chestnut (*Aesculus hippocastanum*).

CHEMICAL STRUCTURES *in* PLANTS

While the chemical structures of these secondary metabolites (terpenes, alkaloids, and phenols) appear very different, the compounds belonging to each of them could look similar to each other yet have completely different pharmacological activities.

The alkaloids caffeine and morphine, for example, have completely different pharmacological profiles even though their chemical structures are related. Each of these compounds is a psychoactive drug, acting on your central nervous system and affecting brain function. But while caffeine is a mild stimulant that's widely consumed in coffee and teas, morphine, the major constituent of opium, is a powerful narcotic (sleep-inducing) drug used to treat and manage moderate to severe pain.

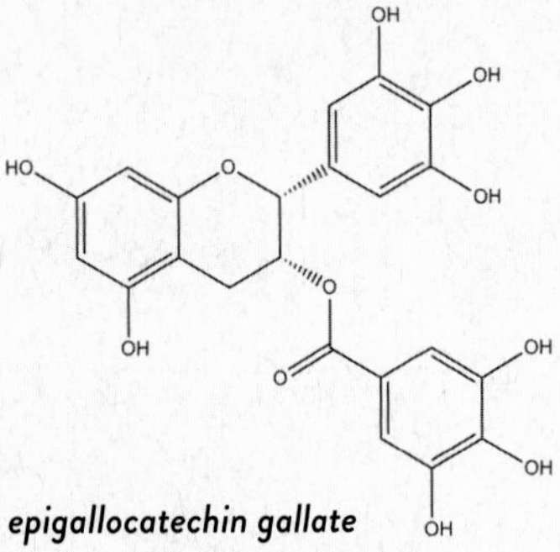

epigallocatechin gallate

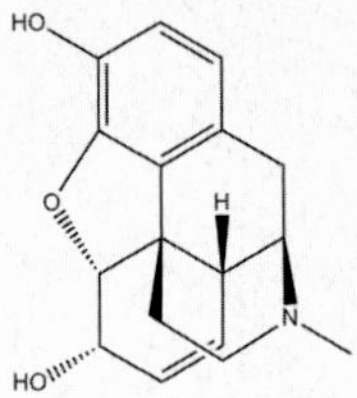

morphine

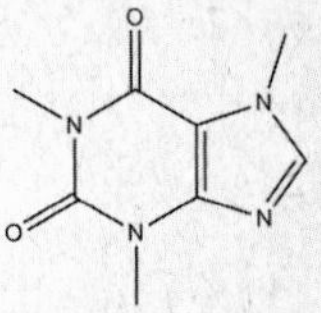

caffeine

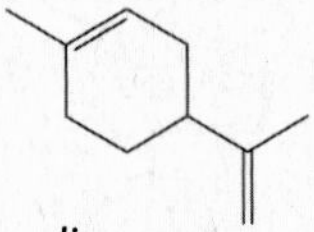

limonene

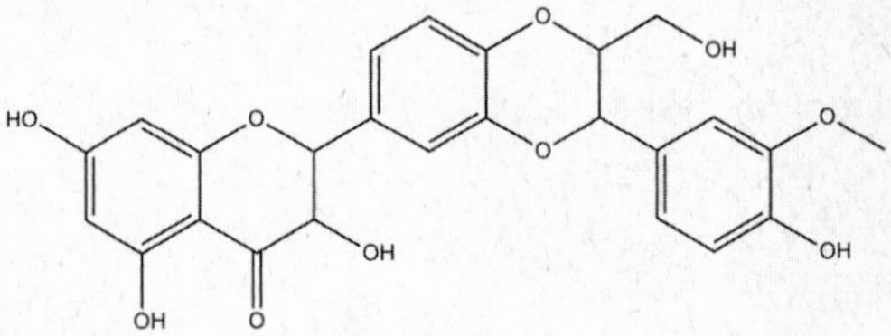

silymarin

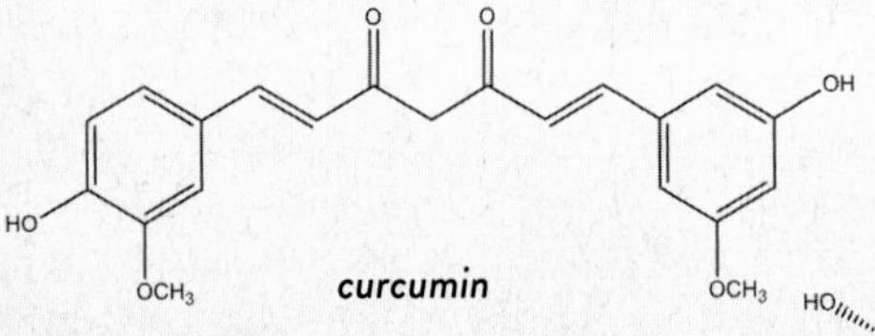

curcumin

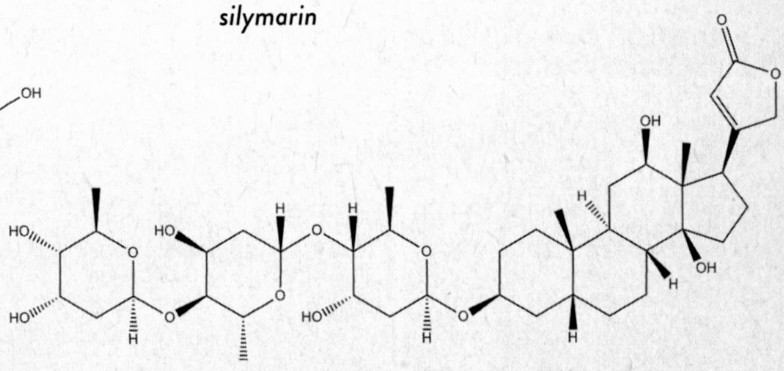

digoxin

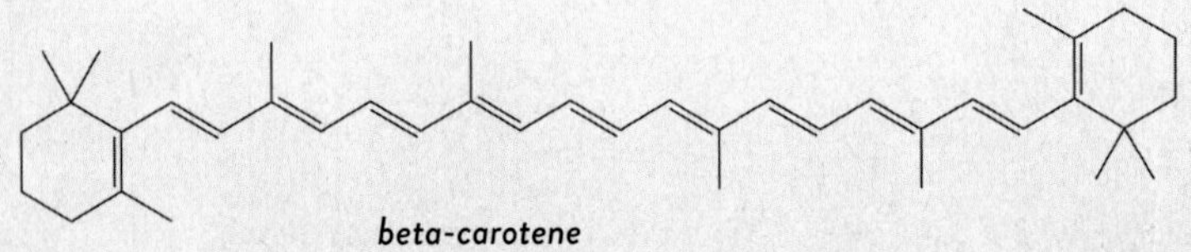

beta-carotene

At least half of all phenols are part of a large subgroup called flavonoids. Flavonoids contain many important antioxidant compounds that help eliminate harmful substances called free radicals from your body. The flavonoid category itself can be divided into numerous smaller subgroups of flavonoid compounds, including isoflavonoids, flavones, flavonols, flavonolignans, anthocyanins, and proanthocyanidins. When several phenol groups are attached to each other, the resulting compound is called a polyphenol.

Green tea (*Camellia sinensis*) is one of many phenol-rich plants with valuable health properties. It contains antioxidant phenols called catechins. Hundreds of studies conducted on these compounds suggest that they could help prevent cancer and heart disease. Many plants in the pea family (legumes) contain isoflavonoids, which also have demonstrated impressive cancer-fighting and hormone-balancing effects in modern studies. Plants rich in isoflavonoids include soy (*Glycine max*) and red clover (*Trifolium pratense*).

Many of the pigments that give plants their coloring are polyphenols. Antioxidant polyphenols called anthocyanins provide the blue and red colors of berries such as blueberries (*Vaccinium angustifolium* and others) and cranberries (*V. macrocarpon*). Red grapes (*Vitis vinifera*) and red wine contain anthocyanin pigments as well as resveratrol, another polyphenol. Studies have shown that berries and red wine, like green tea, could have healthful antioxidant effects.

Tannins are highly astringent polyphenols that can be used not only as tanning agents for the leather industry, but also as medicines. Astringents tone and tighten tissues throughout your body, including mucous membranes and skin; they are responsible for the mouth-puckering sensation you experience when drinking a cup of strong black tea. Oak bark (*Quercus* spp.), witch hazel (*Hamamelis virginiana*), and agrimony (*Agrimonia eupatorium*) are also rich in tannins.

Other important phenols include curcumin (found in turmeric, *Curcuma longa*), a powerful antioxidant that has anti-inflammatory and cancer-preventive properties, and silymarin, a mixture of flavonolignan compounds largely responsible for the health benefits of milk thistle (*Silybum marianum*). Modern studies have shown that milk thistle might protect your liver from the effects of toxins, including pharmaceutical drugs, and help it regenerate damaged cells.

Secondary Metabolites: Alkaloids

This group of plant chemicals can have powerful effects in the human body. Many are potent medicinal compounds that can be toxic in high doses; others are highly addictive.

Caffeine, a naturally occurring stimulant and diuretic found in coffee (*Coffea arabica*), green tea (*Camellia sinensis*), and other foods, is one familiar alkaloid. Other potent alkaloids include ephedrine, a decongestant taken from ephedra (*Ephedra sinica*); theophylline, a bronchial smooth-muscle relaxant present in small quantities in tea; reserpine, a tranquilizer and antihypertensive made from the Indian serpentwood plant (*Rauvolfia serpentina*); and vincristine and vinblastine, cancer-fighting compounds made from Madagascar periwinkle (*Catharanthus roseus*).

Some alkaloids have hallucinogenic effects. Examples include mescaline, which is extracted from the peyote cactus (*Lophophora williamsii*), and psilocybin, which is found in mushrooms of the genus *Psilocybe*. Other alkaloids are highly addictive. They include cocaine, a stimulant and anesthetic taken from the leaves of the South American coca plant (*Erythroxylum coca*); nicotine, taken from the leaves of the tobacco plant (*Nicotiana tabacum*); and morphine, a pain reliever extracted from the opium poppy (*Papaver somniferum*).

Certain pyrrolizidine alkaloids, such as those

found in plants of the borage family, including comfrey (*Symphytum officinale*), can cause liver damage. Other poisonous alkaloids include strychnine (found in *Strychnos nux-vomica*), atropine (found in *Atropa belladonna* and *Datura stramonium*), and coniine (a deadly toxin made from poison hemlock, *Conium maculatum*).

GLYCOSIDES

Phytochemists use the term *glycoside* to describe a plant compound that has a molecule of sugar attached to a noncarbohydrate molecule, called an aglycone.

Glycosides are particularly important in the study of herbal medicine. Many have important medicinal actions; others are dangerous toxins. The cyanogenic glycosides found in apple seeds and bitter almonds, for instance, produce the deadly poison cyanide. But the cyanogenic glycoside prunasin, found in wild cherry bark, is an expectorant when taken in small quantities.

Cardiac glycosides, such as those in lily of the valley (*Convallaria majalis*) and foxglove (*Digitalis* spp.), are extremely potent chemicals that should never be taken during self-treatment. Cardiac glycosides improve your heart's efficiency without increasing its need for oxygen. Plants containing these compounds were once the only treatments for serious heart conditions, such as congestive heart failure (a disease in which your heart loses its ability to efficiently pump blood). However, because cardiac glycosides are eliminated from your body slowly, dangerous levels can accumulate in your blood. To treat congestive heart failure today, doctors prescribe modern pharmaceuticals such as digoxin (isolated from *Digitalis lanata*), which they can monitor and control the dosages of more easily.

Another group of glycosides are the glucosinolates, found primarily in cruciferous vegetables

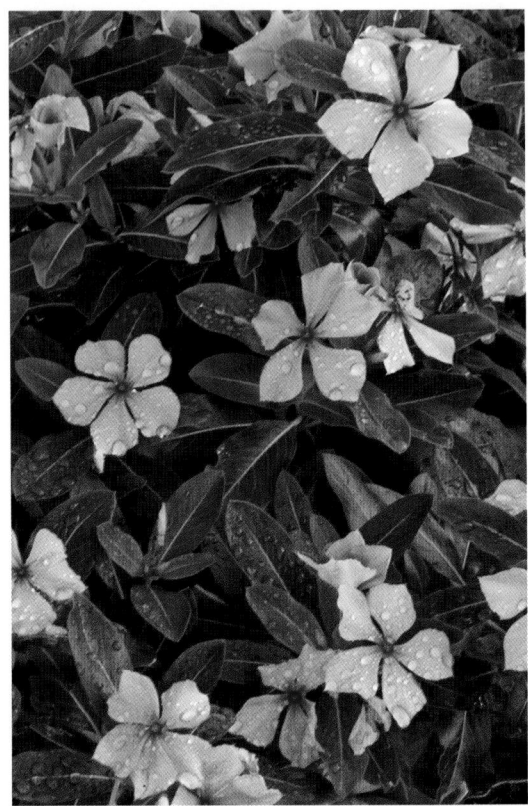

Catharanthus roseus, the source of the chemotherapeutic drugs vincristine and vinblastine.

(members of the mustard family, Brassicaceae) such as broccoli, cabbage, and kale (all *Brassica oleracea*), horseradish (*Armoracia rusticana*), mustard (*B. nigra* and others), and radish (*Raphanus sativus*). When one of these plants is crushed, its glucosinolates undergo a chemical reaction that creates the volatile oil compounds we know as mustard oils. When applied to the skin, mustard oils have a warming, stimulating effect—that's why mustard poultices were traditionally used to relieve chest congestion. Research has shown that indole-3-carbinol might help prevent certain cancers, including colon and breast cancers, and indole-3-carbinol is produced in your body as you break down the glucosinolates in cruciferous vegetables.

Contemporary medical care is filled with new and exciting technologies and approaches. Reports of great advances in our understanding of illness and its treatment appear in scientific journals, newspapers, and other media on a weekly, and sometimes daily, basis. From time to time, reports also appear about the empty pipelines in drug discovery programs, when expectations fueled by modern technology have not been met. Yet many of these programs overlook a rich source of potential therapies—the plant world.

What role could nature, specifically plants, play in contemporary medicine? Some write about the obsolescence and dangers of using plants in healing, while others suggest that the "well" of plants that could be used to improve both health care and the outcomes of disease is far from dry. James S. Miller, PhD, noted in a recent issue of the journal *Economic Botany* that 135 pharmaceutical drugs have been discovered from plants to date and, based on his analysis of the world's flora and conservative historic drug discovery rates, he projects that at least 500 more pharmaceutical drugs remain to be discovered. Delaying the progress toward improved health-care options and outcomes is the fact that as many as 70,000 plant species

have yet to be discovered and, because of habitat destruction and other consequences of global change, many species could disappear before they are identified and evaluated for their chemical composition and medicinal potential.

Here are a few facts to consider. As Dr. Miller points out, many of our most important prescription pharmaceuticals are based on single compounds derived from plants. For example, the compound vincristine, derived from the rosy periwinkle (*Catharanthus roseus*) and approved for use by the FDA in 1963, is used to treat the 3,800 new cases of childhood leukemia diagnosed annually in the United States. It has an impressive record of up to 90 percent remission, based on the type of cancer and age of the patient. A relatively recent example of a whole plant extract being developed as an effective pharmaceutical is from a plant familiar to all—tea (*Camellia sinensis*). In 2006, the FDA approved the prescription use of a topical preparation of tea extract for the treatment of perianal and genital condyloma (warts). When applied as an ointment, Veregen, as this pharmaceutical is called, completely resolved these conditions in 54 percent of patients who used it.

Many herbal remedies prepared as whole-plant extracts and sold as supplements, tinctures, or teas are being incorporated into Western health care through the field of integrative medicine, which is now taught at more than 50 academic medical centers and affiliate institutions in the United States alone. Clinical and preclinical research of these plants and their compounds is underway, and those herbs and formulations with convincing evidence of safety and efficacy will continue to find their way into Western medical care.

Meanwhile, much of the developing world still depends on plants to treat many primary health-care conditions—ranging from respiratory infections, wounds, and colds to diarrheal diseases that could otherwise prove fatal. Nature is the medicine chest for billions of people, and many generations of their traditional healers—the equivalent of our Western physicians—have already carried out human clinical trials.

It turns out that Mother Nature is a brilliant chemist. Hundreds of thousands of compounds have been identified from plants. Some of these are used in prescription pharmaceuticals, others in botanical supplements, and many more remain to be discovered.

UNDERSTANDING HERBAL ACTIONS

Long before scientists began to study how herbs work, traditional healers discovered herbal actions empirically. They used intuition and observed how animals use plants to heal themselves. They experimented, then verified and documented what they learned so that their knowledge could be passed along.

These hands-on healers—folk doctors and village healers, shamans, monks, and nuns, all serving their communities—are the ones to thank for many so-called scientific discoveries about herbs. The indigenous people of northeast Brazil, for example, have long used the jaborandi plant (*Pilocarpus jaborandi*) for medicinal purposes, including the promotion of salivation. Pilocarpine, a pharmaceutical medicine developed from this species, has been used worldwide to treat glaucoma and other conditions. Most recently, it was approved for the treatment of "dry mouth syndrome," which can be a side effect of radiation therapy or certain health conditions. And while laboratory research shows that garlic (*Allium sativum*) has antimicrobial activity, traditional healers knew this through experience and have long used the herb to treat all kinds of infections, from colds and flu to infected skin wounds.

One way to learn how to use medicinal herbs is to learn about their possible effects on the human body. Much like modern pharmaceuticals, herbs can have antispasmodic (muscle-relaxing), analgesic (pain-relieving), and anti-inflammatory effects. Other herbal actions are described with unique terms such as adaptogenic (helping the body defend against physical stress), alterative (slowly restoring efficient body function), and carminative (enhancing digestion).

Herbs appear to have what herb researchers call "affinities" to particular body systems; in other words, herbal actions are more pronounced in some parts of the body than others. Among demulcent (inflammation-relieving) herbs, corn silk (*Zea mays*) comforts the urinary tract, while marshmallow root (*Althaea officinalis*) soothes the digestive tract. Kava (*Piper methysticum*) is an antispasmodic that relaxes muscles all over the body, while wild cherry bark (*Prunus serotina*) acts primarily to relax respiratory muscles. Hawthorn (*Crataegus laevigata*) strengthens the heart and blood vessels, while raspberry leaf (*Rubus idaeus*) tones the tissue of the uterus.

In addition, even though an herb can be especially well known for a certain effect (and so is termed a "specific" for a particular condition), most herbs provide a combination of actions. German chamomile (*Matricaria recutita*), for example, is known as a specific for the treatment of stomach ulcers because it has an anti-inflammatory

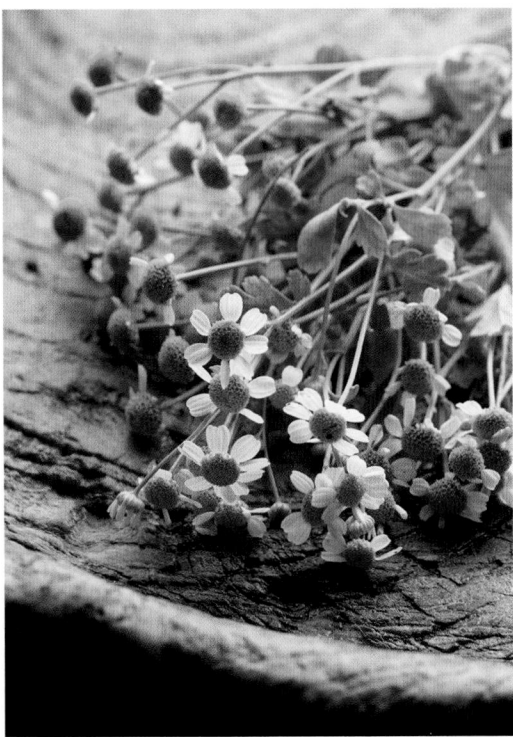

Feverfew (*Tanacetum parthenium*) is best known for helping prevent migraine headaches, but it has also been used to treat arthritis, dizziness, tinnitus, and painful menstruation.

THE TWO FACES *of* PURPLE CONEFLOWER

Current knowledge about the chemistry and pharmacology of purple coneflower (*Echinacea purpurea*) helps show why an herb can have multiple effects on the body. We've discovered that a plant's pharmacological effect depends not only on the chemicals present in the herbal preparation, but also on the different targets of a particular chemical.

Purple coneflower has long been used to prevent and treat the common cold. Traditionally, echinacea preparations were made from roots, but more recently, producers have been using the fresh-pressed juice from the flowers. While analyses of the plant's bioactive constituents are far from complete, scientific studies have consistently shown that different compounds in echinacea preparations stimulated the immune responses of animals—humans included—to viral infections, supporting the traditional use of this herb.

But recent scientific findings show that echinacea preparations could also inhibit some immune cells, possibly adjusting the immune response to an appropriate level. This can be a benefit, since an excess of some immune-regulating chemicals (known as cytokines) in your body after a viral infection can be detrimental to your health.

The bioactive constituents of *Echinacea purpurea* include alkamides, phenolic compounds, polysaccharides, and glycoproteins, among others. In general, alcoholic tinctures contain higher levels of alkamides and phenolic compounds, while aqueous extracts contain more polysaccharides and glycoproteins. In terms of pharmacological activities, polysaccharides and glycoproteins have been identified as having immune-stimulating activity, while alkamides appear to be anti-inflammatory. Phenolic compounds could work both ways.

While studying the effect of *Echinacea purpurea* on

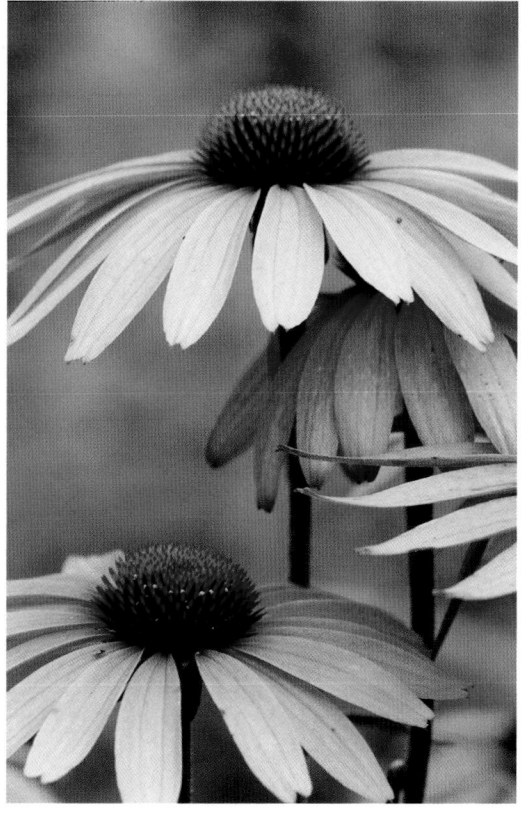

T lymphocytes, a type of white blood cell that fights virus and cancer cells, I found that some of the polysaccharides in the flower tops were able to not only increase, but also decrease the amounts of some cytokines released during a viral attack. Some of our tests suggest that this polysaccharide would be more effective if the preparation were taken before or during the early stage of a viral infection, validating clinical data as well as traditional wisdom about the benefits of early use of echinacea as a plant medicine.

—*Fabiana N. Fonseca, PhD*

effect on the digestive tract. It also soothes frazzled nerves, relaxes tense muscles, alleviates indigestion, and is a valuable anti-inflammatory remedy for skin irritations. Feverfew (*Tanacetum parthenium*) is best known for helping prevent migraine headaches, but it has also been used to treat arthritis, dizziness, tinnitus, and painful menstruation or sluggish menstrual flow.

In other words, from a therapeutic perspective, herbs have both primary and secondary actions. By considering the primary and secondary actions of herbs, as well as their body-system affinities, an herbalist can choose an herbal treatment appropriate not only for relieving an acute problem, but also for improving chronic conditions or heading off future problems.

Catnip (*Nepeta cataria*), for instance, is an antispasmodic herb that also relieves indigestion and acts as a mild sedative, so it's an excellent choice for someone who suffers from stress-related indigestion. And garlic (*Allium sativum*), which relieves infections and aids the circulatory system, could benefit someone who has bronchitis as well as a family history of heart disease.

Tonics and Effectors

Medicinal herbs can be grouped roughly into two very broad categories, according to the intensity of their activity: tonics and effectors.

Tonics are mild herbs that can be taken over the long term as preventive medicines or to gently correct and balance body functions. These herbs, which are more like foods than medicines, are among the safest of plant remedies. Nettle (*Urtica dioica*) is a general tonic herb. Like all herbs, tonics display affinities for particular body systems. For example, hawthorn (*Crataegus laevigata*) and garlic (*Allium sativum*) are excellent tonics for the cardiovascular system, while bitter herbs, such as mugwort (*Artemisia vulgaris*), are effective for the digestive system.

Effectors, on the other hand, have a more immediately noticeable effect upon your body. Herbalists call on these herbs to treat acute illnesses (such as infections) and relieve specific symptoms (such as a cough or sore throat). While many effectors are mild and can even be used as tonics, others contain powerful chemical constituents and must be used with caution. Some can even be toxic in high doses.

Mild effector herbs include feverfew (*Tanacetum parthenium*), saw palmetto (*Serenoa repens*), and turmeric (*Curcuma longa*). Strong effectors include stimulant laxatives such as senna (*Senna alexandrina*) and buckthorn (*Rhamnus cathartica*), as well as powerful, potentially toxic herbs, such as lobelia (*Lobelia inflata*), which some herbalists use in minute doses to relax muscles in people suffering from asthma and bronchitis, and pokeweed (*Phytolacca americana*), which is occasionally used in small doses to treat infection and promote lymphatic drainage.

Synergistic, Additive, and Antagonistic Effects of Herbal Extracts

When herbs are combined in mixtures or formulas, the chemical characteristics of the overall mixture can change, increasing or decreasing the availability and effects of some of the constituents.

Traditional Chinese medicine (TCM) combines herbs within formulas, taking into consideration the synergistic, additive, and antagonistic effects among the constituent herbs. This practice is also common in other herbal systems, such as in Central and South America, where many health conditions are treated with bottled herbal mixtures called *botellas* (in Spanish-speaking countries) or *garrafadas* (in Portuguese-speaking countries).

Advancements in analytical and synthetic chemistry now make it possible to better understand the potential effects of drug combinations on a living system. Scientists are exploring the dose-effect relationships (the change in effect caused by different dose levels) of each drug alone and in combinations to determine whether a given drug or herbal mixture would have an additive, synergistic, or antagonistic effect.

An additive interaction means that the effect of two chemicals taken together is equal to the sum of the effect of the two chemicals taken separately. Synergism, on the other hand, implies an effect that is more than additive—taken together, the two herbs have a greater effect. And antagonism is an effect that is less than additive—taken together, the herbs have a lesser effect.

A combination of herbs in a formula or mix-

In the Dominican Republic, a traditional herbal preparation known as a *botella* contains different plant parts immersed in alcohol. The beverage is used to prevent and treat many health conditions.

ture can target multiple areas of your body and a variety of conditions simultaneously. What's more, combining multiple herbs that have different mechanisms of action also can provide more effective treatment against a disease.

Because of these plant interactions, herbal preparations offer several advantages: They can increase the efficacy of the therapeutic effect; they can reduce the chance of toxicity because less of each herb is needed to achieve the same result; and they can minimize or slow the development of drug resistance.

Addition and antagonism can also be used to perfect an herbal formulation. In a 2006 *Yale Scientific* article outlining the importance of integrating Western and Eastern medical practices to address unmet needs in "conventional" medicine, Yung-Chi Cheng, a professor at Yale Medical School, explained the interaction and roles of different herbs in TCM using the following metaphor:

> The herbs in a typical TCM formulation . . . play different roles. Jun, the emperor herb, is the principal ingredient; chen, the minister herb, aids the jun often by augmenting or broadening its effects or by attending to secondary symptoms; zuo, the assistant, can moderate the activities of the jun and chen or also address secondary symptoms; finally, shi, the ambassador herb, aids in the absorption and transport of all the other herbs to their destinations. Thus, the herbs prescribed in a given formulation must work in concert to achieve a desired effect.

Herb-Drug Interactions

Just as herbs can interact synergistically or antagonistically when combined, so can herbs and pharmaceutical drugs. For example, one in four people in the United States over 45 years of age takes statins, a class of pharmaceutical drug used to lower blood cholesterol levels. Statins work by inhibiting an enzyme that produces cholesterol in your body, so they are considered important in reducing heart disease. The statins are broken down by another enzyme system in your body, leading to their elimination.

But bergamottin, a compound in grapefruit, can block the process that breaks down statins, allowing them to build up to levels that can quickly become toxic, resulting in severe liver, kidney, and muscle damage. That's why physicians advise their patients not to consume this fruit or its juice while taking statins. Now researchers are considering the possibility of using grapefruit compounds to increase the amount and effects of certain drugs in the body so that smaller amounts of these drugs can be used.

In a recent preliminary study, a patient who drank a single 8-ounce glass of grapefruit juice daily increased the absorption of a specific chemotherapeutic drug by up to 350 percent. While much further research is necessary, the study suggests that drugs modulated by plant compounds, such as those found in grapefruit, could be prescribed in smaller amounts.

Many herb-drug interaction charts can be found online. While there are many potentially problematic herb-drug interactions, scientific data has shown that most (but not all) commercially produced herbal products, as well as the herbs themselves (except, of course, for the toxic species) are generally safe when used under the supervision of a knowledgeable health-care practitioner.

The extraordinary chemical diversity of herbs has remarkable potential to improve human health and well-being. To achieve this potential, rigorous clinical trials under standardized, reproducible conditions are needed. Pilot experiments—small-scale clinical trials with herbs and patients—can provide guidance for the design of larger studies. The gold standard for evaluating any new therapy—drug or herb—is the randomized, blind, placebo-controlled clinical trial, where participants are randomly placed into groups receiving the treatment or placebo and they do not know which of the treatments they are receiving. These types of studies will allow medical researchers to determine which herbs are effective for treating specific health conditions and which ones could help us stay healthy as we age, and—of equal importance—which herbs lack sufficient evidence of safety or efficacy, and which might interfere with the proper action of the pharmaceutical drugs we take.

In many ways, medicine is returning to its original roots: using plants to improve the quality of our lives.

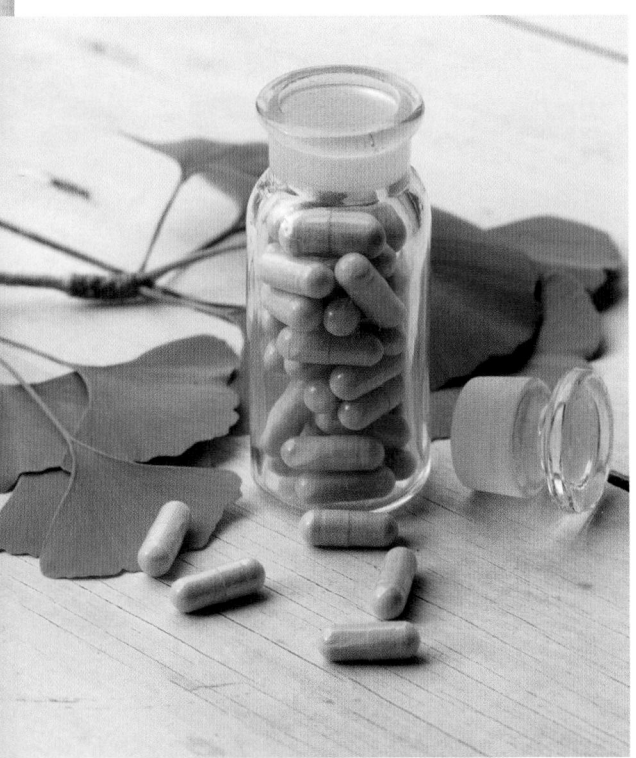

Ginkgo (*Ginkgo biloba*) dilates blood vessels, which helps with cardiovascular conditions, such as high blood pressure. Adverse effects could occur when combining ginkgo with other antihypertensive or certain antidepressant drugs.

A GLOSSARY *of* HERBAL ACTIONS

Many terms are specific to the practice of herbal medicine. The terms on the following pages are not a comprehensive list of herbal actions, but are meant to help explain a few of the basic terms associated with Western herbalism. Other systems, such as traditional Chinese medicine (TCM) and Ayurveda, which are based on completely different concepts, have a terminology all their own. (See pages 8 and 11 for more on these healing systems.)

Adaptogens are compounds found in herbs that can help your body adapt to and defend against the effects of physical stress, such as extreme cold or sleep deprivation. Scientists do not yet understand exactly how adaptogens work. Some theories suggest that they may help control the release and effects of stress hormones and modulate blood glucose levels, which in turn counteracts the damaging effects of stress on your body. Common adaptogenic herbs are ginseng (*Panax* spp.), eleuthero (*Eleutherococcus senticosus*), and reishi mushroom (*Ganoderma lucidum*).

Alteratives are herbs used to gradually bring about fundamental changes in health. Often, they are used to treat chronic skin conditions or autoimmune diseases. Researchers are unsure of how they work, but scientific studies offer a number of possibilities. Some alteratives, such as burdock (*Arctium lappa*), nettle (*Urtica dioica*), and yellow dock (*Rumex crispus*), seem to improve the efficiency of basic body functions, such as digestion, assimilation of nutrients, and elimination of wastes. Others, such as echinacea (*Echinacea* spp.), benefit your immune system. As with many herbs, alteratives probably work by a combination of effects.

Analgesics and anodynes are pain relievers. Examples include willow bark (*Salix* spp.), poplar (*Populus* spp.), and devil's claw (*Harpagophytum procumbens*).

Anticatarrhal herbs help your body eliminate excess mucus. Many of these herbs contain astringent tannins; others are rich in volatile oils. Examples include elecampane (*Inula helenium*), hyssop (*Hyssopus officinalis*), and thyme (*Thymus* spp.).

Anticholesterolemic herbs, such as green tea (*Camellia sinensis*), lower cholesterol levels by either inhibiting your body's production or absorption of cholesterol or by enhancing its excretion.

Anti-inflammatory agents reduce swelling and redness associated with inflammation. Anti-inflammatory herbs for internal use include turmeric (*Curcuma longa*), meadowsweet (*Filipendula ulmaria*), wild yam (*Dioscorea villosa*), and devil's claw (*Harpagophytum procumbens*). Anti-inflammatory herbs used externally include St. John's wort (*Hypericum perforatum*) and arnica (*Arnica montana*).

Antimicrobial herbs contain compounds that kill pathogens, or disease-causing organisms. Herbs with antibacterial, antifungal, and antiviral actions are all considered antimicrobial. Some antimicrobials, such as echinacea (*Echinacea* spp.), also stimulate your immune system. Research has shown that cranberry (*Vaccinium macrocarpon*) and related plants can prevent urinary tract infections because they discourage the attachment of bacteria to the walls of your urinary tract.

Antioxidants protect your body from the damaging effects of free radicals and may help protect against various degenerative diseases. (See "The A-Team: Antioxidants," on page 65.)

Antirheumatic herbs are helpful in the treatment of arthritis and other degenerative conditions that affect connective tissue. These herbs include devil's claw (*Harpagophytum procumbens*), turmeric (*Curcuma longa*), nettle (*Urtica dioica*), boswellia (*Boswellia serrata*), and feverfew (*Tanacetum parthenium*).

(continued)

Antispasmodic herbs relax muscles and ease muscle spasms and cramps. Some may alleviate muscle tension throughout your body, while others are specific to certain types of muscle tissue or organ systems. Many are also relaxing nervines, easing psychological tension as well. Chamomile (*Matricaria recutita*) and valerian (*Valeriana officinalis*) relax spasms in your digestive tract and calm nervous tension. Mullein (*Verbascum thapsus*) relieves spasms in your respiratory tract. Valerian helps ease muscle tension throughout your body.

Astringents tighten and tone tissues, especially mucous membranes, usually due to their tannin content. They also help dry excess secretions. They can be taken internally to treat conditions such as diarrhea or externally, as styptics, to stop bleeding. Examples include yarrow (*Achillea millefolium*) and witch hazel (*Hamamelis virginiana*).

Bitter herbs stimulate digestion, enhancing the flow of digestive juices and peristalsis, the muscle action that moves food through your digestive tract. Some bitter salad greens are eaten before a meal to aid digestion. Gentian (*Gentiana lutea*), mugwort (*Artemisia vulgaris*), and dandelion leaf (*Taraxacum officinale*) are bitter herbs.

Carminative herbs relieve gastrointestinal stress. They also enhance peristalsis, the action that moves food and gas through your digestive tract. Many are also popular culinary herbs and spices; those include thyme (*Thymus* spp.), dill (*Anethum graveolens*), caraway (*Carum carvi*), and ginger (*Zingiber officinale*).

Cholagogue herbs act by stimulating the flow of the digestive enzyme bile, which aids the digestive process. Dandelion root (*Taraxacum officinale*) is a cholagogue.

Demulcent herbs soothe and protect irritated or inflamed tissue and are often specific to one or more body systems. For instance, marshmallow leaf (*Althaea officinalis*) is a urinary tract demulcent; marshmallow root and licorice (*Glycyrrhiza glabra*) are digestive system demulcents. Respiratory demulcents include mullein (*Verbascum thapsus*), licorice, and marshmallow root.

Diaphoretic herbs induce perspiration, helping to "break" a fever and improve circulation. They're also used to treat colds and flu. Examples include yarrow (*Achillea millefolium*), boneset (*Eupatorium perfoliatum*), and ginger (*Zingiber officinale*).

Diuretic herbs stimulate the flow of urine and help your body eliminate excess fluid. Some also have antiseptic actions in your urinary tract, making them useful for urinary tract infections. These could be too irritating for people with kidney problems, however. Examples include dandelion leaf (*Taraxacum officinale*), parsley (*Petroselinum crispum*), and saw palmetto (*Serenoa repens*). Juniper (*Juniperus communis*) is a diuretic with strong antiseptic properties.

Emmenagogue is a term that once referred to herbs that induced menstrual flow, but it has come to be used more loosely to describe herbs that benefit female reproductive health. Herbs thought to stimulate sluggish menstrual flow include yarrow (*Achillea millefolium*) and feverfew (*Tanacetum parthenium*). Black cohosh (*Cimicifuga racemosa*) and vitex (*Vitex agnus-castus*) are believed to help normalize the function of the female reproductive system.

Expectorant herbs promote the elimination of mucus from your lungs. Stimulating expectorants, which commonly contain volatile oils, saponins, or alkaloids, include horehound (*Marrubium vulgare*), elecampane root (*Inula helenium*), and mullein leaves (*Verbascum thapsus*).

Galactogogue herbs help stimulate the flow of milk in nursing mothers. Galactogogues include dill (*Anethum graveolens*) and fennel (*Foeniculum vulgare*). Both are also classic remedies for infant colic.

Hepatic herbs help improve liver function. Examples include milk thistle (*Silybum marianum*) and licorice (*Glycyrrhiza glabra*).

Hypnotic herbs induce sleep and can be taken to treat insomnia. Examples include hops (*Humulus lupulus*), valerian (*Valeriana officinalis*), and passionflower (*Passiflora incarnata*).

Hypotensive herbs help lower blood pressure. These include hibiscus (*Hibiscus sabdariffa*), hawthorn (*Crataegus laevigata*), and valerian (*Valeriana officinalis*).

Immunomodulator herbs affect immune function. Some, such as echinacea (*Echinacea* spp.), stimulate immune cells such as phagocytes, which fight infection by destroying invading pathogens. (See "The Two Faces of the Purple Coneflower" on page 71.) Others are the subjects of ongoing clinical research to determine and clarify their activity. Among these herbs are astragalus (*Astragalus membranaceus*), shiitake mushroom (*Lentinus edodes*), and reishi mushroom (*Ganoderma lucidum*).

Laxative herbs stimulate the action of your bowels. Bulk-forming laxatives are high in fiber; they include psyllium (*Plantago ovata*) and flaxseed (*Linum usitatissimum*). Stimulant laxatives chemically induce peristalsis; they include senna (*Senna alexandrina*), cascara sagrada (*Rhamnus purshiana*), and buckthorn (*R. cathartica*). High doses of these laxatives are not recommended for long-term use. Mild laxatives that work through other actions (by stimulating bile flow, for example) include dandelion root (*Taraxacum officinale*) and yellow dock (*Rumex crispus*).

Nervine herbs affect the function of your nervous system. Nervines can be relaxing, tonic, or stimulating. Relaxing nervines include valerian (*Valeriana officinalis*), passionflower (*Passiflora incarnata*), and chamomile (*Matricaria recutita*). Tonic nervines include oats (*Avena sativa*) and St. John's wort (*Hypericum perforatum*). Herbs that stimulate your nervous system include caffeine-containing plants, such as tea (*Camellia sinensis*), as well as volatile oil–rich plants, such as rosemary (*Rosmarinus officinalis*) and peppermint (*Mentha × piperita*).

Rubefacients are herbs that, when applied externally, draw blood to an area for a localized warming effect. They include ginger (*Zingiber officinale*), black mustard (*Brassica nigra*), and chile pepper (*Capsicum annuum*).

Vasodilator herbs dilate blood vessels, which is useful in the treatment of cardiovascular conditions such as high blood pressure. Examples include ginkgo (*Ginkgo biloba*) and feverfew (*Tanacetum parthenium*).

Vulnerary herbs speed the healing of wounds. Examples include aloe (*Aloe vera*), comfrey (*Symphytum officinale*), calendula (*Calendula officinalis*), and St. John's wort (*Hypericum perforatum*). Some vulnerary herbs can also be used internally.

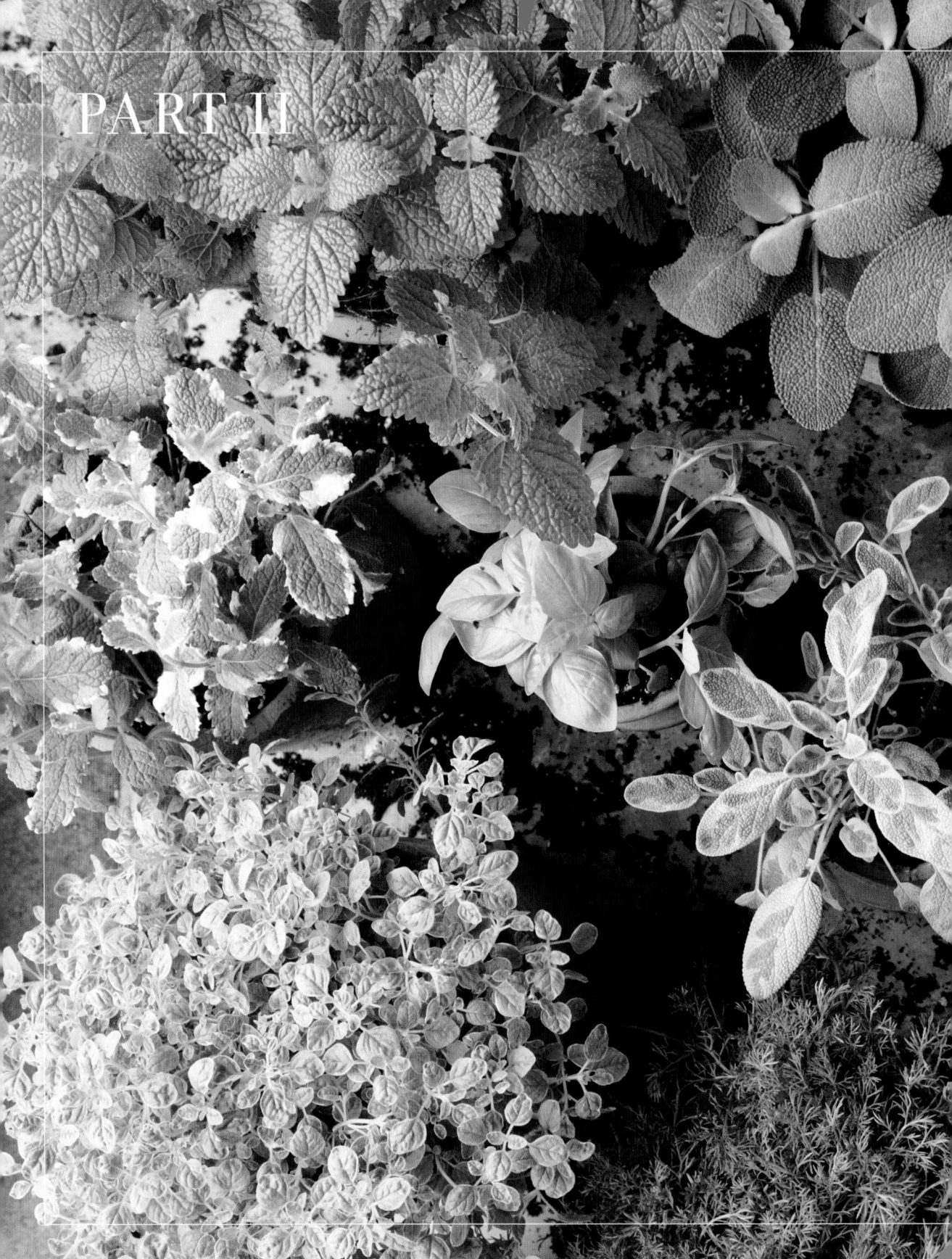

PART II

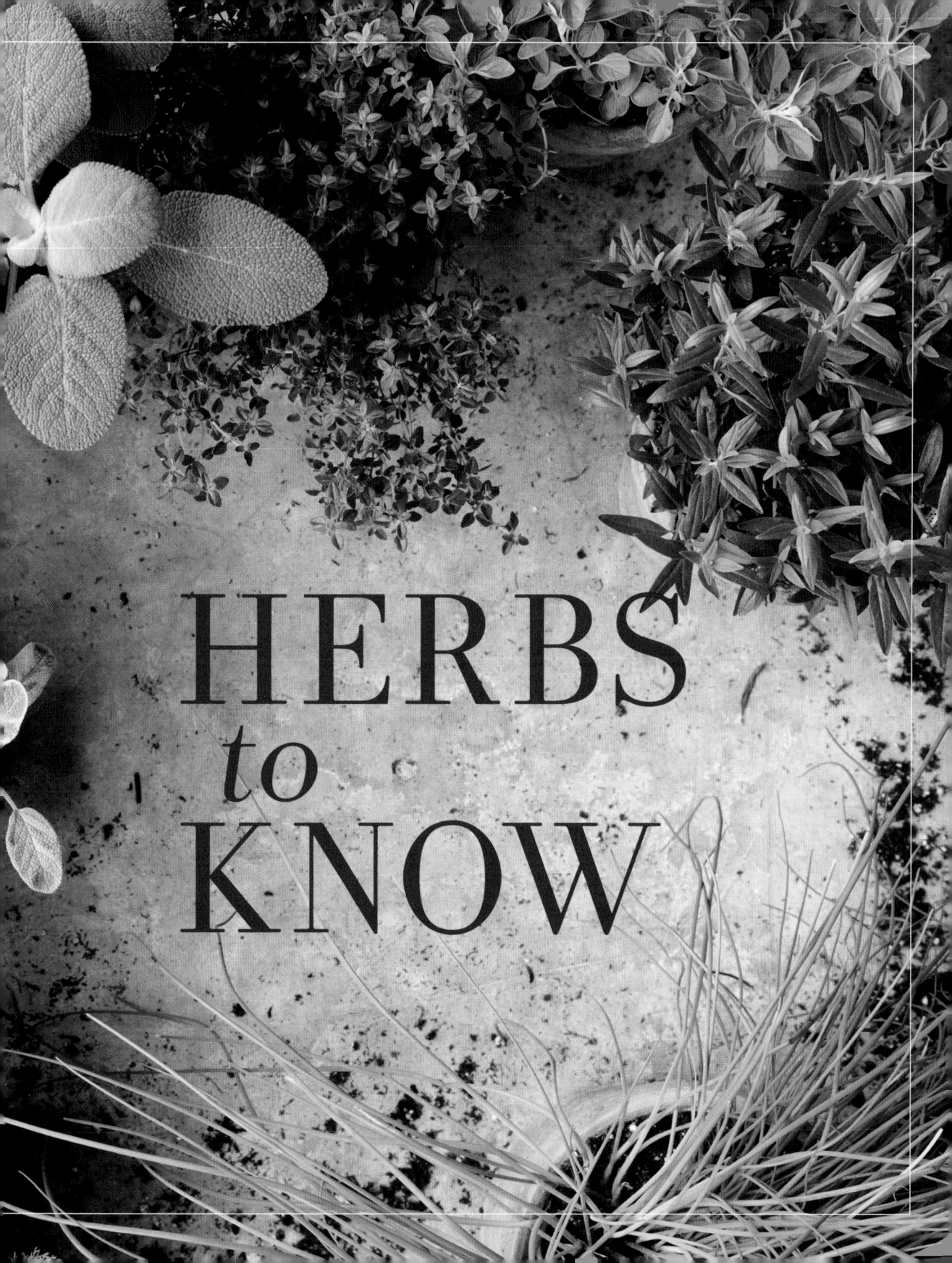

HERBS
to
KNOW

AN ENCYCLOPEDIA
of USEFUL HERBS

Globally, for nearly every traditional culture, herbs have not only helped fulfill basic human needs for survival, but also, in many cases, helped link humankind to the natural world and to the divine.

Tens of thousands of plants have been recorded as having traditional uses by humans, either in areas where they are found naturally or in regions where they have been introduced—sometimes accidentally, as weeds hitchhiking in the hold of a sailing ship or on the bottom of a traveler's shoe, or intentionally, as cultivated plants brought to a new place because of their perceived value.

This A to Z encyclopedia section highlights more than 180 species of herbs from around the world, each with folk or commercial uses. Most can be grown outdoors in the United States or, in the case of tropical and subtropical species, indoors in areas where winters are cold. We've chosen these herbs based on a variety of criteria—some are familiar essentials for the kitchen or medicine cabinet, others are exotics that, until recently, were not well known.

As the world becomes more cosmopolitan, more and more of these unusual plants have begun appearing in our markets. They offer interesting new flavors and healing properties, as well as other uses, from A to Z: exotic aphrodisiacs to plants used in the practice of Zen and other spiritual belief systems. Some can be found in specialty produce markets, others are sold in health food stores as commercial preparations, and many can be ordered as seeds or plants to grow and enjoy in your garden.

WHAT'S IN A NAME?

The herbs in the following section are arranged alphabetically by scientific botanical name—genus and species. In their plant profiles, you'll find as many as five common names. About those botanical names: For some plants, you'll see new names instead of the familiar names you've come to recognize. Why change a plant's name? Remember that botany is a dynamic science, with exciting discoveries made daily, including the identification of new plant species.

Botanists are also gaining a better understanding of phylogeny, the evolutionary relationships between plant groups. As a result, botanists change the names of individual plant species and plant families from time to time as they develop more advanced concepts of plant evolutionary relationships. New and very sophisticated molecular tools are enabling botanists to develop a very clear understanding of how plants evolved and are related and to determine more precise groupings of plant families, genera, and species. So the names of plants change, and new species are added to our knowledge of the plant kingdom at a rate of about 2,000 per year.

Many herbs in commerce—including those in

your local nurseries and seed catalogs—as well as in books, databases, and Web sites, are known by their former names, which are considered "synonyms." While the newly accepted name takes precedence over the synonym, you'll still find lots of good information linked to the older name (or names). So in this encyclopedia, we've recognized the most current scientific name of the individual species of herb, followed by the synonym in parentheses below it. For example:

Senna alexandrina (= Cassia senna)

The first name, Senna alexandrina, is the currently accepted name; Cassia senna is a synonym—a previous name you're likely to find on some product labels and in catalogs, books, and Web sites. As gardeners, cooks, and herbal devotees, the popular and scientific names of a plant are important to know. (See Chapter 2 for more about this.)

USING HERBS WISELY

The herbal profiles also include information about each plant's origin, name derivation, lore, and significant properties, as well as tips for growing and using it. Many of these plants have a long history of traditional medicinal use, and some of those traditional uses are now finding scientific support through rigorous clinical studies, while others are not. (Keep in mind that most herbs haven't yet been studied scientifically—or science hasn't yet explained their effectiveness.) In a very few cases, traditional uses have proven downright dangerous. For these plants, we've included cautionary statements, or we've excluded the plants entirely.

But remember: Anyone can have an unexpected reaction to a plant or any other foreign substance. This can range from a mild skin rash from touching a certain plant to, in very rare cases, a severe or fatal reaction from ingesting a plant substance (which could be a common food). Also, new discoveries in plant pharmacology and toxicology are published daily. So although the following section includes some cautions, it can't cover every possibility. *Please do not rely on the information in this section for self-medication.* Using herbs to achieve and maintain wellness requires the guidance of a health-care professional who's trained in the use of these therapeutic substances and who knows all of their properties, as well as how they will affect you as an individual.

STORIES FROM THE FIELD

Ethnobotanists have many stories. In my case, most are derived from 4 decades of travel and study with traditional cultures—working with people in some of the world's most remote areas. Some stories came from my own backyard— herbal healers within a few blocks of The New York Botanical Garden, located in the Bronx. You can find a few of these stories, called "Field Notes," in this section. They include my personal experiences, as well as interesting anecdotes I've collected and various things I've learned over the years about herbs and their uses.

Feel free to share these notes when speaking with garden club friends or even at a cocktail party. "Informed herbal conversation" is a true art, and this book might help you sharpen this skill. The legendary plant breeder, botanist, and horticulturist Luther Burbank (1849–1926) wrote that "flowers always make people better, happier, and more helpful; they are sunshine, food, and medicine for the soul." Perhaps he was referring to herbs.

Achillea millefolium

Archaeologists have found evidence of yarrow in Neanderthal burial caves, suggesting this herb's association with humans for at least 60,000 years. Native to Europe and Asia, this pungently scented perennial has naturalized throughout North America and other temperate regions of the world. Look for its white, yellowish, or pink flat-topped flower heads and fernlike foliage in sunny, open places, such as along roadsides and in fields.

One of the plant's common names, milfoil (from the French *mille feuille*, meaning "1,000 leaves"), refers to its feathery leaves, which are divided into thousands of tiny leaflets.

The genus name *Achillea* is derived from the legendary Greek hero Achilles, who reportedly used the herb as a styptic to treat his troops' bleeding wounds during the Trojan War, which also explains its ancient name, "military herb."

CULINARY USE

At one time, yarrow was used as a substitute for hops in brewing beer. You can use small amounts of yarrow leaves to flavor salads, soups, and egg dishes.

MEDICINAL USE

Yarrow leaf contains a complex mixture of chemical substances. Two of them, achilletin and achilleine, increase blood coagulation, which encourages the healing of wounds. Flavonoids in the plant stimulate gastric secretions to improve digestion. Yarrow also may have anti-inflammatory and antispasmodic properties, and it has been used to treat menstrual and stomach cramps.

Caution: Yarrow should not be taken during pregnancy. People who are allergic to other members of the family Asteraceae, such as ragweed, may experience skin inflammation and itching when exposed to yarrow.

ORNAMENTAL USE

An excellent garden plant, yarrow attracts butterflies, resists deer, and tolerates drought. The showy, long-lasting blooms add color to perennial borders, cutting gardens, and informal cottage gardens. The flowers also dry beautifully, making them ideal for everlasting arrangements and wreaths. Popular cultivars include 'Apple Blossom' (soft pink blooms), 'Summer Pastels' (burgundy blooms), and 'Paprika' (red blooms with gold centers).

OTHER USES

Valued for its ability to heal and cleanse the skin as well as to firm connective tissue, yarrow is an ingredient in many cosmetic products. The flowers also yield a yellow dye to wool mordanted with alum (see page 397). Use the flowers and leaves together to dye iron-mordanted wool an olive shade.

PLANT PROFILE

Common Names: Milfoil, Yarrow

Description: Perennial, 1 to 3 feet tall, with feathery gray-green foliage and erect stems; broad, flat flower heads composed of numerous white, yellowish, or rosy pink florets; aromatic

Hardiness: To Zone 3

Family: Asteraceae

Flowering: Summer to early autumn

Parts Used: Leaves and flowers

Range/Habitat: Europe and Asia; sunny meadows and roadsides

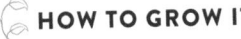

HOW TO GROW IT

Yarrow flourishes in rich, well-drained soil and full sun. Plant root divisions in spring or fall, or sow seeds in spring. Because the long-blooming flowers attract beneficial insects, such as ladybugs, consider planting yarrow in mixed flower borders and in vegetable gardens to help control pests. To propagate yarrow, divide the roots of 3- or 4-year-old plants in either spring or autumn. For medicinal use, harvest yarrow while it's in bloom; the plant's leaves, flowers, and stems can be used fresh or dried.

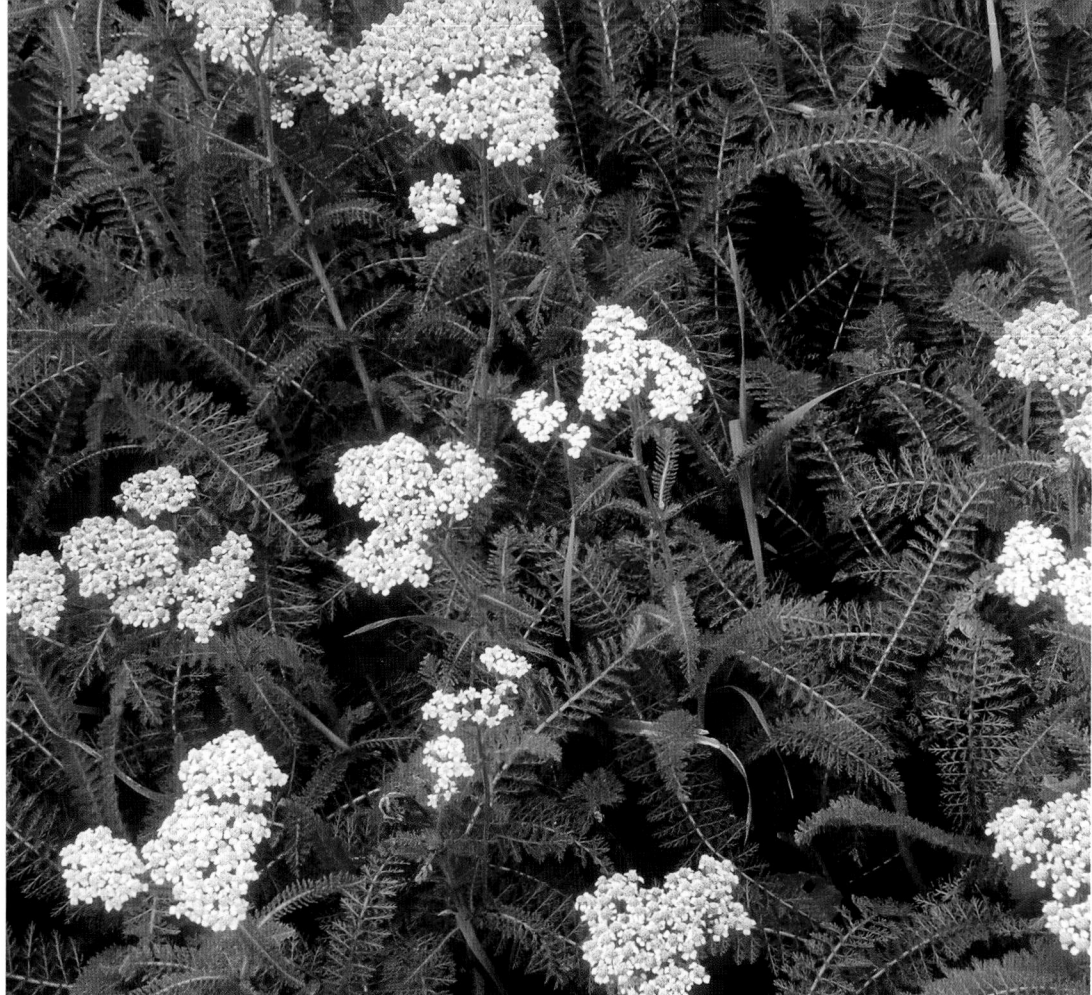

An Herbal Band-Aid

It's possible that an herbalist first brought yarrow to North America, wishing to grow this important plant for its medicinal properties. It certainly has taken root in its new home and is now very common, especially in pastures, meadows, and along roadsides. Native Americans recognized yarrow's ability to heal a variety of conditions. They made an infusion of the whole plant to treat fevers and colds, and they applied the leaves to skin to heal boils, open sores, swellings, burns, cuts, sprains, and eruptions.

Also known as "nosebleed," yarrow at one time was applied inside the nose to stop bleeding. But early European herbalists noted that putting the rolled-up leaves inside the nose had the opposite effect—it caused bleeding, which was a technique used in those days to treat headache.

Next time you are wandering through a field and happen to cut yourself, grind up a few yarrow leaves and apply them to your wound, just as people have done for hundreds of years. Be careful, though: If you are allergic to other plants in this family or if your skin is sensitive to the sun, don't use it.

—M. J. B.

Acorus calamus

Native to India, Europe, and North America, this irislike perennial grows worldwide, especially in wet places. During the Middle Ages, the aromatic yellow-green leaves of calamus were strewn on the floors of churches and houses to ward off fleas, lice, and other pests. In modern India, the powdered rhizome is used as an insecticide to protect stored crops, such as rice.

Although traditional medicine has ascribed many healing properties to this grassy-looking herb, the FDA has judged it unsafe and has banned its use in food and medicines. The essential oil of the root of most varieties contains compounds (asarone and beta-asarone) known to promote tumor formation, although the roots of certain North American and East Asian varieties contain much less of these compounds.

MEDICINAL USE

In traditional medicine, the dried rhizome is chewed or taken as a tea or tincture to stimulate appetite and relieve indigestion, as well as many other conditions of the digestive, nervous, circulatory, respiratory, urinary, and reproductive systems. Calamus has anti-inflammatory and analgesic properties; in Ayurvedic medicine and other therapies, a paste of the rhizome is used externally to treat rheumatoid arthritis, osteoarthritis, and hemiplegia—a type of paralysis that affects one side of the body.

Known in Sanskrit as *vacha* ("vocabulary power" or "speech"), calamus is also thought to bring clarity to the mind and improve spoken language. In Ayurveda, the herb is used to treat stroke victims and epilepsy. Native American tribes chewed pieces of the root to instill energy and focus the mind.

Caution: Depending on its chemical composition and variety, this plant can be very harmful. In animal studies, malignant tumors occurred in rats exposed to high doses of calamus.

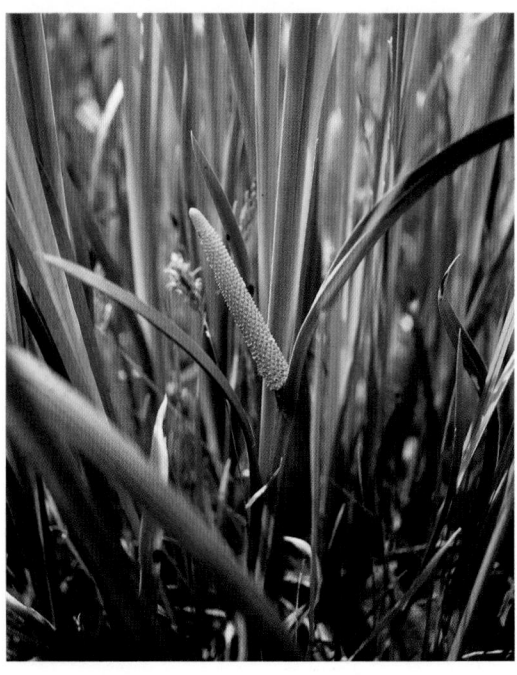

OTHER USES

Sweetly scented calamus has long been used in perfumery. The rhizome can also be added to potpourris and sachets.

 HOW TO GROW IT

Grow this aquatic plant in a sunny location in shallow water or rich, wet soil with a pH of 5.0 to 7.0. In a marsh or at a pond's edge is ideal. In spring or fall, plant the rhizomes 4 to 6 inches deep and 1 foot apart. Harvest large, 2- to 3-year-old rhizomes in early spring or late fall. Propagate by dividing the rhizomes in spring or fall after several years of growth.

Actaea racemosa

(= *Cimicifuga racemosa*)

PLANT PROFILE

Common Names: Black Bugbane, Black Cohosh, Black Snakeroot, Rheumatism Weed, Squaw Root

Description: Grows 4 to 7 feet tall; small, creamy flowers on tall, branching spikes; broad, ovate leaves up to 2 feet long, divided into three-lobed leaflets with toothed margins

Hardiness: To Zone 3

Family: Ranunculaceae

Flowering: Early summer to midsummer

Parts Used: Roots

Range/Habitat: Eastern North America; woodlands

Native Americans called this plant "black cohosh" because of the dark color of its roots; "squaw root" describes its traditional use as an aid in childbirth and as a treatment for women's menopausal and premenstrual symptoms. A member of the buttercup family, black cohosh is native to eastern North America and is one of about 8 *Actaea* species that grow in North America. Another 13 species grow in Asia and Europe.

In the 19th century, black cohosh was a widely promoted herbal remedy and a favorite of Dr. John King (1813–1893), a professor of obstetrics at the Eclectic Medical College in Cincinnati, Ohio. King prescribed it for the treatment of nervous disorders, menstrual irregularities, and menopause. Although the herb fell out of favor with the American medical establishment in the early 20th century, the herb's popularity grew in Europe as German researchers remained interested in its use for treating menopausal symptoms. In recent years, black cohosh has regained popularity in the United States.

MEDICINAL USE

The roots and rhizomes of black cohosh have historically been used for their mild sedative and anti-inflammatory properties. It can be used to treat the pain of arthritis. The herb is best known, however, as a treatment for menopausal symptoms, especially hot flashes and night sweats. It is also used to treat conditions associated with menopause, such as insomnia, nervousness, tension, and depression. The plant contains triterpene glycosides, which may be responsible for its activity. Recent large-scale clinical trials have raised questions concerning the efficacy of this herb for the treatment of certain menopausal symptoms, but other studies are ongoing.

Caution: This herb should not be taken by pregnant women.

ORNAMENTAL USE

The tall, majestic spires of black cohosh add vertical interest to woodland gardens and contrast with lower-growing, rounded plants such as cranesbills (*Geranium* spp.) in borders.

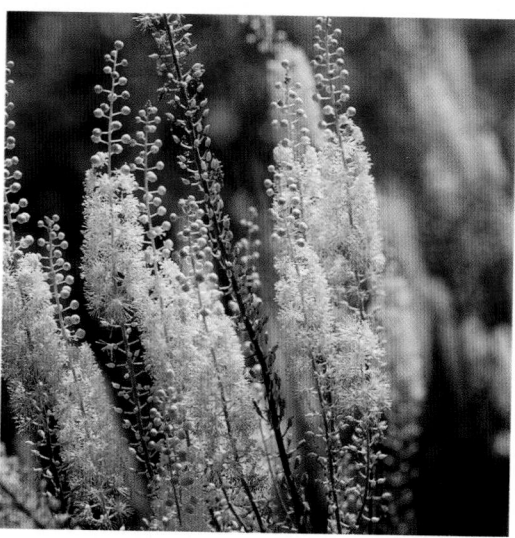

HOW TO GROW IT

Black cohosh grows in moist, humus-rich soil in sun or partial shade. In warmer regions, choose a site with consistent moisture and shade from afternoon sun to keep the foliage from browning. Plant root divisions at any time during the growing season, or sow fresh seed outdoors in fall. The plants grow slowly. Harvest the roots of mature plants in fall, when bioactive compounds are at their highest levels. Divide and replant the remainder of the roots, leaving at least one bud per division.

Aesculus hippocastanum

Native to central Asia, horse chestnut has been grown as a shade tree in North America since the 1700s. The common name "buckeye" comes from the appearance of its shiny reddish brown seeds, known as "conkers," which resemble the eyes of a deer. People sometimes mistakenly think the horse chestnut is an edible species—confusing it with the true chestnut—but it is not, and it can be poisonous. Native American tribes crushed the fresh seeds and scattered them in the water when fishing; chemical compounds called saponins, present in the seeds, slowed or stunned the fish and made them easier to catch.

MEDICINAL USE

Horse chestnut contains a substance called aescin, which helps strengthen and increase vein elasticity.

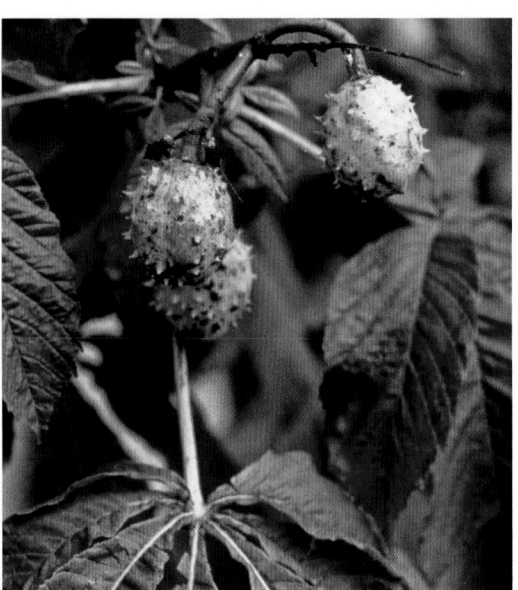

PLANT PROFILE

Common Names: Buckeye, Chestnut, Horse Chestnut

Description: Deciduous tree up to 60 feet tall with a broad, domed crown; palmate leaves; spikes of fragrant white flowers followed by spiny green fruits containing shiny reddish brown seeds

Hardiness: To Zone 3

Family: Hippocastanaceae

Flowering: Spring to early summer

Parts Used: Seeds and bark

Range/Habitat: Native to central Asia, naturalized throughout temperate Northern hemisphere

Studies have shown horse chestnut seed extract to be highly effective for treating varicose veins and chronic venous insufficiency, a condition that causes blood to pool in the veins of the lower legs after standing or sitting. Practitioners also use it to treat hemorrhoids and edema (fluid retention).

Aescin diminishes the number of openings in capillary walls, helping to prevent fluids from leaking into surrounding tissue. For this reason, horse chestnut is a good topical treatment for bruises and sports injuries. Horse chestnut gels can reduce swelling and tenderness after an injury. The herb also has anti-inflammatory properties; herbalists sometimes recommend it to relieve arthritis pain, eczema, phlebitis, and other inflammation.

Caution: Raw, unprocessed horse chestnut bark, stems, seeds, and leaves can be toxic and should not be ingested. Horse chestnut preparations should not be used internally by pregnant women. External preparations should not be applied to broken skin.

ORNAMENTAL USE

The horse chestnut tree has a large, spreading canopy and fragrant white blooms. It makes an attractive shade tree for home landscapes and parks.

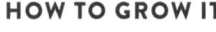

HOW TO GROW IT

Fast-growing horse chestnut trees prefer well-drained, fertile soil in sun or partial shade. Plant the young trees or seeds in spring or fall. To speed germination, soak seeds in water for 24 hours prior to planting. Established trees require little care other than occasional pruning in late winter. Harvest the seeds (inside the prickly pods) and bark in fall.

Agastache foeniculum

This striking member of the mint family takes its botanical name from the Greek words *agan* (very much) and *stachys* (an ear of corn or wheat), referring to the plant's spiky blue-purple flowers. A favorite of hummingbirds and bees, anise hyssop is the source of a delicious, slightly anise-flavored honey. The herb is native to the midwestern United States and has naturalized throughout North and Central America.

PLANT PROFILE

Common Names: Anise Hyssop, Blue Giant Hyssop, Fennel Giant Hyssop

Description: Upright 3- to 6-foot-tall plant with slender stems and maroon-tinted leaves; dense, terminal spikes of bright blue flowers; toothed, opposite leaves; aromatic

Hardiness: To Zone 6

Family: Lamiaceae

Flowering: Midsummer to late summer

Parts Used: Flowers and leaves

Range/Habitat: Naturalized throughout North America and Central America; dry, open areas, such as roadsides

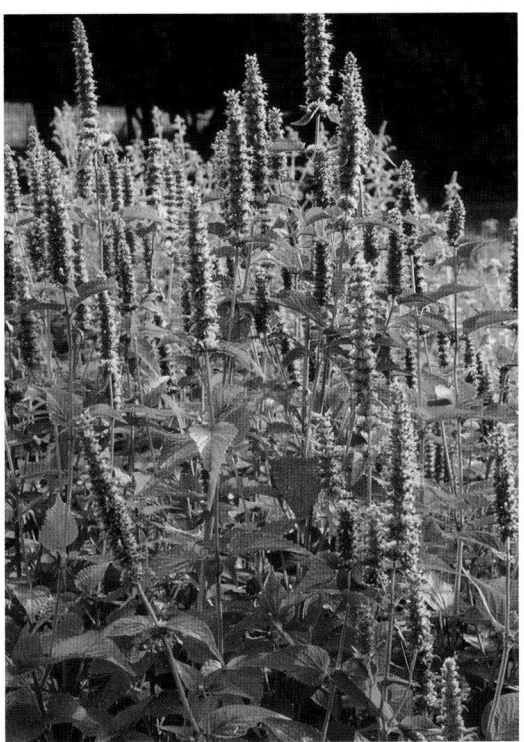

CULINARY USE

Anise hyssop's leaves and flowers have a very sweet, licorice-mint flavor that complements salads, dressings, fruits, soups, stews, and meats. Try adding a tablespoon or two of the fresh, minced leaves and flower buds to fruit desserts, especially those with peaches, nectarines, berries, and melons. Steep the leaves in milk or cream to make delicious ice creams and custards. The herb also makes a delightfully refreshing hot or iced tea.

MEDICINAL USE

Traditionally used by Native Americans to treat colds and coughs, the leaves of anise hyssop contain ingredients that increase perspiration (thus helping "break" a fever) and help clear bronchial congestion. The plant also might contain antiviral compounds useful in treating herpes. A related species, *Agastache rugosa*, has been used in traditional Chinese medicine to treat heartburn, symptoms of gastric reflux, and other digestive problems such as bloating, nausea, and vomiting. *A. rugosa* is also used in a lotion applied to treat ringworm, a skin fungus.

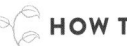

HOW TO GROW IT

An excellent garden border plant, anise hyssop prefers well-drained sandy loam and full sun but will tolerate somewhat poor soil and dry conditions. Plant it in spring. Pinch back plants early in the season to encourage branching. Harvest leaf sprigs just above a leaf joint in spring and summer; the leaves are most flavorful when the plant is in the early stages of bloom. Harvest young flowers in summer. Cut back plants by one-third after they finish blooming to encourage a second flush of bloom. Propagate by division, cuttings, or seed.

Agrimonia eupatoria

Once used as a throat-soothing gargle by speakers and singers, agrimony has astringent properties that make it a useful medicinal herb. Native to Europe, this member of the rose family produces small yellow flowers at the top of tall, slender spikes. The flowers become prickly seed burrs with hooked bristles that commonly attach themselves to passersby. The botanical name may come from the Greek *arghemon,* translating to "albugo," an eye disease once treated with the plant. Another explanation is that the name comes from the Latin *agri moenia,* or "defender of the fields," because of the plant's tendency to grow in groupings near fields.

MEDICINAL USE

The leaves, stems, and flowers contain astringent and antibacterial tannins. Agrimony has been used to treat diarrhea; to staunch bleeding wounds; and to soothe inflammation of the skin, throat, mouth, and pharynx; and for many other therapeutic purposes. It was a component of a special remedy produced in the 14th century to treat the gaping wounds produced by a primitive gun known as the arquebus.

In studies conducted with laboratory animals, agrimony has been shown to have liver-protecting effects, which are thought to be due to its anti-inflammatory and antioxidant properties. A related species, *Agrimonia pilosa,* is used in traditional Chinese medicine to treat nosebleeds, bleeding gums, and blood in the urine.

ORNAMENTAL USE

Agrimony's 5-foot spikes of small yellow flowers add vertical interest to wildflower borders, as well as to woodland and cottage gardens.

OTHER USES

Agrimony is well known for the yellow dye that can be made from its leaves and stems.

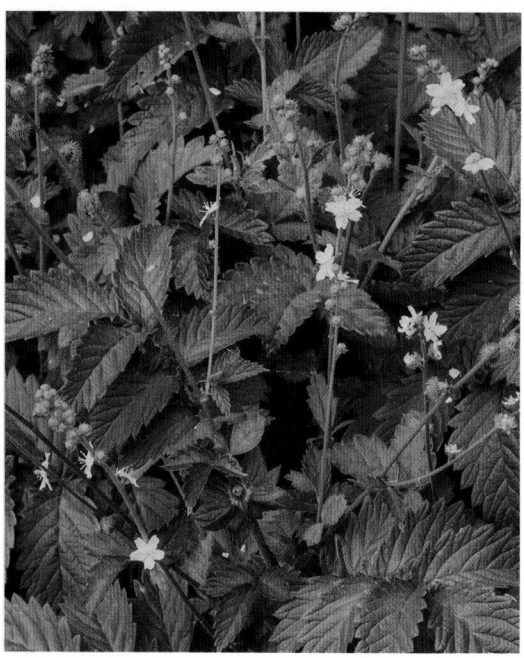

HOW TO GROW IT

Agrimony grows in well-drained, fairly dry soil in full sun. Plant it in groups of six to eight, leaving 6 inches between plants. Harvest blooms in midsummer, before they begin to develop into burrs. To keep the plants from spreading aggressively, cut the stalks before the seeds begin to drop. For yellow dye, harvest the leaves and stems in late fall. For a lighter buff color, harvest in early fall. Propagate by gathering seeds, or divide the roots of established plants.

Allium sativum

Garlic, a powerful cooking and healing herb, can inspire extraordinary passion among people. On any given weekend from July through September, thousands of garlic lovers pay homage to the "stinking rose" at dozens of garlic festivals held throughout the United States and Canada.

A member of the amaryllis family, garlic is generally believed to have originated in Asia. Its edible underground bulb is made up of 4 to 15 "cloves" enclosed in a papery white or pale purple skin. Aboveground, this perennial bears long, flat leaves and an umbel of greenish white to pink flowers. Garlic's name is thought to have originated from the Anglo-Saxon words *gar* (spear) and *lac* (plant), referring to the plant's spear-shaped leaves. *Sativum,* the species name, means "cultivated." Elephant garlic (*Allium ampeloprasum* var. *ampeloprasum*) produces bulbs that lack the plant's characteristic papery skin.

CULINARY USE

One of the world's most popular cooking herbs, garlic adds flavor to an enormous variety of foods, including salad dressings, pasta sauces, soups, vegetables, meat and fish dishes, vinegars, and herb butters and salts. The entire bulb can be baked or roasted, softening the cloves into a paste used as a

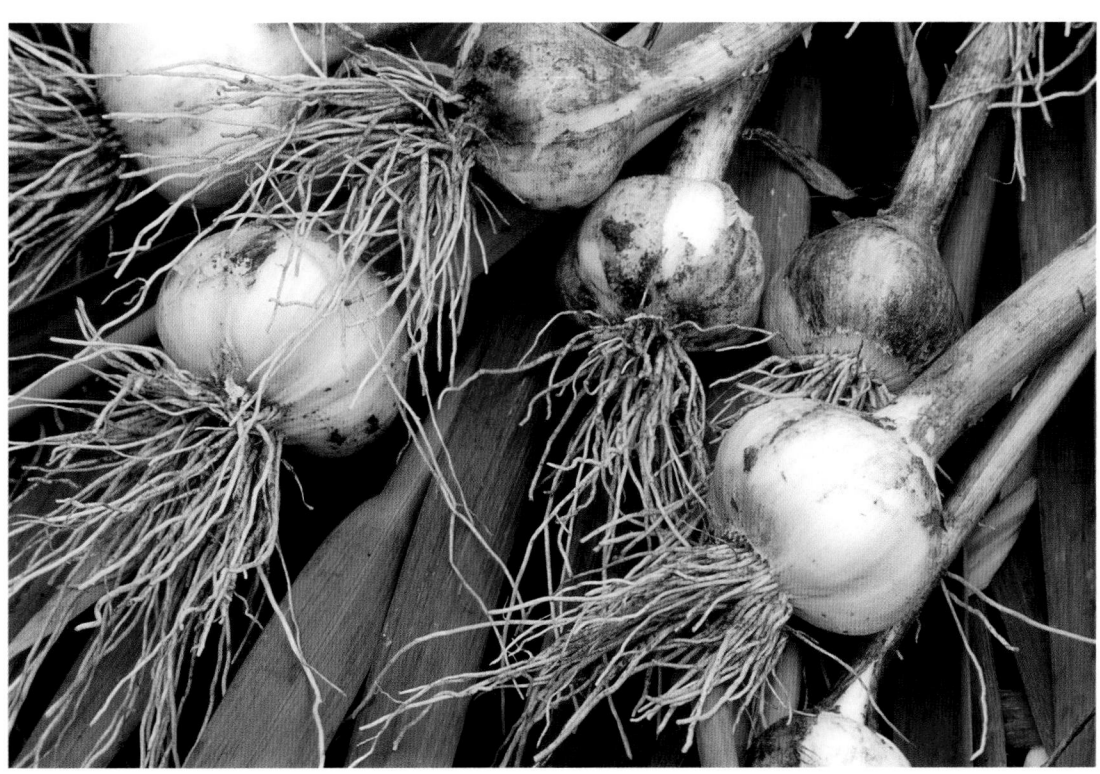

A Clove a Day . . .

Popular folklore suggests that eating garlic will ward off mosquitoes and save you from dousing your body with external repellents, either natural or synthetic. That might be the case. But in a recent study, people who ate large quantities of garlic suffered just as many bites from this irritating pest as they did when they had eaten no garlic. At least the garlic did not attract mosquitoes.

Garlic does have some very positive properties, though. Studies have shown that taking garlic can help lower blood pressure, prevent colds, and reduce the risk of colorectal and stomach cancers. Clinical studies of other reputed health benefits have had both positive and negative results. My take is that you should eat garlic as often as your friends and family will permit.—M. J. B.

seasoning or a spread. For a milder garlic flavor, mince garlic greens and use them as you would chives on soups, salads, pasta dishes, and other savory foods. Tip: To peel garlic easily, use the flat side of a knife blade to lightly crush the clove and loosen its skin.

MEDICINAL USE

People have used garlic for health and healing for more than 5,000 years. In ancient Egypt, the builders of the Great Pyramids ate garlic to prevent colds, bronchitis, and other upper-respiratory conditions. During the Middle Ages, French priests used garlic for protection against bubonic plague. During World War I, soldiers in Europe applied garlic to external wounds as a disinfectant; during World War II, Russian soldiers used garlic so extensively that the herb became known as "Russian penicillin."

The chemistry of garlic is complex, and researchers still don't understand exactly how it works. Garlic contains allicin, a sulfur compound activated when the herb is crushed. Allicin is believed to be responsible for garlic's strong flavor and aroma, as well as its medicinal benefits. Sometimes called the "pungent panacea," garlic has potent antiviral, antibacterial, anti-inflammatory, and antifungal properties. It is commonly used to treat diarrhea, as well as colds and other upper respiratory infections. One clinical study suggested that taking garlic supplements can help prevent the common cold. Regular use of garlic can also gently lower blood pressure.

For the greatest health benefits, use raw crushed garlic—cooking reduces the herb's beneficial compounds—or take garlic capsules with at least 4 to 8 milligrams of allicin. Some health practitioners advise their patients to chew a whole garlic clove twice a day at the first sign of a cold. (Take the clove with olive oil or sauce if plain garlic is too much for you!)

Caution: Consuming large quantities of garlic can cause gastrointestinal upset and might reduce your body's ability to form blood clots. If you're planning to have surgery and you take garlic supplements or eat more than four cloves a day, tell your physician; he or she might want you to stop or reduce your use of garlic before the procedure.

OTHER USES

Some gardeners crush garlic and mix it with water to make a pest-repellent spray. Others report that simply interplanting garlic with vegetable and fruit crops deters pests.

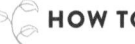

HOW TO GROW IT

Garlic prefers rich, moist, sandy soil and a sunny location. It requires a period of cold (40° to 50°F) to trigger sprouting. In the North, plant garlic in October or November, before the ground freezes; in the South, plant garlic in December or January. Plant the cloves 2 inches deep and 6 inches apart. When the bottom two or three leaves turn brown in early to midsummer, knock the stems over with a rake. Withhold water for a few days, then carefully dig up the plants. Dry them on a screen in a warm, dark, airy location for several days, then brush off any remaining soil.

Allium schoenoprasum

A relative of garlic and onion, chives have been a popular flavoring for nearly 5,000 years. The tender, dark green spears were probably first used in Asia; by the 16th century, the plant had earned a place in European gardens. The name "chives" derives from the French word *cive*, which comes from the Latin name for onion, *cepa*. The cooking and healing properties are similar to those of garlic, but milder.

CULINARY USE

Chives impart a mild onionlike flavor to cheese, egg, and potato dishes. This is due to the presence of sulfur-containing compounds known as disulfides. The herb complements artichokes, asparagus, carrots, corn, onions, peas, spinach, and tomatoes, as well as fish and poultry. Both the minced leaves and whole flowers can be used as a garnish and flavoring in soups, salads, spreads, and dips. The flowers are also attractive and tasty in herb vinegars. For an interesting presentation, tie whole chive leaves around individual servings of baby carrots or asparagus. Chives are an ingredient in the popular French herb mixture fines herbes, which also includes chervil, parsley, and tarragon.

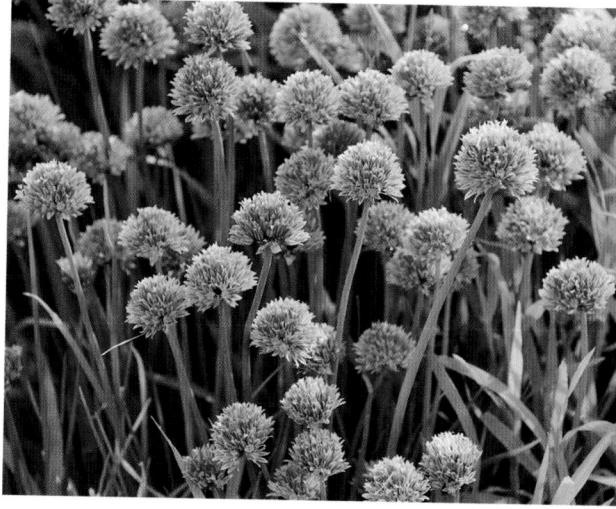

MEDICINAL USE

Historically, chives were used to treat colds, flu, and lung congestion because of the herb's high vitamin C content. The leaves also contain fiber and potassium. Chives are not commonly used in modern herbal medicine.

ORNAMENTAL USE

Rarely bothered by pests, pink-flowered chives make a neat, edible edging for flower, herb, and vegetable gardens. The leaves and flowers also dry beautifully and make lovely additions to dried herb and flower arrangements.

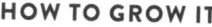

HOW TO GROW IT

Plant clumps of up to six bulbs 5 to 8 inches apart in moist, rich soil and full sun. To harvest, snip blades about 2 inches above the ground, cutting no more than two or three blades from each clump. Divide clumps of established, 3- to 5-year-old plants in early spring or fall.

To bring chives indoors for winter use, pot up the plant in late summer but leave it outside until the tops die back. (A cold, dormant period is needed to initiate new growth.) Then bring the pot indoors and set it on a sunny windowsill or below a fluorescent light. Plants will sprout within a few weeks.

Aloe vera (= *A. barbadensis*)

Aloe has been used to heal wounds, soothe burns, and soften skin for thousands of years. Native to East Africa, aloe was used by ancient Egyptians as an embalming ingredient and to treat skin conditions such as burns. Cleopatra is said to have considered aloe lotions to be the source of her renowned beauty. Legend has it that the Greek philosopher Aristotle (384–322 BCE) told Alexander the Great (356–323 BCE) to conquer the East African island Socotra so that a reliable supply of aloe would be available to Greece.

The plant's name comes from the Arabic word *alloeh*, meaning "bitter and shiny," which accurately describes the gel found inside aloe leaves.

MEDICINAL USE

Aloe contains polysaccharides thought to speed the healing of skin tissue and reduce inflamma-

tion. Aloe leaf juice and gel (a clear, jellylike substance) can be used to soothe burns, superficial skin wounds, sunburn, eczema, and rashes caused by poison oak and poison ivy. Aloe gel has also been applied to fingernails to prevent nail biting. Taken internally, the gel can be soothing to the digestive tract and has been used to treat colitis, Crohn's disease, and peptic ulcers. Studies have shown that aloe could help lower blood sugar levels in people with diabetes.

Aloe latex, or aloin, a brownish yellow gel found under the leaf blades, has traditionally been used as a laxative. Aloe latex is extremely harsh, however, and in 2002, the FDA issued a ban on over-the-counter laxative drug products that contain aloe ingredients. Aloe latex can still be purchased as an herbal supplement.

Caution: Aloe latex is extremely harsh. Do not use it if you are pregnant or nursing, or if you suffer from irritable bowel syndrome, kidney disease, or hemorrhoids. It can cause gastric upset, diarrhea, and abdominal cramping in some people. In addition, long-term use of products that contain aloe latex can lead to dependency. Commercial aloe gel and juice do not contain aloe latex. Externally, aloe gel can cause minor skin irritation.

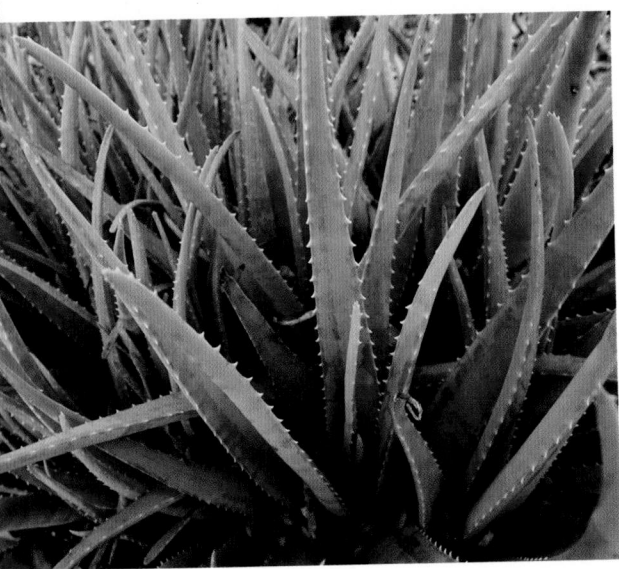

HOW TO GROW IT

Aloe is easy to grow in well-drained soil and full sun to partial shade. In Zone 9 and colder, grow aloe indoors, in a pot filled with a coarse medium. Do not overwater. Potted aloe seems to grow best when slightly crowded; if necessary, repot in late winter or spring. When harvesting aloe gel, cut the outermost leaves first; new growth is produced from the plant's center. To propagate, uproot and replant offshoots that are 2 to 3 inches tall.

Aloysia triphylla
(= *A. citriodora, Lippia citriodora*)

Lemon verbena's attractive leaves and pleasant scent have made it a favorite garden plant since Victorian times, when it was known as the "lemon plant." Native to South America, this tall, deciduous shrub bears small white to pale purple flowers and long, finely toothed yellow-green leaves that have a sweet, lemony fragrance and flavor. Its flavor is the most intense of all of the lemony herbs, including lemon balm, lemongrass, and lemon thyme.

CULINARY USE

Lemon verbena adds bright, lemony flavor to a variety of foods including preserves, marinades, seafood, poultry, salads, dressings, desserts, and wine. To give recipes a lemony lift, combine 7 to 10 leaves with a bit of water in a blender, and substitute the puree for some of the liquid in your recipe. Lemon verbena also makes a delicious hot or cold tea, and it has been used to flavor liqueurs in its native South America.

MEDICINAL USE

Traditionally used as a treatment for settling the stomach, lemon verbena contains a volatile oil (mainly consisting of citral, cineole, limonene, and geraniol) that benefits digestion. A tea of lemon verbena leaves or flowering tops can be used to relieve digestive upset, reduce fever, and improve lethargy. The plant contains flavonoids and iridoids, which give it antispasmodic, sedative, and fever-reducing effects.

Caution: Lemon verbena can cause contact dermatitis in some people.

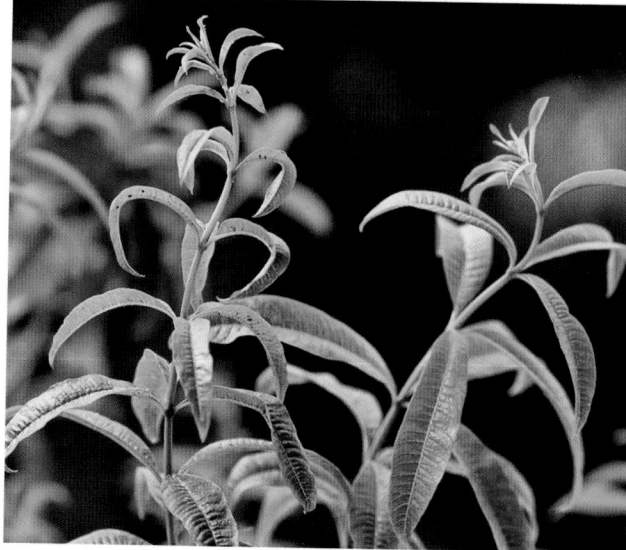

OTHER USES

Commercially, the oil is extracted to make cologne and soap. At home, use aromatic lemon verbena leaves in potpourris, sachets, and cut flower arrangements, or make a simple infusion to scent bathwater.

HOW TO GROW IT

Lemon verbena does best in light, well-drained soil in full sun. It can survive winters in areas where the ground does not freeze; in colder areas, grow it in a pot in a cool sunroom or unheated greenhouse during winter. Pinch back the plant tips to encourage bushy growth. If the plant is very large by fall, cut it back by half before bringing it indoors for winter. (Use the leaves!) Remember that lemon verbena is deciduous, so don't be concerned when it loses leaves in fall. Harvest the leaves in summer, when growth is lush. Dry them on a screen and store them in a jar in a cool, dark location. Start new plants from cuttings taken in summer.

Alpinia galanga

Closely related to ginger, galangal is widely used as a cooking spice and healing herb in Southeast Asia. This 6-foot-tall perennial bears attractive pale green orchidlike blooms and red fruits. Its thick, fragrant rhizome—the part most often used for cooking and healing—is smaller and lighter in color than ginger's. During the Middle Ages, galangal was believed to have aphrodisiac properties.

PLANT PROFILE

Common Names: Blue Ginger, Galangal, Greater Galangal, Thai Ginger

Description: Grows up to 6 feet tall with 20-inch lanceolate leaves; 3- to 4-foot racemes bear pale green, orchidlike blooms and red fruit; rhizomes can have a pink hue

Hardiness: To Zone 9

Family: Zingiberaceae

Flowering: May to August on larger stems

Parts Used: Rhizome

Range/Habitat: Southeast Asia

CULINARY USE

While several different plants are known as galangal, greater galangal (*Alpinia galanga*), which is native to South Asia and Indonesia, is the type used most often in cooking. Galangal has a warm flavor similar to ginger but with notes of black pepper and pine. It is commonly used in Indonesian, Malaysian, and Thai dishes and is an essential ingredient of *nasi goring*, a traditional fried rice dish.

Galangal blends well with lemongrass, garlic, and chile peppers. Use it to flavor curries, soups, stews, vegetables, and fish, but start with small amounts—its flavor is intense.

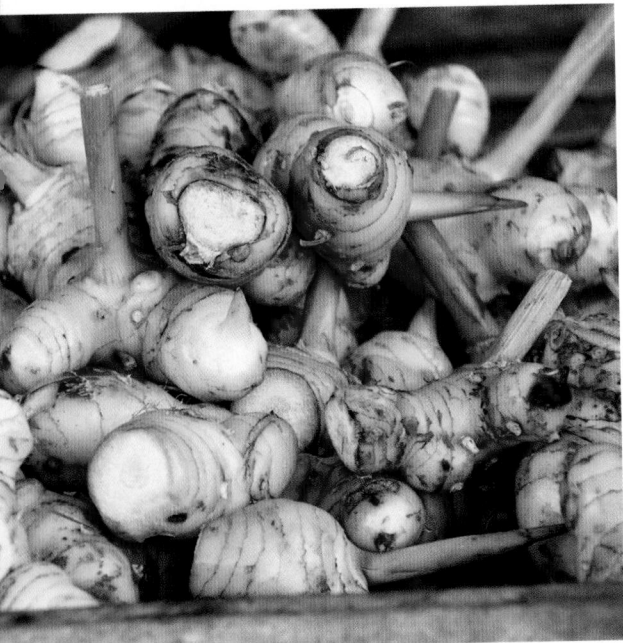

MEDICINAL USE

A stimulant and carminative (an agent that helps dispel intestinal gas), galangal is used extensively in traditional Chinese medicine to treat nausea and digestive problems. Ayurvedic practitioners use the rhizomes to treat arthritis and inflammation of the mucous membranes. Galangal oil is considered an antispasmodic and is suggested for treating respiratory conditions such as asthma. An extract of the rhizome is sometimes used to treat impotence. Galangal can be taken as a tea, extract, or capsule. It can also be applied externally as a poultice.

HOW TO GROW IT

In Zone 8 and colder, grow this tropical plant in a warm greenhouse in rich, well-drained soil and partial shade. Galangal thrives on humidity; mist it often. Begin harvesting rhizomes for fresh use in late summer of the plant's fourth year. Or clean the rhizome of its roots, slice it thickly, and dry it for future use. Reconstitute the dried root in water before using it in recipes.

Althaea officinalis

Before gelatin and other products were used to give marshmallows their pillowy consistency, this herb's roots created the effect. But the plant has a long history of other uses, too. Native to marshy areas of Europe and Asia, marshmallow is a 3- to 4-foot-tall perennial with attractive white or pale pink blooms. It belongs to the genus *Althaea*, a name derived from the Greek word for "heal." Ancient Greek physicians used marshmallow roots to treat wounds, toothaches, and insect stings, while the Romans recommended using the roots and leaves as a laxative. By the Middle Ages, the plant was used to relieve a range of medical conditions, including coughs and lung infections, stomach problems, ulcers, and bladder infections. Externally, the leaves were applied to wounds, bruises, and sprains.

CULINARY USE

The original marshmallow confection was the French *pâté de guimauve*, made from the plant's root. Use the tender young shoots and leaves of marshmallow in spring salads, soups, and stews. The roots have more substance. To prepare them, boil them gently for a few minutes, then drain and sauté them with onions.

MEDICINAL USE

Marshmallow roots and leaves contain mucilage, a substance that soothes inflamed mucous membranes in the mouth, throat, and gastrointestinal tract. Studies have shown that marshmallow root preparations can reduce the duration and severity of coughs. Marshmallow tea and decoction can also be used to treat sore throats, oral inflammations, and gastrointestinal irritations such as ulcers and diarrhea. Externally, marshmallow root compresses and poultices can soothe skin irritations.

> **PLANT PROFILE**
>
> **Common Names:** Mallow, Marshmallow
>
> **Description:** Erect perennial up to 4 feet tall; soft, velvety grayish green leaves; five-petaled pinkish white blooms followed by round, downy fruits; tapering, woody taproot
>
> **Hardiness:** To Zone 3
>
> **Family:** Malvaceae
>
> **Flowering:** July to September
>
> **Parts Used:** Roots, young leaves, and stems
>
> **Range/Habitat:** Native to Europe and western Asia, naturalized in eastern North America; grows in moist places, such as salt marshes and coastal wetlands

Caution: Do not take other drugs for 1 hour before or several hours after taking marshmallow, as it could slow the absorption of those medications.

OTHER USES

Because of its soothing and emollient properties, marshmallow is used in cosmetic preparations to treat irritated skin. Try using a decoction of the root to make a hydrating facial mask.

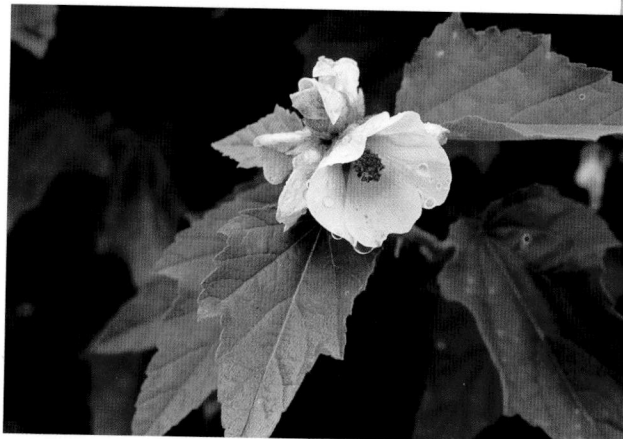

HOW TO GROW IT

Marshmallow is easy to propagate and grow from seed, cuttings, or root divisions. Plant it in full sun and fertile, moist soil with good drainage. In summer, mulch generously with straw, shredded leaves, or compost to retain soil moisture. Harvest young leaves and shoots before the plant begins to bloom in midsummer. Harvest roots in late fall from plants that are at least 2 years old. To prepare the roots for storage, remove the lateral rootlets, wash the roots, peel off the corky bark, and dry them whole or in slices.

Ananas comosus

Known universally for its succulent yellow fruit, pineapple is an exotic member of the family Bromeliaceae, native to South America. This herbaceous perennial has a short, sturdy stem and bears a rosette of spiny green leaves. In the plant's second year, a flowering stalk emerges from the center; the inflorescence resembles a miniature pineapple covered with small red, pink, or pale purple flowers. This slowly develops into what we know as a pineapple, ripening brown on the outside and yellow on the inside.

The plant's common name refers to the appearance of the fruit, which looks like a very large pinecone. Ananas comes from the Paraguayan word *nana*, which means "exquisite fruit." Pineapple is cultivated throughout the tropics, with the largest production in Brazil, Thailand, and the Philippines.

CULINARY USE

Fresh pineapple fruit has a tangy, citrusy flavor that complements fruit desserts and salads. The fruit can also be sautéed, broiled, grilled, or baked. Try pineapple in sorbets, ice creams, relishes, syrups, and sauces. Pineapple salsa gives grilled pork and salmon a tropical twist. Use pineapple juice with brown sugar and mustard as a glaze for poultry. Top burgers with grilled pineapple rings and a sauce made of ketchup, mayonnaise, and chile paste.

MEDICINAL USE

Pineapple fruit is a good source of vitamins A, B, and C. It contains bromelain, an enzyme that aids

---

PLANT PROFILE

Common Name: Pineapple

Description: Stout stem 2 to 5 feet tall, surrounded by long, straplike leaves with spiny edges; small red or purple blooms develop into a single cone-shaped fruit

Hardiness: To Zone 10

Family: Bromeliaceae

Flowering: December to January, when day lengths shorten

Parts Used: Fruit and leaves

Range/Habitat: Native to southern Brazil and Paraguay

---

in the digestion of protein and relieves stomach upset. Other enzymes in pineapple include amylase, which digests starch, and lipase, which digests fat. Bromelain has anti-inflammatory properties, making it useful as a dietary supplement to help your body heal more quickly after surgery and for those suffering from arthritis and stomach or digestive problems. When taken regularly, bromelain may help reduce inflammation and scarring of the arteries that can lead to cardiovascular disease. Fresh pineapple is a good source of fiber, which helps relieve constipation. Its juice has mild diuretic properties. A juice made from the leaves is considered a powerful purgative and antiparasitic in Ayurvedic medicine. In clinical studies, it has been shown to be similar in effect to nonsteroidal anti-inflammatory drugs. Commercially, bromelain is obtained from the stem of the plant.

 HOW TO GROW IT

Pineapple thrives in tropical conditions and fertile, well-drained loam soil with an acid pH. In cooler climates, pineapple can be grown in a pot indoors and moved outdoors during summer, after nighttime temperatures remain above 60°F. Provide at least 6 hours of bright light daily and feed it monthly during the growing season. Avoid overwatering. After about 20 months, when the plant is at least 24 inches tall, flowering and fruiting may occur. Harvest the fruit when at least half of it has turned gold in color. Pineapple is commonly propagated vegetatively from the crown (the leaves at the top of the fruit).

Caution: Wear gloves when handling this plant; its spiny leaves can tear skin.

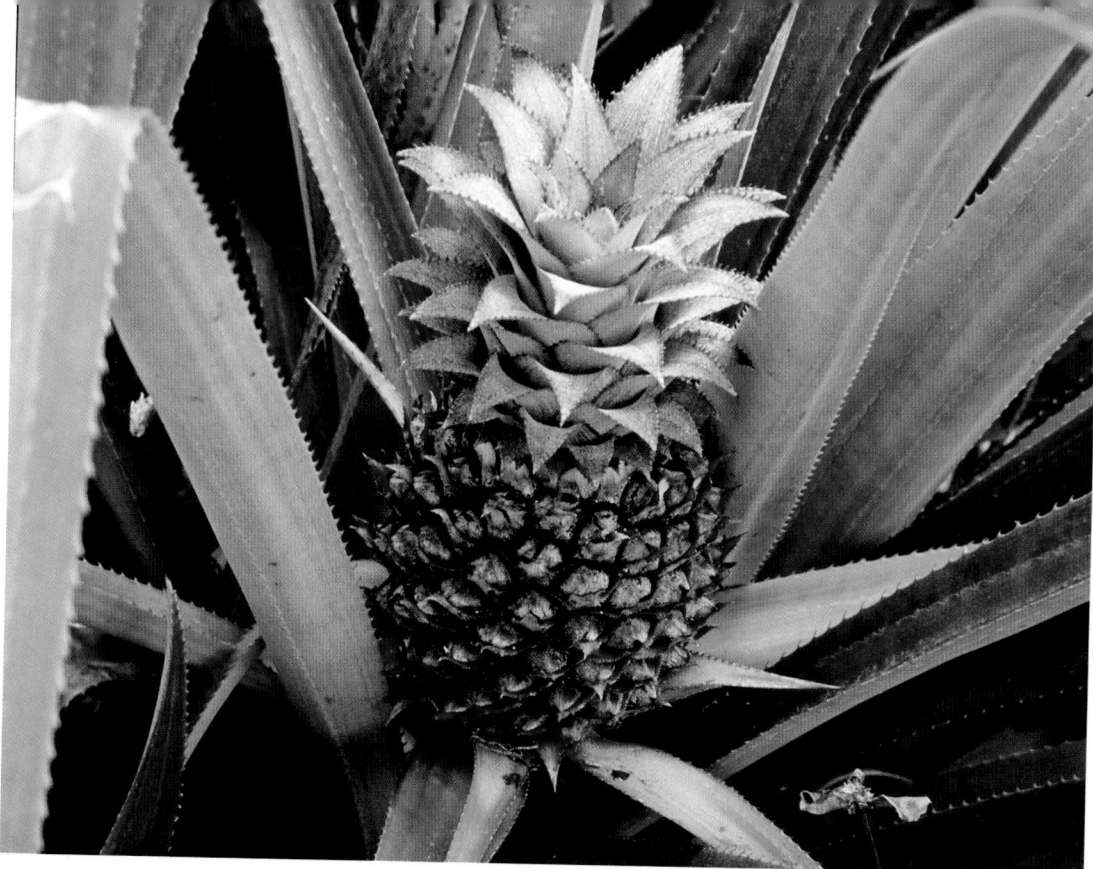

Sweet Healer

The Greek physician Hippocrates (460–377 BCE) suggested, "Let food be your medicine and medicine be your food." Pineapple is a wonderful example of a healing food—delicious and healthful. I first saw a pineapple in a supermarket in Philadelphia. As a young child, this rather massive green fruit was extraordinarily interesting to me—it didn't look like anything I had ever seen before. And when we let it ripen in the house, a wonderful sweet smell filled the air. The rough, almost impenetrable skin had turned a soft golden brown, and it was ready to eat and enjoy.

Fast-forward 40 years later to a scientific expedition in the remote Brazilian rainforest. Coming into an open area, I saw a field of bromeliads with what looked like little pineapples growing from their centers. Here was the center of origin of the cultivated pineapple, and these were the wild relatives that the local people had used as a food many years before. I tasted one—it was fibrous and sour. Many generations of selection and breeding were required to develop the pineapples we enjoy today.

Local people that I stayed with showed me how the leaves of these plants are used to make a fiber that can be woven into a soft cloth or cord. The tender young shoots can be cooked and eaten. And the skin of the fruit grown in the gardens around their homes can be made into a tasty fermented beverage. I've experienced firsthand the remarkable journey made by the pineapple—from a small and mostly inedible wild species to a sweet and succulent fruit cultivated on tens of thousands of acres throughout the tropics.—M. J. B.

Anethum graveolens

PLANT PROFILE

Common Name: Dill

Description: Upright stems, up to 2 to 3 feet tall, topped by yellow-green umbels up to 6 inches across; feathery, bipinnate leaves; flat, ribbed seeds; aromatic

Hardiness: Annual

Family: Apiaceae

Flowering: July through September

Parts Used: Leaves, flowers, and seeds

Range/Habitat: Native to the Mediterranean and southern Russia; naturalized in North America

This herb has graced gardens since the days of ancient Athens and Rome. Native to the Mediterranean region and Asia, dill bears feathery foliage, umbels of yellow flowers, and aromatic seeds. Romans in the 1st century considered the plant a symbol of good fortune. They crowned returning war heroes with fragrant garlands of dill and hung wreaths of dill blossoms in their banquet halls. In the Middle Ages, magicians used dill in spells and charms against witchcraft, as well as in love potions and aphrodisiacs.

CULINARY USE

Dill has a distinctive, tangy flavor. The leaves, known as dillweed, and the stronger flavored

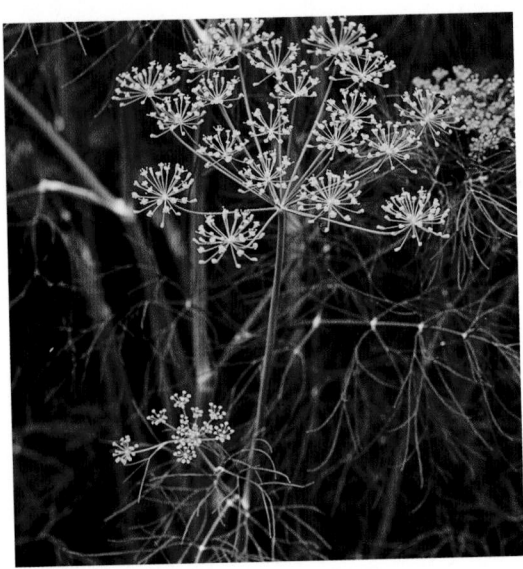

flowers and seeds can be used fresh or dried. Fresh dill leaves pair well with eggs, seafood, salads, and vegetables.

MEDICINAL USE

Both dill seed and dill seed oil have long histories of use in Western and traditional Chinese medicine for the treatment of flatulence, particularly in children. The seeds and leaves contain a volatile oil that acts as a digestive aid, relieving intestinal gas and calming the digestive tract. Dill also retards the growth of *E. coli*, a type of bacteria that can cause gastrointestinal and urinary tract infections. Chewing dill seeds is believed to alleviate bad breath. Dill seed and leaf teas have been given to nursing mothers to increase milk production, and babies have been given the tea, called "gripe water," to relieve colic.

OTHER USES

The flower umbels of dill are a favorite food of beneficial insects, such as lacewings, ladybugs, and hoverflies, which help control aphids and other insect pests. Encourage these insect helpers by interplanting dill with food crops and flowers.

HOW TO GROW IT

Dill grows best in well-drained, slightly acidic soil in full sun. Sow the seeds directly in the garden in spring, after danger of frost has passed; transplanting isn't always successful due to the herb's single taproot. For a steady supply of fresh leaves and flowers, reseed every 3 weeks until midsummer. Begin snipping leaves when the plants are well established, cutting off sprigs where they meet the main stem. Harvest seeds when they turn light brown, 2 to 3 weeks after blossoming. Fresh leaves will maintain their quality for about 3 days in the refrigerator. Leaves and seeds can be dried in a warm, dark location and stored in an airtight container.

Angelica archangelica

PLANT PROFILE

Common Names: Angelica, Archangel, European Angelica, Norwegian Angelica

Description: Long, hollow stems up to 7 feet tall; 2- to 6-inch umbels of greenish yellow flowers, followed by small green fruits, or seeds; pinnate leaves with coarsely toothed leaflets

Hardiness: Biennial

Family: Apiaceae

Flowering: Late spring or early summer of the second year

Parts Used: Entire plant

Range/Habitat: Northern Europe and Asia; found near streams, marshes, and swamps

This tall, robust member of the parsley family was once believed to possess extraordinary powers of healing and protection. The name comes from the Latin *herba angelica*, or "angelic herb," due to its reputation as a magical plant that could ward off witchcraft and illness, including the black death. European peasants placed necklaces of angelica leaves around the necks of their children to protect them, and early European and North American hunters used the herb's aromatic roots to attract wild game and fish.

CULINARY USE

Angelica roots and fruit (commonly called "seeds") are used to flavor vermouth, gin, Benedictine, and Chartreuse. The stems and leaves—which taste like a blend of vanilla and juniper—pair well with almonds, ginger, oranges, and rhubarb. The young stems can be steamed as a vegetable or candied and added to fruit desserts, ice cream, or mousse. (At one time, candied angelica was used as the green candies in fruitcake.)

MEDICINAL USE

One of the most popular herbs in Europe during the 15th century, angelica contains digestion-enhancing volatile oils that support its historical use as a remedy for indigestion. The roots and fruit are used to treat appetite loss, flatulence, and abdominal discomfort. The herb is sometimes used to treat colds, bronchitis, and asthma.

Caution: Angelica can cause a skin rash in some people who are exposed to sunlight after ingesting the herb. This herb should not be taken by women who are pregnant, nursing, or trying to conceive, nor should it be consumed by children younger

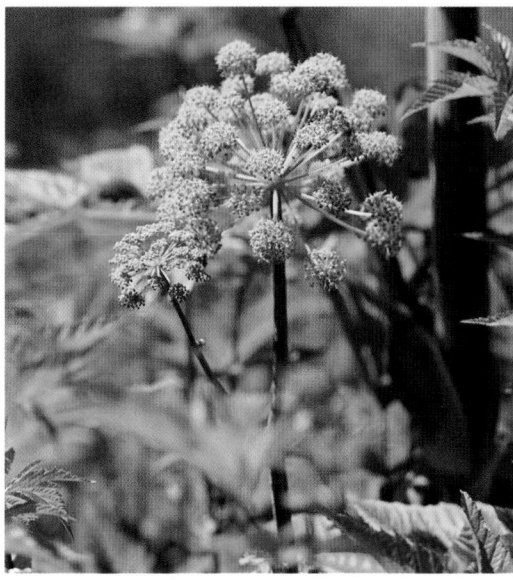

than 2 years old. Some herb–drug interactions are possible; for example, angelica root interferes with warfarin. Angelica roots should be thoroughly dried before use; they are poisonous when fresh.

HOW TO GROW IT

Angelica prefers mild summers and struggles in very hot climates. Give this large plant plenty of room and rich, moist, well-drained soil in sun or partial shade. Plant in either spring or fall, but don't cover the seeds—they need light to germinate. Harvest tender young stems in late summer the first season or in spring the second season, before the plant blooms. Cut stems at ground level. A biennial, angelica self-seeds readily in its second year.

Angelica sinensis

A perennial member of the parsley family, dong quai is best known as a treatment for gynecological conditions. The herb grows at high altitudes in China, Korea, and Japan. Like other angelicas, the plant has lacy flower umbels, hollow stems, and large, lobed leaves. The flowers have a honeylike aroma.

The name *dong quai* means "must return." According to a legend, a young husband had to leave his bride to go up into the mountains. He told her that if he did not return after 3 years, she should assume he had not survived and should remarry. After 3 years, the husband did not return, and the wife reluctantly remarried. Eventually the man did return, however, causing the woman to fall into a deep despair. He gave her a medicine made from the roots of a plant (dong quai) that he had found in the mountains; when she took it, she was restored to health.

CULINARY USE

In China, people add the chopped dried roots to soups. You can also add the fresh roots to salads or cook them as a vegetable.

MEDICINAL USE

Traditional Chinese medicine practitioners use the herb to treat menstrual problems, menopausal symptoms, and a variety of gynecological conditions. The root contains coumarin, which dilates blood vessels, stimulating the central nervous system and increasing blood flow throughout your body. It has been used to treat high blood pressure, poor circulation, and anemia. Researchers have found that dong quai stimulates the production of red blood cells, which carry oxygen throughout the body, thereby increasing energy and combating fatigue. It's commonly referred to as female ginseng.

PLANT PROFILE

Common Names: Chinese Angelica, Dong Quai

Description: Round, hollow, purplish stems up to 7 feet tall; bright green, slightly serrated, pinnate leaves; small white or greenish yellow flowers formed in umbels; honeylike aroma

Hardiness: To Zone 4

Family: Apiaceae

Flowering: Late spring to early summer

Parts Used: Rhizome

Range/Habitat: Native to China, Korea, and Japan; found along stream banks and in ravines

Caution: Dong quai should not be used during pregnancy. Some people could experience a skin rash when exposed to the sun after ingesting the herb. There have been reports of herb–drug interactions when dong quai is used with warfarin.

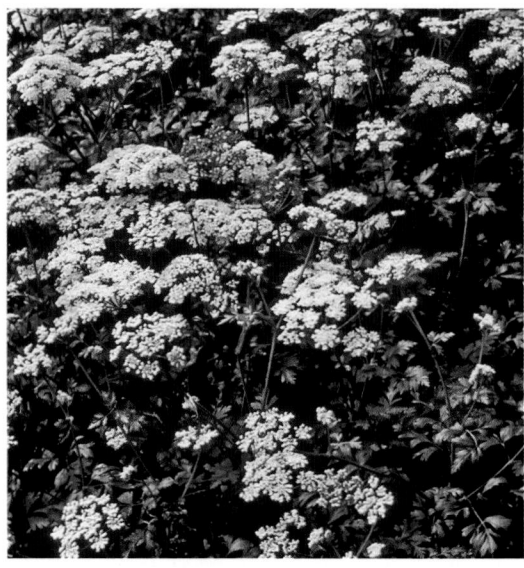

 HOW TO GROW IT

Dong quai thrives in fertile, moist soil in sun or partial shade. Plant the seeds outdoors in fall, or start them in a cold frame or unheated greenhouse during winter, then transplant the seedlings to the garden in spring. After about 3 years, you can dig up the rhizomes, slice or chop them, and then use them fresh or dried. To propagate, collect seed heads after they have dried on the plant. The seed doesn't keep well, so plant it as soon as possible.

Anthriscus cerefolium

PLANT PROFILE

Common Names: Chervil, Garden Chervil

Description: Branched stems up to 2 feet tall with delicate, light green, deeply cut leaflets; small white flowers in compound umbels

Hardiness: Annual

Family: Apiaceae

Flowering: May through July

Parts Used: Leaves

Range/Habitat: Native to Europe and Asia, naturalized in North America

Popular in European gardens and cooking, chervil is an herb with a pleasant, subtle flavor. A member of the parsley family, it resembles parsley in appearance, but its leaves are paler in color and more finely dissected. A basket of chervil seeds was found in the tomb of King Tutankhamen (ca. 1370–1352 BCE), hinting at the importance of this herb in ancient Egypt, although little has been written about its use during this period. In the 1st century, Pliny the Elder wrote about the use of chervil to season food and suggested that it could be used to cure hiccups.

CULINARY USE

Chervil's mild, aniselike flavor is best when the herb is eaten fresh. The flavor does not hold up to prolonged heat, so add chervil to foods just before serving, or use it finely chopped or as a garnish. Chervil enhances the flavor of carrots, cheese, corn, cream, fish, peas, sorrel, and spinach. Bearnaise sauce and classic French vinaigrette benefit from a bit of chervil, too. Together with parsley, tarragon, and thyme, chervil is one of the ingredients in the popular French herb mix fines herbes.

MEDICINAL USE

Chervil's active compounds include coumarin, a volatile oil, and flavonoids. Coumarin is used as the basis for anticoagulant drugs such as Coumadin. The 17th-century English physician Nicholas Culpeper (1616–1654) wrote that eating chervil would "moderately warm the stomach, and is a certain remedy to dissolve congealed or clotted blood in the body" from bruises and falls. Modern herbalists suggest taking chervil leaf tea to aid digestion and for its diuretic effects. The tea can also be applied externally (with a cotton ball) to treat superficial wounds and skin irritations such as eczema. Nutritionally, the herb is a good source of the minerals magnesium, potassium, and selenium.

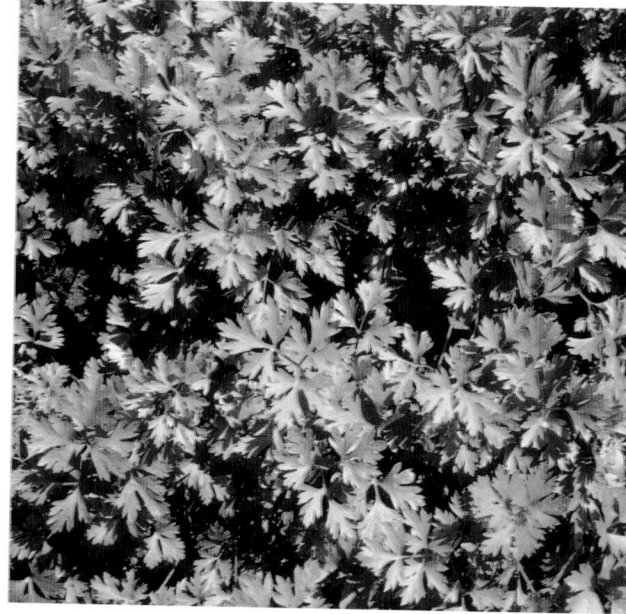

HOW TO GROW IT

Chervil thrives in rich, light soil that retains moisture. The plant will bolt in high temperatures or intense sunlight, so a site in partial shade is best. For a steady supply of leaves, sow seeds every 2 to 3 weeks from early spring to fall. (Seeds sown in fall will germinate the following spring.) Thin seedlings to 8 inches apart. Cut the leaves in 6 to 8 weeks, before the plant flowers. Chervil is also easy to grow in a pot on a cool, sunny windowsill indoors.

Arctium lappa

Love it or loathe it, burdock is a plant that demands to be noticed. Native to Europe and Asia, this weedy biennial grows freely in temperate regions all over the world, bearing long leaves and thistlelike flowers that attract butterflies and bees. Its spiny seed heads are covered with stiff hooks that cling stubbornly to clothes and animals. These burrs are said to have inspired the Swiss inventor George de Mestral (1907–1990) to develop Velcro, which was patented in 1955. The plant's common name comes from "bur," for its tenacious burrs, and "dock," an Old English word for plant.

CULINARY USE

In Japan, burdock root is commonly eaten as a vegetable called *gobo*. The roots are slivered, soaked in water to remove their bitter flavor, and stir-fried with sesame oil and soy sauce. Found in sushi bars worldwide, burdock roots are also eaten raw in salads or cooked like carrots. In Scandinavian countries, the young spring leaves are eaten in salads.

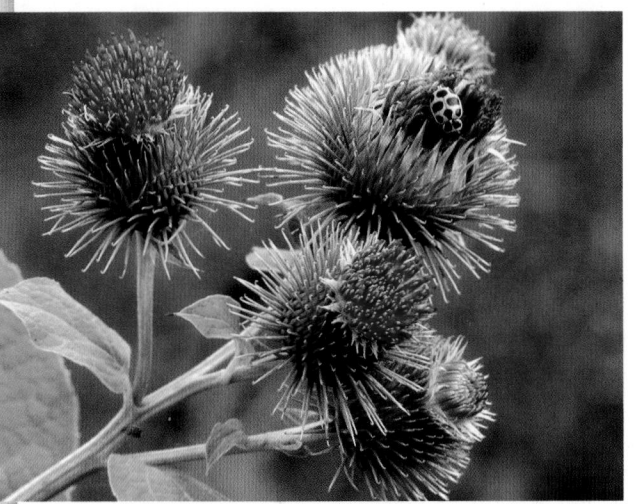

To prepare burdock root, peel, chop, then soak the root for about 30 minutes in several changes of cold water. Try combining the prepared root with shredded carrot, minced fresh ginger, and lemon juice for an appetizer or salad. Young stalks can be peeled, chopped, and steamed, like asparagus.

MEDICINAL USE

Burdock roots and seeds contain bitter glycosides, flavonoids, and tannins. In traditional Chinese medicine, burdock has long been considered an important blood purifier and is included in formulas designed to detoxify the liver and improve digestion. It's also taken internally to treat inflammation. Native Americans used an infusion of the roots or seeds to cleanse blood and applied a poultice of the boiled leaves to sores.

Modern research indicates that burdock may have a liver-protective effect, as well as anti-inflammatory and antioxidant properties. It also contains a substance called arctigenin, which has shown antitumor effects in animal studies. Burdock is a mild antibacterial agent, making it useful in the treatment of skin conditions, including acne and boils, and as an ingredient in some shampoos, creams, and lotions.

🌱 HOW TO GROW IT

Burdock thrives in full sun and fertile, moist, well-drained soil. Sow the seed directly in the garden when the temperature has warmed; thin seedlings to 6 inches apart. Some gardeners mix wood chips or sawdust into burdock beds to loosen the soil, making the 3-foot-long roots easier to harvest in fall or the following spring.

Arctostaphylos uva-ursi

Marco Polo (1254–1324) discovered this herb's uses when he traveled to China, and Kublai Khan learned of it during his invasions. By the 13th century, European herbalists recognized uva-ursi as an important healing herb.

Native to Europe, Asia, and North America, this low-growing evergreen shrub produces sour red berries that are a favorite of bears—explaining both the common name bearberry and species name ("bear's grape" in Latin). The Native American name kinnikinnick (meaning "that which is mixed") refers to the practice of combining the plant's leaves with tobacco and other plants for smoking. Various groups of Native American people ate kinnikinnick berries fresh, dried, or mixed with other edibles.

MEDICINAL USE

Native Americans made a poultice of the plant's leaves, stems, and other parts for treating skin sores and burns, back pain, and back sprains. Some tribes also drank an infusion of the leaves, stems, and berries for back pain, possibly caused by kidney problems.

This herb has long been used to treat urinary tract infections and can reduce inflammation. The leaves contain astringent tannins, as well as the antibacterial compounds hydroquinone and arbutin. Hydroquinone can cause liver damage and other problems, however.

Caution: Pregnant or nursing women and children should not take uva-ursi, nor should those with high blood pressure or certain other conditions.

ORNAMENTAL USE

With glossy evergreen foliage and pink bell-shaped flowers, uva-ursi is a lovely groundcover along a walkway, around a patio, or in a container. Look

---

PLANT PROFILE

Common Names: Bearberry, Kinnikinnick, Uva-ursi

Description: Creeping evergreen shrub with short, dark stems and long fibrous roots; small, glossy, undivided leaves; pink bell-shaped flowers; small, round, glossy red berries

Hardiness: To Zone 2

Family: Ericaceae

Flowering: April and May

Parts Used: Leaves, stems, and berries

Range/Habitat: Throughout the Northern Hemisphere; dry, rocky areas

---

for varieties specially bred for their bright berries or dense foliage.

OTHER USES

An extract of uvi-ursi is used commercially in skin lightening agents. It has replaced pure hydroquinone, which has fallen out of favor for this purpose and is being evaluated as a possible carcinogen. Uvi-ursi can also be used to make a green dye for alum- or iron-mordanted wool or a light brown dye for unmordanted wool (see page 397).

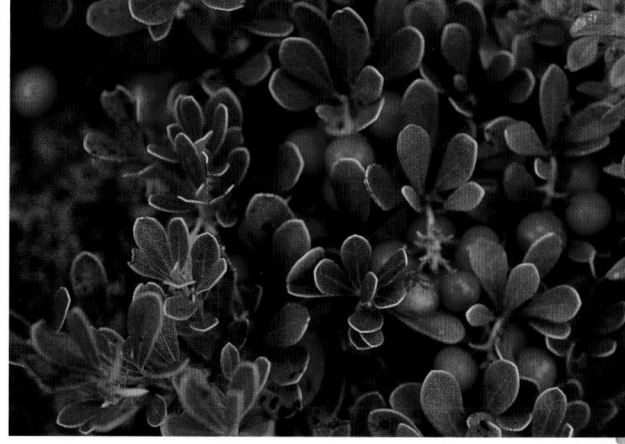

🌿 HOW TO GROW IT

Uva-ursi (often sold as bearberry) needs little care in your garden other than watering when conditions are very dry. Occasionally pinch back the young plants to encourage branching and compact growth. Propagate new plants by layering one of the plant's runners, or start new plants from green stem cuttings.

Armoracia rusticana

PLANT PROFILE

Common Name: Horseradish

Description: Perennial; 12 to 24 inches tall with large, broad, lance-shaped leaves; tiny, white, four-petaled flowers; aromatic

Hardiness: To Zone 3

Family: Brassicaceae

Flowering: Midsummer

Parts Used: Roots and leaves

Range/Habitat: Native to Europe and Asia; widely cultivated

For centuries, this herb was considered a medicine, not a condiment. The French called it *moutarde des allemands*, mustard of the Germans, and indeed, the Germans and Danes were the only Europeans of the Middle Ages to use the root at the dinner table.

This large-rooted perennial has been valued by herbalists as an internal and external medicine, and it has been cultivated since ancient times. The Egyptians used it as early as 1500 BCE, and it is one of the five bitter herbs of the Jewish Passover ceremony.

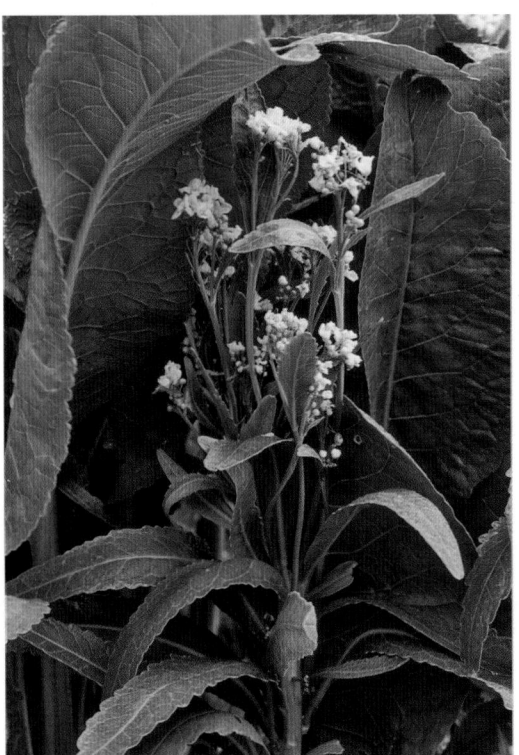

CULINARY USE

Horseradish is best known today for the sharply flavored condiment prepared from its root. To make it, simply grate the fresh root and put a bit of it on food, or combine it with vinegar. The mildly spicy leaves can be added to salads.

MEDICINAL USE

Nutritionally, horseradish is a good source of calcium, dietary fiber, manganese, magnesium, potassium, vitamin C, and zinc. Long recognized for its healthful properties, horseradish has been used to treat disorders such as asthma, coughs, toothache, ulcers, worms, and inflammation of joints and tissues. The root contains isothiocyanates (sulfur compounds also found in garlic and onions), as well as sulforaphane, an antioxidant in broccoli. Released when the root is crushed, both agents clear sinus congestion, open nasal passages, and promote blood flow. Horseradish also has antibiotic properties, making it useful for treating respiratory and urinary tract infections.

Caution: Pregnant and nursing women, very young children, and people suffering from gastrointestinal or kidney disorders should not take horseradish in large amounts. Also, remember not to eat horseradish or other members of the mustard family for at least 3 days before taking a test for blood in the stool, as these foods can cause a false positive.

HOW TO GROW IT

Horseradish prefers loose, rich, well-drained soil in full sun or partial shade. Plant root divisions in early spring or fall. Do not overwater. Harvest the leaves in spring; dig up the roots in fall. Propagate established plants by dividing the rhizomes in early spring or fall.

Caution: In some areas, horseradish spreads easily; consider growing it in a container.

Arnica montana

Arnica's ability to soothe muscle aches, sprains, and bruises has been known for centuries, both in Europe and North America. While European herbalists used their native mountain arnica to make healing remedies, Native Americans used native North American species, such as broadleaf arnica (*Arnica latifolia*) and heartleaf arnica (*A. cordifolia*).

Arnica bears oval, hairy leaves and yellow, daisylike flowers. Its name may be derived from *arnakis*, the ancient Greek word for "lambskin," in reference to the plant's soft leaves.

MEDICINAL USE

A popular remedy around the world, arnica has anti-inflammatory and antiseptic properties, the former ascribed to the compound helenalin and the latter due in part to compounds related to thymol. It is used externally to treat sprains, bruises, swelling, and joint pain, and it is a key ingredient in many first-aid creams and gels.

To make your own remedy for bruises and sore muscles, gently heat 1 ounce of arnica flowers in 1 ounce of oil for several hours. Strain and let the infused oil cool before using it. (For more about making and using infused oils, see page 325.)

Caution: Arnica is toxic if ingested and should not be taken internally except in homeopathic preparations under the guidance of a health-care professional. Arnica ointments or creams should not be applied to broken skin. The herb can cause contact dermatitis in some people.

Because arnica has been overharvested in the wild, choose preparations made from cultivated plants, or use alternative plants such as calendula (*Calendula officinalis*) and yarrow (*Achillea millefolium*) to make your own preparations.

PLANT PROFILE

Common Names: Arnica, European Arnica, Leopard's Bane, Mountain Arnica, Mountain Tobacco

Description: Erect, branching stems, 1 to 2 feet tall, emerge from basal rosettes of oval, downy leaves; yellow-orange daisylike blooms; creeping rhizome

Hardiness: To Zone 4

Family: Asteraceae

Flowering: Midsummer

Parts Used: Flowers

Range/Habitat: Native to Europe, central Asia, and Siberia; mountain meadows, pastures, and open woodlands

OTHER USES

Arnica can be found in a highly diluted form in mouthwash, although it is strictly for rinsing and should not be swallowed.

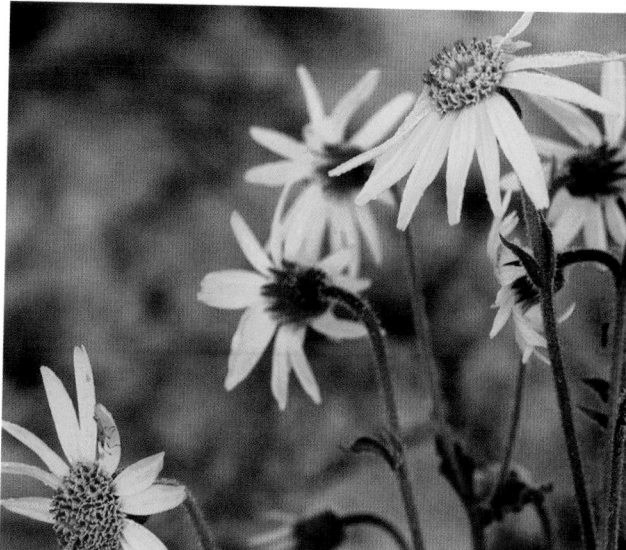

HOW TO GROW IT

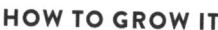

Grow mountain arnica in well-drained, acidic, humus-rich soil in full sun. (The native North American species will tolerate some shade.) Plant root divisions in spring, or sow seeds in fall. In areas where winters are very wet, grow arnica in a raised bed to prevent root rot. Harvest the flowers when they are fully open. Propagate arnica by seed or by dividing the roots in spring.

Artemisia abrotanum

This highly aromatic perennial has had a variety of uses, ranging from aphrodisiac (hence its common name, "lover's plant") to a deworming medication. People even carried the sharply scented herb with them to church to help them stay awake during sermons! A close relative of wormwood, southernwood is native to Italy and Spain.

MEDICINAL USES

Southernwood contains eucalyptol and camphor, chemical compounds that contribute to its strong scent. Herbalists consider this species a "bitter" and use it to treat digestive problems. An extract of the leaf can be applied to small wounds to stop bleeding and promote healing. A homeopathic formulation produced from the young flowering leaves and twigs is sometimes given to livestock.

Caution: This plant should not be ingested during pregnancy.

ORNAMENTAL USE

Southernwood's foliage—fine and feathery in texture, silvery in hue—is an excellent foil for brightly colored flowering plants in beds, borders, and bouquets. Attaining a height of up to 4 feet, southernwood generally works best at the back of a border. Or plant it as a low-growing hedge along a walkway or other location to enjoy its aroma as you brush against its leaves.

OTHER USES

Southernwood is sometimes used as an insect repellent, rubbed directly on the skin or used in closets and in drawer sachets. In crafts, southernwood can be used in wreaths and dried arrangements. The branches make a yellow dye for wool.

PLANT PROFILE

Common Names: Garderobe, Lad's Love, Lover's Plant, Southernwood

Description: Branched; 2 to 4 feet tall; perennial with finely divided, downy gray-green leaves; inconspicuous yellow-white flowers; highly aromatic

Hardiness: To Zone 4

Family: Asteraceae

Flowering: Midsummer to late summer

Parts Used: Leaves

Range/Habitat: Native of Italy and Spain, naturalized in the United States

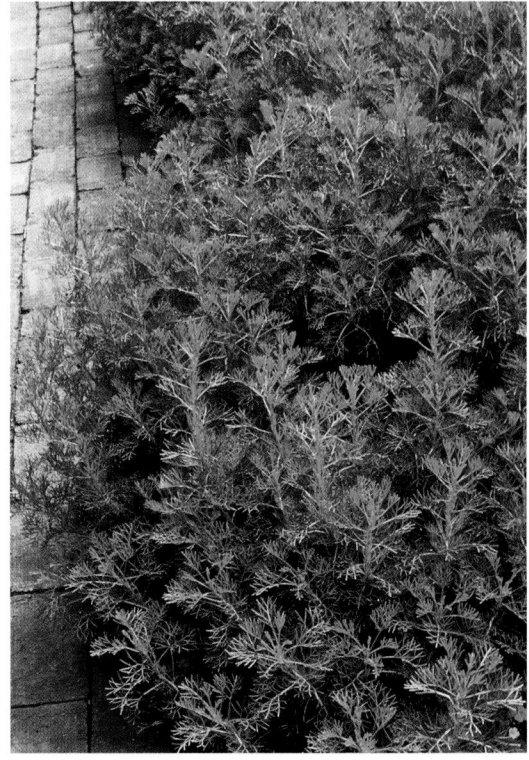

 HOW TO GROW IT

Plant southernwood divisions or cuttings 2 feet apart in average, well-drained soil and full sun. The plants are drought tolerant and easy to care for. In early spring, prune the plants back and remove older, woodier growth from the center. In midsummer to late summer, harvest the leafy branches, cutting back to the woody stems. Dry the branches in bunches, hanging them in a warm, shady location. To propagate, take root cuttings in summer or divide plants in early spring or fall.

Artemisia absinthium

PLANT PROFILE

Common Names: Green Ginger, Wormwood

Description: Many branching stems; 2 to 5 feet tall; small, yellow-green flowers on erect panicles; downy, deeply divided gray-green leaves; aromatic

Hardiness: To Zone 5

Family: Asteraceae

Flowering: Midsummer to late summer

Parts Used: Leaves, stems, and flowers

Range/Habitat: Native to Europe, naturalized in Asia and the United States; found along dry roadsides and in pastures

This bitter-tasting—and smelling—perennial is native to Europe but now grows in Africa, Asia, and the United States. It is distinctive, with silvery stems and green-gray leaves that have whitish undersides. Early herbalists valued wormwood for treating intestinal parasites, as the herb's name implies. In 1597, John Gerard published his classic *Herball, or Generall Historie of Plantes,* and noted that "wormwood voideth away the worms of the guts, not only taken inwardly, but applied outwardly . . . it keepeth garments also from the Mothes; it driveth away gnats; the bodie being anointed with the oyle thereof." Wormwood's pest repellent properties were also recognized by Native Americans, who put pieces of the branches in bedding to repel bedbugs and other pests.

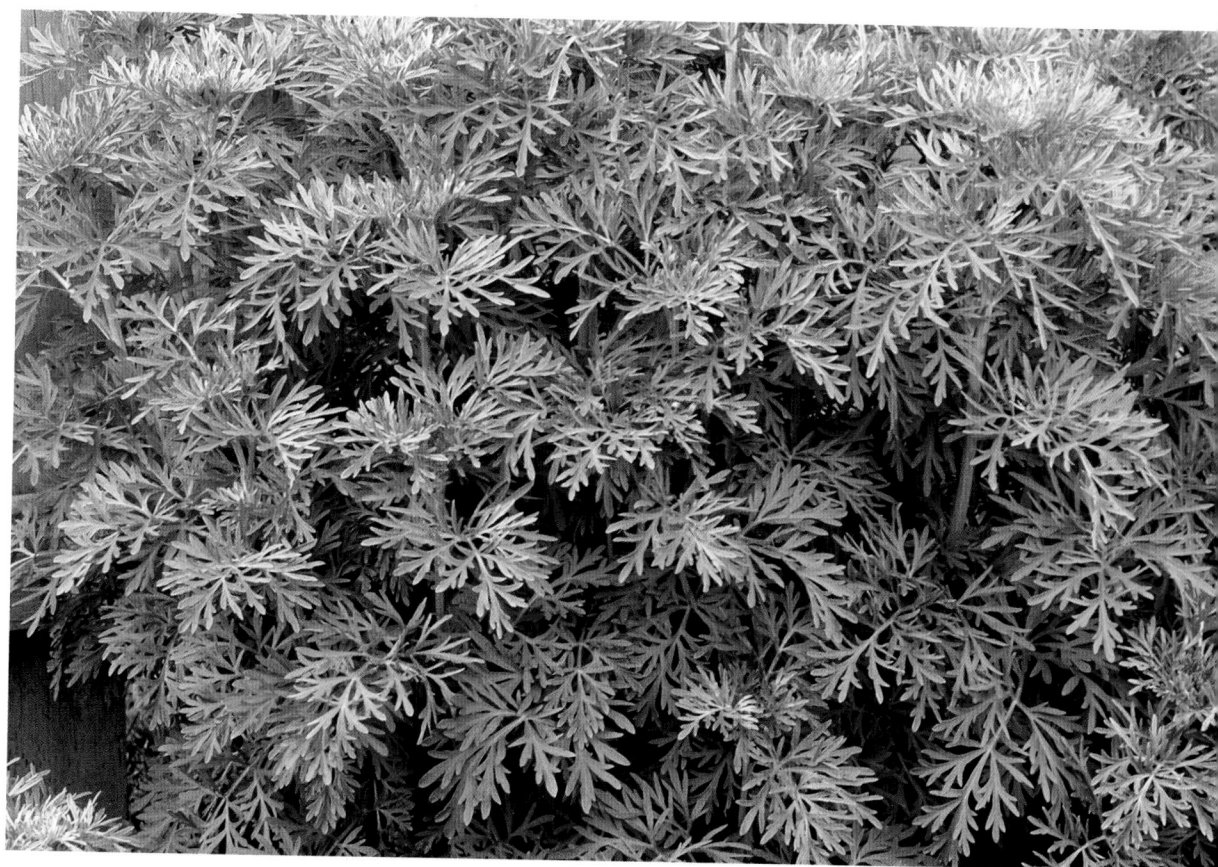

The Green Fairy

Near the end of the 18th century, wormwood began to be used in a digestive tonic developed by Dr. Pierre Ordinaire, a French expatriate living in Switzerland. This 136-proof green liqueur with a bitter licorice or anise flavor possessed powerful psychoactive properties and was all the rage in Europe during the 19th century, when it became an important part of the Parisian Bohemian scene. Vincent van Gogh was among the famous artists of the time who were ardent fans of absinthe, as were writers such as Oscar Wilde and Baudelaire. Absinthe gained the name "the green fairy," and the cocktail hour, between 5 and 7 p.m., became known as the green hour (l'heure vert).

A combination of many herbs, absinthe contained the toxic compound thujone, thought to be responsible for some of its sought-after properties—and also now known to cause brain damage. As the consumption of absinthe increased, a new disease, absinthism, emerged. This form of alcoholism was characterized by delirium, hallucinations, tremors, and seizures. By the 20th century, the drink was banned in most places around the world.

A few decades ago, interest in absinthe reemerged, and versions were made based on the original recipes but without significant quantities of thujone. Since then, consumption of this beverage has increased. If you happen to be in an airport in Europe and wander through a duty-free shop that sells alcoholic beverages, you might find absinthe for sale. Remember, however, that some countries' versions of the drink are mixed with herbs banned for import into the United States, such as Cannabis sativa, or marijuana. Read the labels carefully, and make sure you ask whether or not the drink can be imported legally.—M. J. B.

MEDICINAL USE

In folk medicine, wormwood has been used as an antiseptic, local anesthetic, topical insect repellent, digestive aid, worming treatment and, since the Middle Ages, treatment for gastric irritation. Native Americans, who had many traditional uses for wormwood, gathered and boiled the tops of the plants and applied them as a warm compress to sprains and strained muscles.

Caution: This plant should be avoided during pregnancy and while breastfeeding.

OTHER USES

Planted in the garden, wormwood is said to repel insect pests. The leaves can also be mashed in water to make a botanical pesticide. (Always test homemade pesticides on a small area before treating an entire plant.) Pick some of the stem tips, dry them, and place them in clothes closets to repel moths and fleas.

Wormwood is an ingredient in the spirit absinthe (see "The Green Fairy," above) and is sometimes included in vermouth and bitters.

HOW TO GROW IT

Wormwood is drought tolerant and easy to grow in full sun and well-drained soil. Avoid rich soil; wormwood is more aromatic in poor, dry soils. Keep in mind that wormwood's leaves and roots secrete chemicals that can suppress the growth of nearby plants, and the plant can become invasive. Consider growing it in a large container. Plant wormwood in spring or fall, spacing the plants 15 to 30 inches apart. To harvest, gather the tops of the flowering plants. Hang bundles to dry in a warm, shady location. Store the dried tops in airtight containers. Wormwood can be propagated from semihardwood cuttings taken in late summer or fall, or by division in fall.

Artemisia dracunculus

PLANT PROFILE

Common Names: Estragon, French Tarragon, Tarragon

Description: Upright stems 24 to 30 inches tall; smooth, undivided leaves 1 to 4 inches long; aromatic

Hardiness: To Zone 3

Family: Asteraceae

Flowering: Midsummer to late summer

Parts Used: Leaves

Range/Habitat: Native to southern Europe and Asia

Tarragon bears smooth, aromatic leaves with a distinctive mint-anise flavor that makes it popular for cooking, but this herb also has healing properties. Its name is a corruption of the French *esdragon*, derived from the Latin *dracunculus* ("little dragon"), which could allude either to the herb's sharp taste, its reputation as a treatment for poisonous insect bites and stings, or its purported ability to kill intestinal parasites. Tarragon is native to southern Europe and Asia.

CULINARY USE

Tarragon leaves, widely used in French cooking, enhance egg and chicken dishes, sauces, and salad dressings. The herb is a key ingredient in béarnaise sauce and is included in the popular French herb mix fines herbes. Use tarragon to flavor vinegars, oils, and butters.

Storage note: Tarragon does not hold its flavor when dried; freezing the leaves is a better option for long-term storage. Better yet, grow tarragon indoors throughout the winter to provide fresh leaves for cooking.

MEDICINAL USE

Like other culinary herbs, tarragon has antibacterial properties. The oil contains rutin, which strengthens blood vessel walls, as well as eugenol, which has anesthetic properties. Chewing the leaves can temporarily numb your tongue, an effect the ancient Greeks used to their advantage when treating toothaches. Externally, you can apply the crushed leaves directly to your skin as an antiseptic to treat minor wounds. Tarragon also contains the chemical estragole—a carcinogen when given in large amounts to animals and a suspected genotoxin (harmful to DNA), but the plant also has anticarcinogenic compounds and is generally regarded as safe for culinary use.

Caution: Therapeutic doses of tarragon should not be taken by pregnant or nursing women, although it is safe to consume in small doses in food. Do not take the herb therapeutically for periods exceeding 4 weeks.

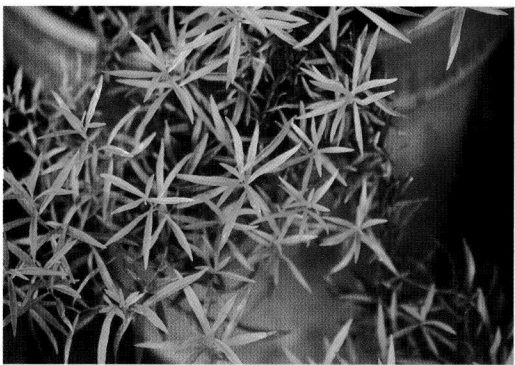

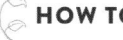

HOW TO GROW IT

For cooking, be sure to buy *Artemisia dracunculus* 'Sativa', not Russian tarragon (*A. dracunculoides*), which is less flavorful. Plant tarragon in rich, well-drained loam in full sun or partial shade. Begin harvesting leaves 6 to 8 weeks later. Pinch off any flowers to encourage lush leaf growth. Tarragon requires a period of winter dormancy for best growth. To grow it indoors during winter, pot a mature plant in summer, then cut it back to the base. Wrap the pot in plastic and set it in a cool location (such as a refrigerator) until fall (2 to 3 months). Unwrap the pot and place it in a south-facing window to break dormancy and encourage sprouting. Harvest sprigs as needed throughout winter. To propagate tarragon, divide established plants in early spring, or take cuttings in late spring. Dividing the clumps every 2 to 3 years will help keep the plants vigorous and flavorful.

Artemisia vulgaris

Found throughout most of Europe, Asia, and North America, this shrubby perennial was once believed to offer protection from evil spirits, wild animals, sunstroke, and fatigue. Ancient Roman soldiers put the dark green leaves of this herb in their sandals to avoid fatigue. (Perhaps the soldiers absorbed mugwort's bioactive compound, thujone, through their feet.) Mugwort was also planted in gardens to repel insects and was used to protect clothing from moths. The origin of its name is unclear, but some think it derives from mugwort's use as a flavoring for drinks, including beer, since ancient times.

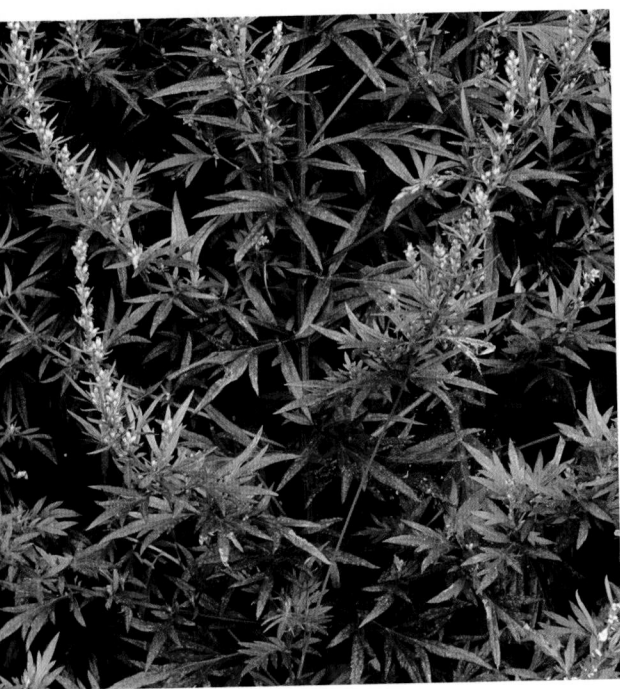

PLANT PROFILE

Common Name: Mugwort

Description: Multistemmed 4- to 6-foot perennial with soft, dark green, deeply divided leaves with whitish undersides; terminal spikes of greenish yellow blooms; aromatic

Hardiness: To Zone 4

Family: Asteraceae

Flowering: Midsummer to late summer

Parts Used: Leaves and buds

Range/Habitat: Europe, Asia, and North and South America; roadsides and wastelands

CULINARY USE

Mugwort is a familiar culinary herb in Europe and Asia, where the young leaves and buds are used in soups, poultry dressings, salads, and stir-fries. In Korea, the herb is used in rice cakes, teas, soups, and pancakes. Use the herb sparingly, as it is strong flavored and bitter.

MEDICINAL USE

Milder in action than other *Artemisia* species, mugwort has been used to treat indigestion, intestinal worms, and anxiety. It is a very important herb in the traditional Chinese medicine practice of moxibustion, during which heat from the burning dried leaves is applied to acupuncture points on the body. Ayurvedic practitioners use mugwort to treat heart problems and general malaise.

Caution: Avoid this plant during pregnancy and while breastfeeding.

OTHER USES

Mugwort is often mixed with other herbs to create dream pillows. The diluted tea can be used as a garden insecticide; be sure to test it on a small area before spraying the entire plant.

HOW TO GROW IT

Mugwort, sometimes considered a weed, is very easy to grow. Plant it in average to poor well-drained soil in full sun. The plant can grow very large (to 6 feet), so a site that provides support, such as near a wall or fence, is best. Harvest leaves and buds before the flowers open in midsummer to late summer. Propagate by division in early spring or fall.

Aspalathus linearis

PLANT PROFILE

Common Names: Red Bush Tea, Rooibos

Description: Shrub, up to 6 feet tall, with needle-like leaves and small, yellow flowers

Hardiness: To Zone 9

Family: Fabaceae

Flowering: Midsummer

Parts Used: Leaves and stems

Range/Habitat: Native to Western Cape of South Africa; high elevations

This member of the legume family is a shrub native to the Western Cape of South Africa. Three centuries ago, the indigenous people of the region began producing a sweet, pleasant tea from the shrub's needlelike leaves and stems. Commercial cultivation of the plant began in South Africa in the 1930s, and today most red bush tea is grown in the country's Cederberg region north of Cape Town. It is called a "red" tea for the color produced through oxidation, which occurs when the green leaves are crushed, bruised, moistened, and put in piles to dry. The Afrikaans name *rooibos* means "red bush."

CULINARY USE

Red bush tea is caffeine-free and is becoming increasingly popular as a substitute for tea (*Camellia sinensis*). When brewed, the leaves produce a brilliant red infusion. South Africans usually drink rooibos with lemon and sugar or honey, although the herb has a natural sweetness. It can be prepared as a hot or iced tea.

MEDICINAL USE

Traditionally, red bush tea has been used to soothe digestion; relieve stomach cramps, colic, and diarrhea; and to treat allergies and asthma. The herb is rich in antioxidants, minerals, and vitamin C and has antiviral properties. It may also enhance immune functions and provide cardiovascular benefits by reducing oxidative stress on the body; studies in this area are ongoing.

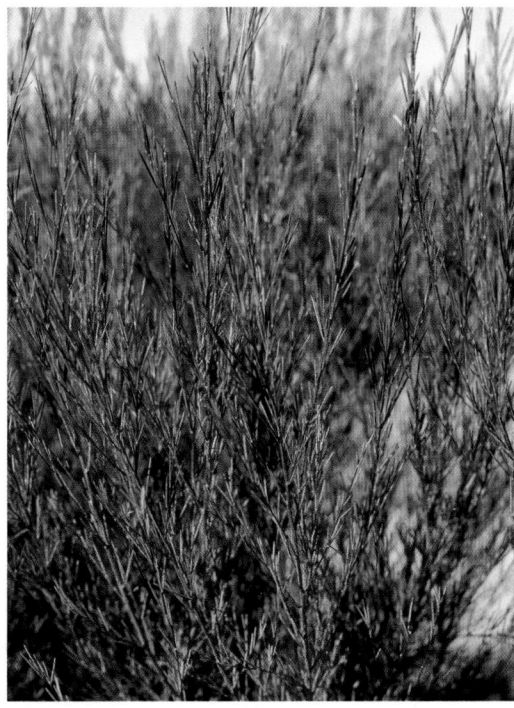

HOW TO GROW IT

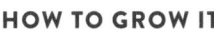

Red bush is difficult to grow outside of its native habitat in South Africa. The shrub requires well-drained, sandy, acidic loam and full sun. If you wish to try growing it, start the seeds indoors (a greenhouse is best) in early spring. Soak the seeds overnight in warm water or scarify them (see page 418) before planting to encourage germination. Plant seeds in a flat filled with a damp mix of compost and sand or perlite, and set the tray in a warm location. In a few weeks, transplant the seedlings to individual pots filled with a 50-50 mix of acidic compost and sand.

The following spring, transplant 1-year-old plants outside, if you live in Zone 9 or warmer. (In colder locations, grow red bush in a large container in a greenhouse.) After 12 to 18 months, the leaves can be harvested. Finely chop them, moisten them with water, and set them in a warm location to oxidize for 24 hours. When the leaves have turned red, spread them out and allow them to dry.

Astragalus membranaceus

The root of this perennial member of the bean family has been used in China as a medicine for thousands of years. Native to Mongolia and northern and eastern China, where it grows in dry, sandy soils, astragalus is considered a very important tonic plant, providing endurance and a feeling of well-being to those who take it.

CULINARY USE

In China, mildly flavored astragalus is a common culinary ingredient. During cold and flu season, add pieces of the sliced root to soups and stews during cooking; remove them before serving.

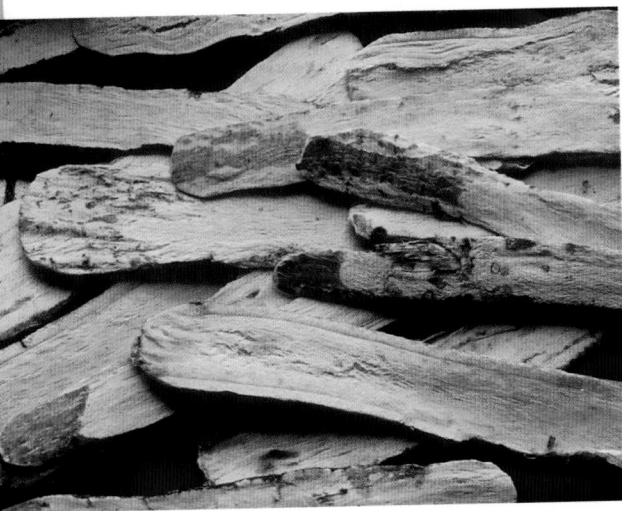

PLANT PROFILE

Common Names: Astragalus, Huang Qi, Milk Vetch, Yellow Leader

Description: Multistemmed, 1- to 2-foot-tall perennial; compound leaves composed of 12 to 18 pairs of bright green leaflets; yellow pealike flowers in long clusters; fibrous branching rhizomes

Hardiness: To Zone 6

Family: Fabaceae

Flowering: Early to midsummer

Parts Used: Root

Range/Habitat: Native to Mongolia and northern China; cultivated in other Asian countries and North America

MEDICINAL USE

Astragalus is one of the most important plants in traditional Chinese medicine (TCM) and is a common ingredient in many Chinese medicine formulas. Its yellow root contains compounds that stimulate your immune system, promoting the formation of antibodies, increasing the production of T cells, and boosting the supply of infection-fighting white blood cells. It is also used in TCM to treat diabetes. It has been shown to be a cardio-protective species and is used to treat heart disease and angina. Combined with other Chinese medicinal plants, astragalus has been studied as an adjuvant to conventional chemotherapy in the treatment of some cancers. Some herbalists suggest using it as part of a treatment for certain viruses and pneumonia.

Caution: Do not use this species if you are pregnant or nursing.

HOW TO GROW IT

Astragalus thrives in very well-drained soil and full sun. To improve germination, scarify the seeds before planting them directly in your garden, after all danger of frost has passed. (For information on seed scarification, see page 418.) If you start the seeds indoors, be careful when transplanting the seedlings—astragalus roots are sensitive to injury. Astragalus is drought tolerant, so do not overwater it. In areas with harsh winters, apply a winter mulch to protect the root. In fall of the plant's third to fifth year, you can begin to harvest the roots. Remove the leafy top growth and lateral roots, then clean the main root and allow it to dry. After several weeks, slice the root into smaller pieces and allow them to dry completely.

Atropa belladonna

As one of its common names implies, this perennial is highly poisonous and potentially deadly! The plant's scientific name comes from the Greek Atropos, one of the Fates who held the shears to cut the thread of human life, suggesting that its toxic properties were well known long ago. The common name belladonna (Italian for "beautiful lady") is derived from its use by women of the Middle Ages. They dropped the sap of this plant into their eyes to dilate their pupils, believing it made their eyes appear more brilliant. (Period paintings of Italian women show them with large pupils, which were considered beautiful.) The practice had a very dangerous downside, however; it impaired their vision for days. Since time immemorial, people have compromised their health in the name of beauty.

MEDICINAL USE

Every part of this herb contains the toxic alkaloid atropine, which relaxes and relieves spasms in the heart muscle and the smooth muscle of the digestive tract. A carefully prepared pharmaceutical formulation containing atropine is still used by physicians to dilate pupils, as well. Today, several prescription medicines use the active ingredients in belladonna to treat intestinal disorders such as diarrhea, irritable colon, and peptic ulcer. This plant is extremely toxic, however, its use can result in rapid heartbeat, delirium, confusion, blurred vision, and many other symptoms. In fact, it was used in poisonings throughout history, as well as to torture prisoners into confessions—often false. It contains scopolamine, once used as "truth serum" in interrogations.

Caution: All parts of this herb are considered toxic.

OTHER USES

Belladonna is thought to be one of the principle ingredients in the hallucinogenic witches' brews of

PLANT PROFILE

Common Names: Belladonna, Deadly Nightshade

Description: Branching perennial, up to 3 feet tall; alternate elliptical leaves with paler green undersides; nodding bell-shaped purple flowers; berries mature from green to deep purple to black

Hardiness: To Zone 6

Family: Solanaceae

Flowering: Midsummer

Parts Used: Leaves

Range/Habitat: Native to Europe, Asia, and Africa; found in woods, thickets, and wastelands

medieval Europe. It has been suggested that some women mixed an extract of this species with fat and other plants to make a hallucinogenic "flying ointment," which they then applied to their skin with a broom or staff. After it was absorbed and had entered the bloodstream, it reportedly caused the sensation of flight—perhaps accounting for the popular image of a witch "riding" a broom. Please don't try this at home!

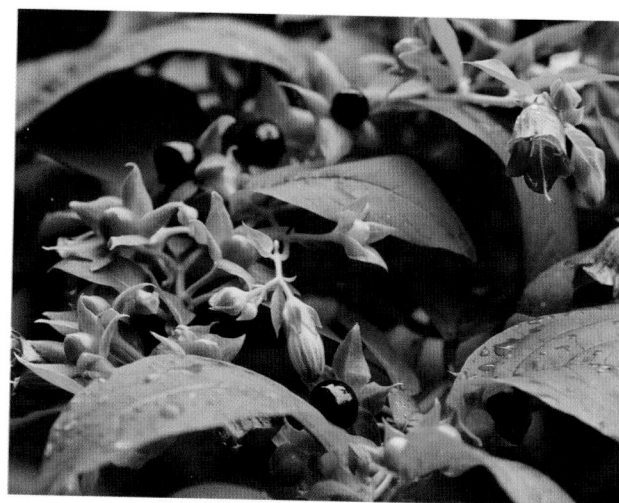

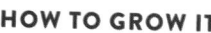

HOW TO GROW IT

Belladonna can sometimes be found cultivated in flower gardens, but it must be kept out of reach of those who might be harmed by its toxicity. Eating as few as two or three of the succulent berries has proven to be fatal to children. Some recommend using gloves when handling this plant, as all parts of the plant are highly toxic, and it is possible to absorb its chemicals through your skin.

Avena sativa

Oats: They're what's for breakfast—and much more. Cultivated throughout Europe since around 2000 BCE, this annual grass is believed to have originated in areas around the Mediterranean. Oats are now grown in temperate areas across the globe, wherever water and humidity are plentiful. The plant has flat leaves and smooth, thin stems. Its pendulous, seed-containing spikes appear in early summer.

CULINARY USE

The hulled seed heads of oats can be eaten whole (as groats, with the nutritious bran intact) or rolled (steamed and flattened). Rolled oats are a common ingredient in breakfast cereals, such as muesli, granola, and oatmeal, as well as in baked goods. For a healthier breakfast, substitute steel-cut oats for instant oats. You can use oat flour, made from ground whole oats, to make breads, cakes, and cookies. You can also substitute oat flour for wheat flour as a thickener for soups and sauces and as a coating for fish and chicken. Oat bran, which is very high in fiber, can be added to many foods. Add sprouted seeds to sandwiches and salads to boost the vitamin and mineral content and add crunch.

MEDICINAL USE

Oat bran contains soluble fiber, which increases the elimination of cholesterol and has been shown to lower cholesterol, triglyceride, and blood pres-

sure levels. When oats are consumed, soluble fiber traps cholesterol in the intestines and eliminates it through the stools. Fiber also helps prevent constipation by attracting water, creating soft, bulky stools that stimulate bowel movements. Oats are used externally in products that help relieve the pain and itching of skin conditions such as dryness and eczema. Oatmeal baths are also helpful in treating these conditions, as well as for treating herpes and shingles. Herbalists sometimes recommend a tonic made from immature oat seeds to treat anxiety and exhaustion, although clinical studies have not proven this use to be effective.

OTHER USES

Oats are commonly grown as animal fodder in temperate areas across the globe. Horses given oats as part of their feed are said to be healthier, leaner, more muscular, and more energetic.

PLANT PROFILE

Common Name: Oats

Description: Grass, 2 to 5 feet tall, with flat leaves and smooth, thin stems; pendulous, seed-containing spikes appear in summer

Hardiness: Annual; dies back after flowering

Family: Poaceae

Flowering: Late spring to midsummer

Parts Used: Seed heads and stems

Habitat: Descended from species native to the Mediterranean

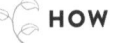

HOW TO GROW IT

Sow in early spring in well-drained soil and full sun. Harvest in summer, before the seeds are fully ripe. Cut the plants near the base when most of the growth has turned brown and the seeds are no longer milky.

Oats can also be used as a soil-building cover crop planted in late summer to early fall. In spring, till under the stubble to add organic matter and nutrients to your soil. Wait 2 to 3 weeks before planting garden crops where oats have grown; a compound in oat residue can inhibit the growth of other plants.

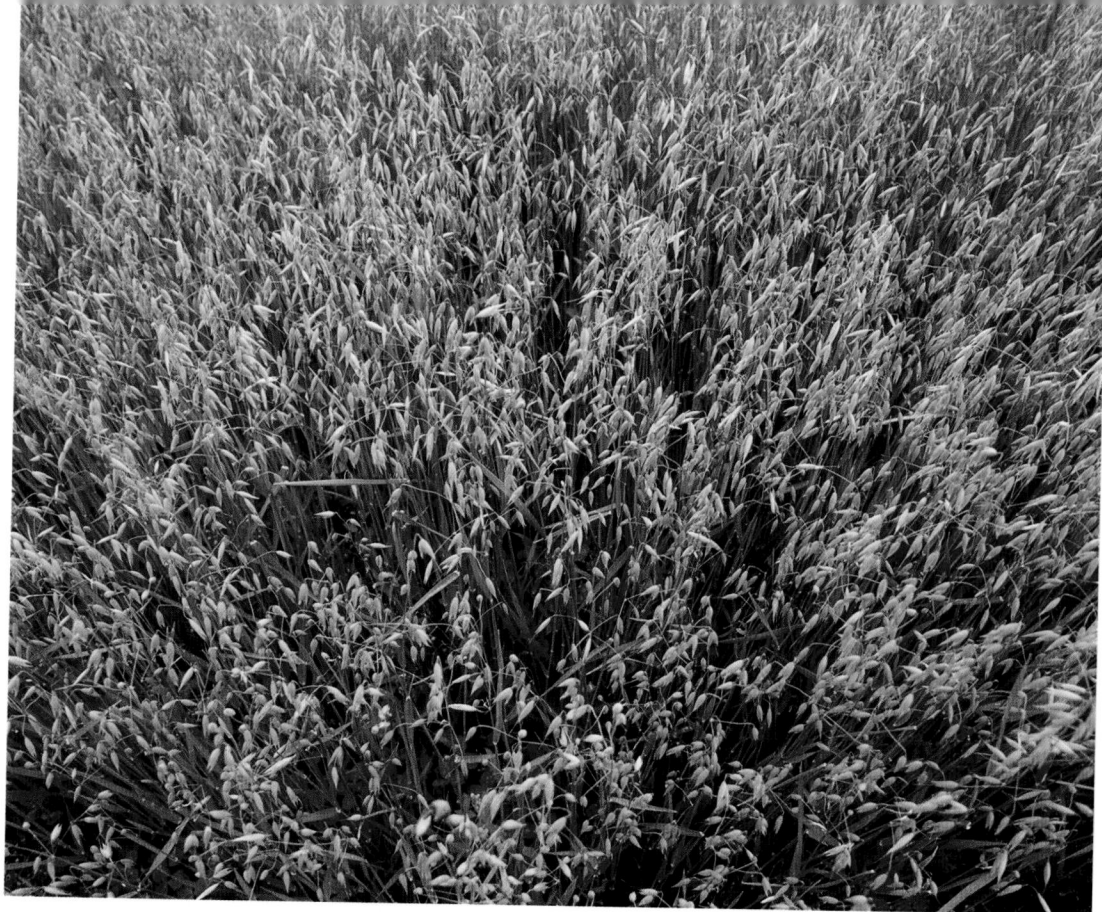

Wild Oats?

While we think of oats primarily as a healthy and nutritious breakfast food, this plant has a long history of medicinal use. To treat colic or a sharp pain in your side, English physician Nicholas Culpeper (1616–1654) recommended putting oats in a bag with bay salt, heating it in a frying pan, and applying it "as warm as can be endured." Boiled oats in vinegar were suggested for the treatment of spots and freckles on the face and body. Culpeper also advised mixing oats with bay oil and applying it as a poultice to treat itches, leprosy, and other ailments.

More than 3½ centuries later, on the Internet, oats are being touted to increase libido, genital sensitivity, and orgasms in men and women. The claims are based primarily on anecdotal evidence, personal testimonials, and a single human trial conducted by a commercial entity. A "buy this product" box usually appears next to the spectacular claims.

What to do? Oats don't seem to cause adverse effects in most people, unless there is a specific food allergy, such as intolerance to gluten and related compounds. Herbalists I know do recommend oat extracts in formulas designed to increase desire and performance, and most of these ingredients are thought to be safe and effective. So eat your oats, work with a knowledgeable medical professional to address any concerns you have about issues related to libido, and experiment with formulas deemed safe.—M. J. B.

Betula spp.

Widely cultivated as landscape trees in the northern regions of the globe, birches have attractive, peeling bark that once was used to make writing paper. But the 30-plus *Betula* species—native to Europe, Asia, and North America—are much more than ornamental. In North America alone, Native American people used birches for many purposes, including canoe making, basketry, dishes, dyes, and medicines. These handsome trees are still valuable sources of medicine, lumber, and more.

PLANT PROFILE

Common Name: Birch

Description: Fast-growing trees, up to 90 feet tall; alternate, ovate leaves with serrated edges; tiny flowers borne on catkins, followed by tiny winged "nuts"; papery black or white bark

Hardiness: To Zone 2 or 3

Family: Betulaceae

Flowering: Summer and fall

Parts Used: Leaves, bark, twigs, and sap

Range/Habitat: Native to Europe, Asia, and North America

CULINARY USE

Birch bark and twigs have a pleasant, wintergreen-like flavor. The bark and sap of sweet birch (*Betula lenta*), which is native to the eastern United States and Canada, can be boiled, sweetened, and fermented to make birch beer.

MEDICINAL USE

Birch oils, distilled from the trees' buds, leaves, and twigs, are rich in methyl salicylate, a pain reliever (and the main ingredient in aspirin) that does not irritate the stomach. Salicylate staves off your body's production of prostaglandins associated with fever and the inflammation of muscles, bones, and connective tissues caused by injuries or arthritis. Birch oil is also used topically in creams and ointments to treat eczema and psoriasis. Birch bark contains phytochemicals that may have astringent, diuretic, antiviral, and antitumor properties.

ORNAMENTAL USE

Birch trees—including the European birch (*B. pendula*), as well as native American species such as sweet birch, paper birch (*Betula papyrifera*), and river birch (*B. nigra*)—are favorite landscape specimens, valued for their interesting bark and bright yellow fall foliage.

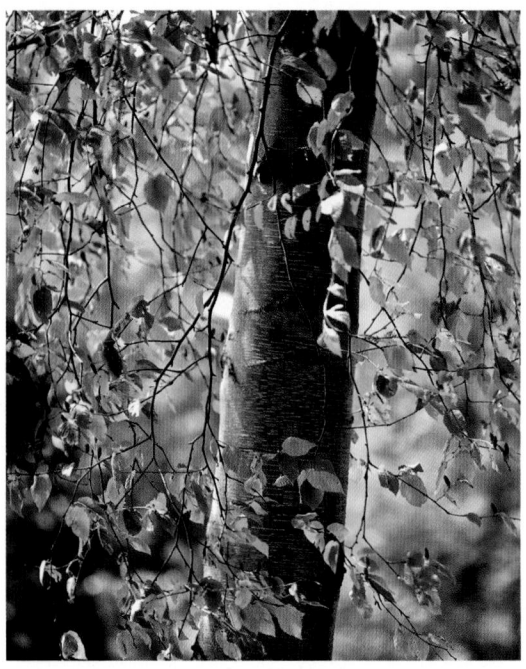

OTHER USES

An extract of white birch (*Betula alba*) is used in cosmetics and to scent soaps, shampoos, and other products, as well as to flavor candy.

HOW TO GROW IT

Birch trees do best in well-drained, sandy or loamy acidic soil and full sun. Prune in summer or fall to avoid excessive "bleeding" (loss of sap), which can occur with late winter and early spring pruning. Harvest leaf buds, young leaves, and twigs in spring. Propagate by planting seeds on the surface of a moistened seed-starting mix. (The seeds need light to germinate.) Mist frequently until germination occurs, in 2 to 3 weeks.

Bixa orellana

Native to the Caribbean region, Mexico, and Central and South America, the annatto tree bears spiny red fruits that contain numerous seeds covered with a waxy red paste. Although the fruits are inedible, the seeds and paste (known botanically as arils) have many medicinal and culinary uses.

One of the plant's common names, achiote, comes from the Nahuatl (an indigenous language spoken in Central America) word *achiotl*. The name lipstick tree is said to refer to the traditional use of the bright red seed paste as body paint. Spanish explorers introduced the plant to Asia in the 17th century, and today, annatto is commercially cultivated in its region of origin, as well as in India. The major exporting countries are Peru and Kenya.

CULINARY USE

Annatto seed paste is used as a coloring for margarine, cheese, microwave popcorn, and other yellow and orange foodstuffs. In its pure form, margarine is a white substance, developed in the 19th century as an inexpensive substitute for butter. In the United States and elsewhere, dairy farmers concerned with possible competition from

---

PLANT PROFILE

Common Names: Achiote, Annatto, Lipstick Tree

Description: Evergreen small tree or shrub, 6 to 24 feet tall; spirally arranged leaves with dark green tops and gray-green undersides; panicles of fragrant pink flowers; greenish brown or red fruits have numerous seeds with bright orange-red fleshy coats

Hardiness: To Zone 11

Family: Bixaceae

Flowering: Late summer or fall

Parts Used: Seeds and seed pulp, leaves, and roots

Range/Habitat: Native to the Caribbean region, Mexico, and Central and South America

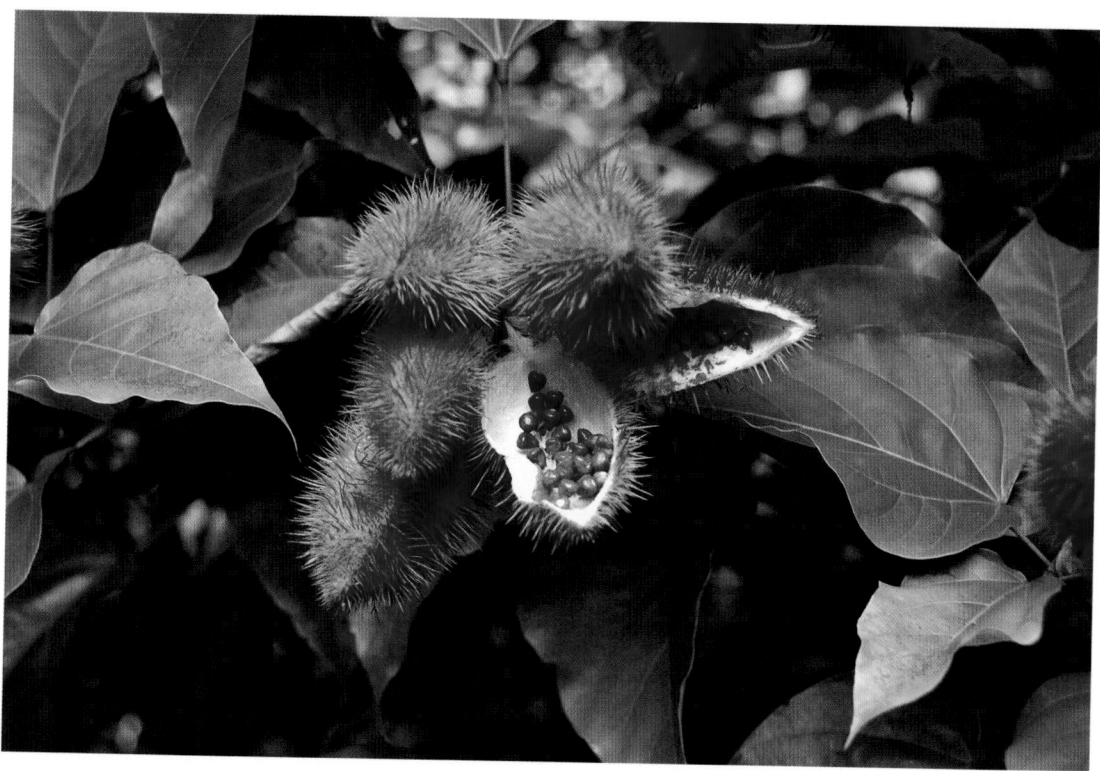

FIELD NOTES

Sunscreen, Insect-Repellent Lip Color

In my first few weeks of graduate studies in ethnobotany at Harvard University, my mentor, Professor Richard Evans Schultes, known as a luminary in this field, suggested I go to the Amazon Valley of Colombia in search of a doctoral dissertation topic. Accompanied by another of his graduate students, James Zarucchi, I traveled to a remote Indian village on the Vaupés River.

There, I became fascinated by Bixa orellana, a small tree known in Spanish as achiote and locally by other names. The people harvested its mature fruit capsules just before they split open, revealing many red-colored seeds. They used the seeds for cooking and to dye the bark clothing they wore for ceremonial purposes. But the most interesting use was as a removable body dye that helps prevent sun damage to the skin and is said to help repel insects, as well. During many years of working with indigenous cultures,

I have observed native peoples use this waxy red dye to color not only their skin, but also their hair, fabric, vessels, and weaponry.

Now cosmetic companies are using the plant to make lip colorings for Western consumers. I've always thought that it would be more fashionable to fully adopt the traditional indigenous use: to cover your entire face with the dye of this plant. But then again, what do I know about trends?—M. J. B.

margarine promoted laws that banned the addition of color to this product, hoping to distinguish it from real butter. When these laws were eliminated, food companies began to enclose coloring packets with their products, and annatto was one of the important ingredients used for this purpose, as it is considered a safe additive to food. Annatto is widely used in Caribbean and Latin American cooking as a dye, flavoring, and spice. The herb's earthy flavor complements many meat dishes, as well as rice and beans. Annatto paste, a popular Mexican flavoring, typically contains annatto, coriander, cumin seeds, oregano, peppercorns, and garlic. The spices are ground together and then blended with bitter orange juice or vinegar to make a marinade.

MEDICINAL USE

The herb may have anti-inflammatory, diuretic, laxative, and expectorant properties. Annatto seeds and leaves have been used internally to treat indigestion, fevers, and intestinal parasites and topically to treat burns. The leaves have also been used to treat heartburn and stomach disorders, and in the Amazon region the sap from the leaves is used to treat eye infections. The astringent red seed pulp is used to treat measles, as a purgative, and for stomachache. A beverage made from the seeds and leaves is reported to be used as a female aphrodisiac, and a drink prepared from the roots was traditionally used to treat dysentery, jaundice, diabetes, and influenza.

OTHER USES

As synthetic colorings face stricter regulation and consumers favor more natural ingredients in their foods and cosmetics, annatto is gaining importance as a dye.

HOW TO GROW IT

This small, tropical evergreen tree or shrub requires a frost-free humid climate, evenly distributed rainfall throughout the year, and full sun. Gardeners in southern Florida or Hawaii can grow annatto outdoors; in Zone 10 and colder, annatto can be grown indoors in a large container. Provide well-drained, neutral to slightly alkaline soil. Under favorable conditions, annatto begins fruiting about 18 months after planting, and full crops of seeds are possible in 3 to 4 years. To propagate annatto, sow seed from freshly gathered ripe seedpods outdoors in fall, or take woody stem cuttings.

Borago officinalis

Borage is an annual that bears bright blue, star-shaped flowers that are loved by bees. The plant's name is thought to derive from the Latin *borra*, meaning "hairy garment," in reference to the herb's bristly leaves. Native to the Mediterranean and naturalized throughout Europe, parts of North America, and parts of Australia, borage has a long history of use in herbal medicine. Nicholas Culpeper's *English Physician* (1652) noted under its "virtues" that borage ". . . leaves and roots are to very good purpose used against putrid and pestilential fevers, to defend the heart, and to resist and expel the poison or venom of other creatures . . . and the seeds and leaves are good to e[i]ncrease milk in women's breasts. . . ."

CULINARY USE

Borage's bright blue flowers make an attractive garnish for cold soups, iced beverages, and cakes.

Caution: Do not consume borage leaves and flowers in large quantities, as they contain compounds toxic to your liver. Oil extracted from the seed is safe to consume, however.

MEDICINAL USE

Borage seed oil is a rich source of gamma-linolenic acid (GLA), a compound that helps balance abnormalities of essential fatty acids. It can be taken to relieve premenstrual discomfort, thrombosis, and chronic inflammation, as in multiple sclerosis. The oil is also used to treat fevers, bronchial infections, oral infections, and chronic nephritis. Borage seed oil has been shown to reduce the symptoms of rheumatoid arthritis during a human clinical trial. According to another clinical study, borage seed oil may reduce the effects of stress on the body by lowering heart rate and systolic blood pressure. It is also recommended for treatment of fibrocystic breast disease.

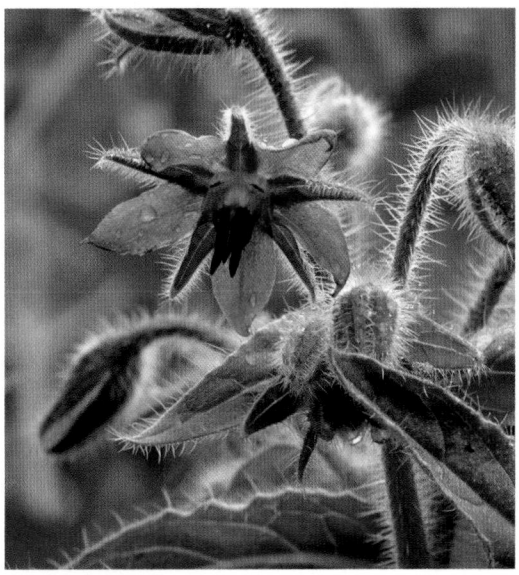

OTHER USES

In addition to its use as a dietary supplement, GLA-rich borage seed oil is used in cosmetic products; its anti-inflammatory and moisturizing properties help heal dried and cracked skin, as well as other skin conditions, such as eczema.

HOW TO GROW IT

Borage grows best in well-drained, moist soil in full sun or partial shade. Plant seeds in spring, and thin seedlings to 18 inches apart. Harvest the young leaves in spring or summer, as the plant begins flowering; pick the flowering tops just as they begin to open. A prolific plant, borage will self-seed rapidly in your garden.

Boswellia serrata

A member of the frankincense family, boswellia is native to tropical Asia and Africa, and it is often found in hilly areas of India. Plants in the family Burseraceae, which grow as evergreen bushes or small trees with small, white, fragrant flowers, are characterized by resin ducts in their thick, aromatic bark. When cuts are made in the bark, a milky fluid emerges and hardens upon contact with the air. The solidified resin of boswellia is made into capsules, tablets, creams, perfumes, and cosmetics.

MEDICINAL USE

Creams containing boswellia extract are used to relieve the aches and pains of arthritis. Boswellia resin contains nonsteroidal anti-inflammatory compounds, including boswellic acids, which may be helpful in the treatment of rheumatoid arthritis and bowel disorders such as ulcerative colitis and

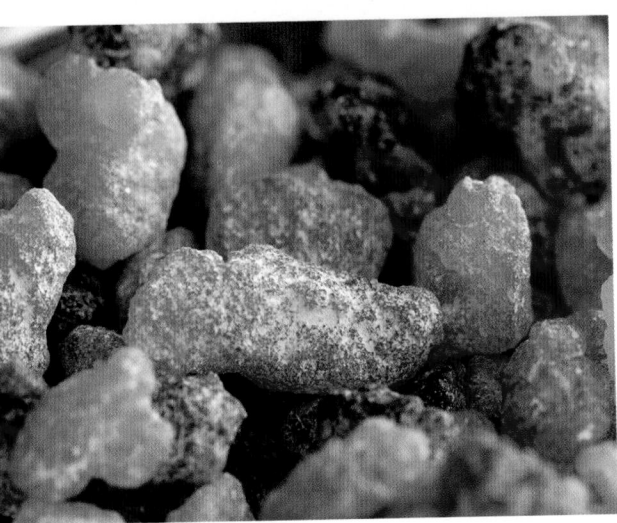

Crohn's disease. Studies have shown that boswellia may be as effective as synthetic drugs in treating these conditions, without the side effects of pharmaceuticals.

In Ayurvedic medicine, boswellia (called *shallaki*) is used as an astringent to treat diarrhea and is included in ointments used to treat sores and boils.

The essential oil of *Boswellia carterii* (the related species known as frankincense) is said to alleviate anxiety.

OTHER USES

Boswellia creams are used to moisturize dry skin and minimize wrinkles. The highly aromatic resin of several *Boswellia* species is commonly used to make perfumes and burned as incense.

HOW TO GROW IT

Boswellia grows in dry, hilly areas in warm climates. In Zone 9 and colder, you can try growing this small tree in a large container in a warm greenhouse. The plant prefers well-drained to dry, alkaline soil in full sun. Water the young plants daily until their root systems are established, then cut back to watering just a few times a week. Trim back the plant from time to time. In the wild, the resin from older plants is harvested by making a slash in the bark and "bleeding" the resin, which then hardens and can be used.

Calamintha nepeta

This peppermint-scented perennial shrub is native to Europe, Africa, and the Middle East and has naturalized throughout parts of eastern North America. The compact plants bear small leaves, which resemble those of oregano, and pale lavender bloom spikes appreciated by bees, butterflies, and hummingbirds. The common name calamint comes from the plant's ancient Greek name, *kalaminthe*, which means "beautiful mint." In legend, this herb was a tall fruit tree until it offended Mother Earth and was reduced to its present small size as punishment. But like many mints, lesser calamint can spread rapidly throughout the garden if not controlled. Perhaps that is its revenge.

CULINARY USE

Lesser calamint is a popular ingredient in Italian cuisine, where it is sometimes called *nepitella*. Tuscan cooks add the herb to sautéed mushrooms, zucchini, and tomatoes. In southern Italy, it is used to flavor goat's milk cheese. Its distinctive flavor— a blend of mint and savory—complements garlic-based sauces, as well as soups and stews.

MEDICINAL USE

Lesser calamint's modern medicinal use is limited: The leaves are used in preparations to treat indigestion and other stomach problems, anxiety, and painful menses. The herb has expectorant properties and may help break a fever by promoting sweating. In ancient times it was used to treat insomnia, expel worms from the body, and promote digestion. It is also said to have been used as a tonic, stimulant, antiseptic, and treatment for flatulence.

Caution: Do not use this herb if you are pregnant. It contains a significant quantity of pulegone, which may cause miscarriage.

PLANT PROFILE

Common Names: Basil Thyme, Lesser Calamint, Mountain Mint

Description: Perennial shrub forms a tidy mound, 15 to 18 inches tall, of small, bright green leaves; lavender-pink bloom spikes last 6 weeks or more; fragrant

Hardiness: To Zone 5

Family: Lamiaceae

Flowering: Late summer to fall

Parts Used: Leaves

Range/Habitat: Native to Europe, Africa, and the Middle East, and naturalized in eastern North America

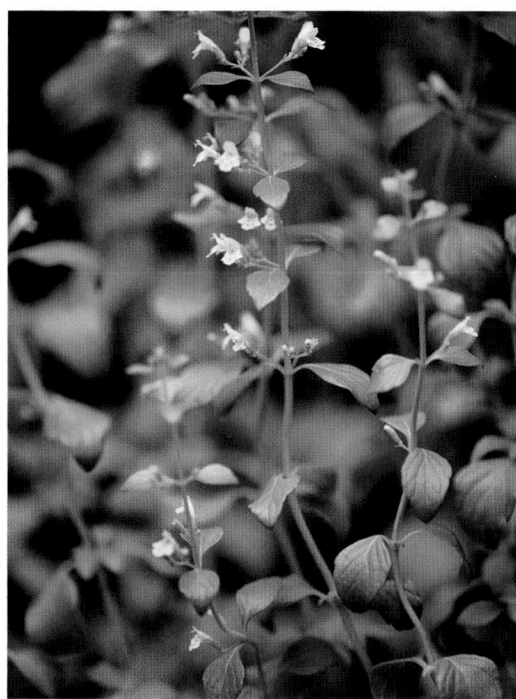

HOW TO GROW IT

Plant lesser calamint in moist but well-drained soil and full sun. Once established, this carefree perennial requires minimal watering. It is rarely bothered by insect pests or disease. While calamint is not invasive the way other mints can be, it does spread readily; to keep this herb in check, grow it in a container and remove seedling volunteers as they appear. Harvest the leaves just as the plants come into bloom. Propagate by division in early spring or fall, or dig up and transplant seedlings.

Calendula officinalis

This bushy Mediterranean annual bears yellow or orange flowers so brilliantly colored that they once were said to be reflections of the sun. Calendula's long bloom period was noted by the ancient Greeks and Romans—the name "calendula" comes from the Latin *calendae*, for "calendar."

The herb has a long history of use. Early Greeks and Romans drank calendula tea to relieve stomach ailments, and they applied the herb externally as a poultice to treat superficial skin wounds. During the Middle Ages, the dried flowers were added to soup and stew pots (hence the name pot marigold) to help ward off illness. Calendula has also been used as a dye for food, fabric, and cosmetics.

CULINARY USE

Calendula petals make colorful additions to green salads and have been used as an economical, though less vividly colored, substitute for saffron in cheese, rice dishes, and soups. Calendula leaves can be eaten raw, but some people find their flavor unpleasant. The dried, powdered herb also can be used as a food coloring.

MEDICINAL USE

Calendula has anti-inflammatory properties, and the herb has long been used to relieve inflammation of the stomach, throat, mouth, and skin. A tea made from the flowers or a tincture made from the entire plant can ease inflammatory digestive conditions such as gastritis, colitis, and peptic ulcers. Calendula tea can also be taken as a mouthwash or gargle to treat mouth and throat inflammation.

Used externally in salves, creams, and oint-

PLANT PROFILE

Common Names: Calendula, Pot Marigold

Description: Branching plant, 1 to 2 feet tall; orange or yellow ray blooms up to 4 inches across; lance-shaped leaves and stems covered with fine hairs

Hardiness: Annual

Family: Asteraceae

Flowering: June to September

Parts Used: Flower petals and leaves

Habitat: Native to areas around the Mediterranean; naturalized in temperate regions worldwide

---

ments, calendula helps heal skin wounds and irritations, such as rashes, insect bites, and burns. A mild infusion can be used as a douche to treat vaginal yeast infections.

Caution: Those allergic to other members of the family Asteraceae, such as ragweed, may be sensitive to calendula.

ORNAMENTAL USE

Calendula is an attractive plant for containers or informal cottage and cutting gardens. Modern cultivated varieties expand the color palette to include peach, apricot, cream, and bicolor single and double blooms.

OTHER USES

This plant, sometimes listed as "marigold," is an ingredient in many personal-care products. Used in hair rinses, calendula brings out gold highlights. Extracts of the flowers are combined with other herbal ingredients in soothing topical creams used to treat inflamed skin conditions, infections, lesions, and ulcers of the leg. Calendula flowers can also be mordanted with alum to make a yellow dye for fabric (see page 397).

 HOW TO GROW IT

After danger of frost has passed, sow seeds in your garden in well-drained soil and full sun. Seeds will germinate in 7 to 14 days. Thin seedlings to 6 to 12 inches apart. Calendula self-seeds readily, so remove the dead flower heads immediately to prevent excessive self-seeding and to extend the flowering period. For culinary or medicinal use, harvest the flowers when the plant is dry, then remove individual petals and dry them on paper in the shade. Spread the petals in a single layer, not touching one another, to avoid discoloration. Store the dried petals in an airtight container.

SUNNY CALENDULA PILAF

Calendula can turn ordinary rice into a vibrantly colored, flavorful side dish that's good for you, too!

2 tablespoons olive oil

1 shallot, finely chopped

2 tablespoons diced celery

2 tablespoons blanched sliced almonds

1 cup long-grain brown rice

2 cups water

¼ cup fresh calendula petals

1 teaspoon chopped fresh lemon thyme

1 teaspoon minced lemon zest

Heat the oil in a medium skillet over medium heat. Add the shallot, celery, and almonds. Cook for about 5 minutes, until the vegetables are soft and the almonds are lightly browned. Add the rice and cook for 1 minute more. Add the water, calendula, thyme, and lemon zest. Bring the mixture to a boil, then cover it and reduce the heat to low. Simmer for 45 to 50 minutes, or until no more steam rises from the pan. Remove the covered pan from the heat and let it sit for 5 minutes. Fluff the rice with a fork and serve.

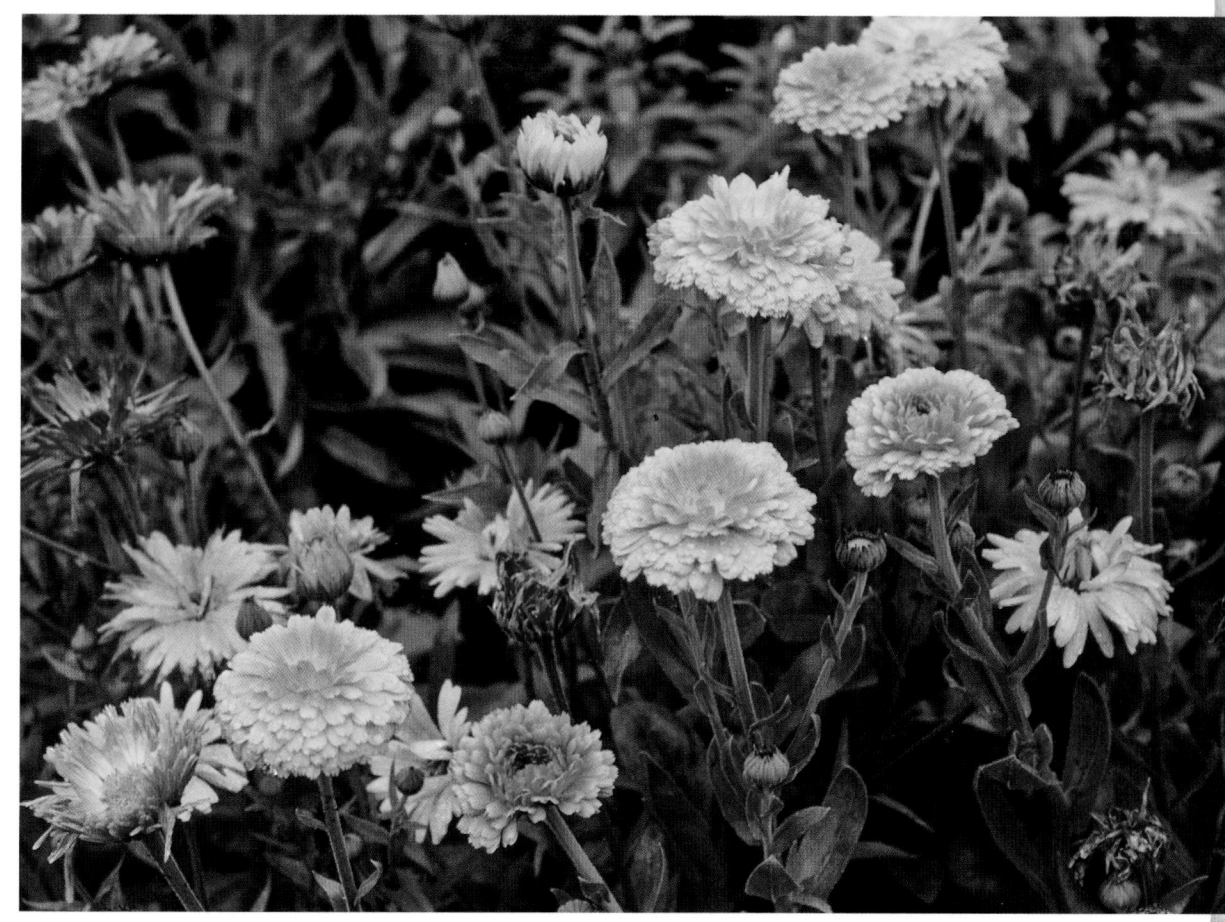

Camellia sinensis

Native to Asia, the tea plant is extensively cultivated in tropical and subtropical countries, including China, India, Sri Lanka, Indonesia, and Japan. Some tea gardens in China have continuously produced this valuable beverage leaf for more than 1,000 years.

Tea has a remarkably long history of use as a beverage in China, Japan, and India, the largest tea-producing nation in the world. These cultures believe that drinking tea optimizes health and ensures longevity. The plant's leaves contain caffeine, a mild stimulant; Eastern religious practitioners once drank this herbal beverage to stay awake during long meditations.

CULINARY USE

Tea is second only to water as the world's most popular beverage. The plant's leaves are used to make four basic types of tea: black, oolong, green, and white. Black tea is fully oxidized (the chlorophyll breaks down and combines with oxygen in the air); oolong tea is partially oxidized; and green tea is wilted but not oxidized. White tea is neither wilted nor oxidized—it is made from the plant's immature leaves and buds, which are steamed and dried immediately after harvesting.

You can impart tea's delicate herbal flavor to prepared foods by replacing some or all of the cooking water with brewed tea. Experiment by adding tea when preparing rice, couscous, and other grains; soups; puddings; and baked goods, such as scones and sweet breads.

PLANT PROFILE

Common Names: Black Tea, Chinese Tea, Green Tea, Tea

Description: Small evergreen tree or shrub, 3 to 30 feet tall; elliptical dark green leaves; fragrant, 1-inch white flowers with yellow stamens

Hardiness: To Zone 8

Family: Theaceae

Flowering: Late summer to fall

Parts Used: Leaves

Range/Habitat: Native to western China and northwestern India; widely cultivated in tropical and subtropical areas

MEDICINAL USE

Both black and green teas are rich in free radical–fighting antioxidants, and both have similar heart health and anticancer benefits. Since the mid-1980s, an impressive number of scientific studies have supported green tea's ability to protect your body against cancer, heart disease, and ulcers. Drinking green tea also invigorates your mind and central nervous system and can help control diarrhea. Externally, green tea has been used as a mouthwash to prevent plaque formation on the teeth. A topical cream produced from green tea and used for the treatment of genital and anal warts caused by human papilloma virus (HPV) was approved by the FDA in 2006. This was the first approval of a whole botanical extract as a prescription botanical drug. Studied in clinical trials of nearly 400 adults, the product (Veregen ointment) proved effective at eliminating the warts.

 HOW TO GROW IT

The tea plant grows best in a warm, humid climate that receives ample rainfall. The soil, altitude, and climate in which the tea plant grows can affect the flavor of the leaves.

In Zone 8 and warmer areas, you can grow tea in your garden as a small evergreen tree or shrub. In cooler regions, grow the plant in a large pot and move it indoors for winter. Provide rich, moist, but well-drained soil with neutral to slightly acid pH and direct sun or partial shade. Water regularly, especially the first year. In midspring to late spring, snip back tips of branches to encourage bushy growth.

Harvest the tender leaves and buds at the ends of the branches in spring, beginning in the plant's third year. After harvesting, spread out the leaves to wilt for a few hours (for oolong tea), or for 2 to 3 days (for black). For green tea, wilt the leaves by cooking them quickly in a skillet or wok for about 2 minutes. To finish drying all three types, spread the leaves on a baking sheet and place it in a 250°F oven for 20 minutes. Store the dried tea in an airtight container.

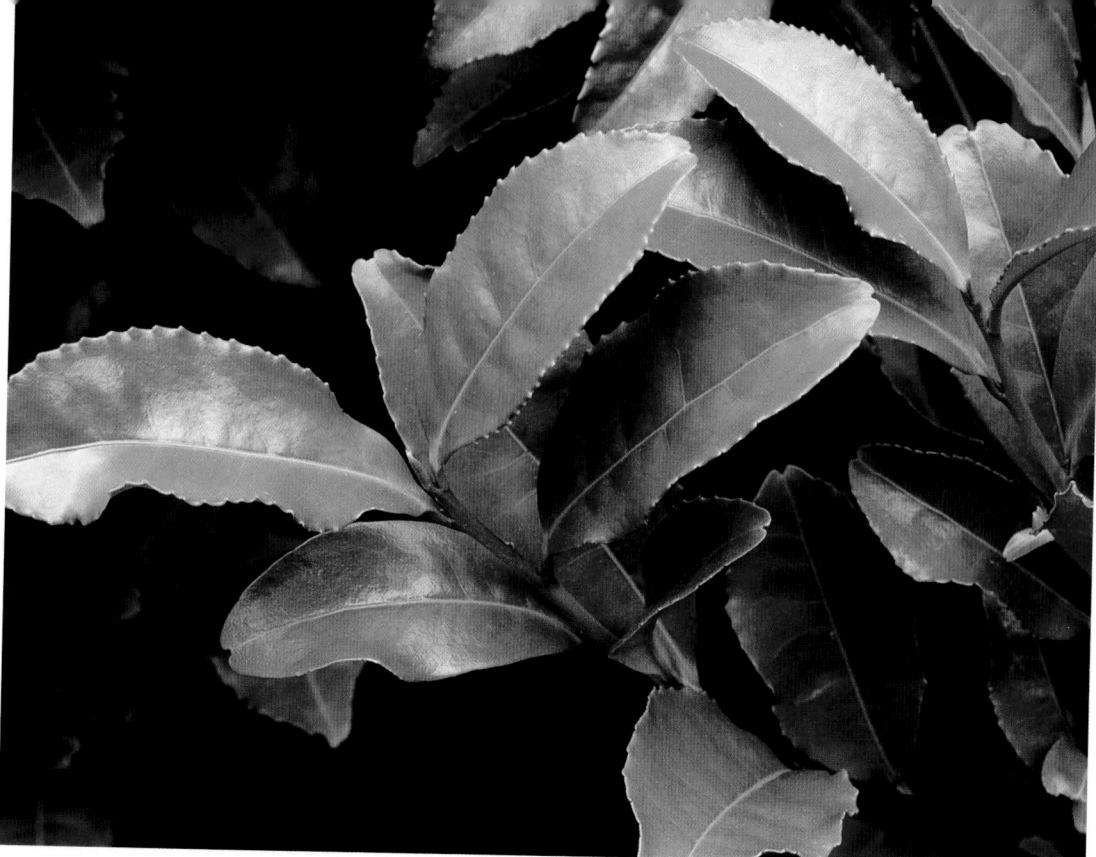

Like green tea, black tea has a stimulating effect on the central nervous system, generally evinced by a feeling of comfort and exhilaration. It also acts as an astringent, which makes it useful for treating diarrhea.

Caution: Tea contains caffeine, which can cause nervousness, heart palpitations, anxiety, insomnia, and digestive disturbances. It should be avoided by pregnant women and by people who suffer from hypertension, anxiety, eating disorders, diabetes, and ulcers.

OTHER USES

Tea is found in many cosmetic products. It is valued for its antioxidant, anti-inflammatory, and skin protective properties.

REFRESH YOUR BODY WITH TEA

Tea is a magical plant with many uses! Here are just a few ways to use this valuable herb to cleanse, soothe, relax, and refresh your body.

- Relieve sore feet and keep them smelling sweet by soaking them for 20 minutes in a bath of strong black tea.

- Mix witch hazel with strong (cool) black tea to make a stimulating scalp toner; massage in the liquid after shampooing. Wait a few minutes, then rinse with water. Follow up with a conditioner.

- Use cool black tea as a mild astringent skin toner; apply with a clean cotton ball.

- Soothe insect bites and cuts by applying a cool, used black tea bag. To reduce inflammation from sunburn, hang four or five tea bags from the faucet when filling your tub; soak in the warm water.

Cananga odorata

Ylang-ylang means "flower of flowers," and indeed, the fragrant yellow flowers of this exotic evergreen tree are highly prized for their essential oil, which is clear with a yellow tinge. A member of the cherimoya (custard apple) family, ylang-ylang is native to tropical lowland forests in areas ranging from India to northern Australia, and it is cultivated in the tropical areas of Africa and Asia. Depending on where the tree is grown, the scent of ylang-ylang oil can vary substantially. As a result, commercially available ylang-ylang oils can have distinctly different aromas, from fresh and floral to sweet and slightly fruity.

PLANT PROFILE

Common Names: Ylang-Ylang

Description: Evergreen tree, up to 100 feet tall (50 to 60 feet when cultivated); drooping branches with long, oblong leaves; strongly scented yellow flowers; dark green oval fruits ripen to black

Hardiness: To Zone 10

Family: Annonaceae

Flowering: Year-round

Parts Used: Flowers and wood

Range/Habitat: Native to tropical lowland forests in areas ranging from India to northern Australia; cultivated in tropical areas of Africa and Asia

MEDICINAL USE

Ylang-ylang's flowers and essential oil have sedative and antimicrobial properties. The oil also has a long-standing reputation as an aphrodisiac. Aromatherapists consider ylang-ylang to be one of the most relaxing fragrances for both mind and body. It is often combined with other oils—particularly bergamot, lemon, and sandalwood—and made into a massage oil or added to a bath to enhance relaxation.

Caution: Use the essential oil of ylang-ylang externally only. Also, use it lightly; the intensity of its scent may cause headache or nausea.

OTHER USES

Ylang-ylang is widely used to scent cosmetics, soaps, candles, and perfumes. Along with rose and jasmine, it is reportedly one of three floral fragrances in the legendary Chanel No. 5 perfume. Its wood is used for house construction in the Pacific Islands, as well as for making cooking fires. The flowers can be woven together to make fragrant garlands and leis.

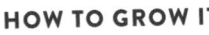

HOW TO GROW IT

A tropical rainforest tree, ylang-ylang grows in well-drained, moist soil and full sun in areas of extreme humidity and minimum temperatures of 50° to 64°F. Established trees will tolerate occasional temperatures of 30° to 32°F, however. Because of these requirements, most North American gardeners cannot grow the standard species.

Dwarf ylang-ylang (*Cananga odorata* var. *fruticosa*) is a good choice for the home garden because it produces the same fragrant flowers as the species but, at 6 feet tall, can be grown in a pot that you can move indoors for winter. Add compost to the potting mix to help retain moisture and provide nutrients. Water regularly. To increase humidity, set the pot on a tray of pebbles, and mist the plant frequently. From spring through summer, fertilize ylang-ylang monthly to encourage bloom, which will begin in 1 to 4 years. Ylang-ylang flowers are most fragrant at night during summer, when both temperatures and humidity are high. Harvest fully mature, deep yellow flowers (about 20 days after blossoming begins) in very early morning, when the essential oil content is highest.

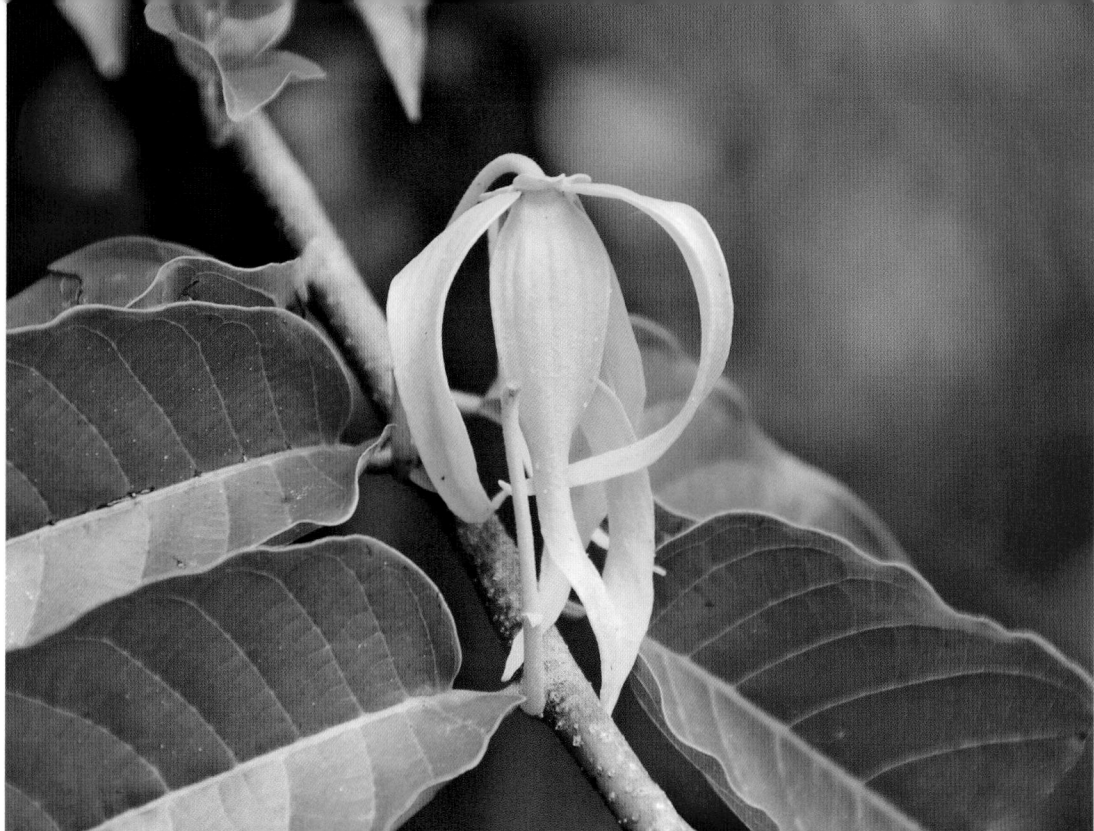

The Essence of Royalty

For more than a decade, I have studied the traditional uses of plants in Micronesia, a very remote area of the Pacific Ocean. On the island of Pohnpei, people cover their bodies with a protective skin emollient made from coconut oil perfumed with essences from local plants—flowers, leaves, and even certain aromatic woods.

I was fortunate to learn the process of making this scented oil from Maria Raza, widely recognized as the maker of the best perfumed coconut oil in her area. Maria uses the flowers of the ylang-ylang tree, locally known as seir en wai. It is the only perfuming ingredient still used for making traditional oil on Pohnpei and the island of Kosrae—the others have been forgotten over time. After the yellow-green flowers are carefully picked, the fragrant petals are removed and then added to heated coconut oil. Throughout the day, the petals' highly aromatic essential oil infuses the coconut oil. The mixture is then cooled and strained. The process is repeated over the next several days—more petals are added, and the oil takes on a delightful yet subtle fragrance.

According to ethnographers who visited the region a century ago, this oil was widely used by the royalty who ruled the island. Commoners also used the "royal oil," but bathed and anointed their bodies less frequently. With the advent of European clothing, the need to protect one's skin from the equatorial sun was reduced, and traditional customs such as the daily use of this oil were slowly lost. Today, visitors to the Micronesian islands can purchase similar oil—infused with ylang-ylang, local gardenia, frangipani, or turmeric roots—in souvenir shops.—M. J. B.

Capsicum annuum

A member of the nightshade family, the chile pepper is a tender, short-lived perennial shrub native to South America and cultivated in warm regions throughout the world. The species, which has been cultivated for thousands of years, includes not only types that bear pungent fruits (like the cayenne, pimento, and jalapeño), but also sweet peppers. The distinction is important because while sweet peppers—particularly ripe red ones—are rich in vitamins and nutrients, they lack the beneficial chemical capsaicin associated with hot peppers.

Chile peppers bear white, bell-shaped flowers that are followed by fruits that turn red, orange, yellow, or other colors as they ripen. The genus name, *Capsicum*, is thought to refer to these hollow fruits; the Latin *capsa* means "box." Used by ancient Maya Indians to treat mouth sores, the chile pepper and its benefits were described in 1493 by a physician traveling with the explorer Christopher Columbus. Before then, the chile pepper was not known beyond the Western Hemisphere. Explorers, in their quest for a western route to the spice lands of the East Indies, called the new plant "pepper" because its fruits were pungent, like those of Indian black pepper (*Piper nigrum*).

CULINARY USE

Chile pepper is among the world's most popular foods and many varieties are available, ranging in flavor from sweet and mild to extraordinarily sharp and burning. (A pepper's heat, determined by its capsaicin level, is commonly measured in

Scoville heat units.) The zesty fruits can be eaten fresh or dried, alone or mixed with other foods. They are especially popular in the dishes of tropical and subtropical countries, including Mexico, Spain, and India, where they are included in curries, chutneys, and bean, egg, and cheese dishes. The plant's leaves are cooked as greens or used in soups in Filipino, Japanese, and Korean cuisines.

Peppers can be preserved by drying, pickling, or freezing. To dry peppers, simply hang them on a string in a warm, well-ventilated location. When they're completely dry, the peppers can be finely ground in a food processor. Store the chile powder in a cool, dry place.

MEDICINAL USE

The fruits of the chile pepper contain antioxidant carotenoids and are rich in vitamin C. Pungent varieties also contain the well-known and -studied constituent capsaicin. In products for external use, such as ointments and creams available over the counter and by prescription, minute amounts of capsaicin irritate body tissues, which increases

HOW TO GROW IT

Chile peppers grow in rich, well-drained soil in full sun. In temperate climates, grow this tender perennial as an annual. Plant seeds in containers indoors about 6 weeks before the last spring frost date. After all danger of frost has passed and the soil has warmed, transplant the peppers to your garden, spacing them about 18 inches apart. Black plastic mulch can help warm the soil in northern areas. Harvest unripe green peppers at any time; harvest ripe peppers when they have attained their full color.

Peppers can also be grown in pots and moved indoors for winter. Ornamental varieties—suitable for containers and even landscape use—are available, as well.

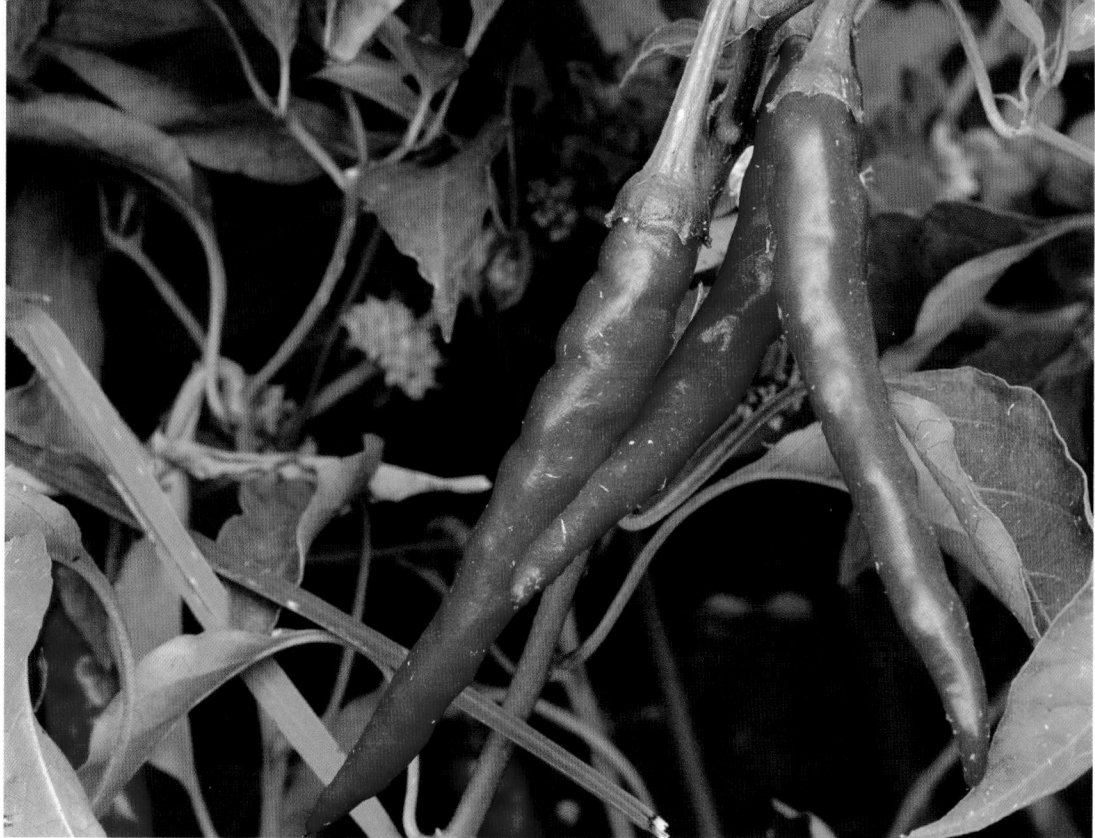

blood supply to painful areas and blocks the transmission of pain impulses throughout the body. Capsaicin is used in this manner to treat conditions such as arthritis, minor sprains, shingles, and carpal tunnel syndrome. Commercially available capsaicin creams—not homemade pepper preparations—should be used for these purposes.

The chile pepper also has antiseptic properties and has been proven to inhibit the growth of *Helicobacter pylori*, the bacteria shown to cause ulcers. It is believed to help warm the body and has been used to treat fevers and to stimulate the digestive and circulatory systems.

Caution: Chile peppers should not be eaten by those who have peptic ulcers or acid indigestion, nor should they be taken in medicinal doses by pregnant or nursing women. The herb is very irritating to the eyes and mucous membranes. It should not be applied to wounds or broken skin. When cutting these hot peppers, wear rubber gloves and do not touch your eyes.

FIELD NOTES

The Chile Grenade

The active compound in chile peppers, capsaicin, is used to produce "pepper spray" for police use and for self-defense against animals or people. In India, a "chile grenade" for police and military use was developed from one of the world's hottest chile peppers, Bhut jolokia. This chile, which is eaten in India and used in traditional medicine, is produced by a closely related species identified as Capsicum chinense and contains genes from another species, Capsicum frutescens. Plant breeders continue to use this species to develop even hotter chile varieties.—M. J. B.

Carica papaya

Papaya is a fast-growing evergreen native to the lowland forests of the American tropics. Although many people think of the papaya plant as a "tree," it's actually an herb, as it does not have a woody stem. The papaya bears seven-lobed, palmate leaves and pear-shaped yellow to orange fruits that can be small or weigh up to 11 pounds. Most of the papaya fruits now sold in supermarkets are produced by a relative of the cultivar 'Solo'; they are a little larger than a pear and perfect for one or two people. Papaya fruits are not only delicious and nutritious, they're also valuable for their ability to support digestive health.

CULINARY USE

Ripe papayas are an excellent source of vitamins A and C. You can eat them as a fresh fruit or include them in desserts. Unripe, green papayas can be steamed, boiled, or roasted like a vegetable. Papaya's black peppery-tasting seeds can be added to salads and salad dressings.

The papaya leaf has a place in the kitchen, too. Hundreds of years ago, native Caribbean people noticed that when they wrapped meat in papaya leaves, the meat became more tender. This is due to an enzyme known as papain; it's found in the white sticky latex of the plant, which is located in the fruit, stems, and leaves. Today, papaya extract is the primary ingredient in many commercially available meat tenderizers.

MEDICINAL USE

Papaya contains the enzyme papain, which is similar to the human digestive enzyme pepsin. Eating the ripe fruit and drinking the leaf tea supports digestion and could help protect your stomach

FIELD NOTES
Papain Usually Stops the Pain

Here's a trick to sweeten papaya fruit: As it ripens, make shallow cuts in the flesh to release its clear, bitter sap.

The sap is interesting for another reason: It contains the enzyme papain, which reduces the toughness of meat by digesting some of the protein. This quality was long ago recognized by indigenous people, who used the latex from the papaya's fruit or stem, as well as the leaves, as a meat tenderizer. The sap is also commonly used to treat stings, bites, rashes, and cuts and to help heal wounds.

I've learned the hard way to always carry a commercial meat tenderizer with papain as a main ingredient in my first-aid kit when traveling to marine regions. When my son was brushed by a jellyfish many years ago and was in great pain, I managed to find a jar of meat tenderizer in a local store on the isolated island we were visiting. Much to my surprise, he screamed out in even more pain when I rubbed the powdered tenderizer on his wound. "What's wrong?" I asked. "This works every time."

"It's burning like crazy now," he replied. I put on my glasses and looked carefully at the label—the highly seasoned meat tenderizer contained chile pepper powder. He never let me forget this incident!—M. J. B.

from ulcers caused by aspirin and steroid medications. (Papain is also available as a supplement that can be taken to treat indigestion and stomach inflammation.) Papaya leaf tea also might stimulate your immune system.

In Central America, people apply a combination of the ripe fruit and crushed seeds to their skin to heal wounds, cuts, and infections. The papaya's round black seeds aren't considered edible (they have a sharp, peppery taste), but people of various cultures have eaten them to treat stomach parasites. The seeds have also been fed to animals as a deworming medication.

Caution: Papaya's seeds, leaves, and unripe fruit should be avoided during pregnancy. In addition, papaya leaf should not be ingested by children younger than 2 years old.

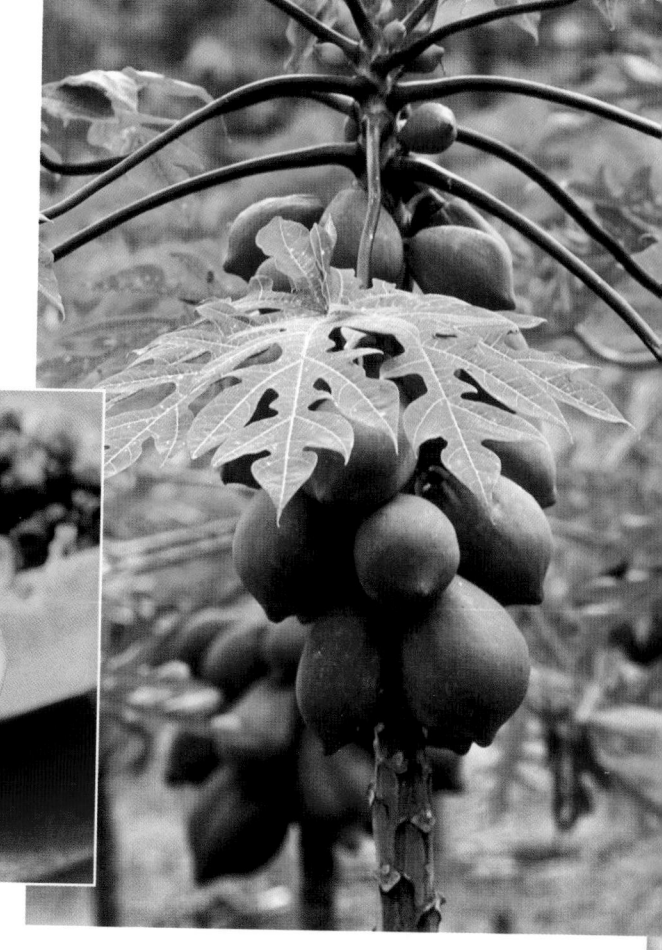

HOW TO GROW IT

Papaya "trees" grow in rich, moist soil in full sun, in areas with high humidity and minimum temperatures of 55° to 59°F. Both male and female trees are needed for fruiting, but the cultivar 'Solo' produces male and female flowers on one plant. You can buy young nursery-grown trees or start this fast-grower from seed.

When temperatures have warmed to about 75°F and all danger of frost has passed, sow the seeds in a sunny, sheltered location in your garden or in a 15-gallon pot. (Plant papaya where you intend it to grow; it does not transplant well.) Plant extra seeds—you will cull most of the non-fruit-bearing male plants. Amend the soil or potting mix with compost, and water regularly. Feed regularly with a nitrogen-rich fertilizer, such as fish emulsion. When the plants are about 3 feet tall, they will begin to flower. Pull out all but one of the males (distinguished by their long, thin stalks and small blooms; female blooms are larger and close to the trunk). The trees should begin fruiting about 10 months after you've planted them. Harvest the leaves at any time; for fresh eating, harvest fully colored, slightly soft fruit.

Carthamus tinctorius

PLANT PROFILE

Common Names: False Saffron, Safflower

Description: Stems, 1 to 3 feet tall, branch toward the top; orange-yellow thistlelike compound flowers, up to 1½ inches wide; alternate ovate leaves; seedlike fruits

Hardiness: Annual

Family: Asteraceae

Flowering: Summer

Parts Used: Flowers and seeds

Range/Habitat: Native to the Middle East; cultivated all over the world

Safflower is a cultivated plant with a long and colorful past. It has been a source of cooking oil since the days of ancient Egyptian pharaohs, and the plant's distinctive orange-yellow blooms were found inside the tomb of the Egyptian pharaoh Tutankhamen (ca. 1370–1352 BCE), woven into a decorative necklace. Ancient Egyptians extracted a yellow dye from the flowers as early as the 12th dynasty (1991–1778 BCE). In Europe and North America, where safflower has naturalized, the plant has been used medicinally to treat constipation, fevers, respiratory problems, and other conditions. Today, safflower's primary use is as a cooking oil.

CULINARY USE

Safflower oil, derived from the plant's seeds, is believed to lower harmful cholesterol levels. Dried safflower petals can be used to enliven the hues of soups, marinades, sauces, salad dressings, basting

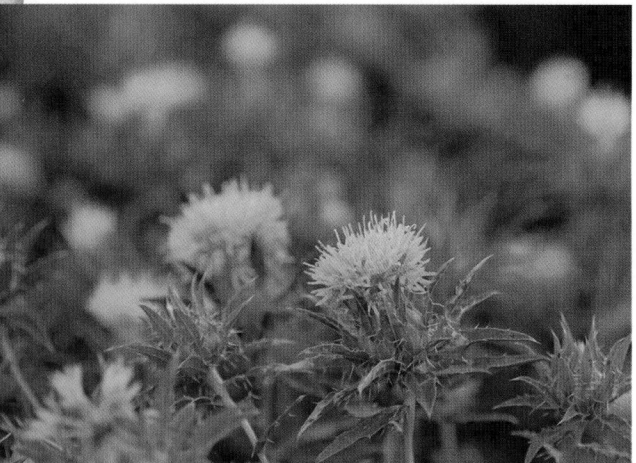

liquids, flavored vinegars, pasta salads, and curries. The dried flowers produce a red color. To heighten the flavor of safflower, crush the flowers lightly with the back of a spoon before use.

MEDICINAL USE

Safflower blossom tea has traditionally been used as a diaphoretic (a substance that causes sweating) and treatment for common children's ailments, such as measles, fevers, and skin problems. Practitioners of traditional Chinese medicine use the dried flowers (called *hong hua*) to stimulate blood circulation, promote menstruation, and reduce pain and bruising. The unpurified seed oil has laxative and purgative properties.

Caution: Do not consume the flowers or seeds if you are pregnant.

OTHER USES

As suggested by its species name, *tinctorius*, safflower is a valuable dye plant. The flowers produce yellow and red pigments used to color cosmetics and textiles, including the robes of Buddhist monks. The oil is added to commercially made cosmetic lotions and salves, as well as to margarine. At home, you can add dried safflower petals to oil infusions to produce a deep orange color.

 HOW TO GROW IT

Safflower is easy to grow in full sun and average soil. Sow the seeds in early spring directly in the garden or in pots; the plants do not transplant well. Thin the seedlings to about 6 inches apart. If you wish to use the fresh flowers, harvest them just as the buds begin to open. If you plan to dry the flowers before use, harvest the fully open blooms.

Carum carvi

A member of the parsley family, this biennial is native to Asia Minor but now grows widely throughout the world. Caraway seed (which technically is a fruit) has been used medicinally and in cooking since at least 3500 BCE. This herb is one of the few whose primary medicinal use (as a digestive aid) has remained the same throughout history. English physician Nicholas Culpeper (1616–1654) mentions that it is one of the most celebrated carminatives (gas-relieving remedies), and herbalist John Gerard (1545–1611) suggests that it be used as part of a mixture of herbs to treat "dropsie," or edema of the soft tissue, such as occurs with congestive heart failure.

CULINARY USE

Every part of the caraway plant is edible. Caraway seeds are popular in the cuisines of Germany, Austria, and Hungary, where they are used to flavor cheeses, breads (especially rye), meats, stews, vegetables, sauerkraut, and pickling brines. The minced fresh leaves, which have a mild flavor similar to the seeds, can be added to salads, soups, and casseroles. Even the root can be used, steamed, pureed, or chopped, and added to winter stews. Caraway seed can become bitter if cooked for too long; add it only during the last few minutes of cooking.

MEDICINAL USE

The volatile oil of caraway smells sweet and peppery; it contains the compounds carvol and carvene, which account for its ability to soothe your digestive tract and help expel intestinal gas. The herb has a long history of use for the treatment of flatulence and colic in babies. Caraway also has antispasmodic properties and may be useful in the treatment of menstrual cramps and diarrhea. The aroma

of the oil is said to be calming and soothing.

Caution: Pregnant or nursing women should avoid medicinal doses of caraway, though small amounts used in cooking are not harmful. If administering the herb to colicky infants, use a diluted infusion.

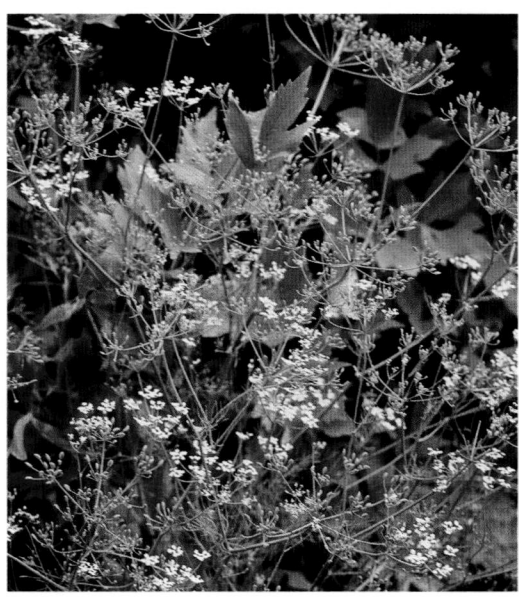

HOW TO GROW IT

Caraway is easy to grow in fertile, well-drained soil and full sun. Plant the seed directly in your garden in spring or early fall; caraway does not transplant well. Gather the ripe seed heads just as they turn brown. Snip entire stems and hang them upside down over a paper-lined tray to finish drying. After a few weeks, when the seeds are completely dry, store them in an airtight container for future use. Propagate new plants from some of the collected seeds.

Caulophyllum thalictroides

Blue cohosh grows wild in much of eastern North America, primarily in forests and other moist, shady areas. It has a long history of use in Native American medicine, particularly for women's health. The seeds and roots are cytotoxic, however. They contain saponins and a nicotinelike alkaloid that give the fruits and roots a bitter flavor. Ingesting them can cause severe gastrointestinal problems and, in some cases, hypertension, sweating, weakness, coma, and paralysis that could lead to death.

MEDICINAL USE

Native American women used a decoction of the root to treat menstrual cramps (by promoting blood flow and easing pain) and uterine inflammation. Some tribes used it to suppress profuse menstruation and to speed childbirth. It was also used by men to treat genitourinary infections.

Scientific reports are unclear regarding blue cohosh's usefulness—and its dangers—but the herb is taken widely by women (and, to a lesser extent, men) for bronchial and muscle ailments. Women ingest the rhizome and root, which contain components that stimulate uterine contractions during childbirth, encourage the onset of delayed menstruation, and alleviate heavy menstrual bleeding and cramps.

Caution: In view of the toxicity of blue cohosh and evidence of its potential adverse effects, be very careful when using this herb, particularly during pregnancy, and take it only under the direct supervision of a trained medical professional.

PLANT PROFILE

Common Names: Blue Cohosh, Squaw Root

Description: Erect, bluish green stems, 1 to 3 feet tall, topped by clusters of small, greenish yellow to brown flowers; dark blue berrylike fruit in fall

Hardiness: To Zone 4

Family: Berberidaceae

Flowering: Late spring to midsummer

Parts Used: Rhizome and roots

Range/Habitat: Eastern North America; deciduous woods and moist stream banks

ORNAMENTAL USE

Although blue cohosh is not a showy plant, its foliage is decorative. The reddish purple leaves of the young plant turn an attractive blue-green at maturity. Long-lasting blue fruits appear in fall. Plant clumps of blue cohosh in a woodland garden.

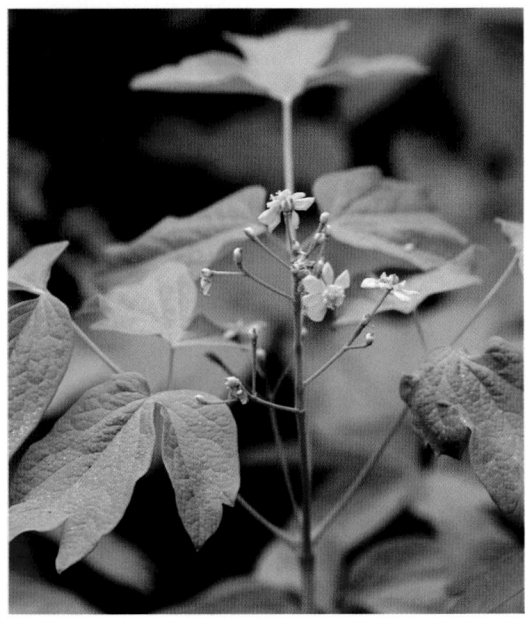

🌿 HOW TO GROW IT

Blue cohosh thrives in partial shade and prefers rich, moist, humusy soil with an acid to neutral pH. Plant seeds or rhizomes in either spring or fall. If planting in fall, sow the seeds in a cold frame or other protected area outdoors. Harvest the roots and rhizomes in fall, when they contain the greatest concentration of active compounds. Divide established plants by cutting the rhizomes and replanting them in fall.

Ceanothus americanus

This ornamental deciduous shrub grows wild in the dry plains, prairies, and open woodlands of the eastern and central United States. Its deep, woody roots allow the plant to survive repeated exposure to wildfires.

Native Americans made a pleasant, healing beverage from its leaves, a healing tea and dye from its reddish taproot, and a fragrant body wash from its saponin-rich flowers. European settlers learned from them to use the shrub's leaves to make a tea, which they substituted for British-taxed black tea during the American War of Independence. New Jersey tea is a favorite food of deer and wild birds, and its flowers provide nectar for many types of butterflies.

MEDICINAL USE

The plant's roots contain antiseptic and astringent tannins, as well as a blood-clotting agent. Native Americans made a tea from the roots and root bark to treat colds, fevers, intestinal problems, mouth sores, respiratory conditions, and skin irritations. Root teas and washes were also traditionally used to treat an enlarged spleen or lymph nodes, hemorrhoids, high blood pressure, nosebleeds, ulcers, and uterine hemorrhaging.

The leaves have been used to make a tea or gargle to relieve sore throats and mouth sores. Modern herbalists recommend preparations of this plant for conditions affecting the lymphatic system or liver.

Caution: Do not use this herb if you are pregnant or nursing.

PLANT PROFILE

Common Names: New Jersey Tea, Prairie Redroot, Redroot, Wild Snowball

Description: Deciduous shrub, up to 3 feet tall; alternate, finely toothed leaves are dark green on top with light green undersides; airy white flowers on racemes; three-lobed seedpods

Hardiness: To Zone 3

Family: Rhamnaceae

Flowering: Early to midsummer

Parts Used: Roots, root bark, leaves, and flowers

Range/Habitat: North America; dry plains, prairies, and open woodlands

ORNAMENTAL USE

The puffy summer blooms of New Jersey tea are a welcome addition to mixed perennial borders or foundation plantings, where they will attract butterflies and birds.

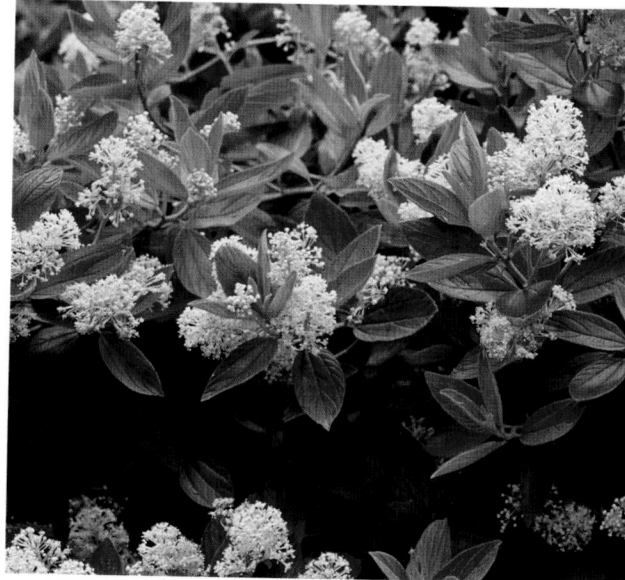

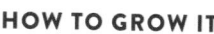

HOW TO GROW IT

New Jersey tea adapts well to either full sun or partial shade and light, well-drained soil. Prune the shrub in late winter to early spring to control its straggly habit. Gather the leaves when the plant is in full bloom, and dry them in the shade. Harvest a small amount of the roots when the shrub is dormant, in late fall or early winter. To propagate, take cuttings in summer and root them in a cold frame or greenhouse.

Centella asiatica

This perennial member of the parsley family produces clusters of scalloped leaves and tiny white or pink flowers on low-growing plants. Native to tropical and subtropical climates in Asia, Africa, North and South America, and Australia, gotu kola has traditionally been used to lengthen life and is one of the most important plants used in Ayurvedic medicine. According to South Asian folklore, the elephant acquired its long life and remarkable memory by eating large amounts of gotu kola leaves.

PLANT PROFILE

Common Names: Gotu Kola, Indian Pennywort

Description: Low-growing, creeping evergreen perennial with round, scalloped leaves; clusters of small white or pink flowers are followed by small, oval fruits

Hardiness: To Zone 9

Family: Apiaceae

Flowering: Periodically

Parts Used: Leaves

Range/Habitat: Tropical and subtropical climates in Asia, Africa, North and South America, and Australia; near water

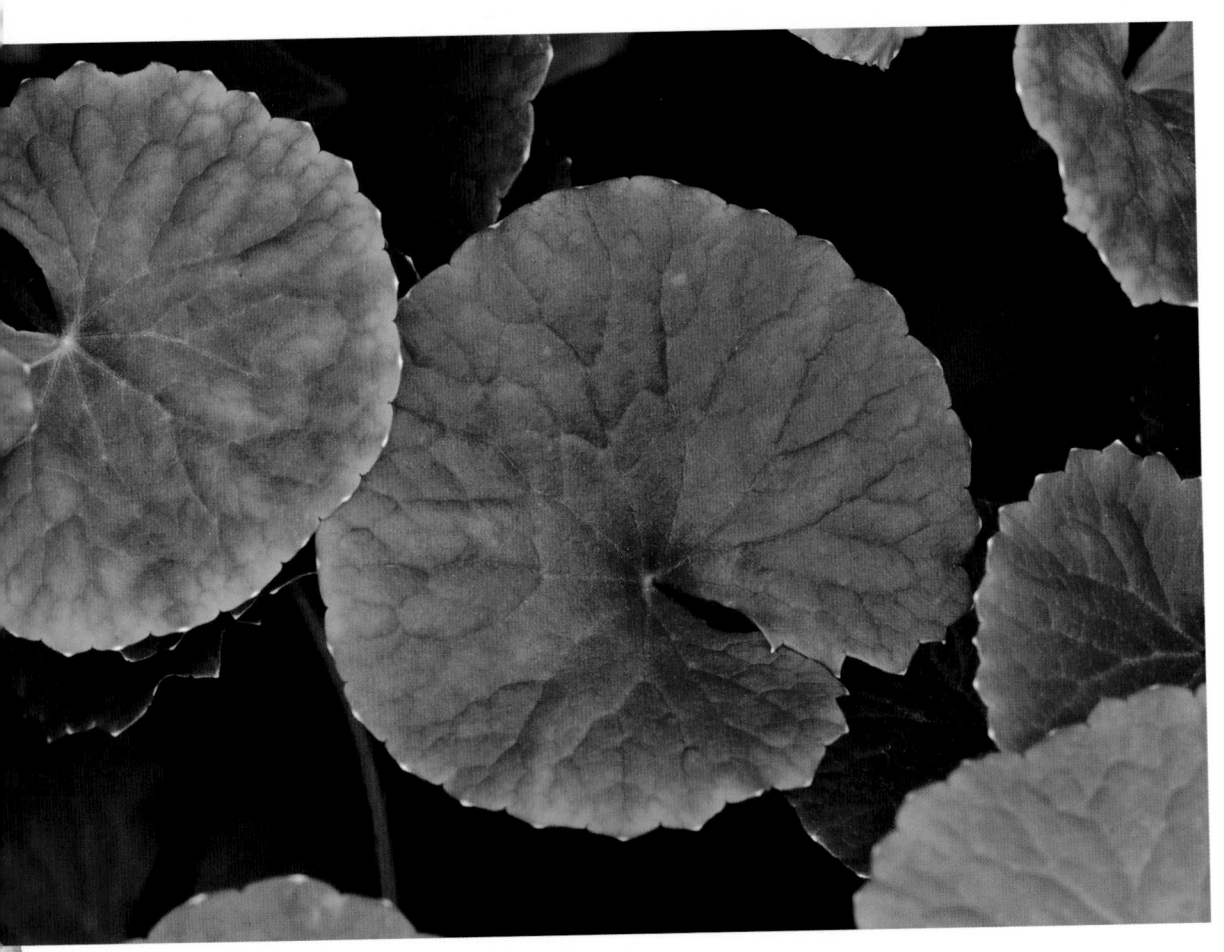

Remember This Herb

I first learned about gotu kola during a trip to India to study Ayurvedic medicine and the plants used in its therapies for thousands of years. This very low-growing species covers the areas it colonizes with a carpet of round, scalloped leaves. Picking a leaf and tasting it, I found it somewhat bitter, but delicious. I understood why it is used not only for healing, but also as a salad green and cooked vegetable in Southeast Asia.

Gotu kola is one of those wonderful herbs that should be used more widely in the United States. Numerous clinical studies have shown how beneficial it can be for various conditions. In one study, people who used a standardized extract of gotu kola had faster reaction times and increased cognitive performance and memory compared with those who took a placebo. The study's authors suggested that this plant might increase alertness and exert a calming effect, improving attention and memory.

Another clinical trial demonstrated gotu kola's efficacy in the treatment of chronic venous insufficiency (a condition where, due to malfunctioning leg vein valves, the leg veins cannot pump sufficient oxygen-poor blood back to the heart), which affects up to 5 percent of the population in the United States. According to another study, gotu kola could also help people afflicted with the leg condition flight microangiopathy, a condition of the blood vessels that includes blood circulation and coagulation problems and which can occur during long air flights.

It was a wonderfully educational journey, and I returned home a great fan of gotu kola and other Ayurvedic herbs, which, in my opinion, deserve more attention and clinical evaluation. —M. J. B.

CULINARY USE

In Thailand, India, and Sri Lanka, gotu kola leaves are eaten raw in salads (often combined with freshly grated coconut and lime juice) or cooked in curries, chutneys, and sauces. The leaves are also juiced and consumed as a beverage.

MEDICINAL USE

Gotu kola is used to help heal superficial wounds and skin problems, such as psoriasis; to reduce scarring after surgery; and to improve circulation and memory. Its leaves contain glucosides—potent healing agents with anti-inflammatory properties. This explains the herb's ability to accelerate the formation of collagen and reduce the formation of scar tissue. Gotu kola, which also has adaptogenic properties, is a common ingredient in topical preparations used to treat burns, sunburn, and wounds.

Gotu kola strengthens veins by stimulating the development of connective tissue, and it can be helpful in the treatment of varicose veins and edema. The herb also contains precursors to the neurotransmitters that are important for memory and learning.

Caution: Gotu kola may cause sensitivity to sunlight. The herb should not be taken by women who are pregnant or nursing, or by children younger than 2 years old.

HOW TO GROW IT

Gotu kola grows abundantly in marshy and wet areas. Plant the seeds in spring in moist to wet soil in partial shade, and allow it space to spread out—this plant produces plenty of runners. In Zone 8 and colder, grow gotu kola in a container and move it indoors when temperatures drop in fall. Indoors, mist the plant often and, if your home is dry, consider enclosing it in plastic to increase humidity. Keep the soil evenly moist indoors and outdoors. Harvest gotu kola leaves year-round. Propagate by root division in spring or fall.

Chamaemelum nobile (= *Anthemis nobilis*)

Native to the Mediterranean region, used by ancient Egyptians, and first recorded in England in 1265, Roman chamomile is cultivated throughout Europe and other temperate areas of the world. Unlike German chamomile (*Matricaria recutita*), a 2- to 3-foot annual with which it is frequently confused, Roman chamomile is a perennial groundcover. The name "chamomile" comes from the Greek *chamaimelon*, meaning "apple on the ground," due to the strong applelike scent that emerges when the plant's foliage is stepped on or crushed. It was used during the Middle Ages as a "strewing herb"—an herb placed on paths to release its pleasant aroma when walked upon.

MEDICINAL USE

Roman chamomile contains a volatile oil that supports the herb's long-standing use to relieve indigestion and stimulate appetite. Chamomile tea (made from the plant's flowers) can reduce stomach cramps, gas, colic, and nausea. Taken before bedtime, warm chamomile tea is also very effective for the treatment of insomnia.

Roman chamomile has anti-inflammatory properties. Used externally in a salve or compress, it helps superficial wounds, skin irritations such as eczema, and puffy eyes. In aromatherapy, the essential oil is used to treat inflamed, irritated skin and nervous conditions, such as anxiety.

Caution: Although Roman chamomile is a very safe, time-tested herb, it can provoke an allergic reaction in people sensitive to ragweed or other members of the aster family. Roman chamomile can also cause contact dermatitis in sensitive individuals.

ORNAMENTAL USE

Roman chamomile is an attractive, fragrant alternative to lawn grass for areas that receive light traffic. 'Treneague', a nonflowering cultivar, is known as lawn chamomile. Space the plants 6 inches apart and water regularly until the plants form a solid groundcover. Set your lawnmower blades on high to mow.

OTHER USES

Essential oil of chamomile is used in perfumes, shampoos, lotions, bath oils, and salves. For a soothing bath, pour boiling water over chamomile flowers and steep them for 30 minutes; strain, cool, and then add the liquid to your bathwater. A chamomile infusion can also be used to add golden highlights to your hair. Roman chamomile flowers make a bright yellow dye.

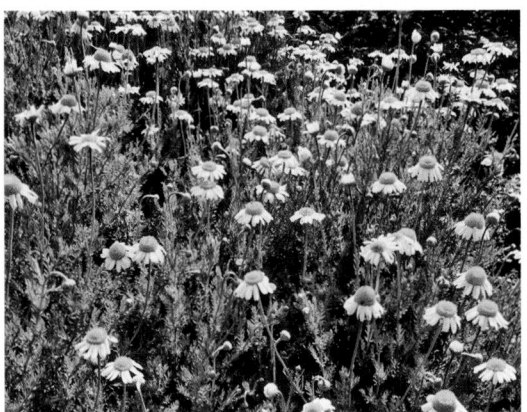

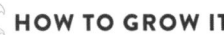

HOW TO GROW IT

Roman chamomile grows in almost any type of soil but prefers moist, well-fertilized loam in full sun. Plant seeds or nursery-grown plants in spring or fall. Propagate by division in early spring. Harvest the flowers just as they begin to open. To dry them, spread out the cut blooms on paper towels. Store the dry flowers in a cool, dark location.

Cichorium intybus

Chicory grows wild throughout much of the world. Its distinctive blue daisylike flowers are a familiar sight in cleared or abandoned areas and fields, as well as along roadsides, where it often spreads aggressively.

Chicory has been used medicinally since ancient times. It is mentioned as a healing herb in the 1st-century writings of the Greek physician Dioscorides, and the ancient Romans used the plant as both a medicine and a food. Thomas Jefferson, who held chicory in high regard, cultivated the herb as a groundcover, cattle fodder, and "tolerable salad" green. In a 1795 letter to George Washington, Jefferson described chicory as "one of the greatest acquisitions a farmer can have."

CULINARY USE

Italian chicory (also known as radicchio) produces heads of red, green, or variegated leaves. Radicchio imparts a pleasantly bitter, spicy flavor to salads and is complemented by sweet fruit, such as oranges and figs. Radicchio can also be brushed with olive oil and grilled, cooked with risotto, or added to pasta sauces and fillings. Chicory roots can be dried, roasted, ground, and then blended with coffee for a flavorful, reduced-caffeine beverage.

MEDICINAL USE

Chicory root is a rich source of inulin, which may encourage the growth of beneficial microorganisms in your intestines. In folk medicine, chicory root is believed to have mild diuretic and laxative effects, similar to dandelion. Ancient Egyptians used the root to treat rapid heartbeat, and they mixed the plant's juice with wine to treat liver and bladder conditions. Native Americans included the roots in nerve formulas and applied a root poultice to fever sores.

Practitioners of traditional Chinese medicine use the aboveground parts of this plant to promote digestion, to increase appetite, and as a diuretic. The crushed leaves can be applied topically to treat skin lacerations, swelling, and inflammation.

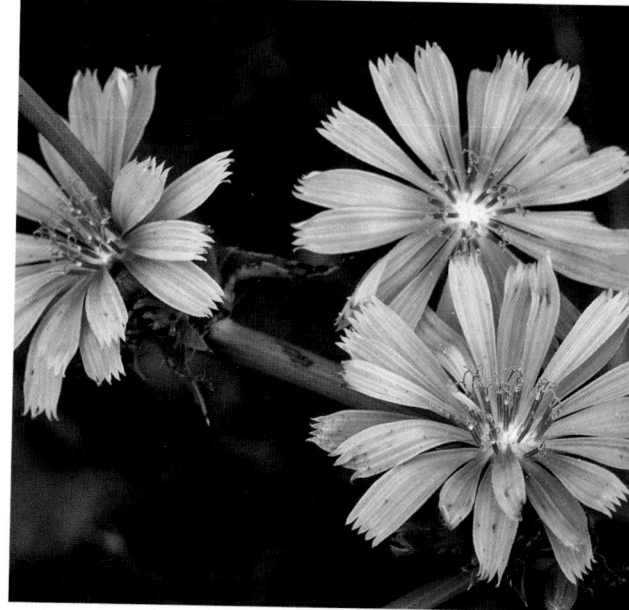

HOW TO GROW IT

Chicory grows best in fertile, well-drained soil and full sun or partial shade. For summer greens, sow seeds in late spring; for fall greens, sow seeds in midsummer. Chicory is very cold hardy, and in all but the coldest regions, it is possible to extend the harvest season into winter with the use of a floating row cover, cloche, or cold frame.

If you plan to harvest the roots, do not allow the plant to go to seed. Harvest roots of 2- or 3-year-old plants in fall.

Cinnamomum cassia and C. verum

PLANT PROFILE

Common Names: Cassia, Cinnamon, True Cinnamon

Description: Tropical evergreen tree, 25 to 50 feet tall; leathery, bright red leaves mature to green; small, yellow flowers followed by purple berries; aromatic, reddish brown bark

Hardiness: To Zone 10

Family: Lauraceae

Flowering: Varies depending on location

Parts Used: Bark

Range/Habitat: Native to humid, tropical forests in southern India and Sri Lanka

Of the genus *Cinnamomum*'s approximately 250 species, two are very important to the spice trade: "true" cinnamon (*Cinnamomum verum*) and "cassia" cinnamon (*C. cassia*). Cultivated in the West Indies, Asia, southern India, and Sri Lanka, these evergreen trees in the laurel family are native to southern Asia. Cinnamon's aromatic, light brown, paperlike bark is harvested from young branches during the rainy season, when it is most pliable. When dry, the bark curls into long quills used, powdered or whole, as a spice. In our supermarkets, whole, unground cinnamon is usually sold in the form of rolled bark (called cinnamon sticks) that's about as thick as a lead pencil.

Cinnamon has a long history of use for a variety of purposes beyond the kitchen. Ancient Egyptians used it in the embalming process, and the Romans used it as an aphrodisiac and perfume. By the 16th century, cinnamon was so valued as a spice that the Portuguese invaded the Indian island of Ceylon (now known as Sri Lanka) to obtain a monopoly on cinnamon production. In the late 1700s, the Dutch began to cultivate cinnamon and the Dutch East India Company became a leading supplier of the treasured bark.

CULINARY USE

A beloved cooking spice, cinnamon is used around the world to flavor sweet dishes, such as cookies, breads, cakes, and pies, as well as savory curries, soups, and stews. Its flavor complements black pepper, cardamom, clove, fennel, ginger, nutmeg, and vanilla. Although the chemical properties of "true cinnamon" and "cassia cinnamon" are similar, their flavors differ. True cinnamon (sometimes called Ceylon cinnamon) is less sweet and has a more complex, citruslike flavor that goes well with fruit dishes. The more familiar cassia cinnamon, popular for baking, is sweeter and more sharply flavored.

MEDICINAL USE

A reference to cinnamon's use in treating diarrhea was recorded in China in 2700 BCE. Hebrews, Greeks, and Romans all used cinnamon to treat indigestion. Cinnamon bark contains volatile oil and tannins, which could explain its effectiveness as a treatment for gastrointestinal disorders, including bloating, flatulence, and vomiting. The bark also contains eugenol, a natural antiseptic and anesthetic compound that can help kill bacteria and viruses, prevent infection, and ease pain. Diluted essential oil of cinnamon is an ingredient in some dental products, such as toothpastes and mouthwashes.

Research has shown that cinnamon powder

HOW TO GROW IT

Cinnamon trees grow in moist, tropical or subtropical conditions in well-drained soil and full sun or bright shade. In Zone 9 and colder regions, grow the plant in a large container in a heated greenhouse, or move it indoors during cold seasons. A sandy, slightly acidic growing medium enriched with compost to retain moisture and provide nutrients is ideal. Keep the soil evenly moist year-round. To obtain the inner bark used for the spice and essential oil, the young shoots are harvested and their outer bark is scraped away. The tree can be propagated by seed or by cuttings taken in summer.

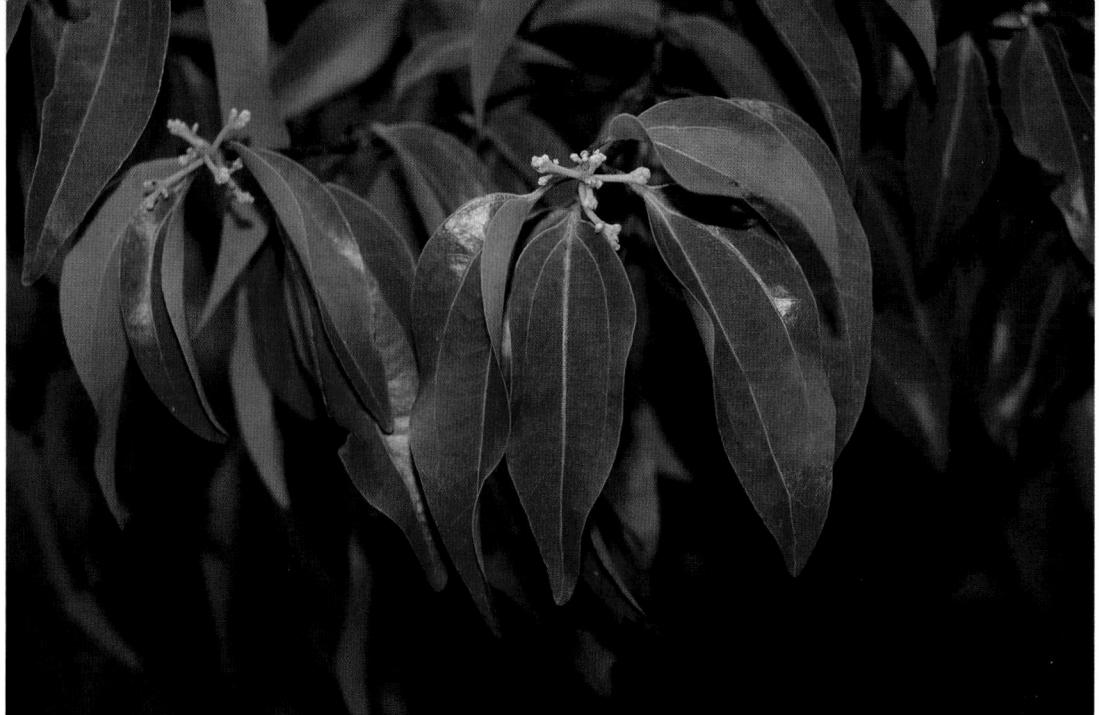

may help lower blood sugar and may be useful in the treatment of type 2 diabetes, although not all studies have proven this effect. Cinnamon is used to warm the body and clear mucous congestion due to colds and flus. It also improves circulation, especially to cold fingers and toes.

Caution: Pregnant women should not use cinnamon medicinally, but the herb is safe to use in small quantities as a spice. Undiluted essential oil of cinnamon is highly irritating to sensitive skin; follow the label directions when using liniments and other products that contain it.

FIELD NOTES
A Case for Conservation

In a volcanic cloud forest on the tiny island of Pohnpei, Micronesia, grows Cinnamomum carolinense, a species found nowhere else in the world. Locally known as madeu, this unique cinnamon has several important uses. Local people carefully scrape off the inner bark of the tree to make a hot tea, which they serve in small glasses to guests. This traditional tea is also used to treat backache, to stem the flow of excessive menstrual bleeding, and for other healing purposes.

Unfortunately, many of the ancient specimens of these very useful trees were cut down and harvested long ago.

During our studies of this forest, we met a local madeu harvester, Yosio Pelep, who expressed great concern that this magnificent tree is disappearing from his island. Yosio— who is participating in a reforestation and tree protection program to ensure that madeu does not go extinct on his watch—showed us the sustainable method he developed to harvest

the tree's valuable bark.

Cinnamomum carolinense is on the verge of extinction, and scientists have not yet had a chance to study its chemical properties and therapeutic potentials. I believe we all have a stake in ensuring the conservation of the world's biodiversity—not only for the benefit of indigenous communities such as on Pohnpei, but also for the benefit of future generations all over the world.—M. J. B.

Coffea arabica

The source of one of the world's most widely consumed beverages, *Coffea arabica* is native to northeastern Africa and cultivated in tropical areas around the world. The genus contains about 90 species of small trees and evergreen shrubs, and while *C. arabica* is the most widely grown, the species *C. liberica* and *C. canephora* also are used commercially to produce coffee. Coffee's red fruits each contain two seeds, known as beans, which are used to make the popular drink. Initially, people made a type of wine from the fermented juice of the plant's ripe berries. The hot beverage we now know as coffee is thought to have been made first by Arabian people, around 1000 CE. (For another account of the drink's origins, see "Field Notes" on page 143.) Until late in the 17th century, Arabia supplied almost all of the world's coffee beans. As the popularity of the beverage grew, the beans were introduced to other favorable climates—the West Indies, Java, India, and Brazil. Today, Brazil and Colombia are leading exporters. Coffee farming and trade support the economies of many developing countries. In the United States alone, more than 100 million people drink coffee daily.

CULINARY USE

Besides being the essential wake-up beverage for millions, coffee is also used to flavor liqueurs and desserts, such as Italy's classic espresso-soaked tiramisu. Espresso is a highly concentrated form of coffee made by forcing water under pressure through finely ground coffee beans. Variations include lattes (served with steamed milk), cappuccinos (with milk and steamed foam), and mochas (with chocolate). The drink can be enjoyed hot or iced.

PLANT PROFILE

Common Names: Arabian Coffee, Coffee

Description: Evergreen shrub, 15 to 40 feet tall; glossy, elliptical leaves; dense clusters of fragrant white flowers and red fruits; fruits contain two seeds, known as beans

Hardiness: To Zone 10

Family: Rubiaceae

Flowering: In the tropics, flower buds form during the dry season and open after the first heavy rains

Parts Used: Seeds and fruits

Range/Habitat: Native to northeastern Africa; cultivated in tropical areas around the world

---

MEDICINAL USE

Coffee contains the bioactive compound caffeine, as well as an abundance of healthful antioxidants. Caffeine acts as a stimulant, a laxative, a diuretic, and an appetite suppressant. Besides keeping you awake and alert, coffee can lift your mood, sharpen your cognition, alleviate asthma, and possibly protect you from Alzheimer's disease and other dementias, various kinds of cancer, type 2 diabetes, and kidney stones.

Recent research has shown that coffee berries—the fruit enclosing the "bean"—are also rich sources of antioxidants. Compounds in the berries are thought to benefit your skin by reducing inflammation, wrinkles, and sun damage. You can buy coffee berry extract as a dietary supplement at health food stores. Many skin-care products include it, too.

Caution: Coffee can cause insomnia, jitteriness, and irritability. Coffee is not advised for people with high blood pressure, gastric ulcers, glaucoma, or heart disease. It should be avoided during pregnancy and when trying to conceive.

 HOW TO GROW IT

Coffee grows in well-drained, moist soil in full sun or partial shade. Although coffee thrives in warm, humid climates with a minimum temperature of 50°F, the shrub can be grown elsewhere in a large container kept indoors during cold seasons. Plant the seeds in rich loam amended with compost. Water regularly and feed with a diluted liquid fertilizer. In a dry environment, such as a heated home, mist often to increase humidity. As a houseplant, coffee will yield few, if any, berries. In tropical climates, the berries are harvested when they turn bright red, signaling that they are ripe. The green seeds (or beans) are then removed and roasted for use. Coffee is easily propagated from seed.

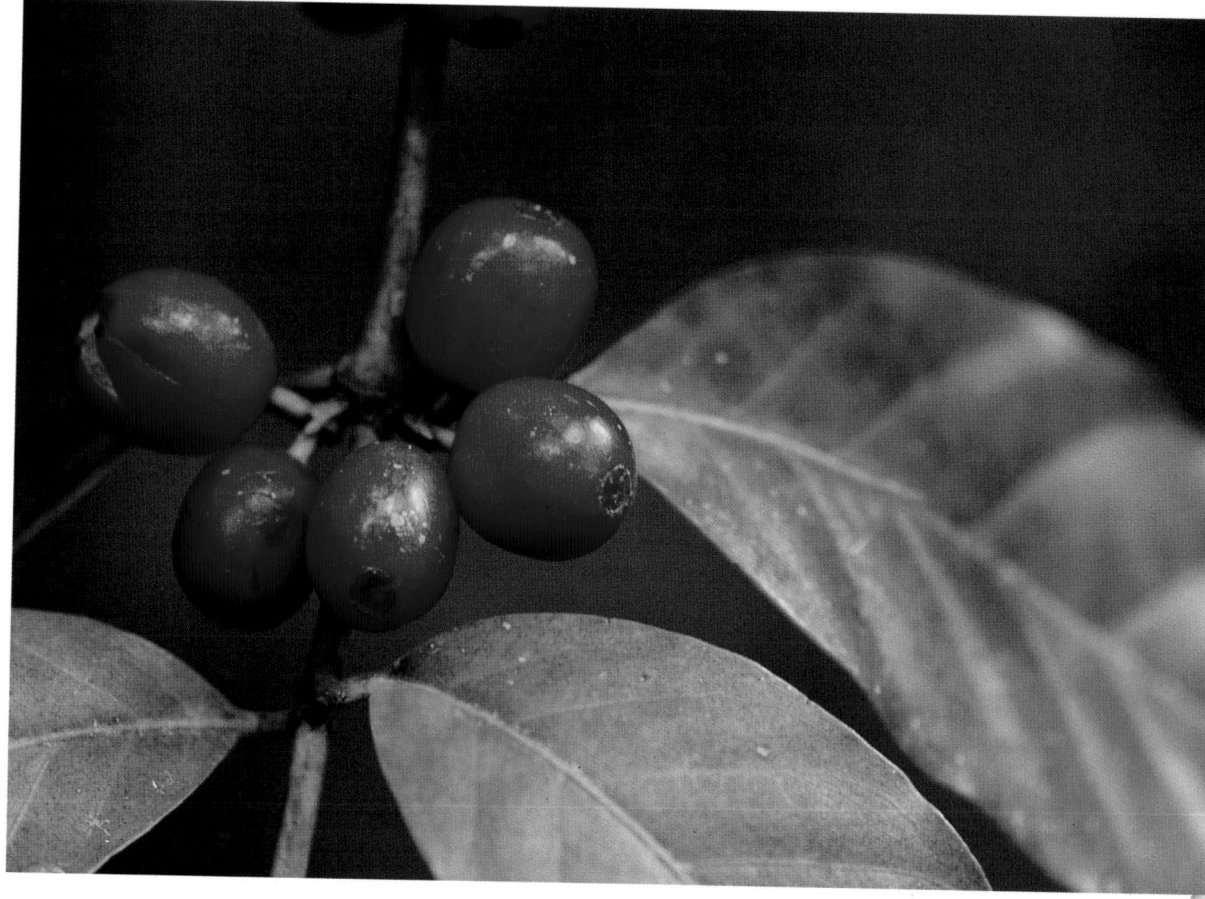

That Heavenly Coffee

Ethiopia is the center of origin of coffee, and a local legend explains its accidental discovery: A goat herder named Kaldi lived in this region 1,000 years ago. One day, the noise and activities of his goats startled him awake from his nap. Normally peaceful, they were jumping on their hind legs. After observing them eating from a low-growing tree with bright red berries, Kaldi chewed a few himself. Soon he felt wide-awake, and the nearby fields suddenly looked much brighter. He no longer wanted to nap. He took the beans to a local holy man and explained what had happened. The priest became angry and threw the beans into the fire, saying they "are the work of the devil." The wonderful aroma that came from the fire drew the attention of everyone in the monastery, who came running to see what was happening.

The chief priest ordered the fire extinguished and the berries to be added to hot water so that their aroma would infuse the liquid. After drinking it, the priest declared that this would become a daily beverage, "keeping us awake during our evening prayers—truly a gift from heaven!"—M. J. B.

Cola nitida

Perhaps best known as an original ingredient in the popular carbonated beverages of the same name, cola is one of approximately 125 *Cola* species native to the lowland and mountain rainforests of west Africa. The tree bears fruits (called "nuts") valued for their stimulatory properties, which derive primarily from caffeine (2.0 to 3.5 percent by weight) and theobromine (1.0 to 2.5 percent by weight).

In Africa, people traditionally chewed the bitter-tasting nuts to lessen fatigue and hunger, or they ground the nuts to make a beverage. Today, cola nuts are still used ceremonially, presented as a sign of hospitality to visiting guests or to mark an important event, such as a wedding ceremony. In some regions, the nuts have sacred significance and are used in divination.

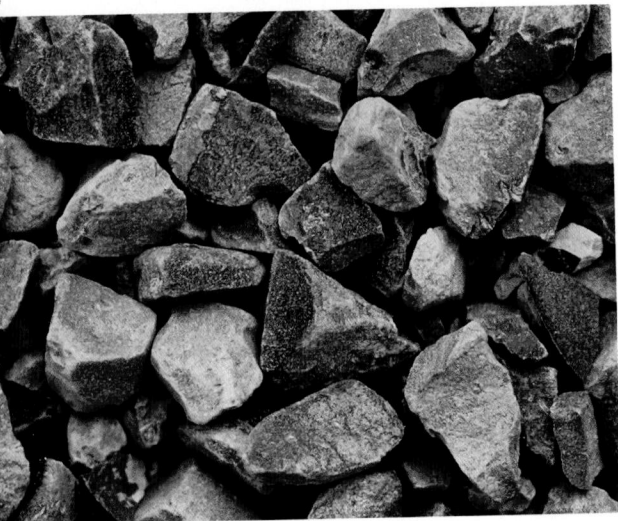

CULINARY USE

Together with the coca leaf, the source of cocaine, the cola nut was a key ingredient in the original Coca-Cola drink, invented in the late 19th century. In 1903, cocaine was removed from the coca leaves used to produce the drink, but the coca leaf and cola nut are still used to flavor this much-loved beverage.

MEDICINAL USE

The cola nut stimulates the production of digestive system acids, speeds up your heart rate, and acts as a diuretic. The herb has been used to suppress hunger, as well as to treat diarrhea and asthma. (Caffeine acts as a bronchodilator, helping to open air passages.) In contemporary European herbal medicine, the powdered nut, liquid extract, and tincture are approved to treat mental and physical fatigue.

OTHER USES

The wood of the cola tree is used for carpentry and construction. The seeds are also used to make a dye, as well as soaps and fertilizers.

HOW TO GROW IT

This tropical tree thrives in full sun or partial shade and wet, humid conditions where the temperature remains above 40°F. In Zone 9 and colder, it can be grown in a large container kept indoors during cold seasons. Cola is easy to grow from seed. To speed germination, soak the seed in water for 24 hours before sowing. Germination occurs best at 85°F. Add compost to the potting medium to help retain moisture and provide nutrients, and water and mist the plant regularly. Cola can be propagated by seed or cuttings. Be patient if you hope to obtain cola nuts: The trees generally require 7 years to begin fruiting.

Coleus forskohlii
(= *Plectranthus barbatus*)

PLANT PROFILE

Common Names: Forskohlii, Hausa Potato

Description: Aromatic, herbaceous perennial grows up to 2 feet tall; bright green, ovate leaves with scalloped margins; clusters of blue-purple blooms on 10-inch spikes

Hardiness: To Zone 9

Family: Lamiaceae

Flowering: Summer to fall

Parts Used: Leaves and roots

Range/Habitat: Dry hillsides and mountain slopes of India, Nepal, Thailand, and Sri Lanka

A relative of mint and lavender, forskohlii grows wild in India on the dry plains and in the foothills of the Himalayas. Other members of this genus of more than 150 species grow in the tropical and subtropical regions of the Indian subcontinent. The leaves are aromatic, with a camphorlike aroma, and have been used to cleanse and deodorize skin.

CULINARY USE

In India, where forskohlii is cultivated on a large scale, people eat the roots pickled or as a condiment.

MEDICINAL USE

This Ayurvedic herb could be beneficial in the treatment of a wide range of conditions, including asthma and other respiratory disorders, angina, congestive heart failure, hypertension, glaucoma, eczema, psoriasis, and insomnia. The leaves and roots of *Coleus forskohlii* are the source of a compound called forskolin, first isolated in the 1970s. Research has shown that it has the potential to lower high blood pressure, relax smooth muscle tissue (such as in the bronchial airways), increase hormone release from the thyroid gland, and stimulate digestion. The compound also holds promise as a treatment for obesity: In recent preliminary clinical research conducted with men, the compound significantly reduced both their percentage of body fat and fat mass.

Caution: Scientific research on this herb is preliminary. What is known relates primarily to its compound forskolin, rather than the entire herb.

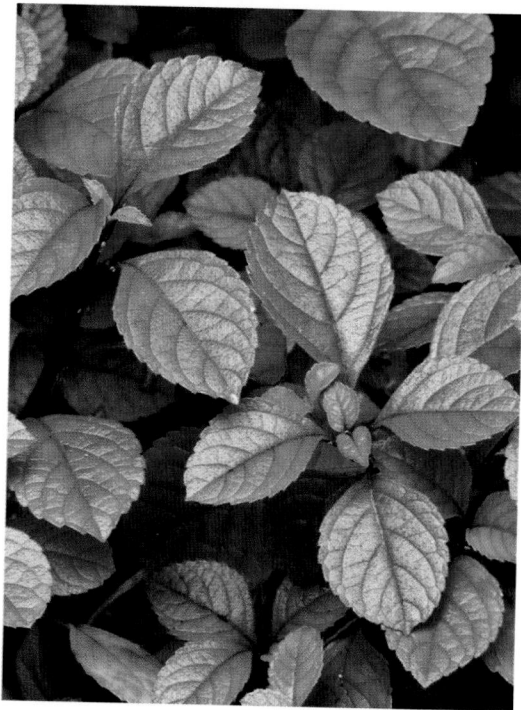

HOW TO GROW IT

Forskohlii thrives in light, well-drained loam in sun or partial shade. In subtropical climates (Zone 9 and warmer), the herb can be grown outdoors as a perennial. In cooler climates, grow forskohlii as a potted plant; in fall, or when the temperatures cool, bring it indoors to a warm, sunny location. Native to arid and semiarid locations, forskohlii is drought tolerant, so avoid overwatering. Indoors, provide the brightest light possible—a greenhouse is ideal. For medicinal use, collect the leaves and roots in fall, when the herb's active constituents are at their highest levels. Propagate established plants by taking cuttings or by dividing the roots in summer.

Commiphora myrrha

Frequently mentioned in the Bible and one of the gifts the wise men brought to the infant Jesus, myrrh is an aromatic, dark-colored resin produced by the *Commiphora myrrha* plant, a shrub or small tree native to the deserts of northern Africa and the Arabian Peninsula. Myrrh has been used in ritual incense and perfumes since prebiblical times. The ancient Egyptians used it both as a fumigant and to embalm their dead. Today, myrrh resin is produced commercially in Somalia, Ethiopia, and the Arabian Peninsula and is sold in lumps of varying sizes.

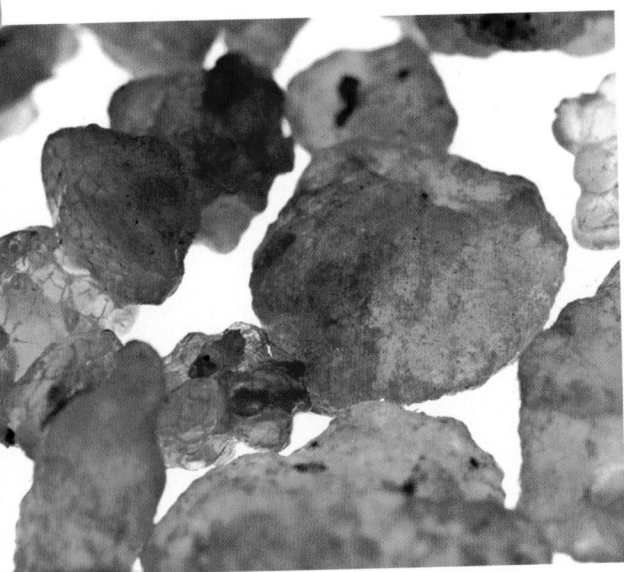

PLANT PROFILE

Common Name: Myrrh

Description: Aromatic shrub or small tree grows up to 12 feet tall, with thorny branches; three-part leaves composed of oval leaflets; small, pointed fruits; aromatic sap

Hardiness: To Zone 10

Family: Burseraceae

Flowering: Blooms repeatedly

Parts Used: Resin

Range/Habitat: Northeastern Africa, Middle East, and western Asia; deserts

MEDICINAL USE

Myrrh has disinfectant properties and acts as an astringent, tightening and drying the body's tissues. The Greek physician Hippocrates (460–377 BCE) prescribed a myrrh liniment for sores. About 500 years later, Dioscorides (ca. 40–90 CE), a Greek physician, suggested a breath-freshening mouthwash that included gum myrrh, wine, and oil. Today, myrrh is an ingredient in many commercial mouthwashes and toothpastes. An analgesic and antiseptic, myrrh also makes a soothing salve for cuts, burns, and wounds.

In Asian medicine, it is used to treat stomach, bone, and abdominal pain; amenorrhea; hemorrhoids; and injuries from trauma. It is also recommended for arthritic and circulatory problems.

OTHER USES

Veterinary medicine has long used myrrh in unguents for wounds, especially for horses. The resin is also used in perfumes and incense, especially for use in religious ceremonies. When burned, myrrh repels mosquitoes.

HOW TO GROW IT

Native to the deserts of Africa and Asia, *Commiphora myrrha* prefers hot, arid conditions, full sun, and very well-drained, sandy soil. It is rarely grown in the United States, and the plants and seeds can be very difficult to obtain. If you are able to obtain seeds, stratify them to improve germination (for more on seed stratification, see page 418). In Zone 9 and colder, grow the plant indoors in a spot that will receive bright light. Water sparingly. To harvest myrrh for commercial use, collectors make small incisions in the tree's bark. The resin that exudes is collected and allowed to harden and is then either distilled for oil or ground into a powder. Plants can be propagated from cuttings taken from young branches or from seeds.

Coriandrum sativum

This annual member of the parsley family has a split personality: The plant's finely cut upper leaves are known as cilantro and the rounded seeds of the fruit are called coriander. Both are used to flavor many foods. Native to southern Europe and nearby areas, coriander has been cultivated there for more than 3,000 years and is now grown throughout the world. The erect plant has pungent leaves and white flowers, followed by pale brown, mildly aromatic fruits. The genus name *Coriandrum* comes from the Greek *koriannon,* which was a type of bedbug thought to have an odor similar to that of this herb.

CULINARY USE

Coriander seeds and cilantro leaves taste very different, but both are used widely in cooking. Whole coriander seeds—which taste like a mixture of lemon and sage—are used in marinades, pickling brines, and in some beverages, such as mulled wine. Ground coriander seed is a popular ingredient in curry blends, soups, and baked goods, especially in Scandinavia and Thailand. Fragrant cilantro has a distinctively pungent flavor reminiscent of parsley and citrus. The leaves are used in the highly seasoned cuisines of Mexico, the Caribbean, India, and Asia. Cilantro root is a popular ingredient in Thai salads and relishes.

MEDICINAL USE

Coriander seeds have carminative properties, so they have been used as a mild digestive tonic to improve appetite and relieve flatulence, intestinal spasms, bloating, and cramps. In ancient Egypt, as well as medieval Europe, coriander was considered an aphrodisiac. In Ayurvedic medicine, dried coriander fruits are made into an infusion, or other preparation, to treat sore throat. The oil is used to treat joint and nerve pain. Coriander seeds can be chewed to sweeten your breath, particularly after eating garlic.

OTHER USES

The flowers of this plant are an important source of nectar for the beneficial insects that prey upon pest insects.

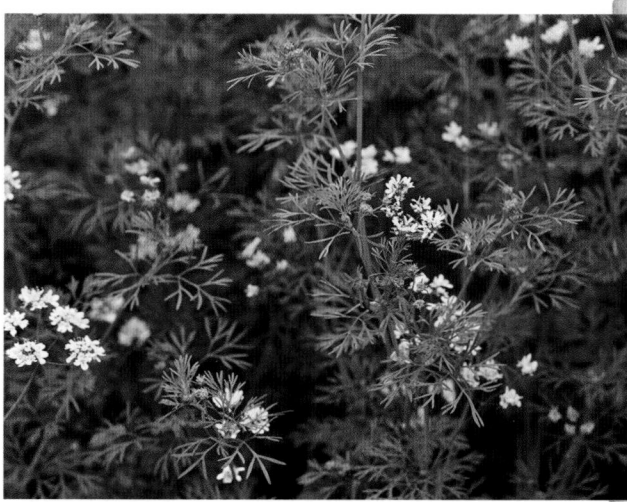

HOW TO GROW IT

Coriander grows best in well-drained soil and full sun. For a summer harvest, plant the seeds of this fast-growing herb in spring; for a fall harvest, plant it in midsummer. Cilantro leaves are usually ready to harvest 1 month after germination, and the seeds develop in about 6 weeks. For the best-flavored cilantro, gather the fresh leaves before the plant blooms. Harvest coriander seeds when they turn brown, indicating that they are ripe.

Crataegus laevigata

A relative of the rose, the hawthorn is a deciduous shrub or small tree that bears clusters of aromatic white flowers followed by dark red, egg-shaped fruits. These fruits, sometimes called haws, resemble rose hips or tiny apples. The fast-growing, thorny shrub is a common sight in old English hedgerows—in fact, the word "haw" is an early Anglo-Saxon term for hedge. The genus name *Crataegus* comes from the Greek word for "strength"—a reference to the hawthorn's hard wood.

PLANT PROFILE

Common Names: English Hawthorn, Hawthorn, May Tree, White Thorn

Description: Deciduous, thorny shrub or small tree, up to 15 feet tall, with dark brown bark; clusters of aromatic white flowers, followed by dark red, egg-shaped fruits

Hardiness: To Zone 4

Family: Rosaceae

Flowering: Spring

Parts Used: Leaves, flowers, and fruits

Range/Habitat: Native to Europe, India, and northern Africa, naturalized in upper Midwest United States and Canada

CULINARY USE

Hawthorn fruits can be made into wines, sauces, and jellies. The edible flowers can be added to salads or steeped to make a tea.

MEDICINAL USE

Hawthorn leaves, flowers, and fruits contain compounds that can dilate coronary vessels and lower blood pressure. The herb has been used to treat a wide range of heart conditions, including hypertension related to a weak heart, angina, arteriosclerosis, the early stages of congestive heart failure, age-related heart disorders, and arrhythmia. Practitioners often encourage the use of hawthorn products for several months or years to reap optimum benefits.

In traditional Chinese medicine, the fruits of the related species, *Crataegus pinnatifida* (known as *shan zha*), are often recommended to stimulate digestion. Both Native American and Chinese medical practitioners have used various species of hawthorn to treat diarrhea, to strengthen the heart, and for other curative purposes.

Caution: Unlike some medicinal plants that act on the heart, hawthorn is relatively nontoxic. However, those taking digitalis should consult with their health-care provider before taking this herb because it necessitates a reduction in the dosage of digitalis.

ORNAMENTAL USE

Hawthorn's attractive foliage, flowers, and berries add year-round beauty to the landscape. Its scented flowers attract butterflies, and the bright red berries persist into winter, providing food for birds such as thrushes and waxwings. Plant hawthorn individually or in hedges. For a more formal look, prune and train the plants espalier-fashion.

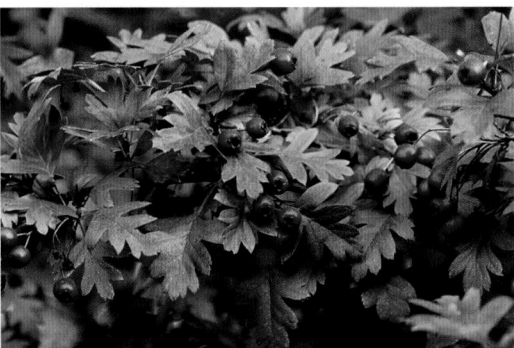

 HOW TO GROW IT

Hawthorn is easy to grow in an open, sunny site with moist, well-drained loam. Plant fresh seed in a cold frame in fall for germination the following spring. If seed is not fresh, scarify it before sowing to speed germination (for more on seed scarification, see page 418). Harvest the flowers and leaf buds in spring; harvest the berries after they ripen in fall. Propagate by seed or by grafts taken in late winter to early spring.

Crocus sativus

Like other crocuses, saffron bears attractive purple or white, cup-shaped flowers and linear leaves—but, unlike most other *Crocus* species, saffron blooms in fall. Saffron has been treasured and traded as a spice and used as a medicine for more than 4 millennia. As early as the 10th century BCE, ancient Persians cultivated saffron and used its threads in textile dyes, perfumes, medicines, and body washes. Saffron (*Crocus sativus*) is often confused with autumn crocus (*Colchicum autumnale*), but the two are very different. Autumn crocus, a highly toxic plant, is the source of the powerful pharmaceutical colchicine, which is used to treat gout.

CULINARY USE

Pungent and aromatic, saffron is the world's most expensive spice. Each saffron flower contains three stigmas, which are the part of the plant used for the spice. Saffron flowers must be handpicked, and it takes more than 14,000 stigmas to make 1 ounce of saffron. But a very little saffron goes a long way in cooking. Saffron adds flavor and color to Mediterranean dishes such as bouillabaisse, risotto, and paella, as well as to baked goods and liqueurs. The spice complements mild cheeses, eggs, rice, lamb, fish, poultry, pork, duck, corn, sweet peppers, onions, garlic, and oranges.

MEDICINAL USE

Saffron is still used in the traditional medicine practices of India and China. Herbal practitioners use saffron to relieve indigestion and colic, to encourage perspiration, and to ease menstrual pain, although equally effective and much less expensive herbs are available. Saffron is also sometimes used to treat high blood pressure and to improve circulation. In Persia, it was traditionally used to treat dementia and depression. Modern scientific studies have supported saffron's potential

for treating conditions such as mild to moderate depression, cancer, and Alzheimer's disease, as well as for improving visual acuity.

Caution: Saffron should not be used in large, medicinal doses during pregnancy.

OTHER USES

Saffron yields an unparalleled yellow dye that is associated with royalty and wealth. One part of crocin, saffron's major pigment, can color up to 150,000 parts of water. Saffron has also been used in beauty-care products since ancient times. Cleopatra is said to have added it to her bathwater to enhance her beauty and increase the pleasure of her lovemaking.

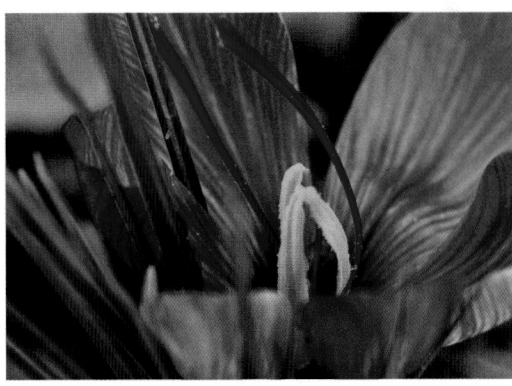

 HOW TO GROW IT

You can grow saffron in a perennial border, container, or rock garden. Plant the corms in fall or spring in well-drained soil and full sun. Set the corms 3 to 4 inches deep and 6 inches apart. Harvest fully open flowers. Pluck and dry the stigmas, spreading them out on paper. Store in an airtight container in a cool, dry location.

Curcuma longa

An aromatic, yellow-flowering perennial with large, glossy leaves, turmeric is native to southern Asia. Its tuberous rhizome, which is golden yellow when cut open, is the source of both a pungent spice and a brightly colored dye traditionally used to color the robes of Buddhist monks in India and Asia. The herb is cultivated commercially in India, Pakistan, Bangladesh, and other countries with tropical growing conditions.

CULINARY USE

Turmeric is a vital ingredient in East Indian, Persian, and Thai cooking. The spice—a powder made from the plant's dried rhizome—gives many popular curry blends and curry dishes their distinctive yellow color and pungent flavor. The fresh rhizome can also be used much like fresh gingerroot, stir-fried with other ingredients or cut into pieces and pickled. Whole, fresh turmeric leaves can be wrapped around fish or vegetables before they are cooked to impart a unique flavor. Turmeric gives the condiment mustard its bright yellow color. It's also sometimes used to color and flavor pickles, relishes, broths, and rice dishes.

MEDICINAL USE

Turmeric is a wonderful example of an edible medicinal used to prevent or treat a broad range of health conditions. Long revered in traditional Asian healing practices, turmeric is considered an excellent anti-inflammatory, antiseptic, and antioxidant. Several compounds, including curcumin—the compound that gives turmeric its bright yellow color—account for this herb's potent

> **PLANT PROFILE**
>
> **Common Names:** Common Turmeric, Indian Saffron, Turmeric, Yellow Ginger
>
> **Description:** Stemless perennial, 16 to 36 inches tall; yellow to orange tubular blooms and large, lanceolate leaves; tuberous rhizome is a bright yellow when cut open
>
> **Hardiness:** To Zone 10
>
> **Family:** Zingiberaceae
>
> **Flowering:** Periodically
>
> **Parts Used:** Rhizome
>
> **Range/Habitat:** Native to southern Asia, widely grown in India, Pakistan, Bangladesh, and other countries

health benefits, and scientists are now investigating turmeric extensively. More than 1,000 scientific papers on turmeric have been published, seeking to understand how it works in the human body and its potential applications in contemporary medicine.

Caution: Turmeric should not be used medicinally by pregnant women or by those suffering from bile duct obstruction, gallstones, stomach ulcers, or stomach hyperacidity.

OTHER USES

Turmeric has long been used as a fabric dye when a rich golden hue is desired. You can experiment with this at home by dissolving the powdered spice in a pot of boiling water, then adding a piece of cloth to the cooled liquid. The longer the cloth steeps, the darker its color becomes. Because of its powerful antiseptic properties, turmeric is added to some cosmetics to improve and protect skin.

HOW TO GROW IT

A tropical perennial, turmeric thrives in bright indirect light, temperatures above 60°F, and high humidity. If your climate is not suitable for turmeric, you can grow this herb indoors in a container. In spring, plant the rhizome (sold in the produce section of some specialty food markets) about ½ inch deep in well-drained, compost-enriched soil. Cover the pot with plastic, then place it in a warm location. When shoots emerge in about 3 weeks, remove the plastic and move the pot to a warm, bright location. Water and mist regularly.

When the leaves begin to die back and growth slows in fall, the plant is entering its dormant phase, which can last several months. During this period, reduce watering and provide brighter light, if possible. This is also the best time to harvest and divide the rhizomes. When new growth emerges in late winter, return the pot to its original location and resume watering.

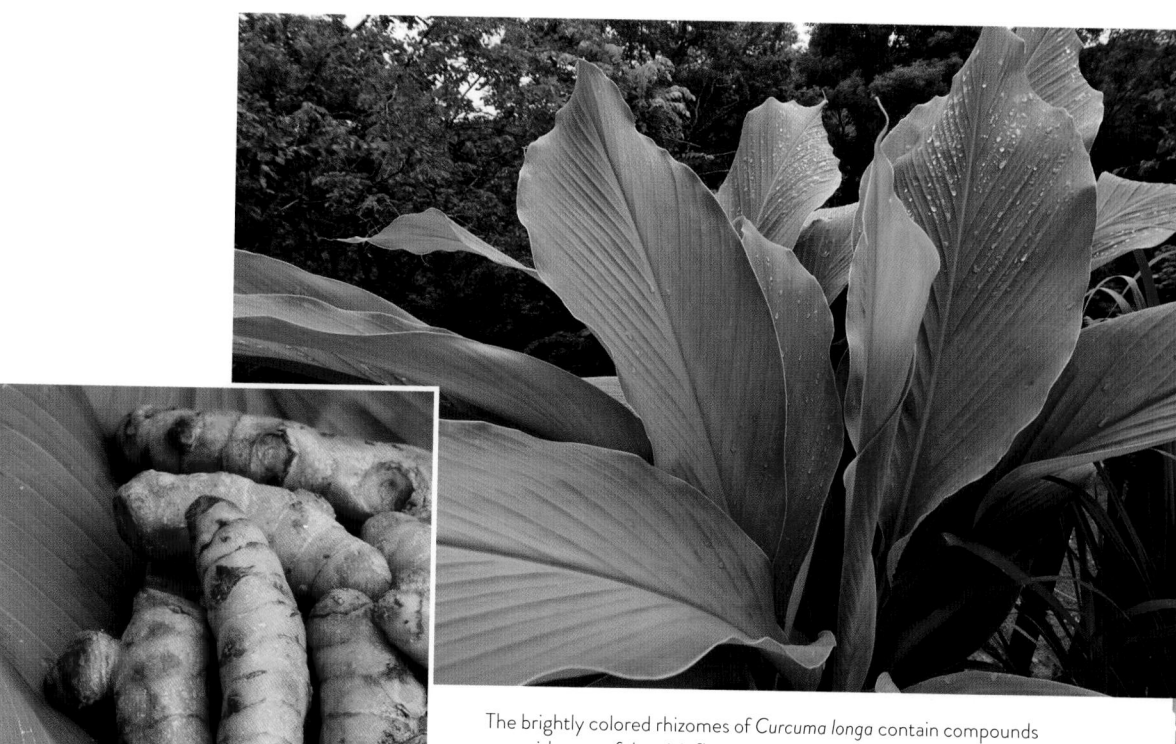

The brightly colored rhizomes of *Curcuma longa* contain compounds with powerful anti-inflammatory and antiseptic properties.

A Golden Healer

From time to time, I stay at Finca Luna Nueva Lodge in Costa Rica, an organic, biodynamic farm and ecotourism hotel surrounded by tropical rainforest. At this farm, the crops are carefully selected to build, not destroy, the soil. One of the farm's specialty crops is turmeric, a plant that I consider to be among the most important healing herbs.

For thousands of years, turmeric has been a premier plant of the Ayurvedic formulary. Its bright orange-yellow roots are used as food and medicine and in rituals. Applied to your skin, turmeric improves and tones your complexion, helps heal wounds, and improves acne. In India, a paste of turmeric root and ground lentils is traditionally used to wash the face and body, ridding the skin of bacteria, cleansing it, and curing skin conditions—all without the drying effects of soap. Skin treated with turmeric takes on a radiant beauty and pleasant golden glow.

As a food or herbal product, turmeric has extraordinary benefits, too. Recent medical research on both animals and humans has validated many of turmeric's traditional uses for the prevention and treatment of conditions associated with inflammation. These include certain cancers, heart disease, and type 2 diabetes. If you have a chance, take an hour to survey the research literature on turmeric via your favorite search engine—you will be astonished at the overwhelming evidence of its benefits. That's why turmeric is an important part of my diet and that of many health professionals whom I know.—M. J. B.

Cucurbita pepo

Native to the Americas and cultivated for more than 10,000 years, the pumpkin is valued for its colorful, edible fruit and healthful seeds. The thick-skinned fruit—borne on long, trailing vines—is commonly associated with holiday pies and Halloween jack-o'-lanterns. But for Native Americans, the pumpkin and other squashes (all members of the genus *Cucurbita*) were a dietary staple that they prepared in many different ways: baked, roasted, and mashed; added to soups and other dishes; or dried and then ground into a meal for use in puddings and sauces. Native Americans also used the pumpkin medicinally. Most widely used to expel worms, pumpkin seed was also employed as a diuretic, a skin cleanser and softener, and a treatment for arthritis.

CULINARY USE

Nearly all parts of the pumpkin—leaves, flowers, seeds, and fruit—can be used in cooking. Pumpkin blossoms, like those of other squashes, can be stuffed, dipped in batter, and then fried, or they can be baked into breads and cakes. Pumpkin leaves are good sources of vitamins A and C, iron, and calcium. Chop the tender young leaves and then steam them, or sauté them alone or with other vegetables. Try cooking them in a bit of canola oil along with chopped onion, garlic, and freshly grated ginger. Finish with lemon juice.

The versatile fruit, an excellent source of vitamin A, can be used in both savory and sweet dishes. Mash or puree the roasted flesh and serve it as a side dish, or use it in soups, cakes, pies, breads, puddings, pancakes, or cookies. Cubed pumpkin can be stir-fried with chiles and basil, added to curry dishes, or combined with coconut milk and spices for soup. To prepare a whole pumpkin as a main dish, slice off the top and scoop out the seeds and fiber; fill the interior with vegetable stew or a stuffing of bread cubes, cheese, garlic, and herbs, and then bake.

MEDICINAL USE

Research has found that pumpkin seeds exhibit antioxidant and anti-inflammatory properties. The seeds are dense in several nutrients, providing protein, fiber, iron, calcium, linoleic acid (believed to help prevent hardening of the arteries), and the minerals zinc and selenium (important for prostate health). Germany's official pharmacopoeia, known as the Commission E monographs, recommends eating 10 grams of ground or whole pumpkin seed daily for the treatment of irritated bladder conditions and the early stages of benign prostatic hyperplasia, a swelling of the prostate that affects urination. Eating pumpkin seeds could also help prevent osteoporosis and reduce the symptoms of inflammatory conditions.

PLANT PROFILE

Common Name: Pumpkin

Description: Herbaceous vine with hollow stems and large, deeply cut leaves; yellow flowers; large, thick-skinned fruits

Hardiness: Annual

Family: Cucurbitaceae

Flowering: Midsummer

Parts Used: Leaves, flowers, seeds, and fruit

Range/Habitat: Central, North, and South America; cultivated worldwide in temperate regions

---

HOW TO GROW IT

Pumpkin is easy to grow in average garden soil and full sun. To speed germination, scratch the seed coat lightly with a nail file. Plant seeds directly in your garden in spring, after all danger of frost has passed and the soil has completely warmed. (In cold climates, you can speed soil warming by using black plastic mulch.) Sow the seeds 1 inch deep, placing four to six seeds per 2-foot-diameter hill; space the hills 5 to 6 feet apart in rows 10 to 15 feet apart. Several weeks after the seeds have germinated, thin to two or three plants per hill. Feed the plants weekly with diluted fish emulsion or compost tea. Harvest pumpkins in fall, before the first heavy frost, when the fruits have attained a deep solid color and the skin has hardened. Use a sharp knife to cut fruit from the vine, allowing 3 to 4 inches of stem to remain attached to the fruit. Store the fruit in a dry location at 50° to 55°F.

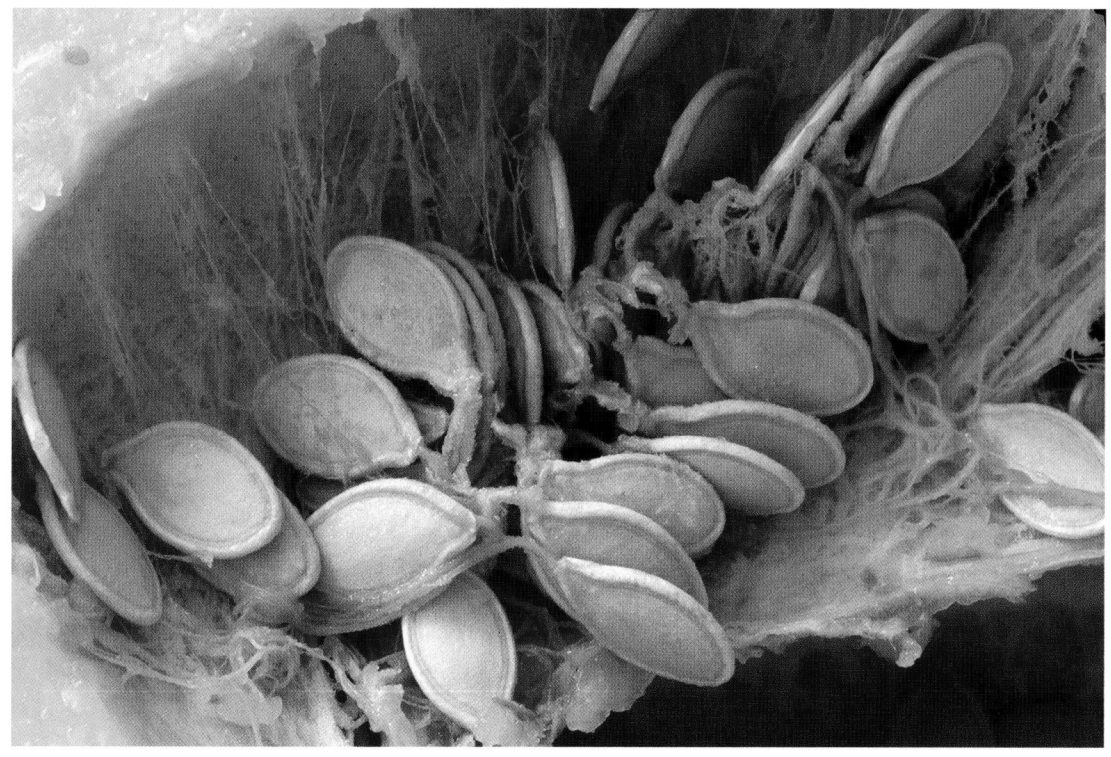

TOASTING PUMPKIN SEEDS

As you prepare a pumpkin for carving or cooking, save the seeds. Rinse off the yellowish fibers that surround the white seeds, then spread out the seeds and let them air-dry. Toast the dry seeds with a small amount of oil in a nonstick skillet, or place them on a nonstick baking pan or foil and toast them in a 250°F oven until crispy. (This usually takes less than an hour.) Lightly salted toasted pumpkin seeds (also called pepitas) make an excellent snack—even the shells are edible and are a good source of fiber. Experiment by adding garlic powder, cayenne pepper, or other herbs and spices for flavor. (If you dislike eating pumpkin hulls, grow 'Lady Godiva'—a variety that produces hull-less, or "naked," seeds.)

Cymbopogon citratus

PLANT PROFILE

Common Names: Fever Grass, Lemongrass, West Indian Lemongrass

Description: Clumping tropical grass, 3 to 6 feet tall, with long, linear leaves; small greenish flowers on curving stems; highly aromatic

Hardiness: To Zone 10

Family: Poaceae

Flowering: Rarely

Parts Used: Leaves, stems, and oil

Range/Habitat: Possibly native to southern India and Sri Lanka, naturalized in other tropical and subtropical regions

This thick-stemmed, dense perennial grass has sharply tapered leaves that emit a strong lemon scent when broken. The name *Cymbopogon* derives from the Greek words *kymbe* (boat) and *pogon* (beard)—a reference to the appearance of the tiny flowers of plants in this genus. Although the precise origin of lemongrass is unknown, scientists believe it could be native to the tropical region of southern India and Sri Lanka, where it has been used for centuries as a treatment for fevers, digestive problems, and nervous conditions.

CULINARY USE

Lemongrass is an integral part of Thai, Vietnamese, and Sri Lankan cuisines. The hearts are eaten as a vegetable with rice, and the chopped leaves are used for sauces, curries, and pastes, as well as in seafood, poultry, and pork dishes. A major source of lemon flavoring and fragrance, lemongrass is used commercially in ice cream, candies, and baked goods. At home, use lemongrass in curries, soups, stews, and seafood dishes—or whenever you want to add a refreshing lemony note to food or beverages without the acidity of lemon juice or lemon peel.

FIELD NOTES

Soothing Lemony Tea

When is a lemon a grass? When it is Cymbopogon citratus, a dense perennial grass found in the Philippines and other tropical regions of the world. Pull up a clump of this grass, close your eyes, and crush the leaves—a wonderful, pleasing, lemony aroma is released. Traditionally, people have made a hot tea from the leaves (sometimes along with the roots) for the treatment of fevers, coughs, and colds. The root was also mashed in local vegetable oil and used to massage sore backs and muscle spasms, as well as rubbed on the forehead to treat headaches. I drink lemongrass tea from time to time when traveling in areas where it is commonly grown and used.

To make the tea, steep a few crushed leaves in hot water for 5 minutes, allow the tea to cool, and enjoy this caffeine-free beverage. It will promote digestion and help you relax. If you can't grow this species outdoors, you can always find the leaves for sale at local ethnic markets or supermarkets—it is widely used in Thai cooking.

Lemongrass is closely related to one of the best-known plant-based insect repellents, citronella oil, which is derived from the leaves and stems of Cymbopogon nardus. Citronella is particularly effective as a mosquito repellent, and it's one of the products I carry in my backpack in the field when insects will be a problem.—M. J. B.

MEDICINAL USE

In East India and Sri Lanka, lemongrass tea (called "fever tea") is traditionally used to reduce fever, and modern herbalists also use the herb for this purpose. Because lemongrass is believed to relax your stomach and intestines, the tea is also used to help relieve flatulence and diarrhea. Lemongrass oil has antifungal and antiseptic properties. To treat skin conditions such as ringworm and athlete's foot, herbalists sometimes recommend a compress of lemongrass oil. You can also apply the leaves directly to your skin to repel insects.

OTHER USES

Highly aromatic lemongrass oil is one of the best-selling essential oils in the world. It is used commercially in perfumes, sachets, candles, cosmetics, and bath products. At home, you can infuse bathwater with this soothing herb: Fill a mesh bag with chopped lemongrass leaves, then place the bag under hot running water in your bathtub.

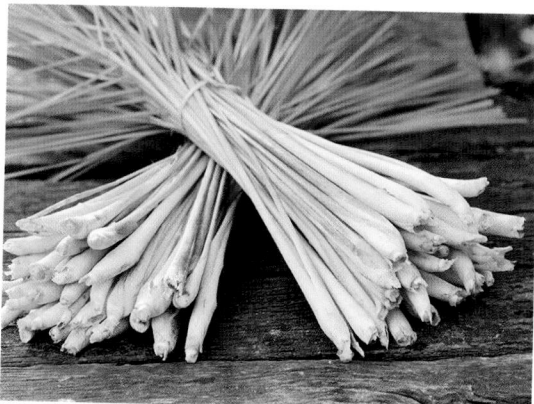

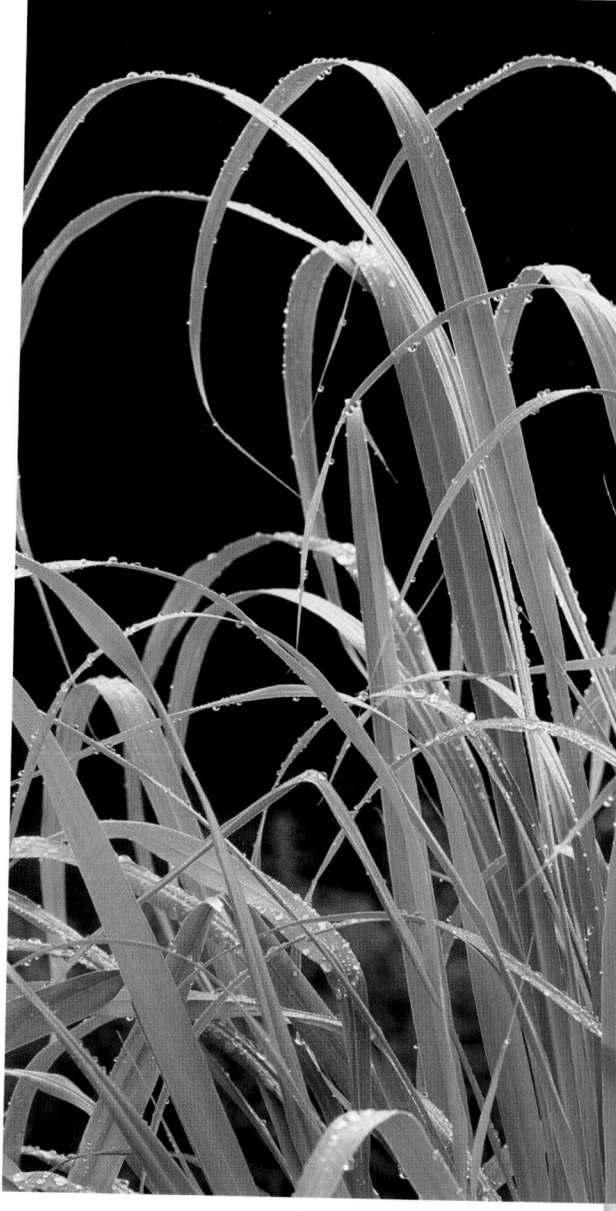

🌿 HOW TO GROW IT

Lemongrass thrives in tropical and subtropical climates in well-drained, fertile soil in full sun. In cold climates, you can try to root lemongrass clumps sold in Asian markets. Place a clump in a shallow container filled with about 1 inch of water. Several weeks later, after roots have formed, plant the lemongrass in a pot filled with a medium rich in organic matter. Or plant it directly in your garden, if all danger of frost has passed. Water regularly. Be sure to bring this tropical species indoors before the first frost, and you can enjoy it all winter. Harvest the bulb and leaves for cooking, or use the leaves to make a soothing tea. To propagate, divide and replant lemongrass roots in spring.

Digitalis purpurea

PLANT PROFILE

Common Names: Digitalis, Foxglove, Purple Foxglove

Description: Produces rosettes of downy leaves in its first year; spikes of 2- to 3-inch pink, purple, or white bell-shaped flowers follow in the second year; flower stalks up to 6 feet tall

Hardiness: Biennial; to Zone 4

Family: Plantaginaceae

Flowering: Late spring to midsummer

Parts Used: Leaves and flowers

Range/Habitat: Native to the Mediterranean region and Europe; woodland clearings and mountain slopes

Native to parts of Europe and Africa, this striking member of the plantain family is naturalized throughout North and Central America. Both the common name foxglove and the genus name *Digitalis* refer to the tubular shape of the plant's flowers, which appear to fit over the fingers like a glove. Digitalis derives from the Latin *digitus*, meaning finger. Although all parts of the plant are extremely poisonous, foxglove has been cultivated for medicinal use for more than 1,000 years. The 16th-century English herbalist John Gerard recommended boiling foxglove in water or wine for use as an expectorant. The herb's main use, for treating a weak heart, was not described until 1785, when English physician and botanist William Withering (1741–1799) published *An Account of the Foxglove and Some of Its Medicinal Uses.* (See "Field Notes" on page 157.)

MEDICINAL USE

Foxglove, a diuretic, contains cardiac glycosides that have been used in traditional and modern medicine to increase the force of the heart's contractions. In the past, the herb was taken in leaf form to treat irregular heartbeat and heart failure. Foxglove is still the source of the widely used pharmaceutical drugs digoxin and digitoxin—important therapies for heart disease—but the plant's leaves are no longer used because the correct dosage is hard to determine. In several cases, ingesting this powerful plant has resulted in death. In one, a closely related species was mistakenly added to a commercially sold internal herbal cleansing product, leading to cardiac arrest and death; apparently it was believed to be plantain leaf. In other cases, people harvest foxglove (confusing it with comfrey or another plant), use it as a tea, and become seriously ill.

Caution: Foxglove is extremely toxic and should *never* be ingested.

ORNAMENTAL USE

Gardeners love foxglove for its beauty. Its tall bloom spikes add early summer color to cottage gardens and mixed perennial borders, and the plants naturalize readily at woodland edges. Select tall cultivars, such as pink 'Giant Shirley' or rose-pink 'Candy Mountain', for a dramatic display in front of a stone wall, hedge, or fence. Foxglove combines well with goat's beard (*Aruncus dioicus*), bugbanes (*Actaea* spp.), and yuccas (*Yucca* spp.).

OTHER USES

Foxglove is sometimes used as a dye. When mordanted with alum (see page 397), the flowers produce a chartreuse color.

HOW TO GROW IT

Foxglove grows in moist, humus-rich soil in full sun or partial shade. Sow seeds indoors in seedling trays in late winter, then transplant the seedlings to the garden after the danger of frost has passed. Seeds can also be sown directly in your garden in late summer. Plants generally bloom the second year. Once established, foxglove needs little attention and will self-seed readily. For a more tidy look, lift the plants after they have finished flowering, remove the faded bloom stalks, and replant the remaining rosettes for next year's bloom.

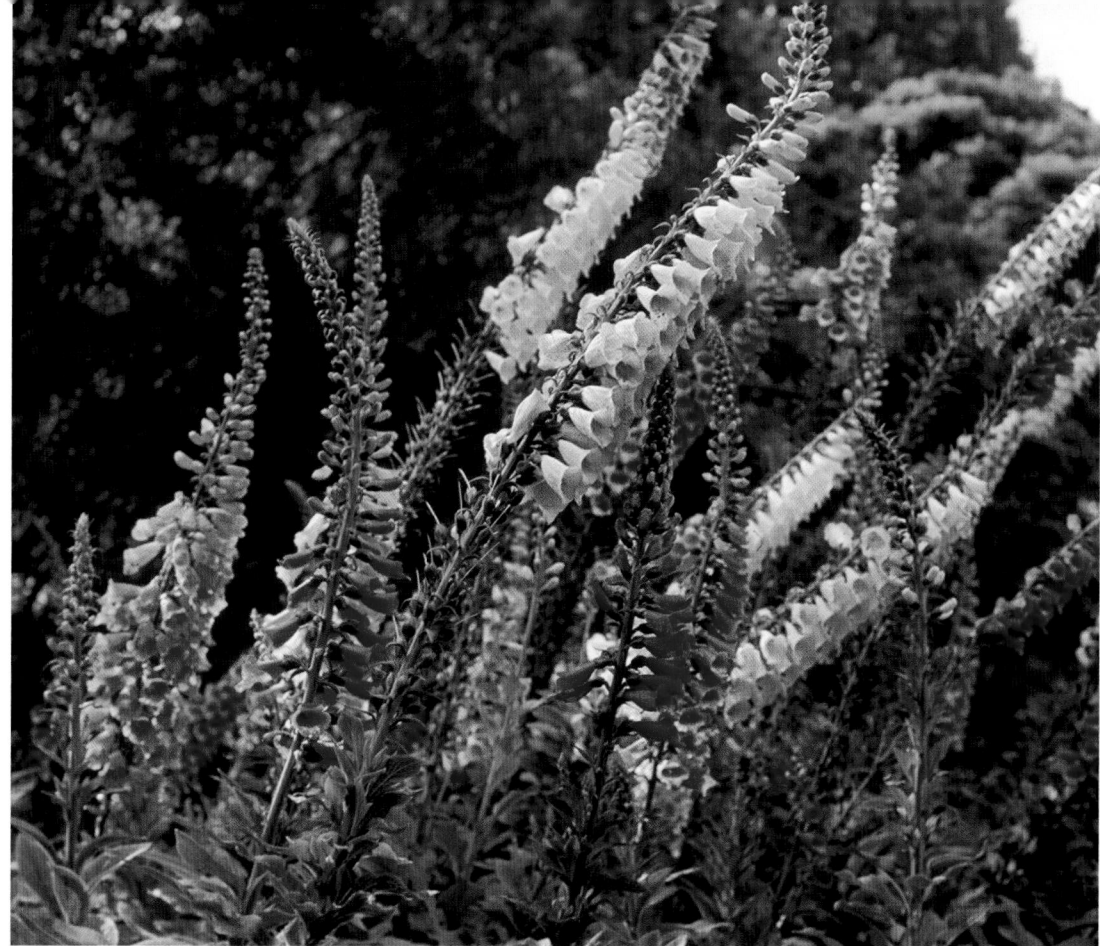

From an English Garden to the World's Pharmacy

In 1775, the English physician and botanist William Withering (1741–1799) was asked to evaluate a folk cure for "dropsy," an ancient name for the swelling caused by an accumulation of fluid (edema) in body cavities or under the skin. This condition produces the characteristic swollen ankles now known to be the result of congestive heart failure, which results when that organ can no longer pump enough blood throughout the body.

Withering found an herbal mixture used by a person he described as "an old woman in Shropshire, who had sometimes made cures after the more regular practitioners had failed." He identified more than 20 different herbs in her mixture and determined that foxglove was the "active herb." Withering then used foxglove to treat his patients with dropsy and observed that the herb controlled heartbeat in a different way than other medicines did. Over time, and with some failures,

his experiments resulted in more standardized foxglove extracts that successfully healed a high percentage of his patients. One contemporary evaluation of his therapies and their results suggested a success rate of 65 to 80 percent! It is remarkable that the plant used by the "old woman in Shropshire" has been, in its various forms, a first-line therapy for centuries. Sometimes, Grandmother knows best. —M. J. B.

Dioscorea villosa

The wild yam is native to North America and naturalized throughout the warmer regions of the world. Approximately 800 species make up the genus *Dioscorea*—a group of tropical and subtropical climbing plants. While some yam species produce tasty, edible tubers, the tubers of *D. villosa* are bitter and used primarily for medicinal purposes, especially to relieve abdominal cramping.

MEDICINAL USE

With strong anti-inflammatory properties, wild yam root has a history of medicinal use for cramping or contractions in the pelvic area, including false labor pains, menstrual cramps, uterine spasms, gallbladder pain, and intestinal spasms and cramps. Wild yam contains a steroidlike compound called diosgenin that once was used in contraceptive hormones such as birth control pills. Though wild yam is now widely promoted for menopausal symptoms, studies have found it to be no more effective than a placebo. Many wild yam creams (mostly marketed to ease menopausal symptoms) contain human progesterone created in a laboratory, often synthetically derived from diosgenin.

Caution: As a precaution, pregnant women, nursing mothers, and women with a history of hormone-related cancers should avoid wild yam.

PLANT PROFILE

Common Names: China Root, Colic Root, North American Wild Yam, Rheumatism Root, Wild Yam

Description: Deciduous vine up to 30 feet long; heart-shaped leaves; small, greenish white flowers; creeping woody roots with tuberous rhizomes

Hardiness: To Zone 6

Family: Dioscoreaceae

Flowering: June to August

Parts Used: Roots and tuber

Range/Habitat: Native to North America, naturalized throughout the warmer regions of the world; edges of woodland areas

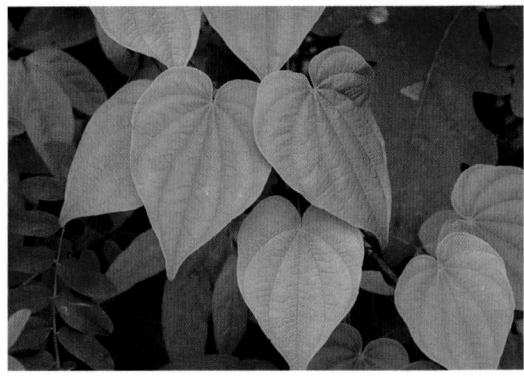

HOW TO GROW IT

Found in damp woodland areas, wild yam thrives in rich, well-drained soil in sun or partial shade. Plant root divisions in spring or fall, or plant seeds or bulbils in spring. Commercial preparations use the dried root, which is harvested in fall.

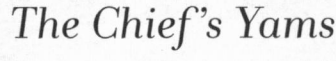

FIELD NOTES

The Chief's Yams

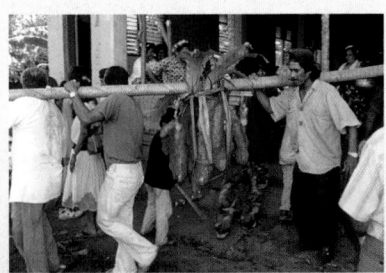

On the island of Pohnpei, in the Federated States of Micronesia, related yam species are a traditional source of food. Yams are also grown on that island for ceremonial presentation to the Chiefs. During the yam feast, tubers of the species Dioscorea alata are dug up, ceremonially presented, and then replanted so that they can continue to grow. I have seen yams of this type that weighed nearly 250 pounds. Local stories tell of the presentation of even larger yams—these yams are said to be the size of small cars and must be carried on poles by 10 or more men!—M. J. B.

Dysphania ambrosioides

(= Chenopodium ambrosioides)

PLANT PROFILE

Common Names: Epazote, Mexican Tea, Wormseed

Description: Multibranched reddish stems up to 4 feet tall; small, toothed leaves; clusters of small yellow-green flowers, followed by many shiny dark brown to black seeds; strongly aromatic

Hardiness: Annual or short-lived perennial

Family: Amaranthaceae

Flowering: Midsummer to late summer

Parts Used: Leaves

Range/Habitat: Native to Mexico and the tropical regions of Central and South America

An annual herb native to Mexico and the tropical or subtropical regions of Central and South America, epazote is widely naturalized in open areas, along roadsides, and around streambeds. In its various forms, this herb is both a medicine and a poison. The essential oil, which contains the compound ascaridole, can be toxic to humans when ingested in excess. Yet the plant has a long history of use as a remedy for intestinal parasites, first in the Americas and more recently in Europe and Asia. Epazote is also a popular culinary herb.

CULINARY USE

Traditionally used in Mexican cooking, epazote has a strong, pungent flavor and distinctive camphorlike aroma. It is a common ingredient in chilis, egg dishes, enchiladas, and tamales. Add the leaves to dishes and soups that include beans, corn, fish, or mushrooms. In bean dishes, it is reputed to help reduce intestinal gas and promote digestion.

MEDICINAL USE

Epazote was an important Native American medicinal plant. The herb was used in many forms to expel intestinal worms; one traditional treatment was to ingest a small quantity of the juice from the herb's crushed leaves, once daily, for several days in a row. To treat children, the herb was mixed with milk. Epazote was also used to treat stomach problems and headaches and was considered a spring tonic.

Caution: Many adverse reactions have been reported from the use of this plant for therapeutic purposes. Be cautious when using this herb medicinally or when handling the plant itself. Epazote has caused photosensitization (resulting in a red, swollen rash) in some people who have harvested it.

OTHER USES

This species is the main active ingredient in a botanical insecticide known as Requiem, used to control aphids, mites, thrips, and other sucking insects on fruit and vegetable crops.

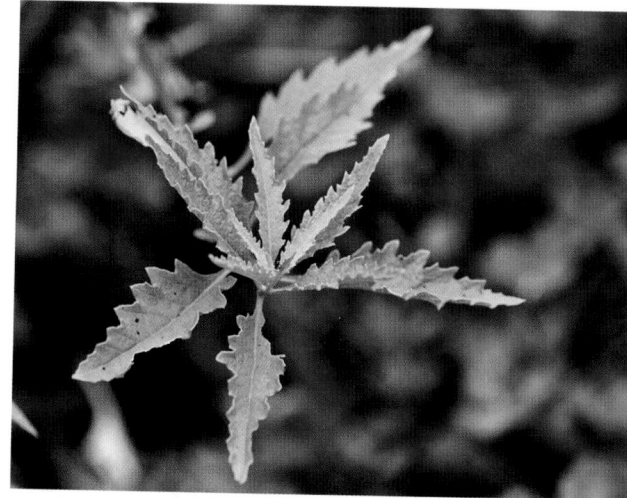

HOW TO GROW IT

Considered an invasive weed in some areas, epazote is easy to grow in well-drained soil and sun or partial shade. Pinch back the plants to encourage leafy growth and prevent flowering and seed formation. For cooking, harvest young leaves from plants that have not gone to seed. Epazote self-seeds readily.

Echinacea purpurea, E. angustifolia, E. pallida

PLANT PROFILE

Common Names: Echinacea, Kansas Snakeroot, Pale Coneflower, Purple Coneflower

Description: Sturdy stems 2 to 3 feet tall; coarsely toothed leaves up to 8 inches long; composite flowerhead with cone center surrounded by purple, pink, or white rays

Hardiness: To Zone 3

Family: Asteraceae

Flowering: July to August

Parts Used: Roots

Range/Habitat: Native to North America; found in open woodlands, roadsides, and fields

This native North American perennial bears showy purple, pink, or white daisylike flowers with large, orange-brown centers. Echinacea, derived from the Greek *echinos*, meaning "hedgehog," refers to the flower's bristly center.

Echinacea is among the most important plants in Native American traditional medicine. Fragments of the plant have been found in archaeological digs of Native American sites dating back to the 17th century. The herb was used as an analgesic to relieve pain and as a treatment for coughs, infections, colds, flus, snakebites, and superficial sores and wounds.

MEDICINAL USE

Three species, primarily, are used in herbal medicine: *Echinacea angustifolia*, recognized by its narrow leaves; *E. pallida*, known by its narrow, drooping petals; and *E. purpurea*, which is also often grown for its ornamental blooms. Echinacea roots, flowers, leaves, and seeds contain polysaccharides and other compounds that stimulate your immune system; the compounds in plants of this genus also have antimicrobial, antibacterial, and antiviral properties.

Clinical studies with some commercial preparations of echinacea have shown its ability to help reduce the symptoms and duration of upper respiratory infections and to prevent the common cold. The herb is most effective if taken during the earliest stage of infection. A tea made by simmering the root in water for 10 minutes, then straining it, can be taken up to three times a day to treat colds and flu. Echinacea salves and tinctures are excellent for healing skin wounds, cuts, canker sores, leg ulcers, and burns.

Caution: People sensitive to other plants in the aster family could experience an allergic reaction to echinacea. When purchasing echinacea products, choose those made with cultivated plants, as some species are endangered in the wild.

ORNAMENTAL USE

In your garden, echinacea is showy and easy to care for. Its deep taproots make it extremely tolerant of heat and drought.

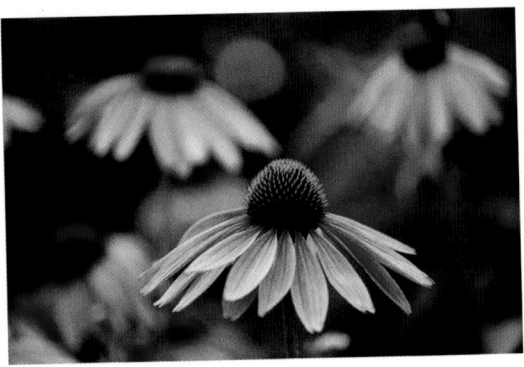

HOW TO GROW IT

Echinacea thrives in average, loamy soil in full sun. Sow the seeds in your garden in fall, or indoors in seedling trays in late winter. If sowing indoors, you can improve germination by refrigerating the seedling trays for 4 to 6 weeks before moving them to a bright place. Harvest the roots in fall; fall is also the best time to propagate echinacea by taking root cuttings. Leave the seed heads on the plants to provide winter food for birds.

Elettaria cardamomum

Cardamom, the seed of a tropical perennial in the ginger family, is one of the oldest spices in the world. Nearly 2,000 years ago, cardamom was considered the "queen of spices" and was sold along the trade routes of the Middle East and Europe. Native to humid forests of South India, the plant bears long, lance-shaped leaves and clusters of white flowers with purple-striped lips. Its fruits, or seedpods, are pale green and contain dark brown, highly aromatic seeds. The fragrance of the seeds is similar to that of eucalyptus, and it dissipates when the seeds are ground. In ancient Egypt, cardamom was used to make perfume.

CULINARY USE

Cardamom is widely used in both Scandinavian and East Indian cooking. It is one of the primary flavorings of the popular herbal beverage known as chai. Use cardamom seed to add a warm, spicy flavor to baked goods, curries, bean dishes, marinades, and fruit dishes. One medium-size pod contains 10 to 12 seeds, which make about ⅛ teaspoon of the ground spice. Use cardamom leaves as a flavorful wrap for fish, rice, or vegetables, or mince them and add them to curry dishes.

MEDICINAL USE

Cardamom contains an essential oil (up to 4 to 8 percent of the seed by weight) that supports the herb's traditional use as a digestive tonic. The herb "warms" and stimulates digestion, and it may relieve intestinal spasms and gas and ease stomach pain. A study in laboratory animals showed that compounds in cardamom helped inhibit stomach ulcers. Cardamom has a pleasant flavor and is often used in herb blends not only to ease digestion

but also to mask the flavor of less-pleasant herbs, such as bitter gentian (*Gentiana lutea*). Cardamom can also help sweeten breath, especially after eating garlic. The herb has been used for thousands of years in Ayurvedic medicine as a diuretic, expectorant, carminative, and energy booster. Some cultures consider it an aphrodisiac.

OTHER USES

Add the seeds to potpourris and sachets for a lovely spicy scent. The highly fragrant essential oil can be added to soaps, perfumes, bathwater, and body-care products.

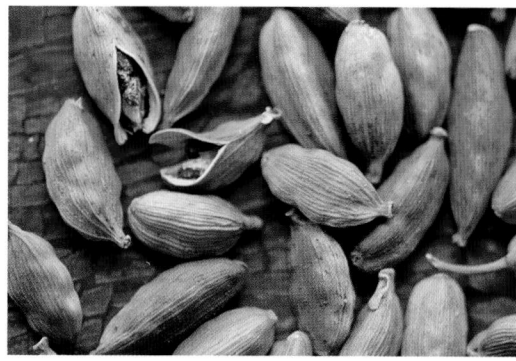

PLANT PROFILE

Common Names: Cardamom, Green Cardamom, True Cardamom

Description: Tropical perennial with stems 4 to 8 feet tall; dark green, lance-shaped leaves up to 1 foot long; small white flowers on trailing racemes; ribbed, light tan seedpods; thick rhizome

Hardiness: To Zone 10

Family: Zingiberaceae

Flowering: Periodically

Parts Used: Seeds and leaves

Range/Habitat: Native to India, Sri Lanka, and Malaysia; rainforests

---

 HOW TO GROW IT

Cardamom grows in tropical areas with rich, moist, well-drained soil and partial shade. In temperate regions, cardamom can be grown in a heated greenhouse or a very warm, humid location indoors. Although it will rarely flower or fruit indoors, you can still enjoy its handsome (and edible) leaves. Mist it daily and feed it with diluted fish emulsion during spring and summer. If seedpods do form, harvest them just before they open in fall.

Ephedra sinica

Ephedra is native to central Asia and is found throughout western China. The low-growing shrub has greenish stems and tiny, scalelike leaves. Ephedra—Greek for "climbing"—refers to the plant's tendency to climb across dry, rocky soil. Traces of the herb were found in a Middle Eastern grave dating back 60,000 years, suggesting that ephedra could have been used as a medicine as early as the Stone Age. Much folklore surrounds this powerfully stimulating plant. Zen monks reputedly used ephedra preparations to stay alert during protracted meditation and prayer. Guards in Genghis Khan's army also are said to have used ephedra—apparently the penalty for falling asleep at one's post was execution.

MEDICINAL USE

Ephedra was mentioned in the classic Chinese herbal *Shen Nong Ben Cao Jing,* written between 300 BCE and 200 AD. It is one of the first Chinese herbs to be widely used in Western medicine. Ephedra derivatives are the main ingredients in many over-the-counter decongestant pharmaceuticals. The herb had been an ingredient in preparations sold to stimulate weight loss and to boost energy and athletic performance, but after serious adverse effects in association with these products were reported, the FDA banned the use of ephedra in botanical supplements in 2004.

Ephedra contains ephedrine and pseudoephedrine, alkaloids that stimulate the central nervous system, elevate blood pressure, dilate the bronchi, decrease intestinal tone and motility, and cause cardiac stimulation and tachycardia. Ephedra is an effective nasal decongestant used to treat the common cold, sinusitis, and hay fever and to relieve the congestion of bronchial asthma and the symptoms of allergies. Side effects, including insomnia and high blood pressure, can occur when the recommended dosage of over-the-counter ephedra products is exceeded.

Caution: Ephedra and its chemical components may cause hypertension, insomnia, and, in large doses, even death. It should not be used by pregnant or nursing women or by people who suffer from anorexia, bulimia, or glaucoma. Ephedra acts as a thyroid stimulant and may increase the effects of pharmaceutical MAO inhibitors.

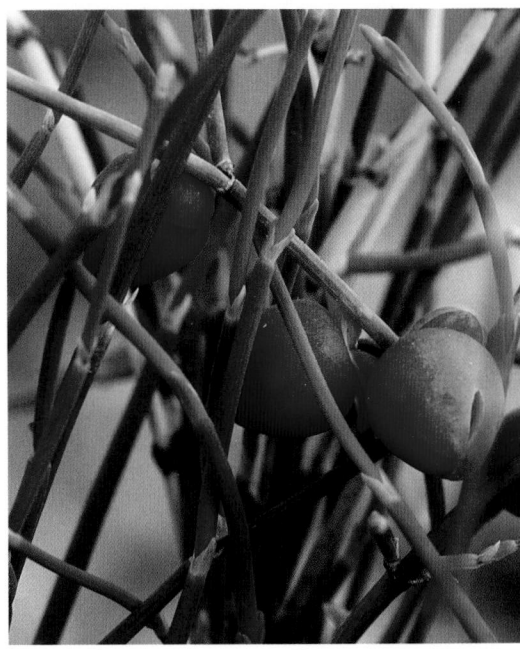

HOW TO GROW IT

Ephedra thrives in full sun and dry, sandy soil. If you wish to grow ephedra as a specimen or ornamental, plant it in well-drained gravelly soil in spring. Divide the roots in either spring or fall.

Epimedium spp.

This low-growing herb, which is native to China, has been used to treat kidney, liver, and joint disorders and to increase sexual desire in both men and women. Legend has it that long ago, a Chinese herder noticed his goats becoming more sexually excited and active after grazing on this plant. The herb's reputed aphrodisiac properties are thought to be due to the flavonoid compound icariin, which is closely related to compounds in at least two erectile dysfunction pharmaceuticals and works in a similar way to these modern medicines.

MEDICINAL USE

In traditional Chinese medicine (TCM), epimedium stems, leaves, and flowers are steeped in wine to make a treatment for impotence. The herb is said to increase sexual activity and the production of sperm and to stimulate sensory nerves. Epimedium appears to lower blood pressure (and could interact with drugs for hypertension). It also slows clotting and has been used in TCM to dissolve blood clots.

Caution: People who take medications that lower blood pressure or slow blood clotting should use this herb with caution.

PLANT PROFILE

Common Names: Epimedium, Horny Goat Weed, Yin Yang Huo

Description: Low-growing perennial up to 20 inches tall; arching stems of delicate rose or yellow blooms; heart-shaped leaves turn a copper color in fall

Hardiness: To Zone 4

Family: Berberidaceae

Flowering: Spring

Parts Used: Leaves

Range/Habitat: Native to China; woodlands

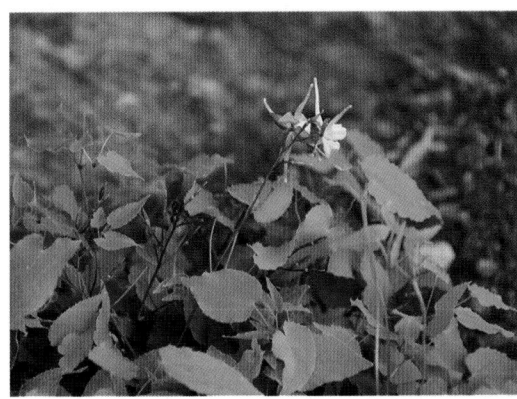

 HOW TO GROW IT

Epimedium, an attractive groundcover, thrives in moist, well-drained, acidic loam and shade. Plant it outdoors in spring after the danger of frost has passed. Mulch your plants with leaf compost to retain moisture. For medicinal use, harvest the leaves in summer or fall, 2 to 3 months after the plants flower. To propagate, divide roots in fall or early spring.

FIELD NOTES

Less Is More

The herbal section of your local health food market contains products with horny goat weed, used to treat impotence or enhance male sexual activity or desire. While the plant does contain a similar compound to those found in pharmaceutical drugs prescribed for this purpose, the plant contains a much lower dose, and other chemicals in the plant may contribute to its activity. On the Internet, I found herbal epimedium products that appeared to be "spiked" with icariin to levels many times that found in nature—closer to being a single compound pharmaceutical. However, pharmaceuticals, such as those for the treatment of impotence, are thoroughly studied before they are approved for sale. Their dosages are established through long-term controlled scientific studies, so these "enhanced" herbal products should be avoided.—M. J. B.

Equisetum arvense

PLANT PROFILE

Common Names: Bottle Brush, Horsetail, Scouring Rush

Description: Sharp-toothed leaf sheaths on jointed stalks topped with flower spikes; later, whorls of needle-like leaves appear on hollow, 18-inch stems

Hardiness: To Zone 2

Family: Equisetaceae

Flowering: Spring

Parts Used: Stems

Range/Habitat: Naturalized throughout most of the world; moist woods and roadsides

Horsetail has been called a "living fossil"—its relatives were abundant in forests more than 100 million years ago, and some of these ancient horsetails grew to 90 feet tall! Those towering species are now extinct, but the smaller descendants of this genus still grow in the wet areas of every continent except Antarctica. These herbaceous plants have hollow stems, scalelike leaves, and brownish cones borne at the ends of the stems. The stems contain silica, which explains the plant's common names "bottle brush" and "scouring rush." The stems can be dried and tied in bundles, then used as an abrasive to scour pots, shine metal, or sand wood. The belief that horsetail can strengthen nails, hair, teeth, and connective tissue is unsupported, however; your body cannot use silica in this form.

MEDICINAL USE

Horsetail contains flavone glycosides and a saponin, which are thought to account for its diuretic properties. Teas and extracts made from the dried stems are taken to treat bladder infections and kidney stones. Applied directly to a wound, the herb can help stop bleeding. Native Americans used *Equisetum arvense* to treat rashes, cuts, and sores; to promote urine flow; and to ease headaches, kidney troubles, and other problems. In China, *Equisetum hyemale* is used for various conditions, including fever and dysentery.

OTHER USES

Horsetail gives a yellowish green color to wool mordanted with alum and a deeper green when an iron mordant is used (see page 397). Although some cultures reportedly eat this plant, this probably isn't a good idea; some species contain a compound that destroys thiamine (vitamin B_1), a vitamin essential to all mammals. A thiamine deficiency can lead to the condition known as beriberi, which can result in severe sickness and even death.

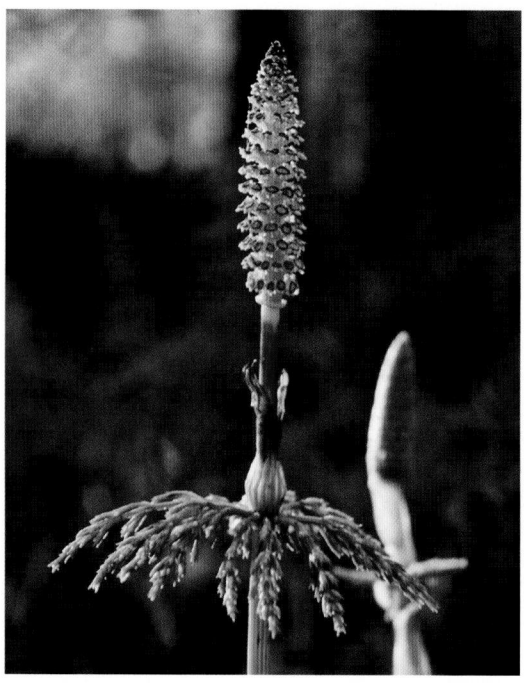

HOW TO GROW IT

Horsetail is rarely cultivated because once it's established, it can be extremely difficult to eradicate. If you wish to enjoy this interesting plant at home, plant it in a container and keep it just below the surface of a pond or water garden. Horsetail thrives in humus-rich, moist soil with an acid to neutral pH and full sun to partial shade. Harvest the stems in fall, when the silica content is highest. Propagate by division.

Eucalyptus globulus

A tall evergreen with large bands of shedding bark and bluish green, highly aromatic leaves, blue gum is the most familiar of the more than 600 eucalyptus species. The species is native to Australia and is commonly cultivated in Europe, Africa, India, and the Americas, including the southwestern United States. Long before it was carried to the West during the 19th century, blue gum was valued in traditional Australian Aboriginal medicine.

Also known as fevertree, blue gum played an important role in halting the spread of malaria in several countries during the 19th century. Planted in mosquito-infested marshes, the trees dried out the swampland through their heavy feeding, destroying the mosquitoes' breeding habitat. Researchers have also discovered that eucalyptus oil contains a compound as effective against mosquitoes that carry and transmit malaria as 20 percent DEET (N,N-diethyl-meta-toluamide, an active ingredient in many commercial insect repellents).

MEDICINAL USE

The tree's leaves contain eucalyptol, an active ingredient in over-the-counter chest rubs used for colds. Inhaling the vapor of a few drops of eucalyptus essential oil placed in boiling water can help clear sinus and bronchial infections.

With antiviral and antibacterial properties, essential oil of eucalyptus can be used to treat diseases such as flu, measles, and typhoid, and as an analgesic, anti-inflammatory rub for muscles and joints. Cooling on the skin, diluted eucalyptus oil also can be used topically to treat insect bites, stings, wounds, and blisters. Eucalyptus oil is used in mouthwashes to treat bad breath, plaque, and inflammation of the gums.

Caution: Never ingest pure eucalyptus oil, and always dilute it before applying it to your skin.

PLANT PROFILE

Common Names: Blue Gum, Eucalyptus, Fevertree, Southern Blue Gum, Tasmanian Blue Gum

Description: Evergreen tree, 50 to 80 feet tall, with large bands of shedding bark and bluish green, highly aromatic leaves

Hardiness: To Zone 8

Family: Myrtaceae

Flowering: Periodically

Parts Used: Leaves

Range/Habitat: Native to Australia, naturalized in North and South America, southern Europe, Africa, and India

Eucalyptus should not be used by those with severe liver disease, inflammatory disease of the bile ducts or gastrointestinal tract, or by children younger than 2 years old. Additionally, eucalyptus preparations should not be used on delicate areas, such as near the nose or eyes.

OTHER USES

Eucalyptus is used to make paper. High-quality honey is made from the nectar of some species of eucalyptus, and the didgeridoo, a traditional Aboriginal wind instrument, is made from eucalyptus stems that have been hollowed out by termites.

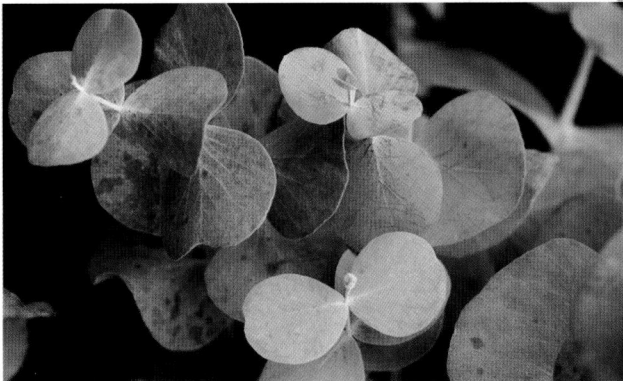

HOW TO GROW IT

Eucalyptus trees grow quickly in areas with warm summers, temperate winters, well-drained soil, and abundant sun. In Zone 7 and colder, grow eucalyptus in a greenhouse where temperatures remain above 50°F. Avoid overwatering; too much moisture causes the leaves to blister. Harvest the leaves before the tree flowers.

Filipendula ulmaria

This hardy perennial is native to Europe and Asia and has naturalized throughout North America. The herb was once called "meadwort," in reference to its use as a flavoring for the honey wine called mead. A member of the rose family, meadowsweet has attractive feathery foliage and creamy white, almond-scented flowers that are the source of the plant's other common name, queen of the meadow.

MEDICINAL USE

Meadowsweet was revered as a sacred herb by ancient Celtic Druid priests as early as 600 BCE and was mentioned in English herbal guide books dating to the 16th century. A tea made from the herb's flowers and leaves was used to treat feverish colds and to alleviate pain in muscles and joints. Aspirin, one of the world's most common and important drugs, was developed from the meadowsweet plant. In 1597, John Gerard recommended this plant, boiled in wine, be consumed to treat bladder pain. In 1839, the compound salicylic acid was identified from its flower buds and

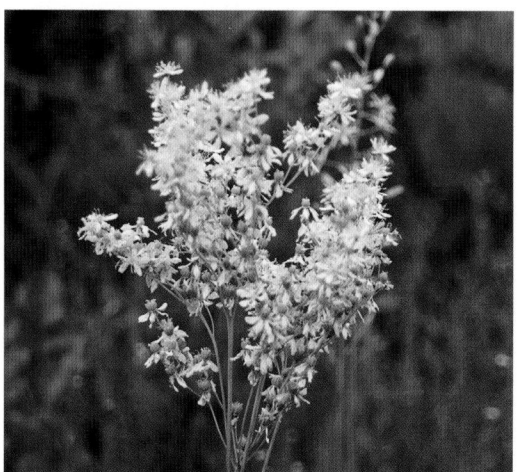

became widely used to treat pain—but one side effect was an upset stomach. In 1899, the company Bayer AG began to sell a synthetic form of this compound known as acetylsalicylic acid, which was more potent but had fewer side effects. The name chosen for the new compound was aspirin—a combination of "a" for acetyl and "spirin" for spiraea, the former name of the meadowsweet plant. Meadowsweet also acts as a carminative and antacid, soothing the digestive tract, reducing acidity, and relieving nausea. It has been used to treat gastritis and peptic ulcers. Because it has a gentle astringent effect, it is useful for treating diarrhea in children.

Caution: People with a sensitivity to aspirin (salicylates) should avoid using meadowsweet.

OTHER USES

Meadowsweet flowers are made into an essential oil with a wintergreen scent and are used in potpourris. When added to cooked fruits and jams, the flowers impart a flavor reminiscent of almonds. The plant's roots yield a black dye.

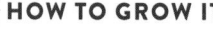

HOW TO GROW IT

Meadowsweet thrives in rich, moist soil in sun or partial shade. If the foliage becomes tattered, cut the plants to the ground and fresh leaves will emerge. Clumps spread rapidly and require frequent division; lift and divide them in fall.

Fragaria vesca

Alpine strawberry, a member of the rose family, is native to Europe and Asia and is widely naturalized in northern temperate areas. Based on archeological evidence, it appears that people have been eating the plant's fruits for at least 10,000 years—perhaps longer. Alpine strawberry was first cultivated in ancient Persia; from there, its seeds were carried and planted in many other areas. Compared to the modern cultivated strawberry, a hybrid, the everbearing alpine strawberry bears smaller, more aromatic fruits. The plants are low-growing, evergreen, and very hardy.

CULINARY USE

Alpine strawberry leaves are frequently used in herbal tea blends. The small, delicious fruits can be eaten fresh; cooked in desserts, preserves, and sweet or savory dishes; or made into wine.

MEDICINAL USE

Alpine or wild strawberry was traditionally used to treat liver and digestive disorders as well as gum disease. Seventeenth-century herbalist Nicholas Culpeper (1616–1654) advised that "the leaves and roots boiled in wine and water, and drank, [will] cool the liver and blood . . . [and] provoke urine."

Today, strawberry leaf tea is used to treat diarrhea and infections of the gastrointestinal and urinary tracts. The fruits, which contain vitamins B, C, and E, have mild diuretic properties. A natural bleach, the fruits can be crushed and mixed with baking soda to clean stained teeth or applied externally as a poultice to lighten skin and soothe sunburn. Strawberry is used as a homeopathic remedy for skin and mouth conditions.

PLANT PROFILE

Common Names: Alpine Strawberry, Fraises Des Bois, Wild Strawberry, Woodland Strawberry

Description: Compact perennial, up to 10 inches tall; evergreen, coarsely toothed, tripartite leaves; flat, white flowers; small, cone-shaped white to red fruit studded with brown seeds

Hardiness: To Zone 4

Family: Rosaceae

Flowering: Spring and summer

Parts Used: Fruit, leaves, and roots

Range/Habitat: Native to Europe and Asia and naturalized in northern temperate areas; found in fields, open woodlands, along paths, and in clearings

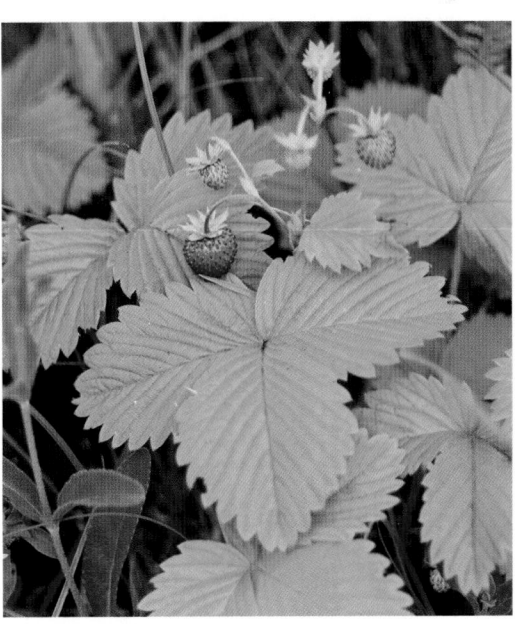

HOW TO GROW IT

Native to woodland areas, alpine strawberries thrive in well-drained, humus-rich, acidic soil and partial shade. Cultivated varieties that produce few or no runners make a neat, attractive groundcover or edging plant. Sow the seeds in your garden in fall or indoors in late winter, directly on the soil surface—do not cover them. The seeds germinate best in consistently moist soil at a temperature of 65° to 75°F. Water plants regularly throughout the growing season; they will slow or stop producing if they receive less than 1 inch of water per week. Harvest the berries when they are fully ripe; gather the leaves as needed throughout the season. Divide 3- or 4-year-old plants in fall.

Frangula purshiana

(= Rhamnus purshiana)

Native to the Pacific Northwest region of the United States, this deciduous tree is a member of the buckthorn family, bearing dark green, serrated leaves and scarlet berries that ripen to black. Seventeenth-century Spanish explorers named it *cascara sagrada* (or "sacred bark"), perhaps because of its value to Native Americans as a medicinal plant. The most important use of the distinctive reddish gray bark was as a laxative. Settlers to the West learned to make a tea by soaking a piece of the dried bark in cold water overnight. In 1877, the pharmaceutical company Parke-Davis first marketed the herb, and a year later, the company introduced a liquid extract of cascara bark as a treatment for constipation.

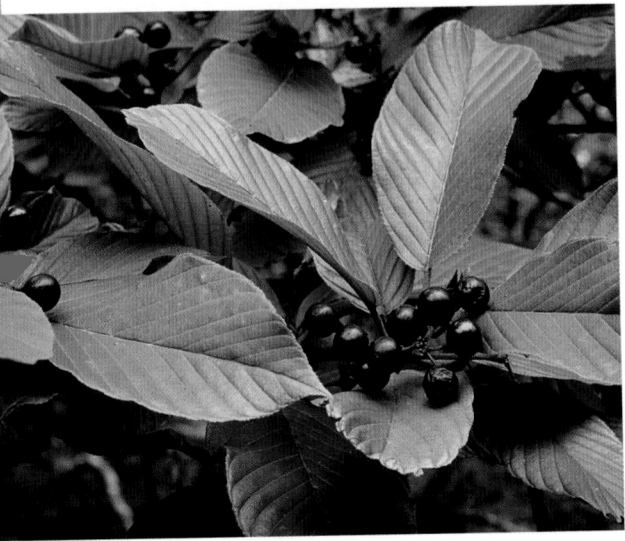

PLANT PROFILE

Common Names: Cascara Sagrada, Sacred Bark

Description: Deciduous tree or shrub, 5 to 25 feet tall; 2- to 6-inch-long veined leaves with serrated edges; umbels of greenish yellow flowers followed by small scarlet to black berries

Hardiness: To Zone 7

Family: Rhamnaceae

Flowering: Spring

Parts Used: Bark

Range/Habitat: Native to the Pacific Northwestern United States and western Canada; high-altitude forests, thickets, and canyon walls

MEDICINAL USE

The tree's bark contains a gentle laxative that stimulates contractions of the large intestine, helping to move food through the digestive system. In 2002 the FDA issued a ban on over-the-counter stimulant laxative drug products that contain cascara sagrada. Today, cascara sagrada can be purchased as an herbal supplement.

Caution: Cascara sagrada should not be used by pregnant women, nursing mothers, or young children; tell your health-care provider that you are using this laxative. Overuse of stimulant laxatives such as cascara sagrada and aloe can create a dependency on their use.

OTHER USES

The bark of cascara sagrada can be used to dye wool various shades of gray, brown, and yellow. The tree's wood has been used for making fence posts and as fuel.

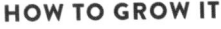

HOW TO GROW IT

A shrub or small tree, cascara sagrada grows in moist, fertile soil and full sun to partial shade in Zone 7 and warmer. It can be propagated by seed, layering, or cutting. For medicinal use, harvest the bark in spring or fall. Before use, cure the bark for at least 1 year. Aging is essential because consuming the fresh bark can cause vomiting and intestinal spasms.

Galium odoratum

Once used as a scenting herb in homes and churches and as a stuffing for mattresses, sweet woodruff is a perennial groundcover native to Europe, North Africa, and Asia. When cut and dried, the plant's leaves and stems smell pleasantly of vanilla and freshly mown grass. The fragrance can persist for years due to the presence of coumarin, a chemical used as a fixative for perfumes.

MEDICINAL USE

Sweet woodruff has diuretic properties and can stimulate perspiration, helping your body eliminate waste through your skin. Coumarin, present at about 1 percent in this species, dilates blood vessels, which increases blood flow. This compound is used as the basis for anticoagulant drugs such as warfarin.

Native Americans traditionally used several related species of *Galium* to treat skin problems such as eczema, poison ivy, and ringworm, as well as gallstones, kidney trouble, and many other conditions. Some tribes considered the plant poisonous.

Caution: In large doses, coumarin can be toxic.

ORNAMENTAL USE

Sweet woodruff forms a lovely, low-maintenance groundcover in shaded locations, particularly beneath azaleas, rhododendrons, and hydrangeas. It establishes quickly and is rarely bothered by pests or diseases. Plant it along pathways, intermingled with spring-blooming bulbs, or under bleeding heart (*Dicentra spectabilis*).

OTHER USES

The flowers and leaves add a sweet vanilla fragrance to potpourris, herbal wreaths, sachets, and perfumes; the dried leaves have also been used to

PLANT PROFILE

Common Names: Sweet Woodruff, Sweet-Scented Bedstraw

Description: Perennial groundcover, up to 8 inches tall; small, white flowers; narrow leaves in whorls of six or eight around each stem

Hardiness: To Zone 3

Family: Rubiaceae

Flowering: May and June

Parts Used: Whole plant

Range/Habitat: Native to Europe, North Africa, and Asia; found in moist, wooded locations

repel moths. The stems and leaves make a tan dye in wool mordanted with alum (see page 397); the roots yield a red dye.

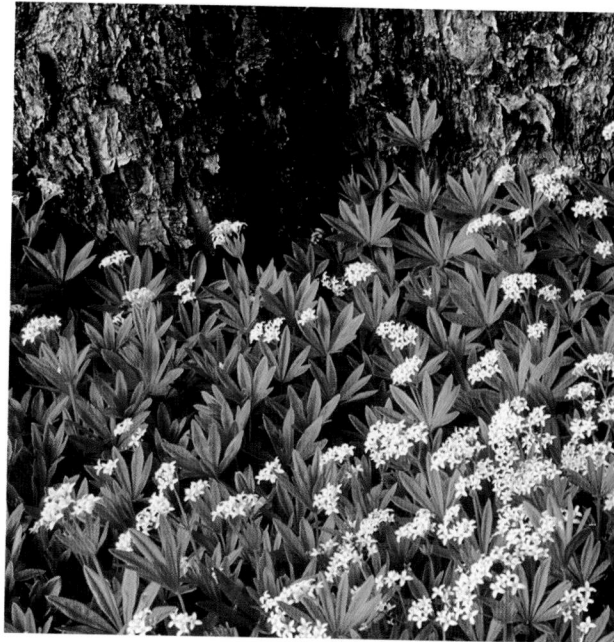

HOW TO GROW IT

A woodland plant, sweet woodruff thrives in moist, well-drained humus and shade. Provide an acidic soil rich in nutrients; leaf mold compost is ideal. After planting in spring, mulch to retain moisture and control weeds. Harvest sweet woodruff foliage as needed. To dry the sprigs, hang them in a warm, dark, airy place, or chop the herb immediately and spread it out to dry in shade.

Caution: There are reports of allergic skin reactions from handling plants in this genus.

Gaultheria procumbens

Wintergreen, known for its stimulating aroma and minty flavor, is a low-growing evergreen native to North America. Although the familiar flavor is now produced synthetically, oil of wintergreen was once used in many popular candies, cough drops, chewing gums, and toothpastes.

Native Americans used wintergreen medicinally to treat a wide variety of conditions. During the American War of Independence, some colonists substituted wintergreen for imported British tea, hence the common name teaberry.

CULINARY USE

Wintergreen's edible berries and leaves—which have a delightful, spicy flavor—are a favorite of foragers from fall through early spring. Clark's Teaberry chewing gum, first produced in the early 1900s, was inspired by the flavor of wintergreen.

MEDICINAL USE

Native Americans such as the Penobscot, Sioux, and Nez Perce traditionally used wintergreen leaf tea to relieve fever, sore throat, upset stomach, and ulcers. They crushed the leaves to make a poultice for treating muscle, nerve, and joint pain, as well as swelling, rash, inflammation, and toothache. Wintergreen stimulates temperature-sensitive nerve endings, temporarily overriding nearby pain signals. The plant contains methyl salicylate, a compound with properties similar to those found in aspirin. Primarily used in over-the-counter topical ointments, methyl salicylate is now produced synthetically.

Caution: Wintergreen oil can be toxic if consumed even in small amounts. People sensitive to aspirin should not use wintergreen or other products containing methyl salicylate in any form

PLANT PROFILE

Common Names: Eastern Teaberry, Teaberry, Wintergreen

Description: Creeping perennial, up to 6 inches tall; glossy, evergreen leaves and tiny, bell-shaped white flowers; round, red berries appear in late summer and persist through winter

Hardiness: To Zone 4

Family: Ericaceae

Flowering: Midsummer

Parts Used: Leaves and berries

Range/Habitat: Native to eastern North America; wooded areas and clearings

(including topical creams), as this compound is absorbed easily into the bloodstream.

ORNAMENTAL USE

With its glossy, evergreen foliage and bright red berries, wintergreen is an attractive, low-maintenance plant for shaded locations, such as woodland gardens. Although it rarely forms a dense carpet, wintergreen mixes beautifully with other woodland plants, such as blueberry and bunchberry dogwood (*Cornus canadensis*).

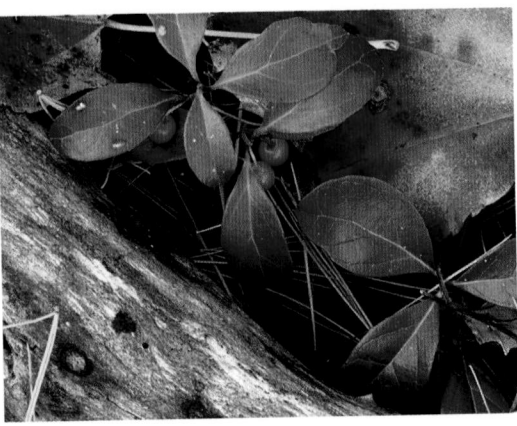

HOW TO GROW IT

Wintergreen grows best in partial shade and evenly moist, fertile soil with an acid pH of 5.0 to 6.0. Native to hardwood and pine forests, wintergreen benefits from pine straw mulch, which will help retain moisture and block weeds. Water it regularly during dry periods. Wintergreen leaves can be harvested at any time; gather the berries when they're red, which signals that they're ripe.

Gentiana lutea

Gentian, a brightly colored ornamental plant with large golden flowers, is perhaps best known for its bitter-tasting roots, which are used to flavor vermouth and Angostura bitters. Native to mountainous regions of central and southern Europe and western Asia, gentian is cultivated commercially in North America and Europe. *Gentiana,* the genus name, derives from Gentius (180–167 BCE), a king of ancient Illyria said to have discovered the herb's medicinal values.

PLANT PROFILE

Common Names: Gentian, Yellow Gentian

Description: Herbaceous perennial, up to 6 feet tall; bright yellow, 2-inch flowers from axils of uppermost leaf pairs; smooth, oval leaves up to 6 inches across and 1 foot long

Hardiness: To Zone 5

Family: Gentianaceae

Flowering: July and August

Parts Used: Roots

Range/Habitat: Native to the mountains of Europe and western Asia; cultivated in Europe and North America

MEDICINAL USE

Gentian's bitter flavor is so strong that it is detectable even at dilutions of 1:20,000. The herb's rhizomes and roots contain components that stimulate the production of saliva, bile, and gastric juices, thereby improving appetite and digestion. Gentian is the major ingredient in dozens of digestive bitters and tonics taken before eating a heavy meal, particularly one rich in fatty foods. It is also recommended as a treatment for anemia and as an appetite stimulant during periods of convalescence. Gentian is said to have anti-inflammatory properties, and herbalists consider it a tonic and energizer.

Caution: Gentian should not be used by those who have gastric or duodenal ulcers, irritation, or inflammation. Pregnant women and people with high blood pressure should also avoid this herb.

ORNAMENTAL USE

Gentians of all kinds are valued for their beauty in rock gardens and informal wild gardens.

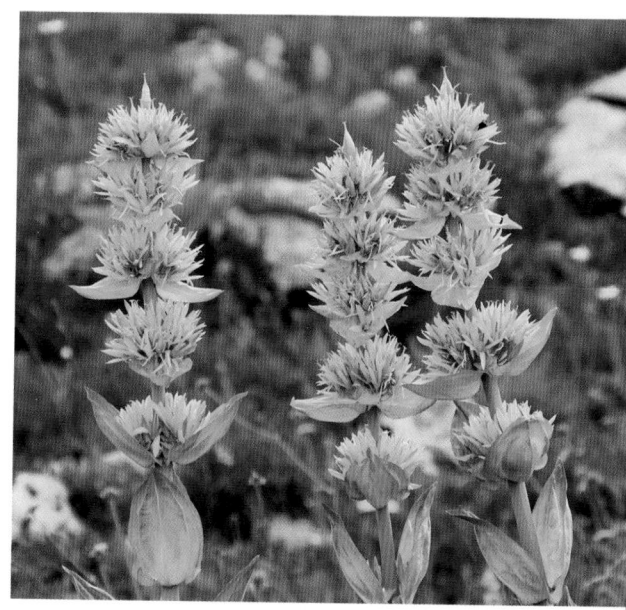

HOW TO GROW IT

Gentian grows best in moist, rich soil with good drainage and bright light, although it will tolerate partial shade. Plant the seeds directly in your garden in fall, or plant crown divisions in spring. (When started from seed, gentian begins to flower in about 3 years.) If you garden in the colder parts of gentian's range and receive little or no snow cover, protect the plants with a winter mulch of straw or evergreen boughs.

Gentian roots take as long as 10 years to reach maturity. The roots, which can be harvested in late summer or fall, must be cured by drying before they can be powdered and used. Good-quality roots are dark reddish brown, tough, and flexible, with a strong odor. They should taste sweet at first, then deeply bitter.

Ginkgo biloba

Ginkgo is the world's most ancient tree and the only surviving member of its genus. Native to China, where it has long been considered a sacred species, the ginkgo was first planted in the United States in 1784 on an estate near Philadelphia. The tree is rarely found in the wild today, and scientists debate whether even these small stands are truly wild.

The name ginkgo comes from the Japanese *gin* (silver) and *kyo* (apricot). Because the plant is believed to have positive effects on memory, brain function, and circulation, it has been called the "antiaging" herb and is one of the best-selling herbal supplements in the United States. Ginkgo is grown commercially in the United States, France, China, and Japan.

CULINARY USE

Although raw ginkgo seeds can be toxic, the cooked seeds (called nuts) are considered a delicacy in China. To obtain ginkgo nuts, remove the fruit pulp, then crack open the nuts' outer shell. (Wear gloves when you do this; the fruits are notoriously foul-smelling, and handling the nuts can cause contact dermatitis in some people.) In China, ginkgo nuts are added to vegetable and rice dishes and are served at weddings and other special occasions. In Japan, the nuts are eaten after meals to aid digestion.

MEDICINAL USE

Ginkgo seeds have been used as medicine in Asia for thousands of years. The Chinese eat cooked ginkgo nuts to increase strength and sexual energy and to restore hearing loss. Boiled as a tea, the nuts are used to treat coughs, asthma, allergies, and wheezing.

PLANT PROFILE

Common Names: Ginkgo, Maidenhair Tree

Description: Large deciduous tree, up to 100 feet or taller; fan-shaped leaves are deeply notched to form two lobes; females bear yellow-orange, odoriferous fruits

Hardiness: To Zone 3

Family: Ginkgoaceae

Flowering: On separate male and female trees, appearing in March and April

Parts Used: Leaves and seeds

Range/Habitat: Native to China; cultivated in Asia, France, and southeastern United States

Modern herbalists primarily use ginkgo leaves. The leaves have antioxidant properties and contain flavonoids (called ginkgo flavone glycosides) and terpenoids (called ginkgolide and bilobalide) that could help improve blood flow to the extremities and to the brain, eyes, and ears, particularly in the elderly. Ginkgo supplements have been researched for the treatment of tinnitus, high blood pressure, and concentration and memory problems, as well as for slowing the progression of Alzheimer's disease. While there are clinical studies that showed promise in this area, several recent studies have failed to substantiate the supplements' effectiveness for these conditions. Because of the plant's ability to dilate blood vessels, the herb is also used to treat intermittent claudication (intense cramping in the calf muscles).

OTHER USES

Ginkgo leaf extract, rich in flavonoids and diterpenes, is used widely in cosmetics, shampoos, and skin creams. The hardy, long-lived trees are often planted along city streets. They're also a favorite subject for bonsai.

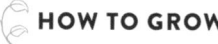

HOW TO GROW IT

Ginkgos are commonly grown for their beauty and ability to withstand cold temperatures, pollution, insect pests, and diseases. Plant ginkgo in full sun and well-drained, fertile soil. Most home gardeners plant only male trees grafted from other males to avoid the smelly fruits borne by females. If you wish to harvest ginkgo nuts, however, you'll need to plant both male and female trees. Prune young trees to a central leader. For making an extract, harvest the leaves in fall and then dry them.

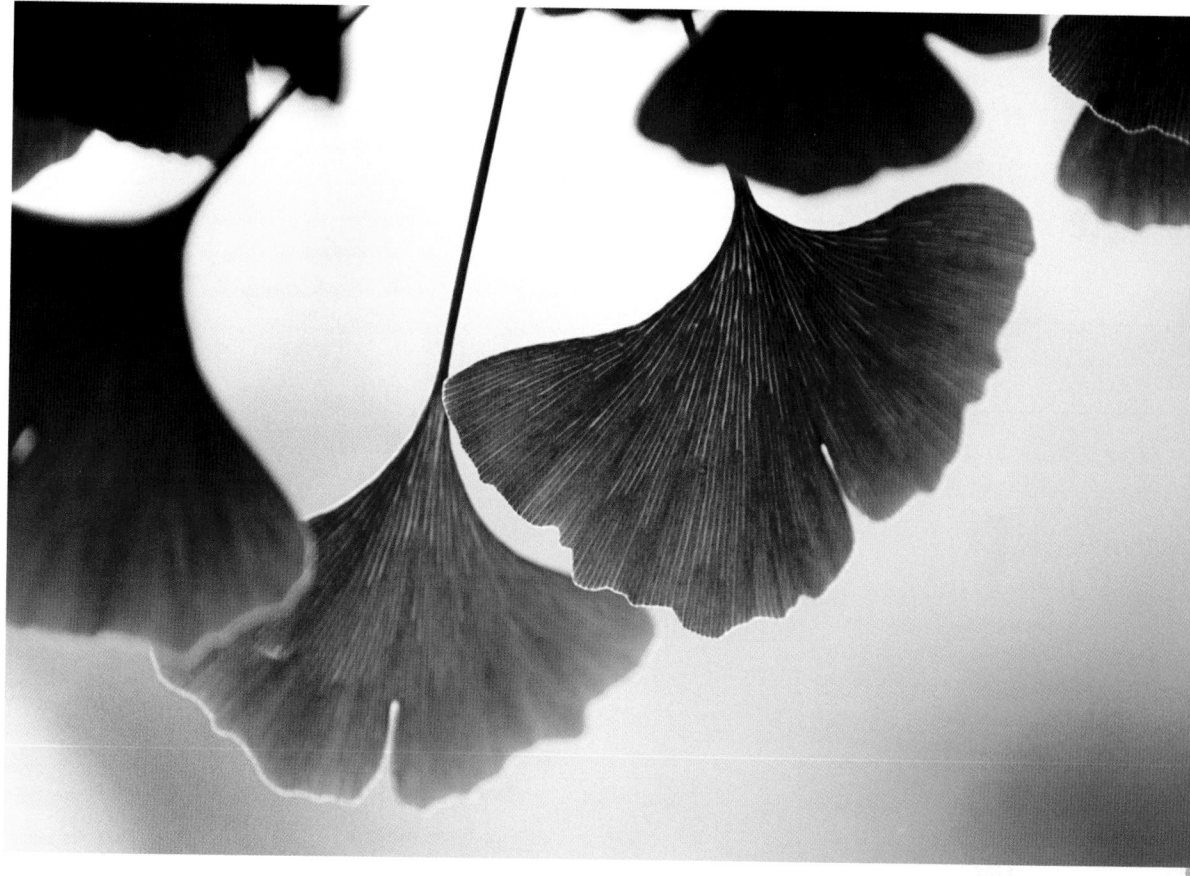

An Ancient Memory

During fall in New York City, I often see families collecting ripe ginkgo fruit beneath the city's female ginkgo trees. Ginkgo seeds—found inside the orange-yellow fruits—are highly valued in the cuisines of China, Korea, and Japan. While some cities no longer plant female ginkgo trees because of the fruits' terrible odor, caused by butanoic acid, the stately ginkgo certainly deserves a place in modern cities.

For me, looking at a ginkgo tree is a humbling experience, as it is considered a "living fossil." The genus Ginkgo is known from Chinese paleobotanical specimens more than 200 million years old. The renowned botanist Carl Linnaeus named the plant in 1771, basing the genus name Ginkgo on the plant's Japanese common name and the species name biloba on the two lobes found on each leaf. Ginkgo arrived in the United

States through the botanist and plant explorer André Michaux in the late 1700s. Today, this ancient Chinese medicine is being studied extensively to evaluate its efficacy in the treatment of conditions ranging from lung problems to memory loss. The next time you see a ginkgo, remember that its ancestors have been around for as long as Mother Nature can remember.—M. J. B.

Glycyrrhiza glabra

A member of the pea family native to the Mediterranean region and Asia, licorice is a perennial with downy stems and pale blue flowers that appear in loose spikes. The plant's deep taproot sends out thin, horizontal rhizomes. The Greek name for the plant is "sweet root" and, in fact, licorice root is about 50 times sweeter than sugar. Although licorice is often associated with a candy flavoring, most licorice-flavored candy today is flavored with anise oil. Licorice has a very long history of therapeutic use, however, and herbalists still value it for its pharmacological properties.

CULINARY USE

Licorice makes a flavorful herbal tea. Commercial producers of beers and soft drinks, pastries, ice creams, puddings, and soy products use licorice extract as a flavoring.

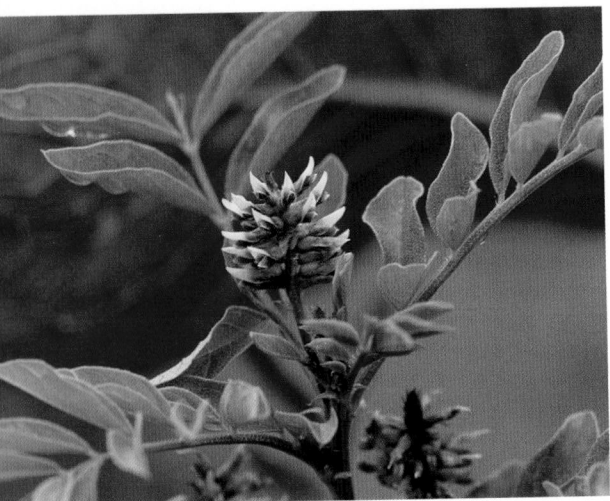

PLANT PROFILE

Common Names: Licorice, Russian Licorice, Spanish Licorice, Turkish Licorice

Description: Erect, branching perennial, up to 6 feet tall; spikes of ½-inch pale blue to violet flowers; alternate, pinnate leaves with 9 to 12 leaflets; long taproot

Hardiness: To Zone 7

Family: Fabaceae

Flowering: Midsummer

Parts Used: Roots

Range/Habitat: Native to the Mediterranean region and central and southwest Asia

MEDICINAL USE

Licorice has anti-inflammatory properties and has traditionally been used as a treatment for arthritis and allergies. Modern herbalists also use the herb as an expectorant and demulcent because it stimulates mucus secretions of the trachea. Its soothing effect on mucous membranes makes it useful for treating sore throats and coughs, as well as for protecting and healing your gastrointestinal tract.

The primary component of licorice root is glycyrrhizin, a compound that acts much like cortisol, stimulating the excretion of hormones by the adrenal cortex. For this reason, licorice is thought to benefit people suffering from adrenal weakness. However, glycyrrhizin can also cause water retention and an increase in blood pressure. To reduce these side effects, researchers have developed a form of the herb called deglycyrrhizinated licorice, or DGL, from which 97 percent of the glycyrrhizin has been removed.

To make licorice tea, simmer 1 teaspoon of the dried and sliced root in 1 cup of water for 10 minutes. Strain. Drink two or three times per day for up to 7 days.

Caution: Do not take this herb if you are pregnant or have heart or liver disease or hypertension.

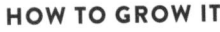

HOW TO GROW IT

Licorice grows in full sun and rich, moist, sandy loam. Plant divisions or cuttings in a prepared garden site in early spring or late fall, and water frequently until plants are established. In Zone 6 and colder, grow licorice indoors in a 12-inch-deep pot. Harvest the roots of 3-year-old plants in late fall. Dig a trench on one side of the plant to expose the roots. New plants will grow from roots left in the soil. Dry the harvested roots in a dark location with very low humidity for 6 months, then store them in an airtight container.

Grindelia spp.

The 60 species of *Grindelia*, a North American perennial, are characterized by the presence of rigid, bristlelike spikes (known as phyllaries) just below the flower petals. Many species have common names that refer to a gummy substance that forms on the flower heads. In some parts of the world, children use this substance as chewing gum. Although the herb didn't come into use in Western medicine until the latter part of the 19th century, Native Americans traditionally used grindelia to treat respiratory and skin conditions.

PLANT PROFILE

Common Names: Asthma Weed, Grindelia, Gum Plant, Gum Weed, Tarweed

Description: Coarse, shrublike perennials or biennials, up to 3 feet tall; slightly toothed, spade-shaped leaves; numerous sticky, yellow disk flowers surrounded by ray flowers, occurring in heads

Hardiness: Varies according to species

Family: Asteraceae

Flowering: Late summer

Parts Used: Flowers and roots

Range/Habitat: Dry prairies from Saskatchewan to Mexico; most species occur west of the Mississippi

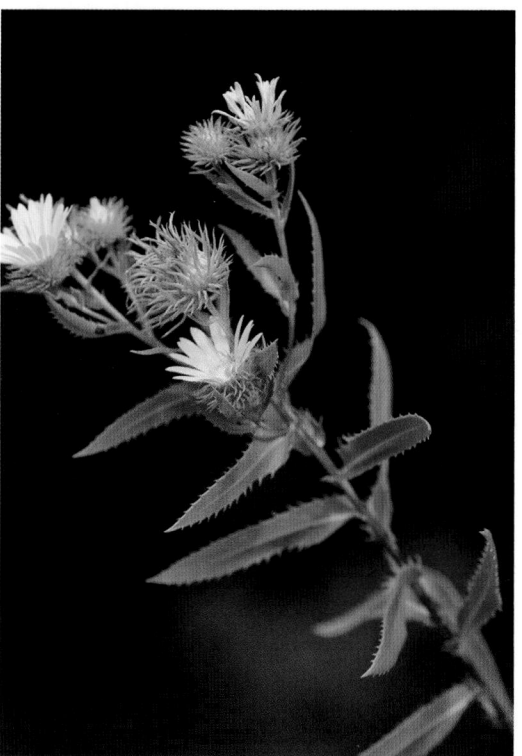

MEDICINAL USE

Grindelia can be used externally to relieve skin irritations caused by poison ivy and poison oak, as well as burns. The yellow flowers produce a sticky resin that contains an anesthetic constituent. *Grindelia squarrosa* is said to be especially effective for this purpose. To make a poultice for poison ivy or poison oak rashes, boil 1 ounce of the plant's leaves, stems, and flowers in 2 cups of water for 10 minutes. Cool, strain, and soak a cloth in the cooled liquid, then apply the cloth to the affected skin.

Taken internally, grindelia has expectorant and antispasmodic properties. The herb helps rid your lungs of excess mucus while relaxing and dilating your airways. It has been used to treat bronchitis, asthma, and whooping cough, although it can be toxic if taken in large doses.

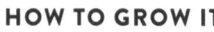

HOW TO GROW IT

A coarse, shrublike plant without ornamental qualities, grindelia is cultivated almost exclusively for medicinal purposes. Grow the herb in full sun and moderately rich, well-drained soil. Start with seeds, cuttings, or divisions. If starting with seeds, sow them outdoors in fall and cover only lightly with soil. Or sow them in a cool greenhouse in early spring, then transplant the seedlings to the garden when temperatures have warmed. Harvest leaves and flowering stems when the plant is in full bloom. Plants can be propagated by seed, cuttings, or division.

Hamamelis virginiana

This large, multistemmed shrub or small tree grows wild in eastern North American woodlands and along stream banks. Although witch hazel appears rather nondescript in summer, it shines in fall, when its leaves turn golden yellow, and its fragrant yellow flowers appear as late as December.

Native Americans found many medicinal uses for this plant—as a pain reliever, cold remedy, treatment for skin irritations, and much more. Some groups also attributed certain supernatural powers to the plant: The Mohegans, for instance, used the shrub's pliable forked branches to locate hidden water supplies and buried treasures. European settlers used the plant in similar ways. The plant's common name derives from the Old English word *wych*, meaning "pliant."

MEDICINAL USE

Witch hazel is valued as an astringent, anti-inflammatory, and analgesic. Native Americans

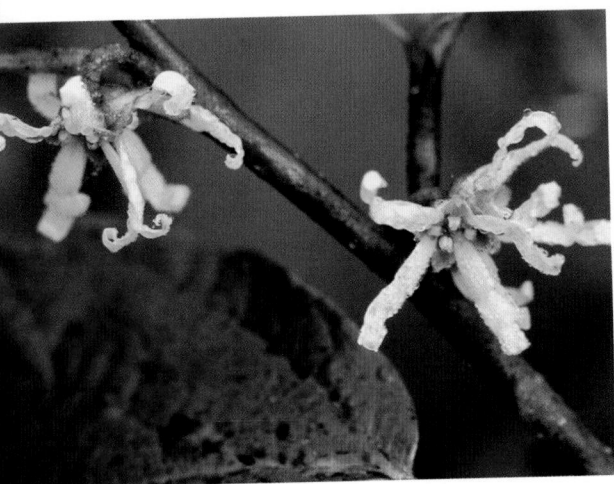

prepared a leaf or bark tea that they used as a general tonic, cough-and-cold remedy, and rinse for mouth or throat irritations. Soaking the leaves and twigs yielded a soothing extract, which they applied as a compress or wash to cuts, bruises, insect bites, rashes, and other skin irritations, as well as for eye inflammation, headache, and muscle and joint pain.

Today, witch hazel is a common ingredient in many personal-care products, including deodorants, aftershave lotions, disposable wipes, soaps, and body creams. Witch hazel is usually applied topically to treat superficial cuts, hemorrhoids, and insect bites.

Caution: Used internally, witch hazel can irritate your stomach.

ORNAMENTAL USE

With fall blooms and bright fall foliage, witch hazel makes a striking addition to naturalistic plantings and shrub borders in your landscape. The Chinese species *Hamamelis mollis* and Chinese–Japanese hybrids (*H.* × *intermedia*) include many outstanding garden cultivars with fragrant golden, copper, or red flowers. Most of the hybrids bloom a bit later (January to March) than the native American species.

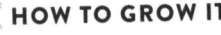

HOW TO GROW IT

Witch hazel flourishes in partial shade and moist, rich soil with a neutral to acid pH. Plant nursery-grown shrubs in spring. Propagate by seed or by layering. To improve the germination of collected seeds, keep them at 70°F for 2 months, then chill them at 40°F for 3 more months before planting.

Helleborus niger

One of a genus of 15 poisonous perennials, this European evergreen takes one of its common names from its beautiful roselike blooms that appear in the depth of winter. What can be seen aboveground is actually the plant's flower stalk, topped with its white or pinkish white flowers; the plant's true stem is underground.

This species was introduced as a garden plant and escaped, naturalizing in the northern United States and Canada. The genus name comes from the Greek *elein* (which means "to injure") and *bora* (which means "food"); the species name refers to the dark color of the plant's root.

In the Middle Ages, people strewed black hellebore flowers on the floors of their homes to drive out evil influences. Pliny the Elder (23–79 CE), a Roman naturalist and philosopher, reported that the healer and diviner Melampus used this plant as a purgative for the treatment of manic conditions around 1400 BCE.

MEDICINAL USE

This plant is toxic and is not used in modern medicine. Black hellebore contains the cardioactive steroids hellebrin, helleborin, and helleborein, which act in a similar way to digitalis, causing irregular heartbeat. Even handling the plant—particularly its roots—can cause severe skin irritation and blistering. In ancient times, black hellebore was used as a powerful purgative for the treatment of parasites and as a treatment for certain mental conditions. But even at that time, using this plant therapeutically was considered very dangerous.

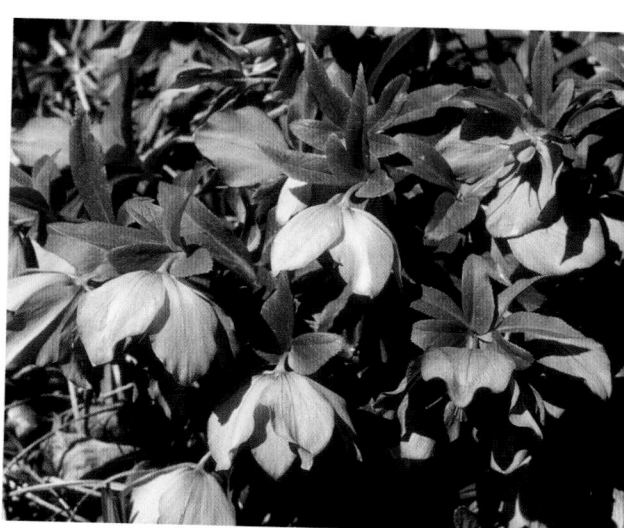

PLANT PROFILE

Common Names: Black Hellebore, Christmas Rose

Description: Perennial, up to 1 foot tall; deep green, evergreen leaves divided into seven to nine toothed leaflets; two or three white roselike blooms produced from an underground stem

Hardiness: To Zone 3

Family: Ranunculaceae

Flowering: January through March

Parts Used: Flowers (ornamental)

Range/Habitat: Central and southern mountainous regions of Europe, naturalized in parts of North America

ORNAMENTAL USE

Blooming in late winter to early spring, black hellebore adds welcome beauty to perennial borders, foundation plantings, rock gardens, and open woodland settings. Grow it alone or in groups.

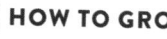

HOW TO GROW IT

Black hellebore thrives in rich, moist, well-drained soil and partial shade. Slugs can become a problem; if so, use diatomaceous earth. Fertilize the plants in spring. Black hellebore can be propagated by seed or division; divide established (6- to 7-year-old) plants in spring, after they have flowered.

Caution: Wear gloves when handling this plant; some people experience severe dermatitis when touching the bruised leaves and roots of black hellebore.

Hibiscus sabdariffa

This Old World plant, native from India to Malaysia, has quite different uses depending on the cultivar. *Hibiscus sabdariffa* var. *sabdariffa* produces edible flowers with red calyces (the outermost flower parts), which are used to make a beverage. The stems of the variety *H. sabdariffa* var. *altissima,* which rise to 16 feet, produce a fiber used to manufacture burlap bags, rope, and string.

Introduced to the southern United States in the late 19th century, hibiscus (*Hibiscus sabdariffa* var. *sabdariffa*) is a bushy plant that grows to 8 feet tall and bears showy yellow blooms. When the flower fades and closes, the reddish calyx begins to swell and becomes fleshy, ripening from the bottom of the plant to the top. Eventually the fruit matures and releases the seeds.

CULINARY USE

Hibiscus flowers can be used to make beverages, syrups, jams, or jellies. *Karkade,* a refreshing Middle Eastern drink served cold, is made from whole flowers that have been soaked for 24 hours. Whole hibiscus flowers can also be floated in drinks or stuffed with cheese and baked.

The red calyces—which contain vitamin C and significant amounts of calcium, niacin, iron, and riboflavin—are widely used in East Africa, Thailand, the Caribbean, and Mexico to make hot and cold drinks. In Mexican markets, bags of dried calyces are sold as "Flor de Jamaica."

To make hot or cold hibiscus tea, harvest the calyces when they have turned bright red. Make a cut on the side of each one and remove the seeds. Steep the remaining part in water—the liquid will turn bright red—and add lemon and sugar to taste. You can also add the chopped fresh calyces to fruit salads, or you can cook them with sugar to make a sauce. For a finer-textured syrup, run the cooked sauce through a sieve. The syrup can be added to puddings or salad dressings, or used as a topping for desserts.

Hibiscus's young leaves taste something like spicy spinach. Add them to salads, or cook them with vegetables, rice, or fish, as they do in Senegal.

MEDICINAL USE

Most parts of the hibiscus plant are used in the traditional healing practices of many world cultures. In East Africa, the heated leaves are applied to wounds and other skin irritations. In India, a decoction of the plant's seeds, which are considered a diuretic, is given to relieve painful urination and indigestion. The calyx tea is also believed to be a diuretic.

Folk traditions suggest that the tea is good for treating anxiety, and numerous clinical trials have shown that those who consumed the tea had lower blood pressure levels than those who took a placebo or drank another type of tea. One study showed that consuming a powder made from the calyces reduced blood glucose levels and total cholesterol, as well as triglycerides.

Hibiscus can also help with constipation. The bitter roots are valued for their emollient properties

 HOW TO GROW IT

Frost-sensitive hibiscus thrives in full sun and moist, fertile soil. It can be started outdoors from seed in Zones 8 through 11. In cooler regions, start the seed indoors and move the plant outdoors after all danger of frost has passed and temperatures have warmed. The plants take up to 8 months to fruit.

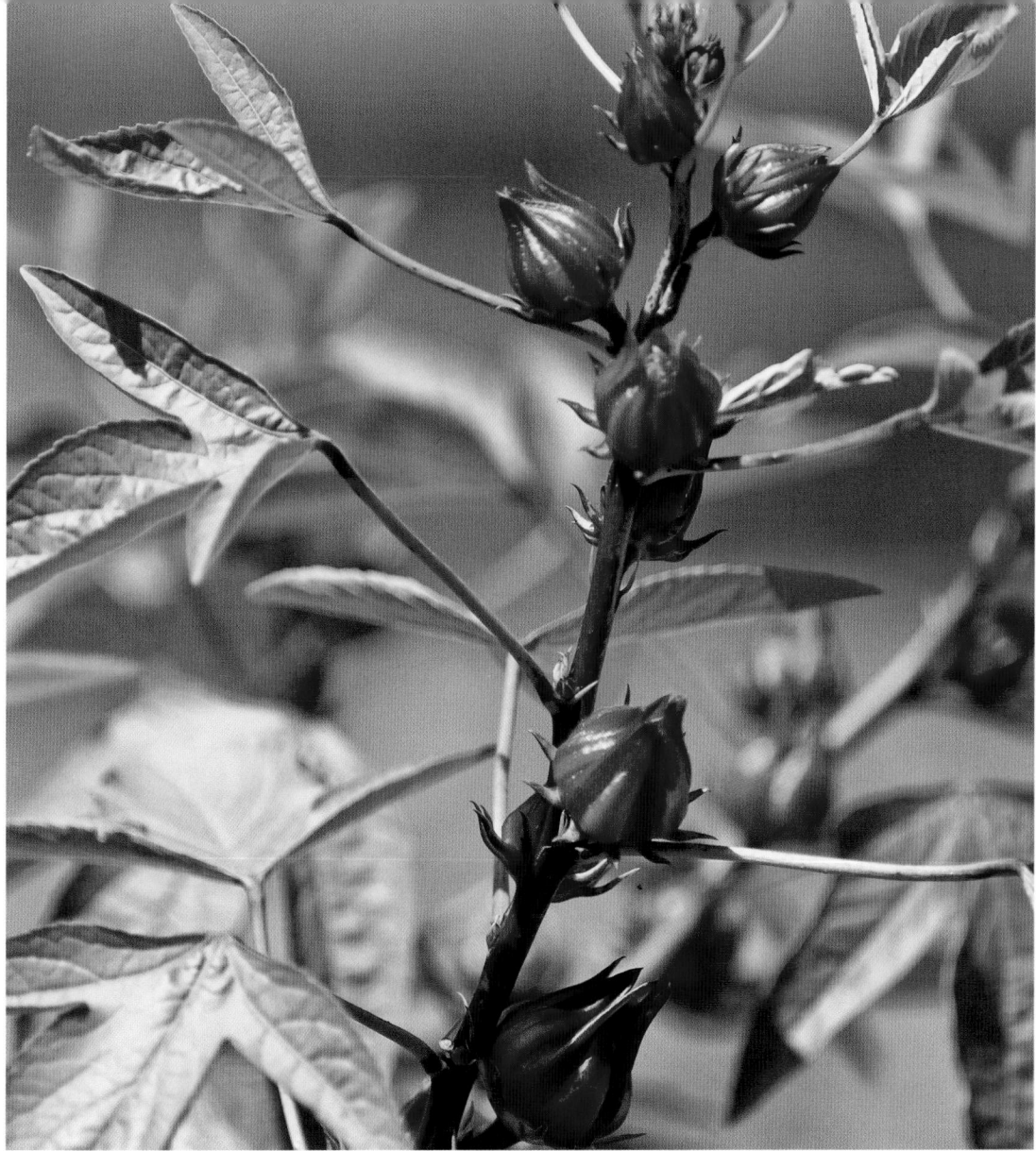

and for toning the stomach and increasing appetite. The plant is rich in anthocyanins (a type of flavonoid), which are thought to provide some of the health benefits.

Caution: Do not consume any part of hibiscus if you are pregnant or taking acetaminophen.

ORNAMENTAL USE

With showy yellow flowers, bright red calyces, and bright red stems with contrasting dark green leaves, hibiscus makes a beautiful addition to the garden—even in areas where the growing season isn't long enough for the plant to set fruits. In subtropical or tropical regions, the bushy plant can be grown in a border or as a hedge. In temperate regions, grow it in a large container on a sunny deck or patio.

OTHER USES

An extract made from the calyx is used as a natural red food coloring. Hibiscus seeds have been used as a coffee substitute, chicken feed, and source of oil. Some consider the seeds an aphrodisiac.

Humulus lupulus

Native to North America, Europe, and Asia, the hops plant is a tall, spindly, clinging vine with bright green, deeply lobed leaves. Its common name comes from the Anglo-Saxon *hoppan*, meaning "to climb." The cone-shaped fruits of the female plant give beer its distinctive flavor. Hops are grown in nearly every country of the world, but especially in the United States and Germany, which are both renowned for their beers. The observation that hops pickers often became unusually tired and sometimes were found napping on the job inspired the creation of sleep pillows, or "dream pillows," containing hops. Today, these sleep-inducing pillows often contain lavender or rose petals, as well.

PLANT PROFILE

Common Name: Hops

Description: Vigorous perennial vine grows up to 25 feet or more, producing new stems from the plant's base each year; bright green, deeply lobed leaves; flowers mature into pale green, papery bracts

Hardiness: To Zone 4

Family: Cannabaceae

Flowering: August to September

Parts Used: Female flower

Habitat: Temperate areas of Europe, western Asia, and North America

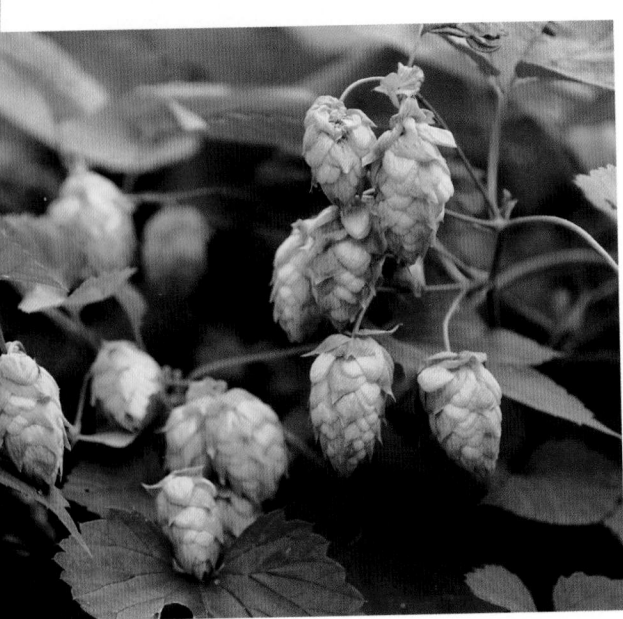

CULINARY USE

Hops provide the bitter elements used to brew beer. The young shoots can also be boiled, steamed, or eaten raw and served like asparagus.

MEDICINAL USE

The fruit of the hops plant contains resinous bitter substances, essential oil, and flavonoids that have sedative and spasmolytic properties. Herbalists use hops tinctures, teas, and capsules to relieve anxiety, insomnia, restlessness, and lack of appetite.

Caution: Avoid using hops if you have been diagnosed with depression.

OTHER USES

In the landscape, the hops vine makes an attractive cover for a fence, arbor, or pergola. You can also cut and dry the flower heads to make beautiful wreaths or everlasting arrangements.

 HOW TO GROW IT

Plant hops vines in spring in full sun or light shade in deep, moist soil enriched with compost. Choose a site that receives good air circulation to prevent mildew, and provide strong support for the vigorous vines. Vines begin bearing during their third year. Harvest the papery cones in early fall. For best flavor and effectiveness, use fresh hops quickly. If you must store hops, dry them immediately in a 125° to 150°F oven, then keep them in a cool location, away from light. Propagate hops from young softwood cuttings taken in spring (6- to 8-inch cuttings should have at least two sets of buds each), or from leaf bud cuttings taken in early summer.

Hydrastis canadensis

A member of the buttercup family, goldenseal bears deeply toothed leaves and red, raspberrylike berries. The plant's common name refers to the golden marks on the rhizomes, thought to resemble the wax seals once used on envelopes.

Native Americans used the bright yellow roots as a dye and as a remedy for a wide range of conditions that included skin inflammations, digestive problems, and ailments of the eye, ear, lung, heart, and liver. Goldenseal quickly became a popular home remedy among European settlers, as well.

At one time the plant grew throughout the moist, rich woodlands of eastern North America, but goldenseal's popularity as a medicinal led to the overharvesting of the wild plants; today this species is considered endangered. Goldenseal remains one of the top-selling botanical products sold by the health-food industry, and some commercial suppliers now cultivate it.

MEDICINAL USE

Goldenseal root contains the alkaloids berberine and hydrastine, which stimulate digestion, increase bile flow, and lower blood pressure. Believed to have antibacterial, antiseptic, and astringent properties due to the presence of berberine, the herb is used to treat diarrhea, respiratory infections, colds, eye infections, and (as a mouthwash) sore gums and throats. Commercially prepared goldenseal salves and ointments (sometimes blended with comfrey or plantain) are available for treating sores, cuts, and other skin irritations. While clinical studies have shown that the compound berberine could be beneficial for treating some infections, clinical studies have not been conducted using the whole plant extract.

> **PLANT PROFILE**
>
> **Common Names:** Goldenseal, Orange Root, Yellow Root
>
> **Description:** Perennial, 6 to 12 inches tall, with deeply divided, five-lobed leaves; oblong orange-red berries with two shiny black seeds inside; golden roots
>
> **Hardiness:** To Zone 5
>
> **Family:** Ranunculaceae
>
> **Flowering:** Spring
>
> **Parts Used:** Rhizomes and roots
>
> **Range/Habitat:** North America; moist woodlands, meadows, and open highlands

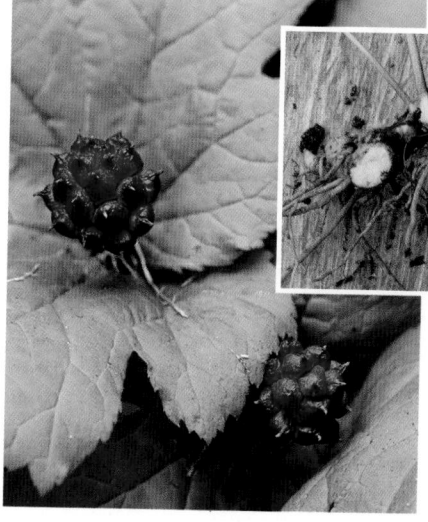

Caution: Goldenseal should not be used during pregnancy or by very young children.

OTHER USES

With mordants (see page 397), the root produces permanent dyes ranging from pale yellow to orange. Mixed with indigo, it produces an attractive green.

 HOW TO GROW IT

Goldenseal thrives in rich, moist, well-drained soil in dappled shade. The genus name *Hydrastis* is Latin for "water," referring to goldenseal's affinity for a damp growing environment. Budded rhizomes (available from specialty suppliers) are easiest to grow. Plant them in soil enriched to a depth of 10 inches with compost, leaf mold, and sand. In winter, mulch with shredded leaves. Harvest the roots of established plants (at least 4 to 5 years old) in late fall.

Hypericum perforatum

PLANT PROFILE

Common Name: St. John's Wort

Description: Erect perennial, up to 2 feet tall; spreads by underground runners; small, oblong leaves; bright yellow, flat flowers; turpentine-like smell

Hardiness: To Zone 5

Family: Hypericaceae

Flowering: Midsummer

Parts Used: Flowers

Range/Habitat: Native to Europe, North Africa, and Asia; naturalized in North America in woods, meadows, and along roadsides

St. John's wort, a perennial, bears bright yellow, five-petaled flowers and red, pink, orange, green, or brown berries. The flower petals have tiny black dots near the margins that give the plant its species name, *perforatum*. The common name possibly comes from the plant's bloom time—around St. John's Day (June 24)—or from the reddish color of its crushed flowers, symbolizing the saint who is often depicted in a red robe. For more than 2,000 years, people have used St. John's wort to treat insomnia, anxiety, and mild depression. The Greek physician Hippocrates (460–377 BCE) was an early proponent of the plant's therapeutic value.

MEDICINAL USE

Many scientific studies have confirmed the safety and effectiveness of St. John's wort for treating mild to moderate depression, along with accompanying

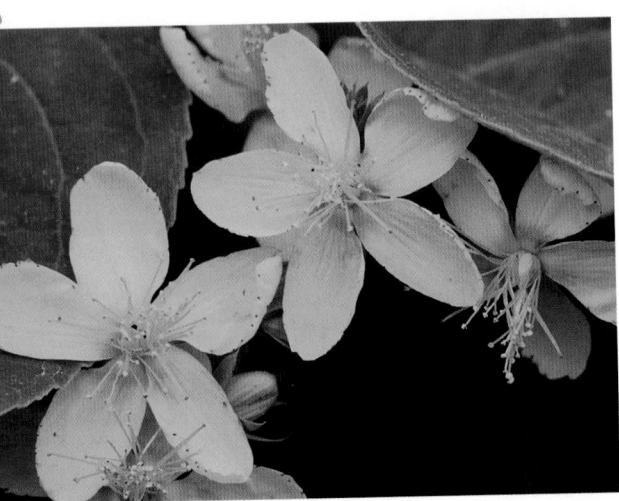

fatigue, anxiety, and insomnia. The compound or compounds responsible for the herb's antidepressant activity are not yet known. Its flowers and unopened buds contain hyperforin (a compound that has antibiotic properties) and hypericin (a substance that gives St. John's wort oils and tinctures a deep red color). When used externally, St. John's wort seems to help nerve pain, wounds, burns, and insect bites. It is a common ingredient in skin cleansers, as well as face, body, and hand creams.

Caution: Fair-skinned people using St. John's wort should avoid excessive exposure to sunlight because this herb can increase sun sensitivity. Talk to your physician or pharmacist before using St. John's wort if you are taking prescription medications, as the chance for herb-drug interaction is high. Do not use this herb if you are taking prescription antidepressants.

OTHER USES

The stems can be used to dye alum-mordanted fabric a brownish red (see page 397). The flowers produce a yellow, orange-red, or mauve dye, depending on the mordant and dyeing method used.

HOW TO GROW IT

St. John's wort grows best in full sun and well-drained, fairly dry soil. Plant the seeds or root divisions in spring or fall. St. John's wort spreads by runners; pull out unwanted plants to control their growth. For medicinal use, cut the flowering stems just as they begin to bloom; use the flowers fresh or dried.

Caution: St. John's wort can become invasive and can be toxic to cattle if consumed in extremely large quantities.

Hyssopus officinalis

A member of the mint family, hyssop bears soft, hairy gray leaves and double-lipped blue flowers that are highly attractive to bees and butterflies. In times past, people placed branches of this strongly aromatic and antiseptic herb on the floors of sickrooms and kitchens. It was so highly regarded as a medicinal panacea that, according to an old saying, "Whoever rivals hyssop's virtues, knows too much." The ancient Greek physician Hippocrates (460–377 BCE) named the plant hyssopus, from the Hebrew *ezob*, meaning "holy herb"—although it is not the same hyssop mentioned in the Bible. The biblical hyssop is believed to be another member of the mint family, *Origanum syriacum*.

CULINARY USE

Hyssop tastes like a combination of sage and mint. Traditionally, people used it to flavor soups and meat dishes. Try adding small amounts of this strong-flavored herb to bean dishes, salads, and fruit dishes. Hyssop is an ingredient in Chartreuse liqueur and a renowned flavoring for honey in France.

MEDICINAL USE

Hyssop contains flavonoids, tannins, resins, and terpenes, including marrubiin, which is a strong expectorant. The plant also contains compounds that have antiviral, antibacterial, antispasmodic, and anti-inflammatory properties. Herbal practitioners use hyssop to relieve the symptoms of colds, flus, and other respiratory infections, as well as asthma in both children and adults. It is also useful for treating indigestion, gas, bloating, and colic. Externally, a poultice of crushed hyssop leaves can soothe skin inflammations, cuts, and bruises.

Caution: Hyssop should not be used during pregnancy.

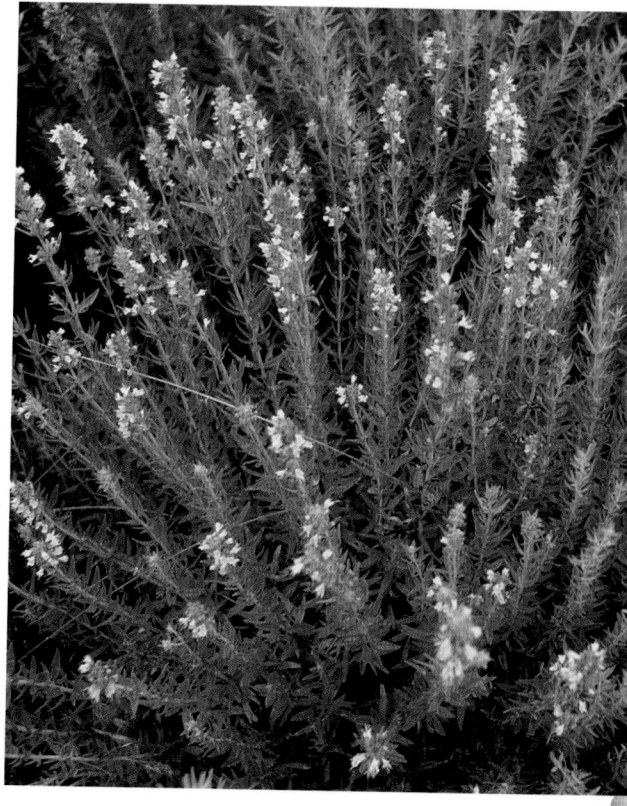

PLANT PROFILE

Common Name: Hyssop

Description: Compact perennial, 2 to 3 feet tall, with opposite gray leaves and dense spikes of blue double-lipped flowers; highly aromatic

Hardiness: To Zone 4

Family: Lamiaceae

Flowering: Early to midsummer

Parts Used: Flowers and leaves

Range/Habitat: Grows freely in the Mediterranean region, especially in the Balkans and in Turkey

HOW TO GROW IT

Hyssop is easy to grow in a sunny, dry location. In early spring, sow seeds ¼ inch deep; thin seedlings to about 1 foot apart. For medicinal use, harvest the flowering tips just before the blooms begin to open. Propagate hyssop by seed, root division, or cuttings.

Ilex paraguariensis

PLANT PROFILE

Common Names: Maté, Paraguay Tea, Yerba Maté

Description: Evergreen shrub or small tree, 15 to 50 feet tall; oval, leathery leaves with serrated edges; small, greenish white, four-petaled flowers and red berries

Hardiness: To Zone 9

Family: Aquifoliaceae

Flowering: Late winter to early spring

Parts Used: Leaves

Range/Habitat: Native to South America; grows wild near streams

A member of the holly family found in subtropical South America, maté is a caffeine-containing evergreen shrub or small tree used most commonly to produce the slightly bitter tea of the same name. After the leathery leaves are harvested, they are heated, ground, and then stored in sacks for approximately 1 year before being used to make the beverage.

More than 300 years ago, indigenous people taught Jesuit missionaries about the stimulant properties of this tea, and the missionaries then introduced maté tea to European colonists in Brazil, Paraguay, Argentina, and elsewhere. The Jesuits named the herb from the Spanish word for "gourd," a reference to the gourds from which the South American indigenous people drank their tea.

In parts of South America, people still drink maté from a small gourd (*cuia*), using a straw

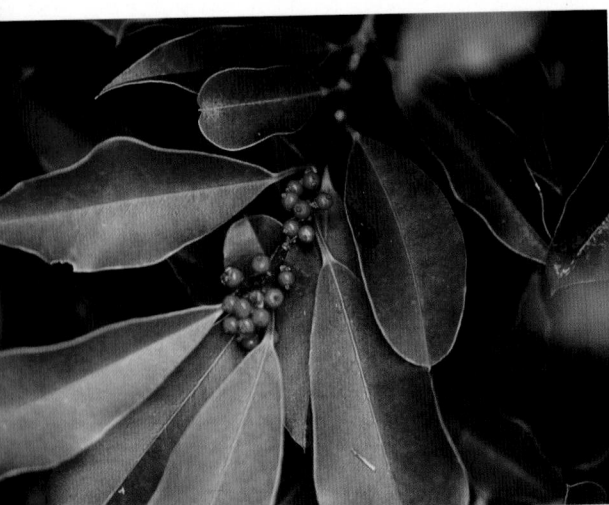

(*bombilla*). Those who enjoy maté sip their beverage throughout the day, reusing the ground leaves and refilling the gourd with hot water.

CULINARY USE

Maté is so popular in South America that more than 200 brands of the tea are sold in Argentina alone. Maté is usually enjoyed plain, although milk, lemon, or sugar are sometimes added for flavor. A cup of maté contains about half as much caffeine as a cup of brewed coffee; it also contains vitamins A and C, along with minerals, including iron, calcium, potassium, and zinc. In South America, the herb is used to flavor foods ranging from bread to soft drinks.

MEDICINAL USE

In addition to caffeine, maté contains astringent and antiseptic tannins similar to those in green tea (*Camellia sinensis*). The herb stimulates the nervous system, relieving mental and physical fatigue, and it has diuretic and anti-inflammatory properties. In South America, maté is taken as an appetite suppressant and used to relieve mild depression, nervous tension, migraine headaches, and joint pain.

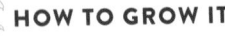

HOW TO GROW IT

Maté thrives in moist, well-drained soil in full sun or partial shade; it requires a minimum temperature of 20°F. As a houseplant, it will reach a mature height of 2 to 4 feet. For best growth indoors, provide full sun and a minimum temperature of 50°F. Harvest the leaves when the berries ripen to red. Propagate from seed or semiripe cuttings.

Illicium verum

Chinese star anise is a small evergreen tree native to China and Vietnam. Shaped like an eight-pointed star, the fruits (or seedpods) have a warm, sweet licorice flavor similar to that of aniseed. After a heavy meal, you can chew the pods to freshen your breath and stimulate digestion. But first, be sure you have the right star anise: Chinese star anise is sometimes confused with Japanese star anise (*Illicium anisatum*), a related species with highly toxic fruit. The fruit of the Japanese species is slightly smaller, tastes somewhat bitter, and lacks a sweet smell. Some people who unknowingly consumed the Japanese species have been accidentally poisoned.

CULINARY USE

Chinese star anise is a key ingredient in Chinese five-spice powder and is used to flavor many Asian dishes. Use a pinch of the ground pods to flavor Asian soups or Peking duck. It is also an important source of flavoring for liqueurs, such as anisette.

MEDICINAL USE

This herb has carminative (gas-relieving), stimulant, and diuretic properties. In traditional medicine, the fruit has been used as an expectorant and to treat constipation and dysentery, upset stomachs, spasms, and toothaches. In traditional Chinese medicine it is used as a tea to relieve colic and has been used to treat arthritis.

Shikimic acid extracted from Chinese star anise was used to produce the antiviral medication Tamiflu, originally developed to lessen the severity and duration of common colds and influenza. This drug has become the first line of defense against more serious viral infections, such as H5N1 avian influenza (bird flu). Limited supplies of this herb and the worldwide threat caused by influenza epidemics have resulted in a search for

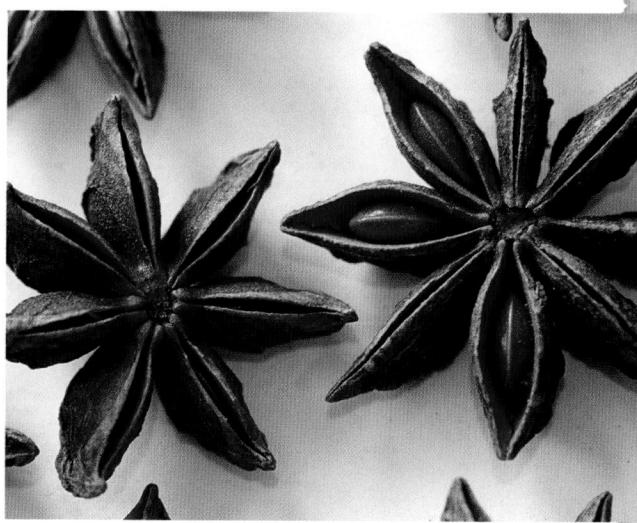

PLANT PROFILE

Common Name: Chinese Star Anise

Description: Small, rounded, evergreen tree, up to 15 feet tall and 9 feet across; small, greenish white or red flowers and glossy foliage; aromatic seedpods open to a star shape when ripe

Hardiness: To Zone 9

Family: Schisandraceae

Flowering: March to May

Parts Used: Fruit (seedpod)

Range/Habitat: Native to South China and Vietnam

other methods of obtaining shikimic acid, such as bacterial fermentation.

OTHER USES

Chinese star anise is a flavoring in some medicines and toothpastes. The essential oil adds a licorice scent to soaps and cosmetics. Use the attractive pods decoratively in potpourri or as part of handmade holiday ornaments and garlands.

 HOW TO GROW IT

Provide a humid environment, filtered sunlight, and moist but well-drained soil with a neutral to acid pH. In Zone 8 and colder, grow Chinese star anise in a container, and move the potted plant indoors when the weather turns cold. This slow-growing plant may take several years to begin flowering and fruiting. Harvest the fruits just before they ripen. Propagate by taking semiripe cuttings.

Impatiens capensis

Touch the ripe fruits of this North American orange-flowered annual and they will burst open, releasing seeds in all directions. Also known as "touch-me-not," jewelweed grows along creek beds, in moist woods, and in other locations where there is plenty of moisture. It has a beautiful translucent, succulent green stem, which is all the more apparent when held up to the light. The name jewelweed comes from the way rain forms silvery beads—reminiscent of jewels—on the plant's leaves. The species is related to garden impatiens, and it bears bright orange trumpet-shaped blooms that are highly attractive to hummingbirds, bees, and butterflies.

Jewelweed is a very important medicinal plant that's been used by Native Americans for a variety of purposes, both internal and external. It grows in the same environments as poison ivy, which is helpful, because jewelweed can be used to treat rashes and hives caused by contact with skin irritants such as poison ivy and poison oak, as well as stinging nettles.

MEDICINAL USE

The most common traditional Native American use for this plant was as a dermatological aid, applied as a poultice, ointment, or wash. The people of various groups used the crushed plant or its parts to treat burns, cuts, bruises, skin rashes, eczema, poison ivy, nettle stings, sprains, and sore limbs. Some tribes also used infusions of this plant to ease childbirth, as a diuretic, or to treat fevers.

PLANT PROFILE

Common Names: Impatiens, Jewelweed, Touch-Me-Not

Description: Annual, 3 to 5 feet tall, with oval, toothed leaves; trumpet-shaped 1-inch orange flowers with red spots; long seedpods pop open when touched

Hardiness: To Zone 2

Family: Balsaminaceae

Flowering: July to October

Parts Used: Entire plant

Range/Habitat: Native throughout most of North America; found in moist woodland areas

OTHER USES

Native Americans used this plant to make an orange-yellow dye for cloth. The whole plant was chopped and then boiled together with the cloth in water; rusty nails were sometimes added to the pot.

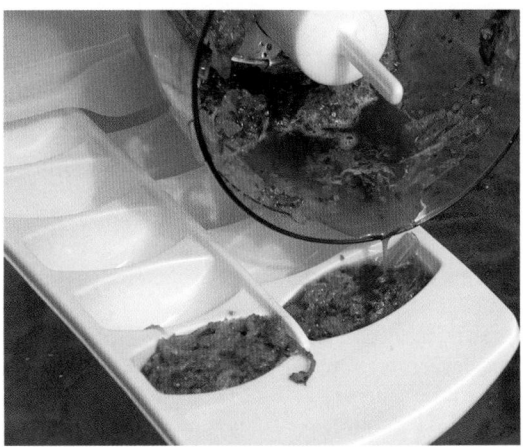

HOW TO GROW IT

Considered a weed in some areas, jewelweed grows easily in moist, fertile soil and partial shade. The seeds need light to germinate, so sow them directly on the soil surface (without covering them). For best results, plant fresh seeds of jewelweed outdoors in late fall for germination the following spring. Or give the seed 4 weeks of cool stratification (see page 418) before you sow it outdoors in spring. Keep the soil moist until plants become established. The plants self-seed freely.

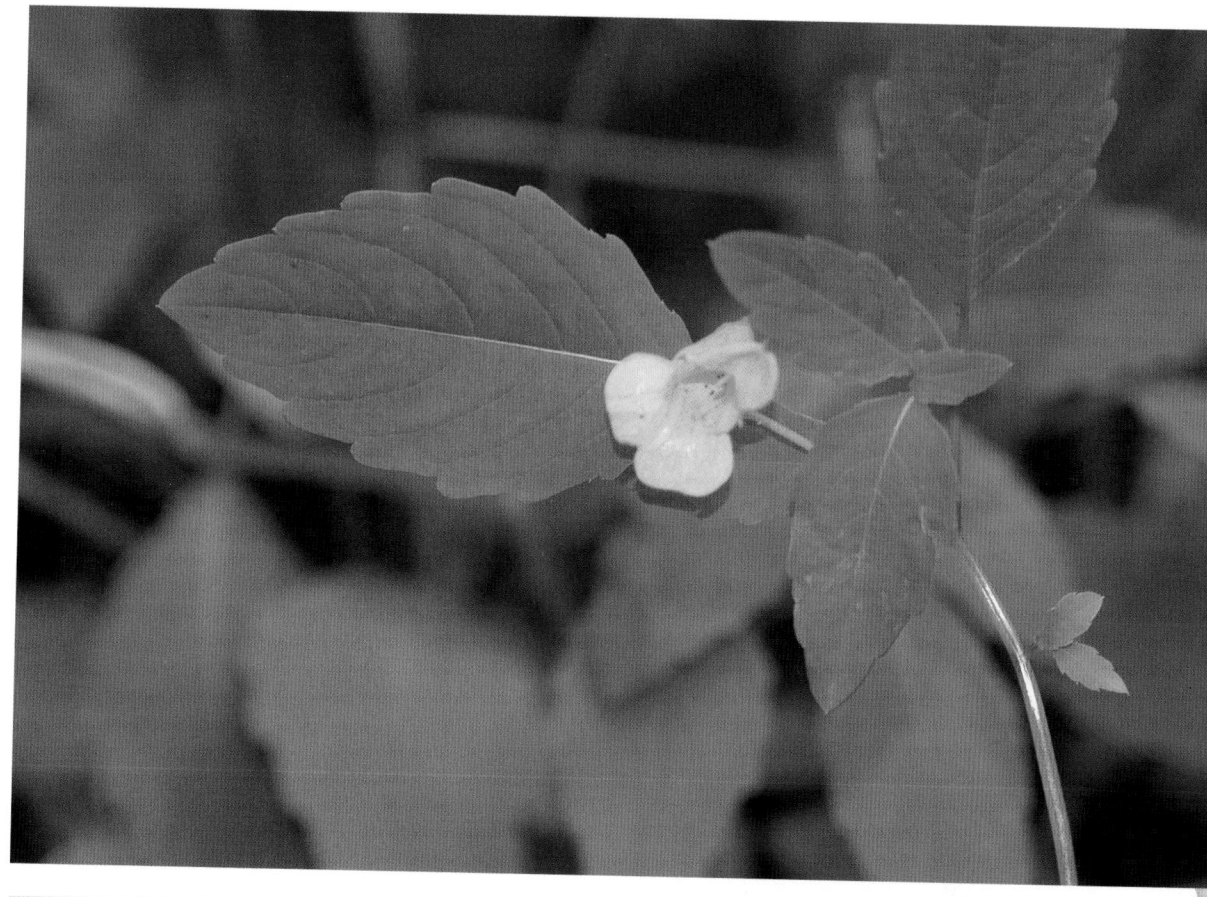

Put Skin Troubles on Ice

Growing up, I spent a lot of time hiking and camping in Northeastern forests, surrounded by massive trees and picturesque outcroppings. During these walks, I learned a great deal about native plants and their uses. One of my favorites was jewelweed, a plant that often grows in moist areas near two hiker's scourges—poison ivy and stinging nettle. When I brushed against a stinging nettle and irritating hives began to form almost immediately, my guide grabbed a handful of jewelweed stem, crushed it in his hand, and told me to rub it on the painful, burning area. Almost immediately the stinging disappeared, as did some of the redness. Native Americans used jewelweed the same way to treat poison ivy and poison oak rashes, as well.

I still use this plant today, but because it is an annual with a short life (and I am not always by a stream or wetland when I need it), I preserve it for future use. After harvesting the stems, I rinse off any soil, then chop the stems in a blender for a few seconds to produce a sticky, fibrous, clear green liquid. Then I freeze the liquid in an ice cube tray (see photo). Whenever I need to soothe poison ivy or another skin rash or irritation throughout the year, I apply a cube to the area several times daily until the problem is resolved.—M. J. B.

Indigofera tinctoria

Indigo, a member of the pea family native to India, is a tropical deciduous shrub that bears small reddish pink flowers. Although the leaflets and branches of many *Indigofera* species yield a natural blue dye, *I. tinctoria*—which was used at least 6,000 years ago in China—is used most commonly today. Approximately 660 pounds of *I. tinctoria* are required to produce about 2.2 pounds of dye. The ancient Greek word for the dye, *indicon*, means "blue dye from India." Ancient Romans used the word *indicum*, which later became

PLANT PROFILE

Common Names: Indigo, True Indigo

Description: Deciduous shrub, 2 to 6 feet tall; small reddish flowers produced in racemes; opposite leaflets

Hardiness: To Zone 9

Family: Fabaceae

Flowering: June and July

Parts Used: Leaves, stem, and roots

Range/Habitat: Native to India, naturalized in Hawaii and the southern United States

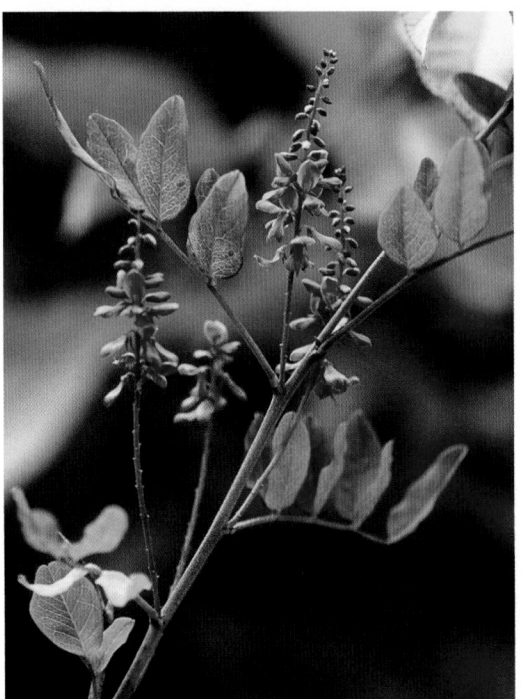

"indigo" in English. The worldwide cultivation of indigo declined sharply with the advent of synthetic dyes in the 20th century.

MEDICINAL USE

Although not often used in contemporary Western herbal medicine, indigo root and stem are thought to cleanse the liver and blood, relieve pain, reduce inflammation, and fight fever. In one animal study with rats, indigo was shown to have liver-protectant properties. In Ayurvedic medicine, indigo has a broad range of uses: It promotes hair growth, acts as a purgative, treats intestinal obstructions, and can be used in a poultice to treat skin conditions such as scabies, wounds, and sores. Fresh leaf juice is used to treat whooping cough, asthma, and heart palpitations. The herb known as wild indigo (*Baptisia tinctoria*), also of the pea family, is used medicinally as an astringent, anti-inflammatory, antiseptic, and fever reducer, but it contains several compounds that are quite toxic.

OTHER USES

The fermented leaves of this species can be used to produce a blue dye for fabric. To ferment the leaves, steep them in water for 12 to 48 hours, stirring frequently. The blue sediment that forms is the dye.

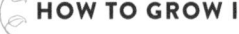

HOW TO GROW IT

This frost-tender tropical plant prefers a hot, humid climate, full sun, and well-drained sandy loam. It will not thrive in clay. In colder regions, grow it as an annual. To improve germination, scarify (see page 416) the seeds gently with sandpaper, then soak them in warm water for 24 hours before sowing. Prune hard to encourage the new growth that produces flowers. Propagate by cuttings taken in summer. A nitrogen fixer, indigo enriches the soil where it is grown.

Inula helenium

The species name of this sunflower look-alike is said to reflect its association with Helen of Troy: Elecampane either sprang from her tears, or she was holding a branch of it when Paris stole her away. Two of the plant's common names come from its early use by veterinarians to treat pulmonary disorders in horses and skin diseases in sheep. The ancient Romans used elecampane's roots to relieve the symptoms of post-banquet indigestion. "Let no day pass without eating some of the roots of elecampane . . . to help digestion, to expel melancholy, and to cause mirth," wrote the Roman scholar Pliny (23–79 CE) many centuries ago.

CULINARY USE

Elecampane roots can be candied or used to flavor desserts. To make an aperitif, infuse the roots in wine, along with other herbs or fruit.

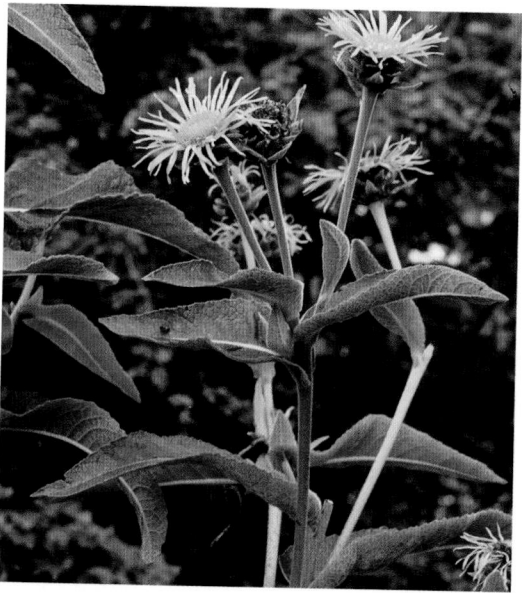

MEDICINAL USE

Herbalists throughout the world have used elecampane's thick, fleshy root to treat diseases of the chest. Rarely used alone, the dried, crushed root is said to be an effective ingredient in many compound medicines. Native American herbalists used elecampane root in combination with spikenard and comfrey roots to treat bronchial and other lung ailments. In China, where the native species of the plant is known as *hsuanfu-hua*, elecampane syrup, lozenges, and candy are used to treat bronchitis and asthma.

Besides relieving lung problems, elecampane is also thought to relieve stomach cramps and other digestive ailments. Taking a mixture of the powdered root with sugar or steeped in tea is believed to help regulate menstrual cycles. The root also works as a diuretic; at one time, it was used as a treatment for water retention due to congestive heart failure, then known as dropsy.

Elecampane root tea is still sometimes used as a remedy for coughs and other minor respiratory ailments.

Caution: Avoid using this herb if you are pregnant or nursing or are allergic to ragweed.

HOW TO GROW IT

Grow elecampane in moist but well-drained clay loam and partial shade. Harvest the roots in fall during the plant's second or third growing year, after a hard frost or two. (The roots of older plants are too woody for use.) To propagate the plant, take offshoots or 2-inch root cuttings from a mature plant during fall. Cover the cuttings with moist, sandy soil, and keep them at 50° to 60°F until growth occurs, which should happen by early spring.

Isatis tinctoria

This perennial or biennial species, native to Asia and Europe, was once a dominant source of blue dye. One of the earliest recorded uses was by the ancient Egyptians, who used it to dye the cloth used to wrap mummies. In the British Isles, ancient warriors painted their bodies with woad to frighten their opponents, and according to folklore, the herb was one of the dyes used to color the green tunic of Robin Hood. The plant was cultivated as a major industry and trade item until the mid-17th century, when it was largely replaced by indigo. Both woad and indigo have been eclipsed by synthetic dyes.

MEDICINAL USE

Woad is a very astringent herb and is believed to have antiviral properties. Ancient herbalists considered it useful for reducing the inflammation of external wounds and sores and used it as a styptic by applying it as a poultice or plaster. A woad

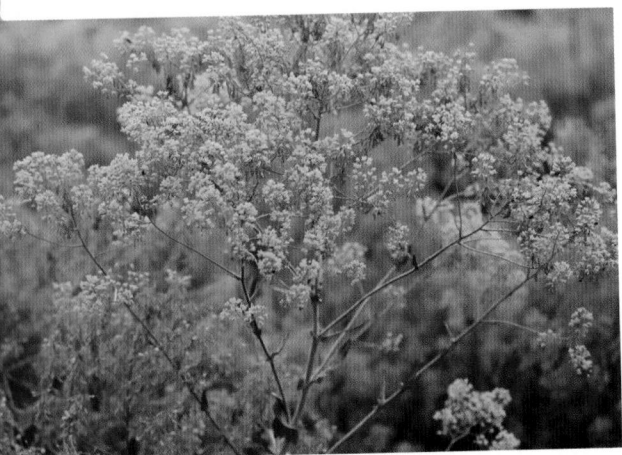

PLANT PROFILE

Common Name: Woad

Description: Biennial or perennial; 3 to 5 feet tall; bluish green oblong leaves up to 4 inches long; stalks topped with small yellow flowers appear in second year; black seedpods

Hardiness: To Zone 5

Family: Brassicaceae

Flowering: Spring

Parts Used: Leaves

Range/Habitat: Native to Asia and Europe, naturalized throughout North America

poultice was also thought to help alleviate an enlarged spleen. Contemporary herbalists use woad topically to treat skin rashes and abscesses.

Caution: Although woad may have astringent properties, it is toxic and should not be taken internally.

OTHER USES

To produce the blue dye, fresh leaves are macerated, rolled into balls, and sun-dried. Following this, the balls of woad are crushed, mixed with water, fermented, and then made into a powder for use as a dye. It is the lengthy fermentation process that can produce a strong and offensive odor, reminiscent of the smell of sewage. For that reason, Queen Elizabeth I, Queen of England, would not allow the manufacture of this dye within 5 miles of her royal palaces. There were also issues of woad cultivation taking up too much arable land in England at a time when there was a serious food shortage. Queen Elizabeth I also issued the 1585 edict "By the Queene. A Proclamation against the Sowing of Woade" that forbade new plantings of this dye crop in areas where food plants could otherwise be produced.

HOW TO GROW IT

Grow woad in rich, well-drained soil and full sun. Avoid growing woad near other members of the family Brassicaceae, such as cabbage or broccoli, to reduce the chance of disease and pests. Sow seed directly in the garden in either spring or late summer. To make dye, gather leaves just before the plant blossoms, beginning during the second season. Established plants self-sow freely.

Caution: Woad is considered an invasive weed in some western states, and its growth is prohibited or quarantined in several places. Check with your local extension office before planting it if you live in the West.

Larrea tridentata

Chaparral is a thorny, olive green or yellow ever-green shrub with a strong odor of tar, or creosote. The plant dominates the landscape of the desert regions of North America, forming vast populations. For many Native American groups, chaparral was a panacea, useful for treating a wide range of conditions that included dandruff, snakebite, and low energy. The wood was used to make arrows and tools, and the fiber was used as a building material.

MEDICINAL USE

Traditionally, Native American people made a chaparral leaf wash or poultice to treat arthritis, bruises, and wounds, and to treat aching or sore areas of the body. An infusion of the leaves was considered to be an antiseptic and was used to wash and cleanse the skin. It was also used to treat the sores on domesticated animals caused by the rubbing of a collar or strap. Chaparral tea was taken internally to relieve asthma, colds, sore throats, diarrhea, and many other conditions.

Chaparral contains nordihydroguaiaretic acid (NDGA), a powerful antioxidant formerly used by the food industry to preserve cooking oils. This compound is known for its anti-inflammatory properties. The herb also has antimicrobial, antiviral, and hyperglycemic properties. According to a study published in the *Journal of Dental Research*, using chaparral mouthwash reduced cavity formation by 75 percent.

Caution: Do not take chaparral internally; internal use of this herb has been known to cause severe liver and kidney damage. Do not use chaparral internally or externally if you are pregnant, nursing, or have liver or kidney disease.

PLANT PROFILE

Common Names: Chaparral, Creosote Bush

Description: Thorny, olive green or yellow ever-green shrub, up to 6 feet tall; dark green leaves with opposite leaflets; bright yellow flowers up to 1 inch across; highly aromatic

Hardiness: To Zone 8

Family: Zygophyllaceae

Flowering: Midsummer

Parts Used: Leaves, flowers, and stems

Range/Habitat: Found throughout desert regions of the southwestern United States and parts of Mexico

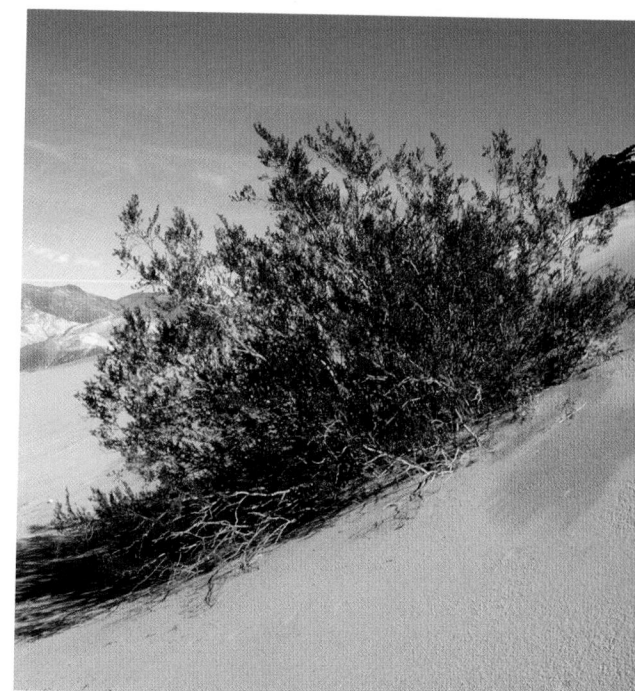

HOW TO GROW IT

A desert plant, chaparral thrives in dry conditions, sandy or gravelly soil, and full sun. Consider growing it in a large container because its roots contain chemicals that can kill nearby plants. To improve germination, scarify the seed (see page 416), then soak it in water for 24 hours before sowing it in a flat indoors. Cover the seed with a small amount of soil. After the second set of true leaves appears, transplant the seedlings. Water periodically for the first 2 years, but allow the soil to dry out completely before watering again. Allow seed heads to dry on the plant before collecting them for propagation.

Laurus nobilis

The leathery, dark green leaves of this small Mediterranean tree symbolized success to the ancient Greeks and Romans, who wove its branches into crowns to honor scholars, poets, generals, and Olympic victors. Derived from the Latin *laus*, meaning "praise," *Laurus nobilis* is still used to signify victory or achievement. Herbalists of the past used bay leaves and berries to treat various conditions—including hysteria, flatulence, and colic. Today, bay is most valued in the kitchen.

PLANT PROFILE

Common Names: Bay, Bay Laurel, Grecian Laurel, Sweet Bay, True Bay

Description: Dense pyramid-shaped evergreen shrub or tree, up to 50 feet tall; shiny, dark green, leathery leaves up to 3 inches long; umbels of inconspicuous flowers; dark purple berries

Hardiness: To Zone 8

Family: Lauraceae

Flowering: Spring

Parts Used: Leaves

Range/Habitat: Native to the Mediterranean region and Asia Minor; widely cultivated

CULINARY USE

Dried bay leaves are very popular in French, Spanish, and Creole cuisine and are used to flavor poultry, stews, vegetables, and meat dishes. Bay is an ingredient in bouquet garni, a group of herbs (usually parsley, thyme, and bay) tied together or placed in a cheesecloth bag and used to flavor soups. Always remove bay leaves before eating; they have very sharp edges and, if swallowed, can injure your throat.

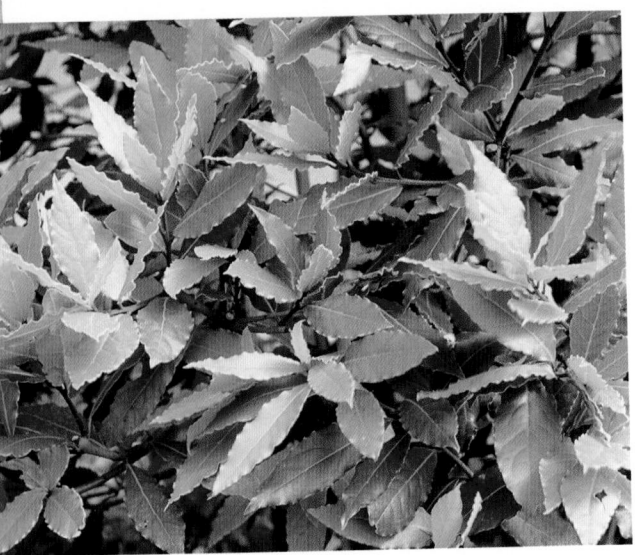

MEDICINAL USE

Though bay is primarily a culinary herb, it is also used as a digestive tonic to stimulate appetite, increase the secretion of digestive juices, and settle your stomach. When used in cooking, bay leaves help break down foods, especially meats, making digestion easier. Liniments and salves containing essential oil of bay can be used externally to ease arthritis pain, sprains, and bruises.

Caution: Essential oil of bay may irritate the skin of sensitive individuals and should be applied only in dilute (approximately 2 percent) concentrations.

OTHER USES

An infusion of bay leaves can be added to bathwater. The fatty oil extracted from the fruits is used in some skin-care products, shampoos, and soaps.

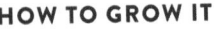

HOW TO GROW IT

Bay is an ideal container plant and can be easily pruned and maintained at a mature height of about 5 feet. Provide well-drained soil and full sun or partial shade, and shelter the plant from cold and frost. Propagate by taking semiripe cuttings, and plant them in fall. Bay leaves can be collected year-round and dried for future use. Flatten the drying leaves with a board or other object to prevent curling. Store them in an airtight container in a dark location.

Lavandula angustifolia

PLANT PROFILE

Common Names: Lavender, True Lavender, English Lavender

Description: Bushy branching shrub, 2 to 3 feet tall; narrow, gray-green leaves; spikes of small purple, blue, or pink flowers; highly aromatic

Hardiness: To Zone 5

Family: Lamiaceae

Flowering: Early to midsummer

Parts Used: Flowers, leaves, and stems

Range/Habitat: Native to France and the western Mediterranean, naturalized in Europe, the Middle East, and India; dry, stony soils

Vast fields of cultivated and wild lavender color the countryside of southern France, Spain, and other areas of the western Mediterranean region. One of the world's most beloved herbs, this highly aromatic plant in the mint family bears narrow, gray-green leaves and purple or pinkish flowers. The genus *Lavandula* includes several dozen species and hundreds of cultivars. *Lavendula angustifolia*, sometimes called true or English lavender, is a favorite garden species.

The common name lavender comes from the Roman *lavare* ("to wash"), a reference to the herb's use as a scent for bathing and washing clothes. But the versatile herb has had many other uses, too. During the Middle Ages, people believed lavender to be an aphrodisiac, and they sprinkled lavender water on a lover's head to keep him or her faithful. In the 19th century, women prone to fainting revived themselves with lavender-scented handkerchiefs. English farmers even tucked lavender under their hats to prevent sunstrokes and headaches.

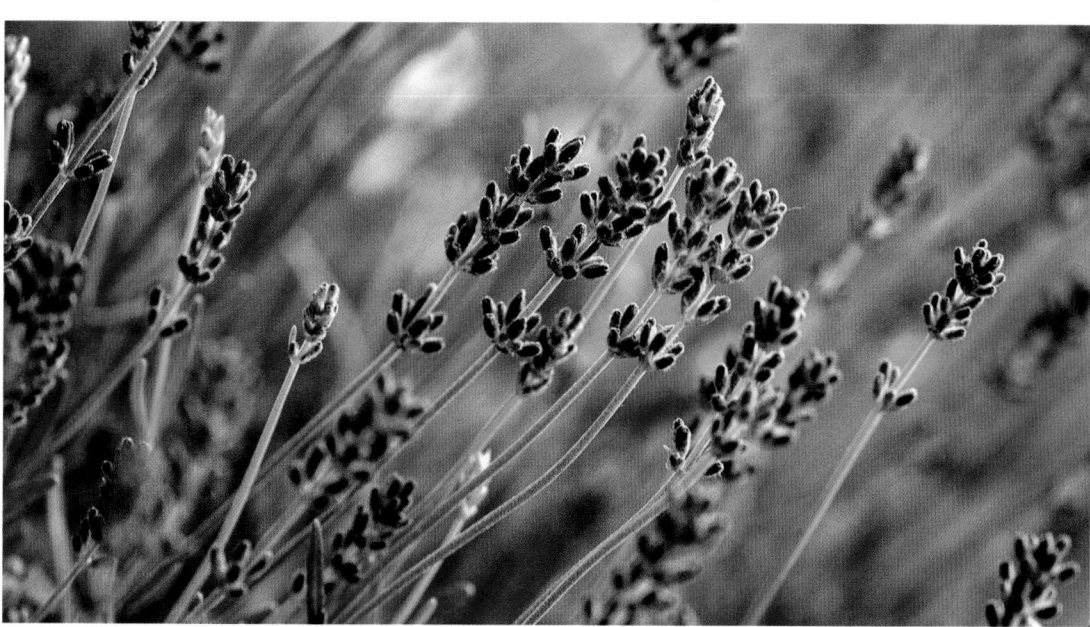

 HOW TO GROW IT

Plant lavender in well-drained, neutral to alkaline soil in full sun. Cut the bloom spikes just as they begin to open. Dry them in small bunches inside paper bags. Strip the dry buds from the stems, then store them in an airtight container. Replace woody, overgrown plants with new ones every 4 to 5 years. Propagate by taking semiripe cuttings in summer.

CULINARY USE

Lavender flowers and leaves add color and a pungent, slightly bitter flavor to salads. The plant is sometimes used to flavor oil, vinegar, cheese, jam, honey, sugar, and ice cream and other desserts. The flowers can be candied and used to decorate cakes. On its own or in tea blends, lavender makes a delicious hot or cold beverage.

MEDICINAL USE

Well known for its soothing effects, lavender contains chemical compounds that appear to have anti-inflammatory, muscle-relaxing, pain-relieving, and sedative properties. It benefits digestion by stimulating the secretion of gastric juices, including bile. Lavender's long-standing reputation as a powerful antiseptic has been supported by many studies, and recent research suggests that it has antifungal and antiviral properties, too.

The flowers are often used in sleep pillows—small sachets tucked under pillows to help ensure restful sleep. Lavender flower tea has been used to relieve anxiety, depression, indigestion, insomnia, and restlessness. It's also been used as a mouthwash for halitosis and as a douche for vaginal yeast infections.

Undiluted lavender oil can be used to reduce pain and speed the healing of minor burns, insect bites, and other wounds. Try adding the fragrant oil to massage oil or bathwater to relieve sore muscles and tension. Inhaling the diluted oil, as in aromatherapy, promotes calmness.

Caution: People with sensitive skin could experience contact dermatitis when exposed to lavender oil. Test a small amount of the oil on your skin before applying it to a large area, or dilute it with a carrier oil or water.

ORNAMENTAL USE

Lavender is an excellent choice for borders, rock gardens, and hedges. The herb releases its scent when touched, so it is often planted in entryways, along paths and decks, and in other areas where passersby will brush against it. Lavender's gray-green foliage and purple or pink flowers pair attractively with roses, yarrow, and echinacea.

OTHER USES

Aromatic lavender is used to scent skin lotions, shampoos, soaps, perfumes, potpourris, and herbal sachets. Lavender "wands" (made by weaving the bloom spikes) can be hung in closets or placed in drawers to scent clothing and deter moths.

FIELD NOTES

Essential Antiseptic

If you have a dissecting microscope, you can look at the underside of a lavender leaf and see its many small round glands. These glands are filled with the powerful substance known as lavender oil.

From earliest times, lavender was recognized not only for its wonderful aroma, but also for its remarkable disinfectant powers. The Romans filled their communal baths with lavender flowers, and during the Middle Ages, houses were scrubbed with lavender extract to cleanse and disinfect them.

During the Great Plague of London (1665–1666), glove makers scented their wares with lavender to ward off disease. (Lavender repels fleas, now known to have transmitted the plague.)

René-Maurice Gattefossé, a French chemist, discovered the healing powers of lavender after being burned in a laboratory accident in 1910. His hands started to develop gas gangrene, but he rinsed them with lavender oil and within a day or so they started to heal. Gattefossé is known as the father of aromatherapy; not only did he coin the term, but he also spread the word about the medical use of essential oils, such as lavender, through his research, teachings, and writing. During the First World War, lavender oil was employed as an antiseptic and is said to have saved many lives by preventing infection. Today, many scientific studies and clinical trials support the traditional uses of lavender oil for healing and improving health. —M. J. B.

Lepidium meyenii

A perennial related to mustard, maca grows at very high elevations—to 15,000 feet—in the Andes Mountains. It withstands conditions that many other species cannot—freezing temperatures; intense sunlight; high winds; and poor, rocky soil. Maca grows low to the ground. Its flattened taproot—the part used as food and medicine by Andean farmers in Peru and Bolivia—is about the size of a radish. In ancient times, this traditional crop was traded for cassava, rice, quinoa, and other tropical crops grown by lowland-dwelling peoples. It's said that when the Spanish came to the high Andes, their horses suffered from the elevation, but after foraging on maca they recovered and became energetic.

CULINARY USE

Maca is an excellent source of carbohydrate (60 to 75 percent), protein (11 to 14 percent), and fiber (8.5 percent). In its native growing regions, the taproot is roasted in a pit oven and eaten as a cooked vegetable, boiled and mashed into porridge, or made into a type of flour. The delicious porridge includes sugar and milk and has been said to taste similar to butterscotch. A beer known as Kuka is also made from maca by the Andean Brewing Company.

MEDICINAL USE

Maca is traditionally known as a food that increases stamina and energy, as well as fertility, virility, and libido. Studies of animals as well as humans seem to confirm these traditional beliefs. Herbalists use maca to treat male impotence and erectile dysfunction, as well as menstrual disorders, menopausal symptoms, hot flashes, and fatigue.

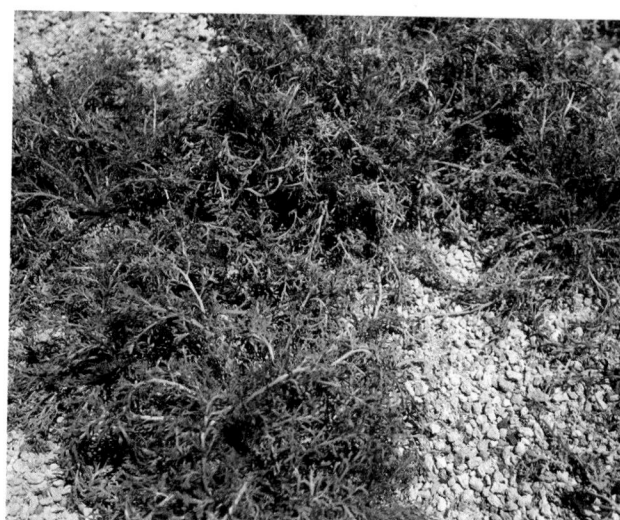

Caution: Not enough is known about possible problems associated with maca use during pregnancy and breastfeeding, so avoid using it under these circumstances.

 HOW TO GROW IT

Maca thrives in well-drained, alkaline soil, cool temperatures, and full sun. Little is known about growing this high-altitude mountain plant in North America, but it is believed to do best as a winter crop planted in early fall. Sow the seeds directly in your garden (try a cold frame or cool greenhouse in Zone 6 and colder), covering them lightly with soil. Harvest the roots the following spring. Propagate by seed.

Levisticum officinale

The only plant in the genus *Levisticum,* lovage is native to the mountainous areas of southern Europe and southwestern Asia. It produces celery-flavored leaves in early spring—often before other fresh herbs are available—followed by tiny yellow flowers and aromatic seeds. Both its common and genus names come from the Latin word *ligusticum,* or Ligurian, for the Italian province where this herb once grew abundantly. The species name *officinale* refers to its value as an herbal medicine.

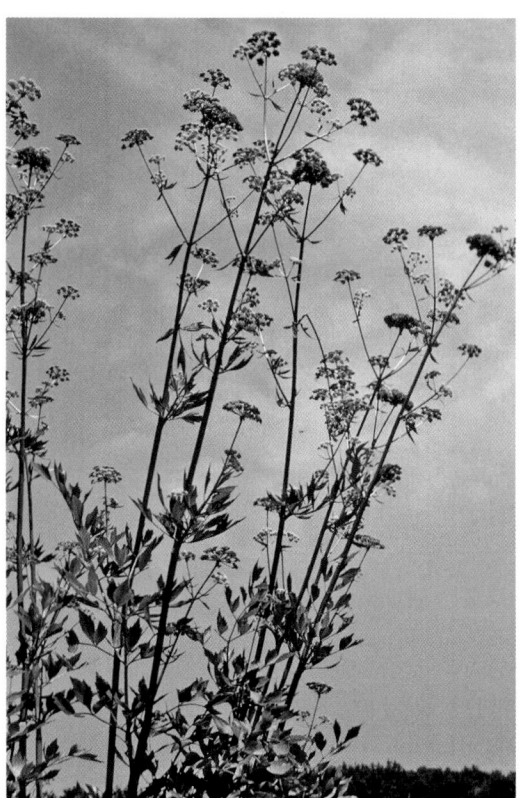

CULINARY USE

You can eat every part of the lovage plant. In the Lombardy region of Italy, lovage leaves are made into a traditional stuffing for capons, with sautéed giblets, walnuts, Parmesan cheese, fresh bread crumbs, eggs, cream, and nutmeg. The leaves, which have a celerylike flavor, can also be steamed or blanched and eaten as a vegetable or added to soups, stews, salads, and omelets. You can cook lovage roots as a vegetable and add the sweet-flavored seeds to desserts and liqueurs. Use the fresh, hollow stalks as straws in cocktails, including the tomato juice and vodka beverage called a Bloody Mary.

MEDICINAL USE

In medieval times, this herb was thought to have aphrodisiac properties, and in the early 17th century it was used to scent bathwater. Lovage contains a volatile oil that has sedative and anticonvulsant properties, so it would provide a relaxing bath. A tea made from the leaves has been used as a tonic for the digestive system to treat conditions such as indigestion, gas, colic, and poor appetite. An oil distilled from the root is used in aromatherapy for these conditions, as well. Lovage could also be helpful in the treatment of upper respiratory conditions such as bronchitis.

Caution: Lovage should not be used during pregnancy or by those with kidney disease or weak kidneys.

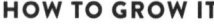

HOW TO GROW IT

Lovage grows well in deep, rich, moist soil in full sun or partial shade. Choose a site at the back of a border for this tall plant, and amend the site with compost before planting the seeds in spring or fall. Harvest leaves and young stems before the plant flowers. Propagate by dividing the roots of established plants in spring.

Ligusticum porteri

Osha is a perennial herb native to the mountains of western North America, from Montana to northern Mexico. The entire plant, including its dark brown, fibrous roots, has a strong, camphorlike scent. Osha root was, and continues to be, an important Native American healing herb. Some say people learned of the plant's healing powers by observing bears (an animal associated with healing) digging up the roots and chewing them or rubbing them on their fur. The Zuni in New Mexico made an infusion of the root and rubbed it on their bodies to treat aches and pains; they used the crushed root to treat sore throats. Other groups, such as the Apache, ate raw osha as a vegetable. Commercial demand for this herb, combined with the difficulty of cultivating it, has led to the overharvest of some wild populations. To help protect it, moratoria on its wild harvest have been implemented from time to time. Osha is easily confused with poison hemlock, which grows in similar areas, so collectors must be sure to identify the plant correctly.

MEDICINAL USE

Osha has antibacterial and anti-inflammatory properties and may be useful in the treatment of sinus, throat, and upper and lower respiratory system infections. Osha helps loosen respiratory secretions and relaxes smooth muscle tissue, making it beneficial for treating coughs and asthma. This is due, in part, to the plant's chemical compounds known as phthalides, which have sedative and muscle-relaxant properties. The herb also helps with wound healing. Recent research has shown that the roots and shoots of the plant have significant quantities of melatonin and serotonin, human neurotransmitters involved with conditions such as depression and seasonal affective disorder (SAD).

> **PLANT PROFILE**
>
> **Common Names:** Osha, Bear Root, Mountain Lovage
>
> **Description:** Perennial, up to 3 feet tall; finely dissected leaves; flat heads of white umbel flowers followed by ribbed, oblong fruits; dark, fibrous root with a yellow-white interior
>
> **Hardiness:** To Zone 6
>
> **Family:** Apiaceae
>
> **Flowering:** Late summer
>
> **Parts Used:** Leaves, roots, and stems
>
> **Range/Habitat:** Native to the Rocky Mountains and high elevations of northern Mexico; moist wooded areas and meadows

Caution: Do not take osha if you are pregnant or nursing.

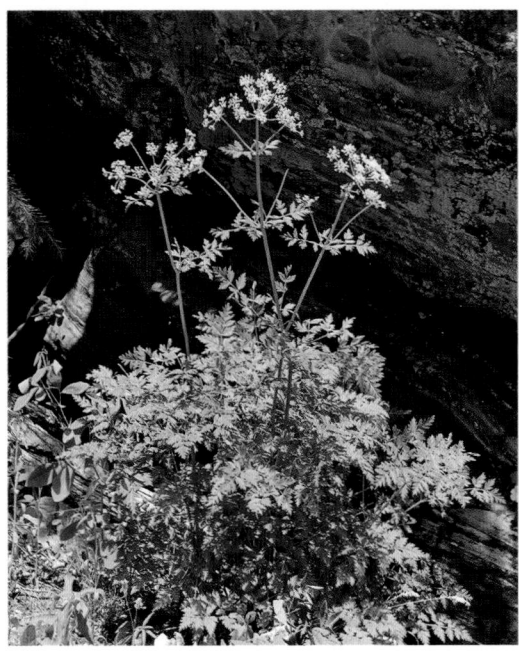

HOW TO GROW IT

Osha is considered difficult to cultivate, especially outside of its native range, perhaps due to specific soil requirements. If you wish to try growing this plant, sow fresh seeds in fall in a cold frame, or stratify the seeds (see page 418) by chilling them in your refrigerator for up to 10 weeks before planting in a flat indoors. In spring, transplant the seedlings to a fertile, well-drained site that receives full sun. Osha is slow growing and can take up to 10 years to produce large roots for harvest.

Linum usitatissimum

PLANT PROFILE

Common Names: Flax, Flaxseed, Linseed

Description: Slender, branching annual, up to 30 inches tall; delicate, five-petaled blue flowers followed by fruits containing up to 10 glossy brown seeds

Hardiness: Annual

Family: Linaceae

Flowering: June to August

Parts Used: Stems and seeds

Range/Habitat: Believed to be native to Egypt

Flax—a slender, branching annual that bears delicate, five-petaled blue flowers—is one of the world's oldest cultivated plants and certainly the oldest textile fiber. Although its origins are not fully known, flax is presumed to be native to Egypt, where it has been used since ancient times to make linen. In Biblical times, three grades of linen were made, ranging from coarse to extremely fine.

CULINARY USE

Flaxseed adds a subtle nutty flavor to salads, baked goods, and cereals. Try adding the nutritious seeds to breakfast smoothies, or mix them with honey for a tasty breakfast spread. The seeds are most easily digested when they're ground—but ground or whole, they should be stored in an airtight container in the refrigerator or freezer. Use flaxseed oil in salad dressing. Flaxseed oil is highly perishable, so store it in an opaque bottle in your refrigerator.

MEDICINAL USE

Flaxseed oil is a rich source of the essential fatty acid alpha-linolenic acid, which is required for the formation of cell membranes in your body. Fatty acids are converted into prostaglandins that may help reduce inflammation and allergies. Flaxseed oil has been shown to be effective in lowering blood cholesterol levels. It may offer a protective effect against cancer, particularly breast cancer. The seeds have a long history of use in treating chronic constipation. Applied externally, flaxseed may help draw toxins from your blood, reduce inflammation, and speed the healing of superficial wounds.

Caution: Flaxseed should be taken with at least 6 ounces of liquid; otherwise, it can promote constipation. Do not take flaxseed if you believe you have a bowel obstruction.

OTHER USES

Flax fibers can be woven into fabric, called linen, or used for making baskets or crafts. Obtaining the fiber involves soaking the flax stems in water, drying them, and then crushing them so that the stem's woody core separates from the usable fibers. To make linen, the fibers are combed, spun, and then woven.

Raw, unprocessed flax oil is used as a nutritional supplement, while processed oil from the seeds of this plant, combined with additives, is known as linseed oil. Linseed oil is used in paints, putty, and finishes for wood.

HOW TO GROW IT

Flax thrives in deep, fertile, well-drained soil and full sun. It prefers relatively cool temperatures and should be sown outdoors at the same time peas and other cool-weather crops are planted. For the best-quality fiber, cut stems about 3 months after planting—after they've flowered but before seedpods form. To obtain seeds, pull up the entire plant when the lower leaves turn yellow and the seedpods are golden. Hang the plants in a warm, dry location. When the seedpods are dry, place them in a bag and crush them with a rolling pin or other hard object; separate the broken pods from the seeds with a sieve or colander.

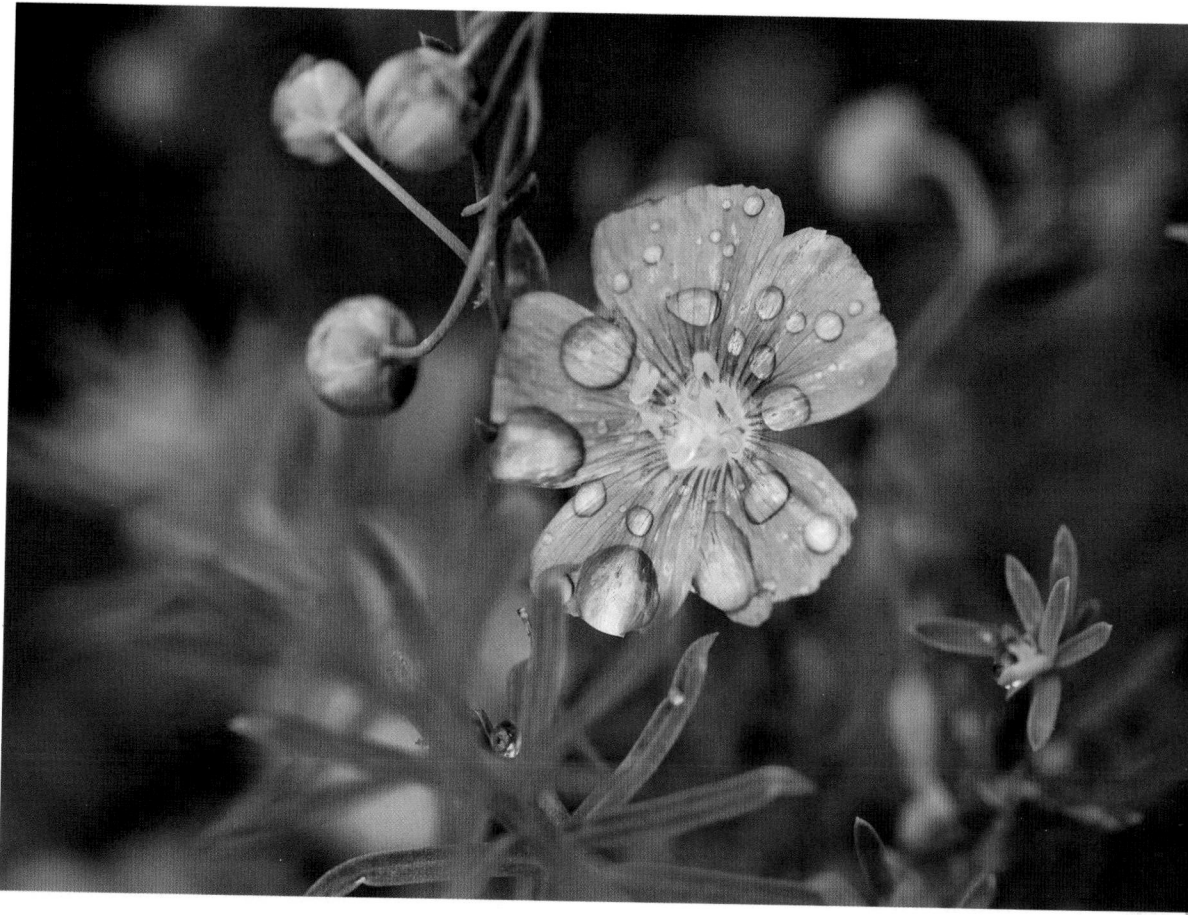

More Than Fiber

In the past, flax was much more than a food, medicine, and fiber plant. In parts of Europe, it was a good luck charm with the power to ward off evil. Flax was planted around houses and graves, added to coffins, and suspended above doorways to protect against spirits from the underworld.

Curiously, in many of these legends, the spirits were distracted from their evil deeds because they stopped to count the plant's small seeds, fibers, or threads. Flax garments also had great religious and spiritual significance; for Israelite priests, for example, linen was the proscribed clothing.

To me, a field of blue flax flowers, waving with every wind, is a beautiful sight. When the plants are ready to harvest, the field is a sea of brown capsules ready to release their tiny seeds. And while we can't evaluate the veracity of some traditional beliefs about flax in today's laboratories, we do know that including flaxseed in our diets can help provide protection against some serious diseases and promote good health.—M. J. B.

Lobelia inflata

The genus *Lobelia*, named for the 16th-century Flemish botanist Matthias de L'Obel, contains more than 400 species. Native to eastern North America, *Lobelia inflata* was well known to the Cherokee, Iroquois, and other Native Americans, who used the powerful plant to treat a variety of conditions. Samuel Thomson, an American herbalist-physician of the early 19th century, recommended lobelia as a muscle relaxant during childbirth; as a poultice for healing abscesses; and for the treatment of epilepsy, tetanus, diphtheria, dysentery, and whooping cough. Many herbalists of the time believed that the vomiting induced by lobelia cleansed the patient.

The herb's powerful and toxic effects on the central nervous system have caused it to fall from favor in recent times. Lobelia is not an herb for home experimentation—confine it to the "history" portion of your garden, and keep it far away from children. All parts of the plant contain toxins; ingesting it can be fatal.

MEDICINAL USE

Native Americans smoked lobelia leaves to relieve asthma and bronchitis (hence the common name Indian tobacco). The herb contains a muscle-relaxing alkaloid called lobeline, which is related to nicotine. By relaxing the muscles of the smaller bronchial tubes, lobeline opens airways, stimulates breathing, and promotes the loosening of phlegm. It has also been used to induce vomiting in people who have been poisoned. The plant is highly toxic, however, and should never be used internally for its traditional purposes. Some herbalists still use it externally to relieve muscle tension and to soothe bruises and bites.

Caution: Even a miniscule amount of this herb, alone or in an herbal preparation, can cause paralysis, coma, and death.

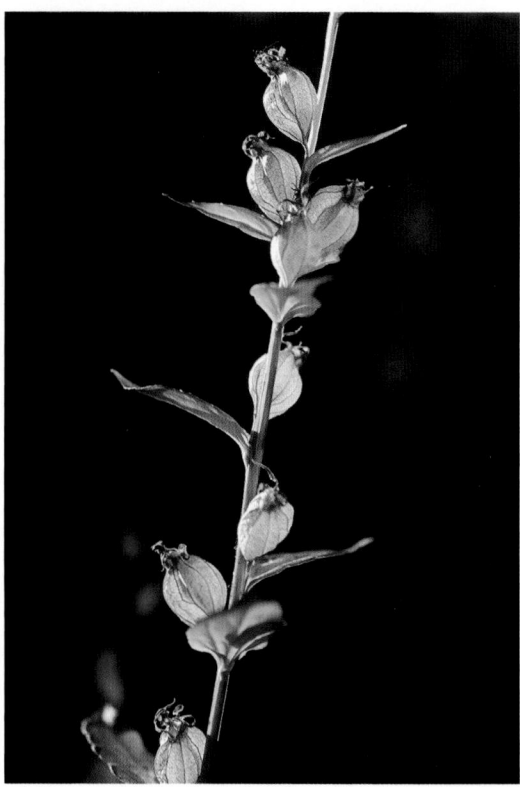

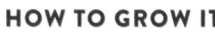
HOW TO GROW IT

An attractive garden border plant, lobelia thrives in well-drained, fertile soil and full sun to partial shade. Sow the seeds in moist soil, either directly in your garden in spring or in seed flats indoors in late winter. The seeds need light for germination; do not cover them with soil. Space plants 8 to 12 inches apart, and water during dry spells. Propagate by gathering seed in fall.

Lycium barbarum

The oval red fruits of this 9-foot-tall woody perennial are a rich source of amino acids, vitamin C, and antioxidants. In recent years, goji berry has gained a worldwide reputation as a superfood, often packaged and sold commercially as juice, dried berries, or a supplement. Native to southeastern Europe and Asia, the plant is a member of the same family as the tomato, pepper, and potato. Its preferred common name is derived from the Chinese name for the berry, *Ningxia gouqi*. During the 19th century, Chinese railroad workers introduced the plant to parts of western North America, where some wild stands still grow.

CULINARY USE

Goji berries have a sweet, tomatolike flavor. In China, the fruit is used to make tea and other beverages and is added to stews, soups, jellies, and rice congee, and to pork, chicken, and vegetable dishes. The mildly bitter-tasting leaves can also be added to soups or cooked with meat.

MEDICINAL USE

In traditional Chinese medicine, goji berries are believed to "brighten the spirit" and promote long life. Both the dried fruits and root bark of this plant are used to treat impotence, backache, weakness, dizziness, and diabetes. The root bark is also used to relieve sore throats, joint pain, and pneumonia. The berries are considered an aphrodisiac.

The goji berry contains antioxidants, including the carotenoids beta-carotene and zeaxanthin, which some believe protect our eyes from macular degeneration (although recent research has not substantiated this). A few studies have supported other benefits, however. In a recent clinical study, people who consumed goji berry juice had increased feelings of well-being and indicators of immune response compared to a placebo group. Another

clinical study of a small group of people showed that drinking goji berry juice increased feelings of well-being and improved neurological and psychological performance, as well as bowel function.

Caution: Taking this herb regularly in combination with blood thinners or diabetes and blood pressure drugs could interfere with or increase the activity of the pharmaceutical drugs.

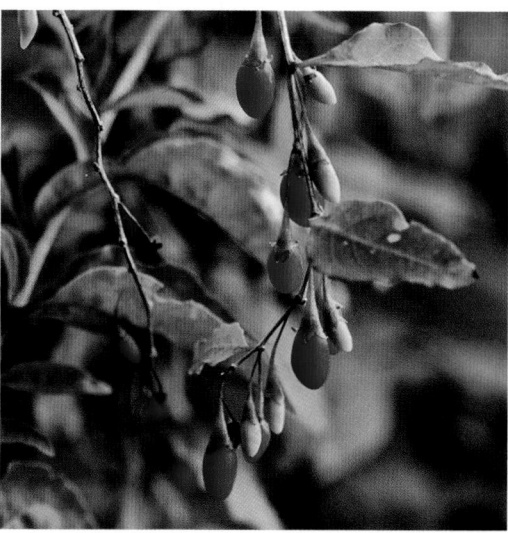

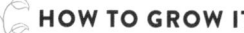

HOW TO GROW IT

Grow goji berry in full sun and well-drained, alkaline soil that's been amended with compost. Space the plants several feet apart, and pinch new growth occasionally to encourage bushiness. Fruiting begins in the plant's third year. Cover ripening fruits with netting to shield them from birds and other wildlife. Pluck the berries by hand when they are bright red (like cherry tomatoes) and sweet. Propagate by seed or cuttings.

Marrubium vulgare

PLANT PROFILE

Common Names: Horehound, White Horehound

Description: Herbaceous perennial, 2 to 3 feet tall, with branching stems and soft, hairy leaves with serrated edges; white flowers in dense whorls

Hardiness: To Zone 4

Family: Lamiaceae

Flowering: Spring to early summer

Parts Used: Leaves

Range/Habitat: Native to southern Europe, central and western Asia, and North Africa, and naturalized in North America; dry, sandy places

This woolly leaved perennial thrives in dry, sandy areas across Europe, Asia, North America, and Africa. The genus name *Marrubium* is thought to derive from *marrob*, the Hebrew word for "bitter juice," and horehound may have been one of the original bitter herbs of the Jewish Passover tradition. The herb's common name possibly comes from the ancient Egyptians, who called it the Seed of Horus, or from the ancient Greeks, who were said to have used it to treat the bites of mad dogs. Folk legend held that horehound could break magic spells.

Horehound was said to relieve chronic hepatitis, tumors, tuberculosis, typhoid, paratyphoid, snakebite, worms, itches, jaundice, and bronchitis. But it was especially valued for its actions against coughs and lung troubles. Horehound cough syrups and drops were used as early as the 1600s; the English herbalist John Gerard (1545–1611) wrote that "a syrup made of the fresh green leaves and sugar is a most singular remedie against the cough and wheezing of the lungs." While horehound remains an ingredient in some over-the-counter and prescription drugs, especially cough syrups, today it is known best as an old-fashioned candy flavoring.

CULINARY USE

Horehound's menthol-flavored leaves are used to make confections and throat lozenges. To make horehound candy, add sugar to an infusion of the leaves, then boil until the mixture reaches a thick consistency. Pour it into a shallow pan and cut it into squares after it cools.

Horehound seed can be added to iced tea and lemonade. In England, horehound has been used as a substitute for hops in beer, and horehound ale is still sold in Europe.

MEDICINAL USE

Horehound's primary medicinal constituents include tannin and marrubiin. (Marrubiin does not exist in the living plant but is formed during the extraction process.) Marrubiin has expectorant properties, which might contribute to the herb's value as a cough soother. The herb also has a high concentration of mucilage, which eases sore throats. Traditionally, the leaves have been used to make a soothing tea for coughs, colds, and sore throats.

Sometimes horehound was infused with other herbs. One old-fashioned cold remedy that could be taken several times a day was a tea made from equal parts horehound, licorice root, marshmallow root, and hyssop. Mothers also gave children horehound syrup to settle an upset stomach.

Horehound tea is sometimes taken as a bitter to produce gastric action and aid digestion. Scientists

HOW TO GROW IT

Horehound is a useful addition to any garden, as its flowers are a favorite of bees. Plant it in full sun and well-drained, sandy loam in early spring. Horehound tolerates dry conditions and can survive on as little as 12 inches of water a year. Harvest lightly the first year, cutting no more than the top third of the plant. The plants should begin to bloom in their second year. For the highest oil content, harvest the leaves just as the flower buds begin to form. The plant loses flavor quickly; to preserve the leaves, remove them immediately from the stems and chop them. When they have dried, place them in airtight jars and store them in a cool, dark location.

have found that marrubic acid, formed from marrubiin, stimulates the flow of bile in rats. Horehound also serves as a mild laxative.

A small-scale human clinical trial involving this species showed that it had some positive effects on patients with type 2 diabetes, lowering plasma glucose levels slightly, with more substantial reductions in cholesterol and triglycerides. Further studies are needed to determine whether horehound could be used as a treatment for this condition.

Caution: Do not use this herb if you are pregnant or nursing. Also, be cautious if you have a history of heart or gastrointestinal trouble; reported side effects from using large amounts over a long period include arrhythmia, low blood pressure, and diarrhea. Do not confuse this plant with black or stinking horehound (*Ballota nigra*), which may be toxic in large quantities.

OTHER USES

In the past, horehound stems and leaves were used as insect repellent. The 1st-century Roman agriculturist Columella recommended horehound for "cankerworm" in trees; others have suggested that the herb repels grasshoppers and flies. In a 2004 lab experiment comparing the effect of eight different herbs on the feeding activity of Colorado potato beetles, an extract of *Marrubium vulgare* was found to be "strongly repellent."

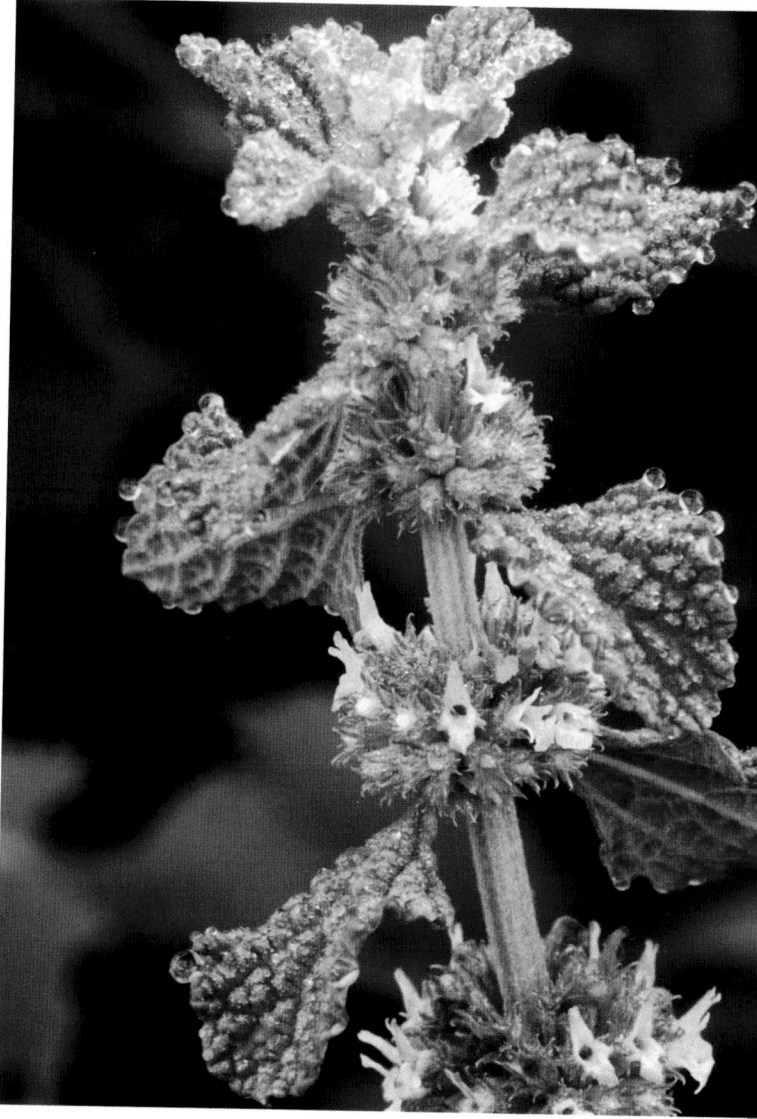

HOREHOUND COUGH SYRUP

You can make an old-time cough remedy by mixing horehound tea with honey. Boil 1 ounce of fresh or dried horehound leaves in 2 cups of water for 10 minutes. Strain off the leaves, then measure the remaining liquid. Add twice as much honey as liquid, and mix well; if necessary, warm the mixture over low heat until it is a uniform consistency. Pour the syrup into a clean bottle with a tight-fitting lid. Store the syrup in your refrigerator for up to 2 months. To soothe a cough, take 1 teaspoon up to four times a day.

Melissa officinalis

PLANT PROFILE

Common Name: Lemon Balm

Description: Loosely branched perennial up to 2 feet tall; opposite toothed leaves on square stems; clusters of tiny white flowers, highly attractive to bees; lemon scented

Hardiness: To Zone 4

Family: Lamiaceae

Flowering: Summer to fall

Parts Used: Leaves

Range/Habitat: Native to the mountains of southern Europe, northern Africa, and western Asia, widely naturalized

This powerfully lemon-scented perennial in the mint family bears toothed, oval leaves and tiny white flowers that are highly attractive to honeybees. (*Melissa* is the Greek word for honeybee.) At one time, people rubbed beehives with lemon balm to encourage the bees' productiveness. The chemical composition of lemon balm oil is very similar to a pheromone found in worker bees; this pheromone helps them locate their colony and sources of nectar.

Native to southern Europe and western Asia, lemon balm has been grown for more than 2,000 years. It has a long history of use in traditional medicine, especially as a sedative and antispasmodic. In potpourris and perfumes, it adds a fresh, lemony scent.

CULINARY USE

The fresh leaves impart a citrusy flavor to salads, soups, sauces, vinegars, and fish dishes, as well as hot and cold teas. Try adding the chopped fresh leaves to a pound cake. Or stuff sprigs into poultry or whole fish before cooking.

MEDICINAL USE

Lemon balm has been used since ancient times to lift mood and reduce fever; the Greek physician Dioscorides (ca. 40–90 CE) prescribed it in the 1st century. In the Middle Ages, people used the herb to reduce stress and anxiety, promote restful sleep, improve appetite, lower fever, and ease the pain and discomfort of indigestion. Lemon balm is one of the ingredients in Bénédictine and Chartreuse, healing liqueurs developed by monks hundreds of years ago. The 16th-century physician Paracelsus (1493–1541) also added this herb to his famous elixir that promoted revitalization.

In modern aromatherapy, herbalists recommend essential oil of lemon balm to promote relaxation and rejuvenation, especially in cases of depression and nervous tension. The herb is believed to have carminative, nervine, antidepressant, sedative, and diaphoretic properties. It contains caffeic and rosmarinic acids, which offer antiviral effects against herpes simplex 1 and 2. In Europe, lemon balm ointment is widely used to treat herpes blisters. Due to its pleasant flavor and soothing nature, this herb is especially suitable for treating children.

To make a tea, pour 1 cup of boiling water over five or six fresh leaves or 1 teaspoon of dried leaves. Steep for 5 minutes. Strain and sweeten, if desired. Drink several times per day.

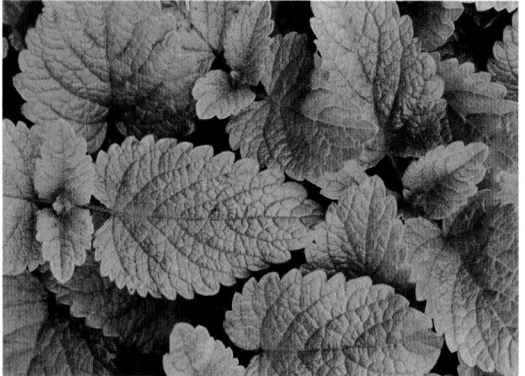

HOW TO GROW IT

Lemon balm thrives in moist, well-drained soil in full sun or partial shade. Harvest the leaves before the plant flowers, beginning in early summer. Lemon balm is a prolific self-sower; pinch off blooms to discourage its spread. Propagate by seed, cuttings, and root division.

Mentha spp.

The genus *Mentha*, named for the mythological nymph Minthe, includes many species used for flavor, fragrance, or medicinal purposes. Most are native to Europe and Asia and have naturalized widely—the spreading roots send up new plants that can quickly overtake other plants in the area. All have square stems; spikes of tiny purple, pink, or white flowers (loved by bees); and highly aromatic leaves.

Peppermint (*Mentha × piperita*) bears smooth, purple-tinged leaves and spikes of lilac-pink flowers. Ancient Greeks and Romans not only used the herb to flavor sauces and wine, but also wore peppermint crowns during feasts. Popular varieties include lemon or orange mint (*M. × piperita* var. 'Citrata'), lime mint (*M. × piperita* 'Lime'), and chocolate mint (*M. x piperita* 'Chocolate'). Spearmint (*M. spicata*) bears spikes (or "spears") of pale pink-violet flowers and wrinkled, bright green leaves favored for teas and cocktails, such as the mint julep and mojito. Pineapple mint (*M. suaveolens*), also known as apple mint, has purple-pink flowers and light green leaves with a fruity aroma and flavor.

CULINARY USE

Add mint to desserts, salads, sauces, and jellies, and to hot and cold teas and cocktails. For a refreshing complement to hot or spicy foods, combine chopped fresh mint with chopped cucumbers and plain yogurt. Also try fresh mint in tuna salads; dress it with lime vinaigrette. Mint pairs especially well with peas (including split peas), carrots, and new potatoes.

MEDICINAL USE

Spearmint and peppermint can be used to treat gastrointestinal disorders such as stomachaches and nausea, as well as fatigue. Peppermint's main constituent is a volatile oil, which is generally about 50 percent menthol. Both the fresh and dried

---

PLANT PROFILE

Common Name: Mint

Description: Square-stemmed perennials, up to 2 feet tall; terminal spikes of tiny purple, pink, or white flowers; opposite toothed leaves; highly aromatic

Hardiness: To Zone 4

Family: Lamiaceae

Flowering: Midsummer to late summer

Parts Used: Leaves

Range/Habitat: Native or naturalized along streams and in other moist areas in temperate regions throughout the world

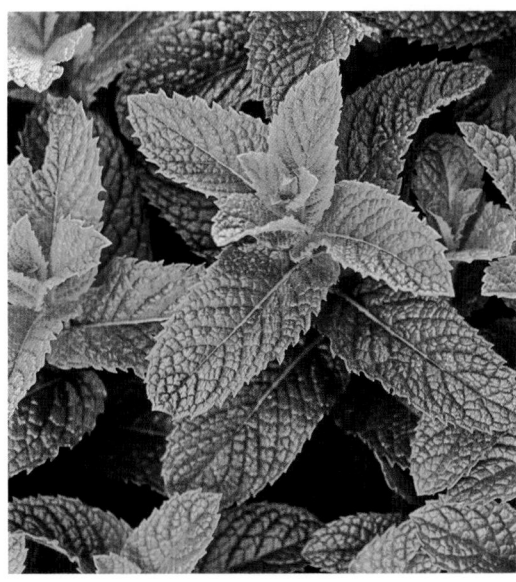

Many mints, including spearmint (*Mentha spicata*), aid digestion.

---

leaves of the plant, as well as its essential oil, generate an antispasmodic effect on the smooth muscles of your gastrointestinal tract. By stimulating digestive flow and the production of bile, peppermint may help relieve gastrointestinal conditions such as flatulence, painful digestion, intestinal cramping,

---

HOW TO GROW IT

Popular in kitchen herb gardens, mint grows best in moist soil in full sun or partial shade. Most mints spread readily, so consider planting them in large containers or a confined area of your garden. Harvest the leaves several times per season, before the plant flowers. Mints are easy to propagate by root division or cuttings.

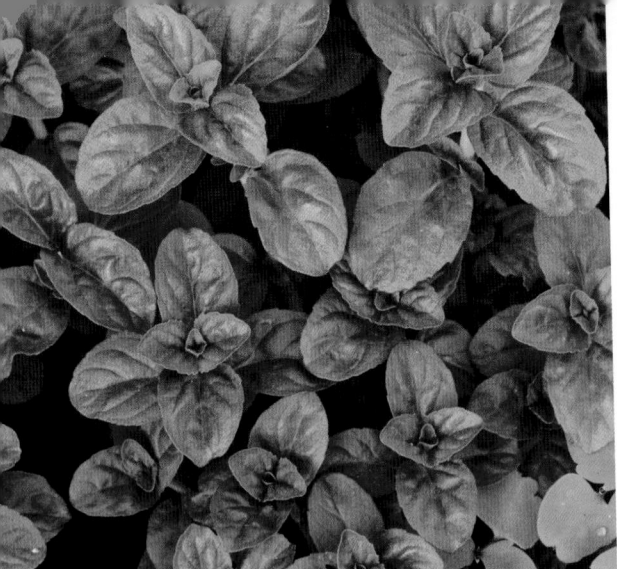
Pennyroyal (*Mentha pulegium*) is a traditional flea repellent.

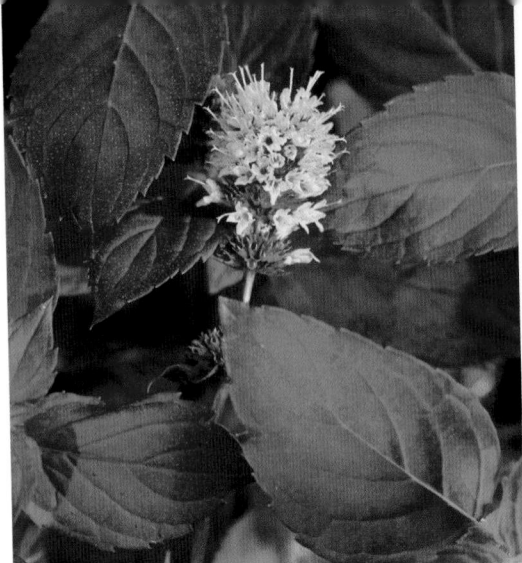
Perk up salads with leaves and blooms of peppermint (*Mentha × piperita*).

irritable bowel syndrome, and nausea due to stomach upset, motion sickness, or pregnancy.

Peppermint oil is used to treat the symptoms of irritable bowel syndrome and is most often recommended as an enteric-coated pill that will open and release the oil in your intestines, rather than in your stomach. In aromatherapy, peppermint oil is used as a stimulant to increase concentration and reduce sleepiness. Placing a drop of the essential oil in a pan of hot water and inhaling the steam may help relieve lung and sinus congestion.

Spearmint oil is considered gentler than peppermint oil (it contains much less menthol than peppermint does), but it also can be used to treat digestive complaints. In aromatherapy, it is used to treat fatigue as well as respiratory conditions such as colds, coughs, and bronchitis.

In the past, pennyroyal (*Mentha pulegium*) tea was used to treat stomach problems and to promote menstruation, but consuming tea of this species has been linked to cases of acute liver damage and infant death. Pennyroyal should be used *only* under the supervision of a highly qualified healthcare practitioner.

Caution: Pennyroyal should not be used by people with liver or kidney disease, or by pregnant or nursing women. The essential oil is highly toxic.

OTHER USES

Mint oil is used commercially to flavor candies, chewing gum, cough drops, breath mints, digestive aids, dental products, and cold and flu remedies. Many skin-care, hair, and beauty products contain mint because it has a cooling and stimulating effect.

Pennyroyal was traditionally used as an insect repellent: The species name, *pulegium*, derives from the Latin word for flea. But the essential oil of this plant is extremely toxic; never apply it to your pet's skin or fur.

MAKE YOUR OWN MINT TOOTHPASTE

The refreshing flavor of mint makes it a natural for toothpaste and other dental products. To make your own minty mouth cleanser, bring ¼ cup of water to a boil along with 1 tablespoon of chopped fresh peppermint leaves. Remove the pan from the heat and steep for 20 minutes. Meanwhile, mix together ½ teaspoon of baking soda, ½ teaspoon of cornstarch, and ½ teaspoon of grapeseed oil; stir until smooth. Strain the cooled mint tea, then add the liquid to the baking soda mixture. Bring the mixture to a boil again, stirring until it's slightly thickened and smooth. Cool completely and store in an airtight container.

Mitchella repens

This delicate-looking evergreen vine with bright red, dimpled berries can be found creeping over woodland floors in eastern and central North America. In late spring, the vines produce pairs of white or pinkish tubular flowers that are fused together at their bases. The fruits, which persist through winter, are a favorite of ruffed grouse, bobwhite, and other wildlife. Also called squaw vine, the herb has long been used by Native American women to alleviate menstrual problems and ease childbirth.

CULINARY USE

The fruits have a slight wintergreen flavor and can be used in jams; frost is said to improve their flavor. Native Americans dried the raw, mashed, or cooked fruits and stored them for later eating. The Iroquois prepared them as a sauce or added them to corn bread.

MEDICINAL USE

Partridge berry contains alkaloids, glycosides, mucilage, and tannins. Native American women made a tea from the leaves and fruit of this herb to treat menstrual pain and cramps, to regulate menstrual cycles and relieve heavy bleeding, and to induce childbirth and ease delivery. Lactating women used a salve made from the herb to soothe sore nipples.

Native Americans also used the plant for urinary and intestinal disorders, fever, joint pain, and swelling. European settlers adapted the Native American uses, and some modern herbal practitioners still use it in similar ways. In addition, the fruits have been used to make a sedative tea and an astringent skin wash.

PLANT PROFILE

Common Names: Partridge Berry, Squaw Vine, Twinberry

Description: Creeping evergreen perennial with small, rounded leaves; tubular pinkish white flowers in pairs, fused at their bases; scarlet berries have two small indentations

Hardiness: To Zone 4

Family: Rubiaceae

Flowering: Late spring to early summer

Parts Used: Fruit, leaves, and stems

Habitat/Range: Native to eastern and central North America; woodlands, slopes, and stream banks

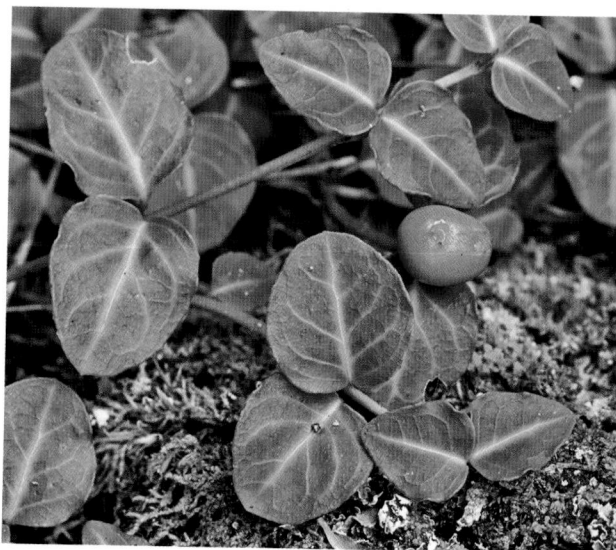

Caution: Do not use this herb if you are pregnant or nursing unless you are under the care of a health professional.

 HOW TO GROW IT

Partridge berry thrives in fertile, acidic soil and partial shade. Try growing this woodland native as a low-maintenance groundcover beneath evergreen trees or acid-loving shrubs, such as azaleas, where the plants will not be disturbed. Water during dry spells. Harvest the leaves and stems from late spring through early summer. If you wish to use the berries, harvest them when they ripen (turning bright red) in midsummer to fall. Propagate by softwood cuttings.

Momordica charantia

Bitter melon, a vining herb that can reach 6 feet or more, grows in tropical areas, including parts of Africa, Asia, the Caribbean, South America, and the Pacific Islands. The species includes two basic forms: a wild type with very small (about 1½-inch-long) inedible fruits and a cultivated form with much larger fruits reminiscent of a ribbed cucumber, covered with warts or bumps. When ripe, the fruit turns yellow-orange and splits open to reveal seeds covered with red pulp. Despite its extremely bitter flavor, the fruit is eaten as a vegetable—raw, pickled, or cooked—in its native regions, and it is commonly sold in Asian markets in North America. Bitter melon has a long history of use in Asian traditional medicine, as well.

CULINARY USE

Usually, bitter melon fruit is harvested and eaten when green; as it ripens, it loses its distinctive bitterness. The fruit is often cooked in soups and with meat, stuffed, or cut into pieces and boiled. In India, the peeled fruit is soaked in salt water before cooking to reduce some of the bitterness. Thai cooks fry the fruit with eggs. Asian cooks also stir-fry the shoots and young leaves, which are a rich source of vitamins A and C, as well as calcium. The people of the remote Pacific Islands of Micronesia even cook and eat the plant's roots.

MEDICINAL USE

This plant is used as a healing herb wherever it grows. In Thailand it is used as a tonic and to treat skin diseases. Ayurvedic medicine recommends the fruit, leaves, and roots for the treatment of type 2 diabetes. Laboratory studies with animals have shown that both a fruit extract as well as the fried fruits improved glucose tolerance, one of the goals of treating type 2 diabetes. A small study with humans showed an increase in glucose tolerance in 73 percent of patients who consumed the fruit juice.

In India, the fruit of the wild plant is used to lower fevers, while the cultivated fruit is eaten to treat arthritis, gout, and liver and spleen conditions. In Belize, where this is one of the most important medicinal plants, people boil the leaves and vines of the wild plant to make a beverage that they drink to treat parasites, amoebas, and constipation. The plant is also added to bathwater to treat skin infections, tick and chigger bites, sores, and wounds.

Caution: This herb should not be used by pregnant women, nursing mothers, or young children.

 HOW TO GROW IT

Bitter melon is easy to grow in fertile, well-drained soil and full sun. Start the seed indoors 4 to 6 weeks before your last frost date, then transplant the seedlings to your garden after all danger of frost has passed. Provide support for the climbing vines, and water them regularly. Fruiting should begin about 60 days after transplanting; harvest when the fruit are light green. Propagate by seed.

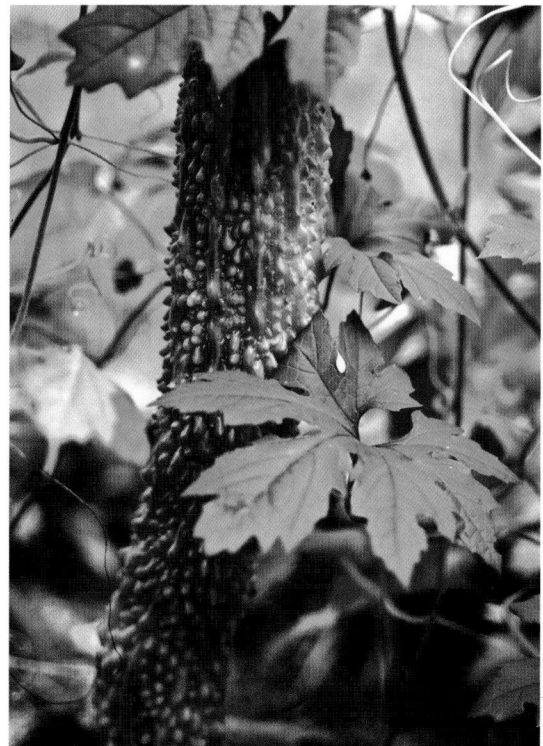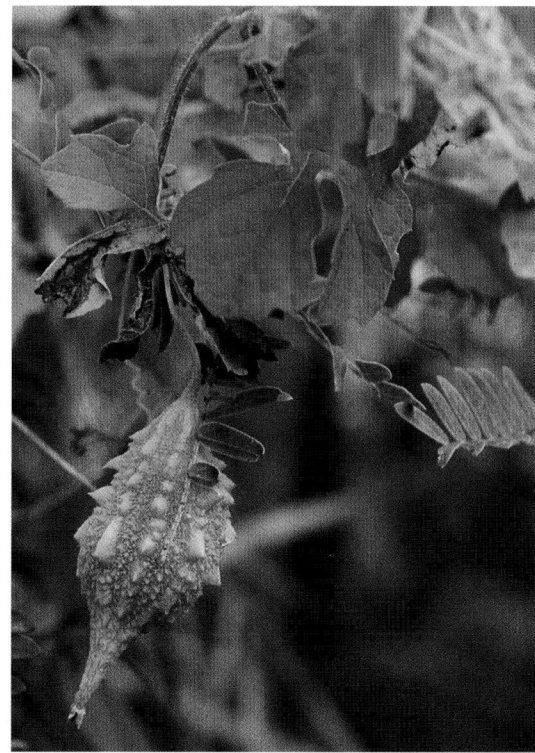

The fruit of the cultivated bitter melon (left) is edible and much larger—8 to 12 inches or more in length—than the fruit of the wild type (right)—1 to 2 inches long—which is not eaten and is used for its medicinal value.

Bitter Melon and Type 2 Diabetes

In many of the places I've traveled throughout the tropics, a curious little fruit-bearing vine can be seen climbing over fences and rocks and along the ground. The plant has two forms: this wild species, and another that has been domesticated to produce a larger, edible fruit known in commerce as bitter melon. Both forms are used medicinally to treat type 2 diabetes, and in several places, the plant is even called "vegetable insulin" (referring to its use, not its composition). At my local Asian market, imported packages of the sliced dried fruits are sold to make what is said to be a blood sugar–lowering tea.

Now many scientists are investigating bitter melon's potential. For her recently completed doctoral dissertation, a student I worked with, Amy Keller, PhD, studied the antidiabetic activity of the cultivated fruit of Momordica charantia both in laboratory assays using living cells and with animals. She found one component of the fruit to be rich in saponins—a class of chemicals in many plants traditionally used as natural soaps. Dr. Keller also discovered that the saponins were able to stimulate insulin secretion in a lab assay—the first time this has been observed with bitter melon. Recently, Egyptian scientists announced their intention to make a bitter melon extract into a therapy for type 2 diabetes. Where this path will lead is unknown, but it could someday be another example of the healing powers of nature.—M. J. B.

Monarda spp.

Monarda is a genus of 17 native North American aromatic perennials related to mint. Their showy flower heads—which range in color from bright red (*Monarda didyma*) to lavender (*M. fistulosa*) to yellow (*M. punctata*)—are extremely attractive to bees. The common name "bee balm" refers to its use as a poultice for the treatment of bee stings. Named for Nicolas Monardes (1493–1588), a 16th-century Spanish physician who documented many New World plants, herbs in this genus are also known as bergamots because their fragrance is similar to that of bergamot orange (*Citrus bergamia*).

The monardas, which grow wild throughout North American woodland edges, prairies, and along stream banks, were widely used by Native Americans and early European settlers. Native Americans prepared infusions and poultices from the plants to treat fevers, colds, flus, respiratory and kidney conditions, abdominal discomfort, skin infections, wounds, and many other ailments. During the American War of Independence, Colonial Americans dried the leaves of *Monarda didyma* and used them as a substitute for British-imported tea. The common name "Oswego tea" was coined by the renowned 18th-century botanist John Bartram (1699–1777), who encountered the herb at Fort Oswego, New York, where it grew abundantly.

CULINARY USE

A blend of *Monarda didyma* leaves, mint, and orange peel makes a delicious iced tea. The plant's flowers are also edible and can be added to salads or used to decorate cakes, fruit punches, or iced teas. Use *M. fistulosa* leaves in teas or to flavor bean and meat dishes. *M. citriodora*, known as lemon bergamot, also makes a tasty tea and flavorful accent for fish and meats. Try mincing the fresh leaves of any type and adding them to plain yogurt with a bit of honey as a topping for fresh fruit. Or include a handful of the fresh leaves when making jelly. Strain the leaves before boiling down to the gel stage.

MEDICINAL USE

Plants in this genus contain a compound with antiseptic and expectorant properties. *Monarda punctata* has been used to treat digestive ailments such as indigestion, nausea, and vomiting and upper respiratory conditions such as cold and flu. It also helps to reduce fever by increasing sweating, and it encourages the onset of menstruation. Combined with other herbs, *M. didyma* is helpful in the treatment of urinary tract infections and indigestion, and laboratory studies have suggested that it may inhibit the growth of certain viruses.

Caution: Monarda species should not be taken during pregnancy.

HOW TO GROW IT

Plant *Monarda didyma* in rich, moist soil in full sun. *M. fistulosa* and *M. punctata* prefer dry, light, alkaline soil in full sun. Pinch back the tops of your plants in late spring to encourage bushier growth. Harvest leaves for tea just before the plant flowers in midsummer to late summer, and again after flowering has finished. To obtain the best flavor for tea, strip the leaves from the stems and dry them in a warm, shady place for 2 to 3 days. Longer drying periods tend to produce less-flavorful teas. Store the dried leaves in an airtight container in a cool location.

After 3 to 4 years, bee balm clumps tend to die out in the center. To rejuvenate your planting, dig up the roots in fall and replant only the outside sucker shoots. Space the new plants about 2 feet apart.

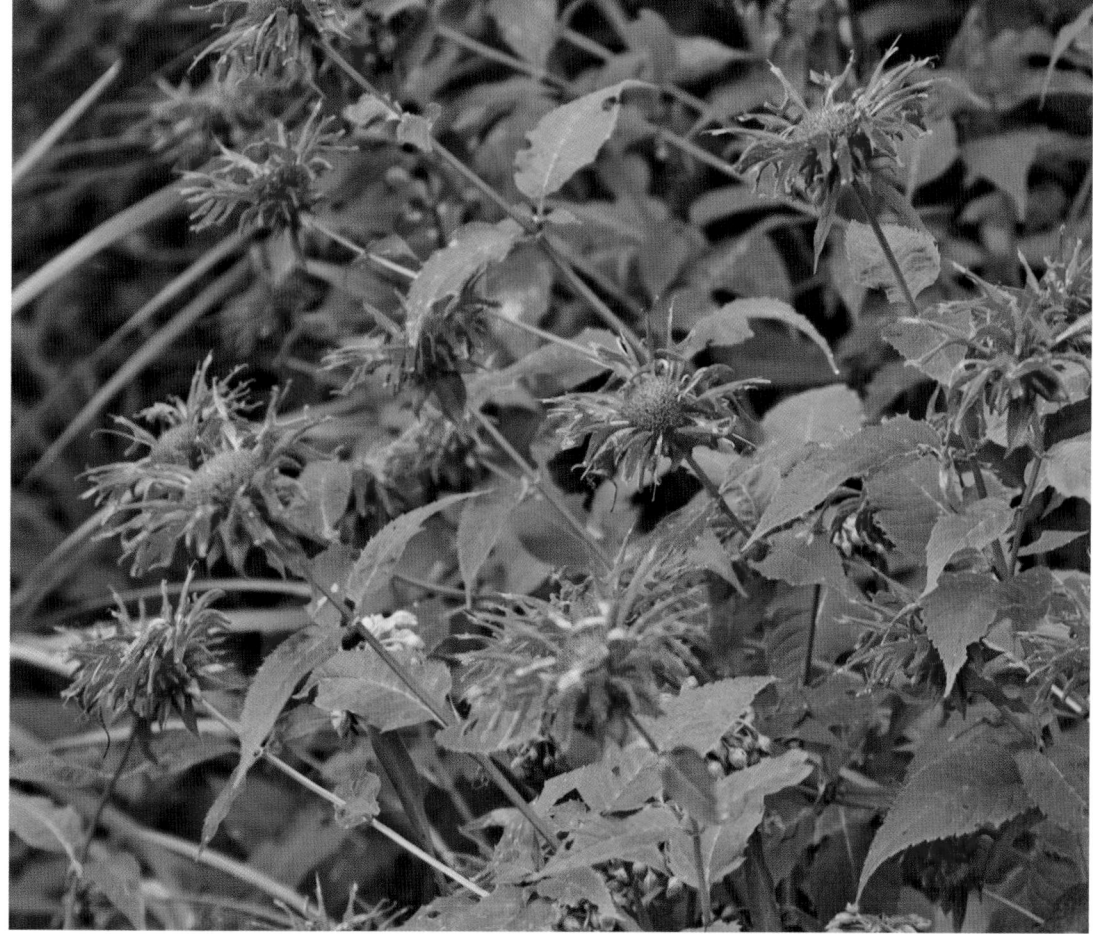

ORNAMENTAL USE

Long blooming and deer resistant, monardas make excellent garden plants. Their bright blooms attract hummingbirds, bees, and butterflies and add color to cottage gardens, informal borders, and cut flower arrangements. Recommended cultivars include 'Blue Stocking' (violet-purple blooms), 'Cambridge Scarlet' (bright red blooms), 'Croftway Pink' (rosy pink blooms), and 'Snow Maiden' (white blooms).

FIELD NOTES
Learning from the Birds, Bees, and Butterflies

With a profusion of blood red flowers that glow in the late summer sun, bee balm (Monarda didyma) can transform the landscape into a spectacular palette of color. Large numbers of bees, butterflies, and hummingbirds congregate around each planting to feed on the refreshing nectar. But not every creature can procure the saccharine treasure—they must have long tongues that can reach down into the floral tubes. We can enjoy this essence, as well: Pour a cup of boiling water over a teaspoon of fresh bee balm flowers or leaves, allow the tea to steep for 10 to 15 minutes, and then sweeten it to taste. Try this wonderful tea in the evening before sleeping, particularly if a cold is coming on.—M. J. B.

Morella cerifera

(= *Myrica cerifera*)

PLANT PROFILE

Common Names: Bayberry, Candleberry, Southern Bayberry, Wax Myrtle

Description: Shrub, 15 to 20 feet tall, with long, leathery leaves and inconspicuous flowers; females bear clusters of waxy, blue-gray berries in fall; leaves and berries aromatic when crushed

Hardiness: To Zone 7

Family: Myricaceae

Flowering: March to April

Parts Used: Berries and root bark

Range/Habitat: Southeastern United States; coasts, wetlands, and forests

The long, leathery leaves of this native American evergreen shrub contain aromatic compounds that release a pleasant fragrance when crushed. Both Southern bayberry and the similar Northern bayberry (*Morella* [*Myrica*] *pensylvanica*) belong to the family Myricaceae, which derives its name from the Greek *myrike,* meaning "fragrant plant."

Bayberry male and female flowers occur on separate plants. Females yield small, blue-gray waxy berries that are an important food source for several birds. A wax extracted from the berries of this and related species was used to make the fragrant candles popular during the winter holiday season, but today many of these products have been replaced with synthetic substitutes. The wax was obtained by boiling the fruits in water, then skimming the thin layer as it collected on top of the water. After the wax was filtered, candles were made by dipping a wick into the collected wax, or by molding the wax.

MEDICINAL USE

Native Americans traditionally used the root bark, leaves, and stems of bayberry for healing. The Choctaw boiled bayberry leaves and stems in water and used the decoction to treat fevers; they prepared the root similarly to relieve sore throats. European settlers used bayberry to treat pain, convulsions, and other conditions. Herbalists in the 18th and 19th century commonly prescribed it for colds, flu, diarrhea, and fever.

Bayberry contains the antibiotic and antioxidant compound myricetin. As an astringent and tonic, the root bark is believed to tighten and dry mucous membranes. Modern herbalists sometimes recommend decoctions and tinctures of the root bark for nasal congestion, colds, sore throats, and diarrhea.

Caution: There are reports of toxicity with this plant, and the wax of bayberry may have carcinogenic effects. This plant should not be used by pregnant women.

ORNAMENTAL USE

Southern bayberry is an attractive, fast-growing landscape shrub that makes an outstanding evergreen screen or hedge. The plant is rarely bothered by insect pests, diseases, or drought.

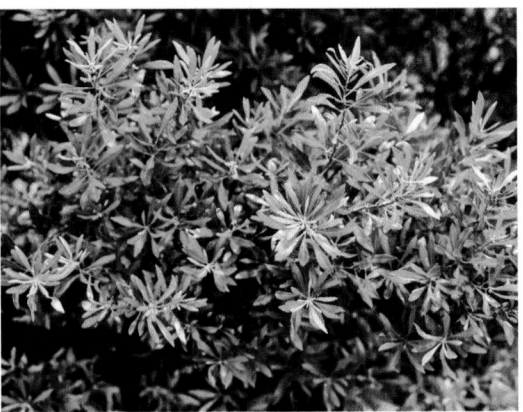

HOW TO GROW IT

Bayberry is easy to grow in moist, rich, well-drained soil in full sun to partial shade. Plant 1- or 2-year-old nursery-grown shrubs in spring or fall. Both male and female plants are needed to produce fruit. Bayberry responds well to pruning. Harvest the blue-gray berries when they ripen in early fall. Harvest the root bark from mature shrubs in spring. To propagate, take softwood cuttings in early summer to midsummer.

Myrrhis odorata

An aromatic perennial native to Europe and naturalized in North America, sweet cicely was once believed to offer protection against bubonic plague. There is evidence of its use in ancient times, too; Roman herbalist Pliny the Elder (23–79 AD) may have mentioned it in his writings about local plants. Like other members of the parsley family, the herb has lacy, fernlike foliage and bears numerous white flowers in umbels that are attractive to bees. Versatile sweet cicely is both a food and a medicine. In earlier times, the leaves were commonly cooked as a "potherb" with other vegetables, and the entire plant was valued for healing digestive disorders. A related plant also known as sweet cicely, *Osmorhiza berteroi*, is native to North America and has been used in similar ways.

CULINARY USE

Sweet cicely tastes like a combination of celery and anise. The plant is naturally sweet, and both the leaves and green seeds make an excellent, calorie-free substitute for sugar in fruit or vegetable salads, jams, desserts, syrups, or anywhere else a sweet accent is needed. You can also press the leaves into fish before grilling. The root can be steamed, simmered, or cooked and pureed, just like parsnip. Try adding the grated fresh root to breads and muffins.

MEDICINAL USE

The leaves, stems, and seeds of this plant are used to treat intestinal gas, increase appetite, and aid digestion. Sweet cicely tea has long been used as a mild laxative. The boiled root can be used to prepare an antiseptic ointment to help heal bites and wounds. To freshen your breath, simply chew the leaves.

PLANT PROFILE

Common Names: Anise, Sweet Cicely

Description: Perennial, up to 3 feet tall; lacy, fern-like foliage that's spotted underneath; umbels of white flowers, followed by shiny, dark brown, ridged seeds

Hardiness: To Zone 3

Family: Apiaceae

Flowering: June to August

Parts Used: Leaves, seeds, stem, and roots

Range/Habitat: Native to Europe, naturalized in North America; grassy areas and woodland edges on mountains and hillsides

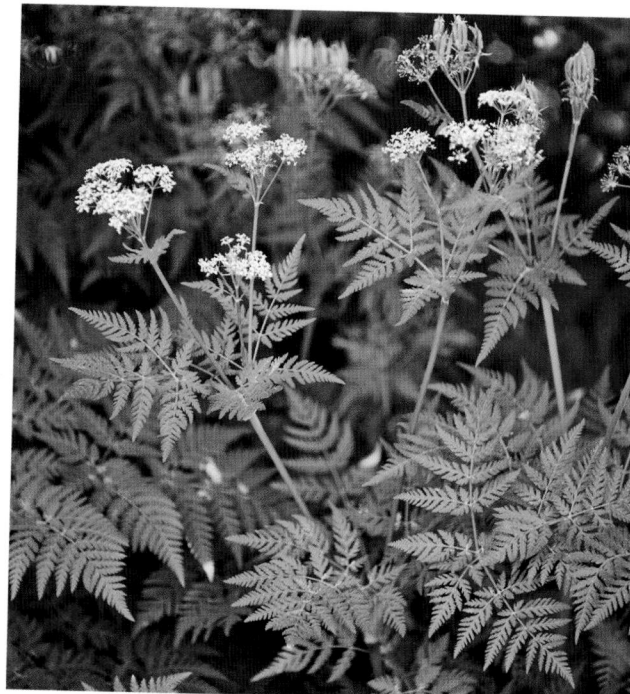

HOW TO GROW IT

Start from purchased plants, if possible. Sweet cicely seeds require a period of cold and moisture to germinate. To provide this, sow the seeds in a container filled with moist seed-starting medium. Enclose the container inside a plastic bag, then store it in a refrigerator for about 8 weeks. After 8 weeks, move the container to a warm, bright location. Seedlings should appear 2 to 3 weeks later. Outdoors, plant sweet cicely in moist, well-drained, humus-rich soil and partial shade. Harvest the herb's leaves as needed throughout the growing season; the leaves are best when they're fresh and do not dry well. Harvest seed heads when the seeds are still green. Hang the stems upside down to dry; store the dry seeds in an airtight container.

Nepeta cataria

A relative of mint, catnip is a unique herb—it's stimulating and intoxicating to cats but relaxing to humans. Early Greeks and Romans cultivated the plant not only for cats, but also for their own use as a culinary and healing plant. It was mentioned in *Apicius*, a collection of recipes used in ancient Rome. In medieval times, catnip leaves and young branches were used in salads and as a seasoning. A Middle English herbal recommended catnip tea for "evils that a man has about his throat." The herb came to America with the colonists, and in 1796 it was listed as a commercial crop. Early American writers Washington Irving, Nathaniel Hawthorne, and Harriet Beecher Stowe all mentioned catnip in their writings.

CULINARY USE

In the past, catnip was a popular kitchen herb, valued for its mintlike flavor and ability to aid digestion. Try adding a small amount of minced leaves to salads, sauces, and stews. It also makes a pleasant tea.

MEDICINAL USE

This gentle herb has been used medicinally for at least 2,000 years. It contains nepetalactone isomers, components similar to the sedative compounds found in valerian. Like valerian, catnip has traditionally been used as a mild tranquilizer and sedative. When taken after a meal, catnip tea can help relieve indigestion and heartburn. Because this herb stimulates perspiration, it's also used to treat fevers. The Chinese use the related herb jing jie (*Nepeta tenuifolia*) to treat skin infections, colds, sore throats, and fevers.

Caution: Catnip should not be ingested during pregnancy because its volatile oils could irritate the uterus. Drink the tea in moderation; large amounts can cause nausea.

PLANT PROFILE

Common Names: Catnip, Catmint

Description: Perennial, 2 to 4 feet tall, with opposite, coarsely toothed, gray-green leaves; spikes of tubular ¼- to ½-inch spotted white or blue blooms; aromatic

Hardiness: To Zone 4

Family: Lamiaceae

Flowering: June to August

Parts Used: Leaves and flowers

Range/Habitat: Native to Eurasia; naturalized in North America; rocky, mountainous areas and dry roadsides

ORNAMENTAL USE

Long blooming, deer resistant, and tolerant of dry conditions, catnip is an excellent choice for your ornamental garden. As a bonus, the brightly colored flowers draw butterflies and hummingbirds.

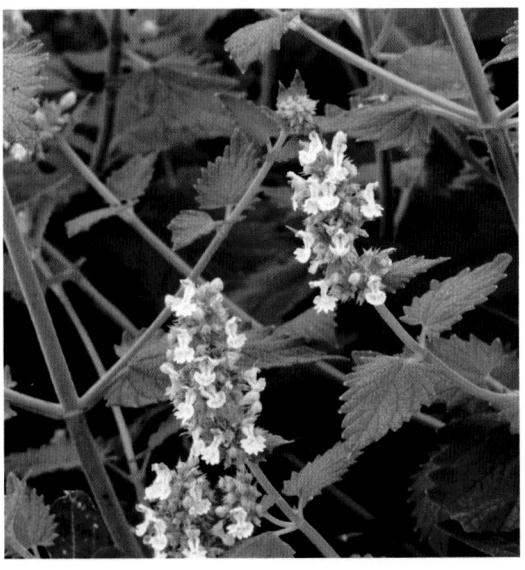

HOW TO GROW IT

Catnip flourishes in well-drained soil in full sun or partial shade. The herb is drought tolerant, but it grows best with consistent watering. Harvest the leaves as needed throughout the season. To encourage a second flush of bloom, cut back the faded flower stems in midsummer. (Dry the leaves from the cut stems for later use in teas.) Propagate catnip from seed or by root division; established plants self-seed freely.

Ocimum basilicum

This star of the summer garden and kitchen is believed to be native to India, tropical Africa, or Asia. A member of the mint family, basil has been cultivated and used in the Mediterranean region for thousands of years. Ancient Egyptians used the herb in embalming preparations and burned it (with myrrh) in ceremonies to appease the gods. They also used it to scent water for washing their hands and faces. Curiously, the ancient Romans associated basil with love, while the Greeks considered it a symbol of mourning.

The genus name *Ocimum* is derived from the Greek "to smell," acknowledging the plant's powerful aroma. Important varieties include 'Anise' (purplish leaves and a sweet licorice scent); 'Cinnamon' (pink flowers and a strong cinnamon scent); 'Genovese' (considered by many to be the best-flavored basil); 'Purple Ruffles' (an ornamental variety with dark purple, fringed leaves); and 'Lemon' (citrus-scented leaves).

CULINARY USE

Basil's strong fragrance and flavor—sometimes described as a cross between licorice and cloves—make it a favorite in many cuisines. Basil is a primary ingredient in Italian pesto sauce and the French *pistou,* both of which are made with olive oil and garlic. It is also a key flavoring in many Asian dishes.

Use basil with tomatoes and in tomato-based dishes, or in place of lettuce on sandwiches. It can be used in soups, stews, and seafood dishes, as well as with cooked squash, eggplant, potatoes, carrots, and other vegetables. Add it near the end of cooking to preserve its fresh flavor. Italians often place fresh basil on the table in a

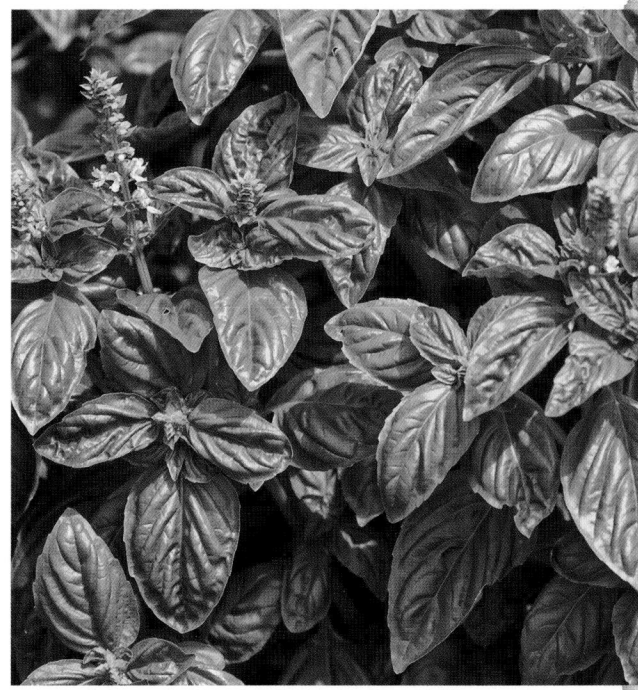

Large-leaf sweet basil (*Ocimum basilicum*), favored for cooking.

HOW TO GROW IT

Basil prefers light, rich, well-drained to slightly dry soil in full sun. Plant seeds or set out transplants only after all danger of frost has passed and soil temperature is at least 50°F. In areas where the growing season is short, seeds can be started indoors 4 to 6 weeks before the last frost date. For the strongest flavor, harvest sprigs before flower buds form. Pinching back the stem tips every 2 to 3 weeks will encourage strong, bushy growth. Keep the cut stems in a vase with a little water on your kitchen counter; the leaves will remain in good condition for up to 5 days. To enjoy fresh basil throughout the winter, root cuttings in water, then grow the potted cuttings in a bright, warm location.

small vase of water to be used as a seasoning, like salt and pepper, during meals. Basil loses much of its flavor when dried. To enjoy the herb throughout the winter, chop the leaves of freshly harvested basil and put them in an ice cube tray. Fill the tray with water and freeze for later use in soups, stews, and sauces.

MEDICINAL USE

Basil is a good source of vitamins A and C. The leaves, rich in volatile oils, are used to improve digestion. The herb may help relax intestinal spasms and relieve gas, bloating, and nausea. It is also useful as a treatment for intestinal parasites.

Basil has antiseptic and antibacterial properties. A poultice of the crushed leaves can be used to treat acne or applied to insect bites to relieve itching. Several commercially available topical healing preparations contain extract of basil.

This herb is also used to help reduce fevers and relieve colds, coughs, and flu symptoms. It has mild sedative properties, as well, and has been used to treat anxiety, depression, and insomnia. In aromatherapy, essential oil of basil can be added to massage oil and used externally to relax muscles.

Caution: Basil essential oil should not be used internally, nor should it be used in any form during pregnancy. It should *always* be heavily diluted in a carrier oil and never applied directly, in its pure form, to your skin. It contains the compound estragole, which evidence shows may be a carcinogen and mutagen (causing mutation). If used in excess, the oil can be stupefying—causing confusion or worse.

OTHER USES

Basil essential oil is used in some soaps, perfumes, and cosmetics. Many people believe that its scent is uplifting. In Italy and Greece, the aromatic herb is commonly grown in pots on porches or windowsills to help repel flies and mosquitoes. Try rubbing the fresh leaves on your clothing to do the same. Or apply a few drops of a diluted tincture of basil leaves to your clothing, being careful to avoid contact with your skin. You can also try filling your aromatherapy diffuser with basil oil and putting it outdoors on a balmy summer day when mosquitoes are around.

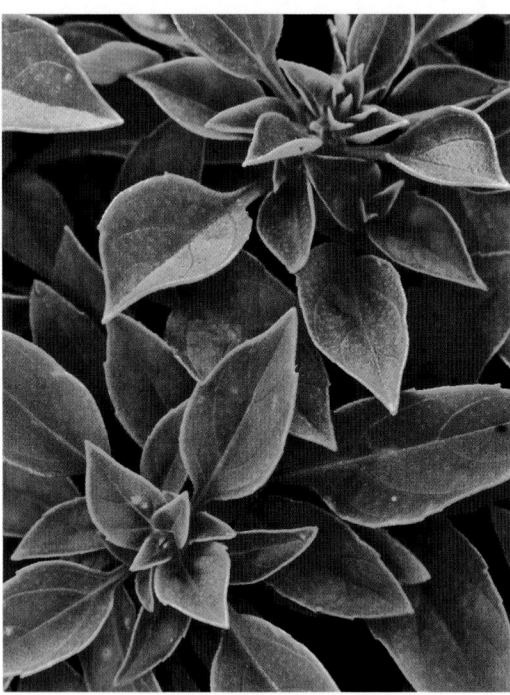

Bush basil (*Ocimum minimum*) is perfect for pots.

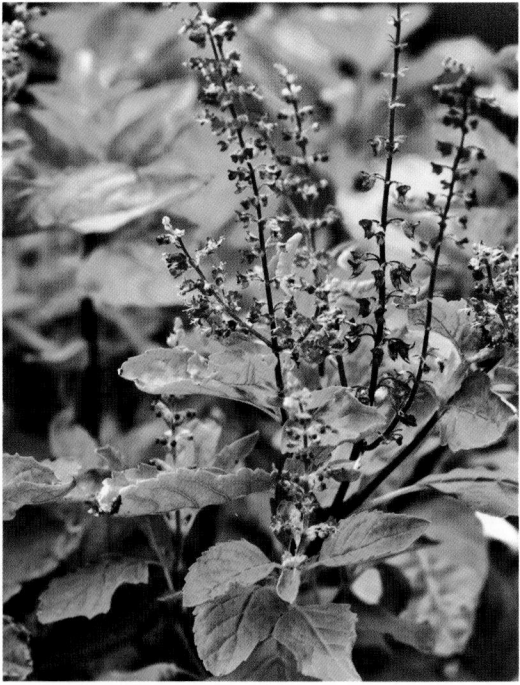

Tulsi or holy basil (*Ocimum tenuiflorum*) is an Ayurvedic adaptogen.

Oenothera biennis

Native to eastern and central North America, evening primrose is widely naturalized throughout the world. This tall plant bears beautiful, fragrant yellow flowers that open each day at dusk. The genus name is derived from the Greek term for "wine-scenting," referring to the ancient use of the roots of related species to flavor wine. Native Americans ate the seeds of *Oenothera biennis* as food and made a poultice from the whole plant for treating skin conditions such as bruises. Early American settlers used evening primrose to treat gastrointestinal upset, sore throats, and rashes.

Today the herb is valued mainly for its seed oil, which is used medicinally and as an ingredient in some cosmetics. As many as 5,000 seeds are needed to produce one capsule of evening primrose oil.

CULINARY USE

Harvested at the end of the first season, the thick roots have a sweet flavor, similar to that of parsnips. Add the young leaves and shoots to soups and stews; you can also add the flowers to salads. Roast the ripe seeds in the oven and use them in breads, cereals, or other foods.

MEDICINAL USE

The oil pressed from ripe evening primrose seeds is a good source of gamma linoleic acid (GLA), an unsaturated fatty acid that reduces inflammation and ensures the health of cell membranes. Some studies have shown that evening primrose oil may help reduce joint pain from rheumatoid arthritis, and it could be useful in the treatment of eczema. People also take the herb for nerve damage associated with diabetes, high blood pressure, high cholesterol, breast pain or tenderness, and other

PLANT PROFILE
Common Names: Evening Primrose
Description: Herbaceous biennial, up to 6 feet tall; crinkled, lance-shaped leaves form a rosette the first year, grow spirally on a stem the second year; fragrant yellow flowers open at dusk
Hardiness: Biennial; to Zone 3
Family: Onagraceae
Flowering: Late spring to late summer
Parts Used: Seeds, flowers, and roots
Range/Habitat: Native to North America, widely naturalized

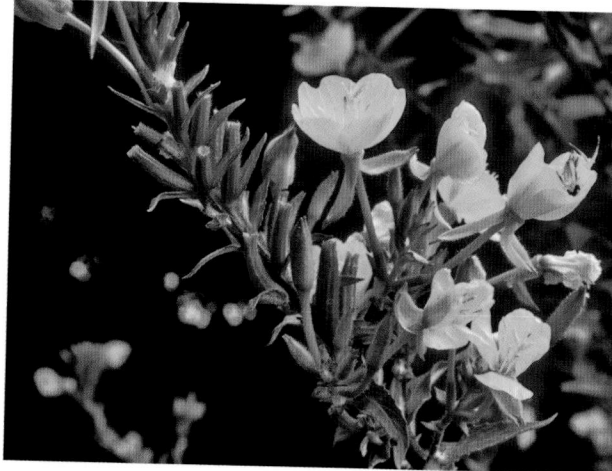

conditions, but additional clinical studies are needed to support these uses.

ORNAMENTAL USE

Grow evening primrose at the back of an informal border, along a fence in a cottage garden, or in a wildflower meadow. Its bright yellow blooms attract sphinx moths and bees; the seeds draw goldfinches.

HOW TO GROW IT

Evening primrose grows well in poor, dry soil, including coastal sandy areas, in full sun or partial shade. Plant the seeds directly in your garden, scattering them on the surface of the soil, in either spring or fall. Or start seeds indoors in early spring, then transplant seedlings to the garden 6 to 8 weeks later. Harvest the young leaves in early summer. To harvest the seeds, look for the seedpods in midsummer to late summer, after the flowers have faded. Collect the pods when their tops turn brown; inside the pods, the mature seeds should be dark brown and hard. Harvest the roots in fall. Considered an invasive weed in some areas, the plant self-seeds freely.

Origanum majorana

Origanum, the genus name for both oregano and marjoram, comes from the Greek *oros*, which means mountains, and *ganos*, which means joy—a reference to the cheerful appearance these plants give to the Mediterranean hillsides where they grow. The genus, which includes more than 40 species, was valued primarily for its healing properties before it became popular for cooking. *Oreganum majorana*, marjoram, is thought to be native to North Africa, the Middle East, and parts of India and has naturalized in southern Europe. The ancient Greeks also used this aromatic herb as a spice, a tea, and a hair pomade. In ancient Crete, distinguished leaders wore a sprig of marjoram as a badge of honor. Today, oil of marjoram is used as a fragrance in soaps, creams, lotions, and perfumes.

CULINARY USE

This herb, which has a much more subtle flavor than its close relative oregano, is excellent for use in Mediterranean meat or seafood dishes, soups, tomato sauces, and pasta dishes. It also combines well with carrots, cauliflower, mushrooms, peas, potatoes, and squash.

Oil of marjoram is a common flavoring for commercially produced beverages, ice creams, baked goods, soups, and condiments. The herb is also used as a food preservative.

MEDICINAL USE

An ingredient in ancient "sneezing powders" used to treat rhinitis, marjoram can relieve symptoms of the common cold. When taken into the respiratory system through steam inhalation (the herb's volatile oil is vaporized by boiling water), marjoram may help unblock sinuses and relieve laryngitis. Essen-

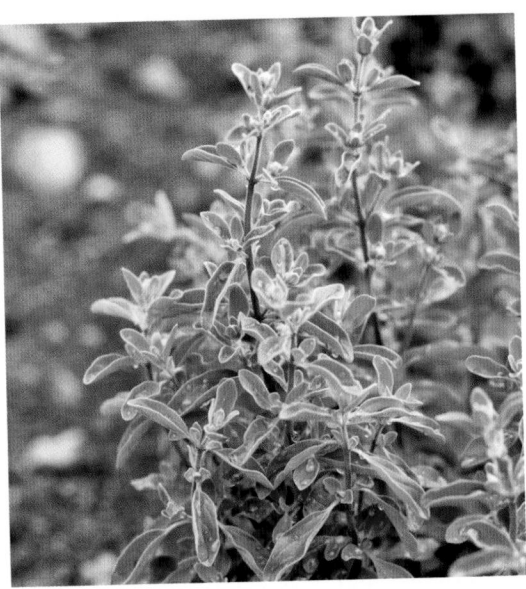

tial oil of marjoram can be added to a bath to encourage relaxation and to alleviate the symptoms of a cold or flu. Marjoram oil is included in massage oils to help relieve muscle cramps, including those brought on by menstrual and joint pain.

HOW TO GROW IT

Marjoram thrives in rich, well-drained dry soil and full sun. Start seeds indoors 6 weeks before your last spring frost date. Space seedlings 18 inches apart in your garden after danger of frost has passed; avoid overwatering. Just before the plants bloom, cut the stems to within 1 inch of the ground. Dry the stems in a warm, dark place, then rub them on a screen to remove the leaves. Discard the stems and store the leaves in an airtight container. Propagate by cuttings or root division.

Origanum vulgare

This fragrant, bushy perennial grows to 2 feet tall, bearing hairy oval leaves and branched clusters of pink flowers that attract bees and other beneficial insects. Native to Europe, central Asia, and the Mediterranean regions, oregano has been used since prehistoric times as a food and medicinal plant. The ancient Greeks considered it a sign of happiness when the plant was found growing on the grave of a loved one. Before hops plants were introduced to England (probably in the late 15th century), oregano's flowering tops were added to ale and beer as a preservative and flavoring. In medieval times, the plant was strewn, along with rushes, on stone floors to release a sweet scent when walked upon.

CULINARY USE

Fresh or dried, oregano is popular in Italian, Greek, and Mexican cuisines. It complements cheese, tomato, bean, pasta, meat, and egg dishes. Also called the "pizza herb," oregano imparts a flavor that is universally known. Commercially, it is used to flavor some alcoholic beverages, baked goods, and meat products.

MEDICINAL USE

The essential oil of oregano contains thymol and carvacrol, chemicals that have powerful antiseptic, antibiotic, and antifungal properties. The herb is used to improve digestion, to kill intestinal worms, and as an expectorant to treat inflamed bronchial membranes. To relieve a cough, you can take oregano as a tea or inhale it by steam. (The herb's volatile oil is vaporized by boiling water.)

Externally, the leaves can be applied as a hot compress—as the ancient Greeks did—for treating skin conditions, swellings, joint pain, and colic. Diluted oregano oil can be applied to insect bites and athlete's foot.

PLANT PROFILE

Common Name: Oregano

Description: Fragrant, bushy, 2-foot-tall perennial; opposite, hairy, oval leaves; spikes of pink, purple, or white flowers

Hardiness: To Zone 5

Family: Lamiaceae

Flowering: Midsummer to late summer

Parts Used: Leaves and flowers

Range/Habitat: Native to Europe, central Asia, and the Mediterranean region

Practitioners of traditional Chinese medicine use oregano to treat gastrointestinal and respiratory conditions, childhood malnutrition, and fevers.

OTHER USES

Oregano leaves and flowers are fragrant additions to potpourris; the dried flowers can also be used in wreaths and crafts. Essential oil of oregano is an ingredient in some men's colognes.

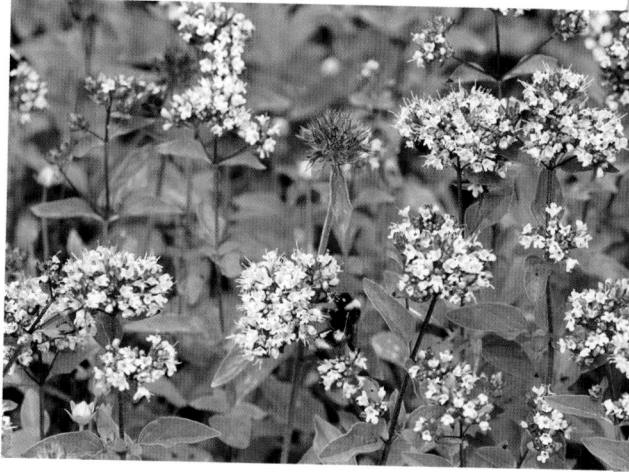

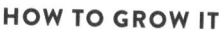

HOW TO GROW IT

Oregano thrives in well-drained to dry soil in full sun. Start with nursery-grown plants; if possible, taste the herb before purchasing because individual plants can vary in flavor. Beginning during the second year, cut back the stems almost to the ground just as the plants begin to bloom. Dry the stems in a warm, dark place, then rub them on a screen to remove the leaves. Discard the stems and store the leaves in an airtight container. Propagate by cuttings or root division.

Panax quinquefolius; P. ginseng

PLANT PROFILE

Common Names: American Ginseng; Asian Ginseng

Description: Single stem, up to 16 inches tall; glossy green, lobed leaves; mature plants bear umbels of green flowers, followed by bright red berries; wrinkled roots

Hardiness: To Zone 3

Family: Araliaceae

Flowering: June to August, depending on location

Parts Used: Root

Range/Habitat: *Panax quinquefolius* is native to hardwood forests in eastern North America, *P. ginseng* is native to northern China and Korea

Ginseng, one of the most important and widely used herbal remedies of our time, has a long history of use for healing. The genus name, *Panax*, comes from the Greek word for panacea, or cure-all. Six species are used in traditional medicine around the world. The best known are *Panax quinquefolius* (American ginseng) and *P. ginseng* (Asian ginseng). (Eleuthero, *Eleutherococcus senticosus*, the so-called Siberian ginseng, is not a true ginseng.) A perennial, ginseng bears single stems with three to six leaves and a flowering stalk that produces bright red berries. The fleshy root is the part most often used medicinally.

American ginseng (photo opposite) is native to the cool, hardwood forests of eastern America, where it is still wild harvested. (Some American ginseng is cultivated in North America and China.) Native Americans used the root of this plant in many medicinal compounds, including a remedy that induces sweating to lower a fever.

Asian ginseng is native to northern China and South Korea but is nearly extinct in the wild. The herb is widely cultivated in China, Korea, Russia, and Japan, and it is considered very important in traditional Chinese medicine (TCM). If you go into an Asian herb shop or grocery, you might see ginseng roots on display in bottles—their thick, gnarled shapes sometimes have an uncanny resemblance to the human form.

CULINARY USE

Ginseng root has a sweet, slightly bitter flavor. It is used in teas and soups, as well as in some commercial soft drinks and chewing gums.

MEDICINAL USE

Ginseng has an impressive history of medicinal use dating back 2,000 years. Herbalists use the herb to relieve and prevent mental and physical fatigue, and studies have shown that it can also reduce the frequency and severity of colds. The root contains stimulating compounds known as ginsenosides, which might gradually improve your body's response to stress, minimize the effects of depressants such as alcohol and barbiturates, and lower blood sugar levels.

In TCM, Asian ginseng is considered a warming herb, which means that it benefits the blood and circulatory system. Practitioners use it to treat exhaustion, impotence, lack of appetite, and diseases that sap strength, such as cancer.

American ginseng, which is considered less potent than Asian ginseng, is considered a cooling herb that benefits the respiratory and digestive systems. Healers use it to treat nervous indigestion, weak stomach, loss of appetite, and mental exhaustion. Some herbalists believe American ginseng to be especially beneficial for people who are overstressed and overworked.

HOW TO GROW IT

Ginseng prefers cool and shady hardwood forests. The plant flourishes in areas with ample moisture in summer and freezing temperatures in winter. Because it is susceptible to fungal diseases and rodent predation, it can be difficult to grow, and the seed is not readily available. If you are able to obtain seeds, plant them in fall. When the plants are 5 to 6 years old, you can begin harvesting the roots, although ginseng plants are not considered fully grown until they are about 20 years old.

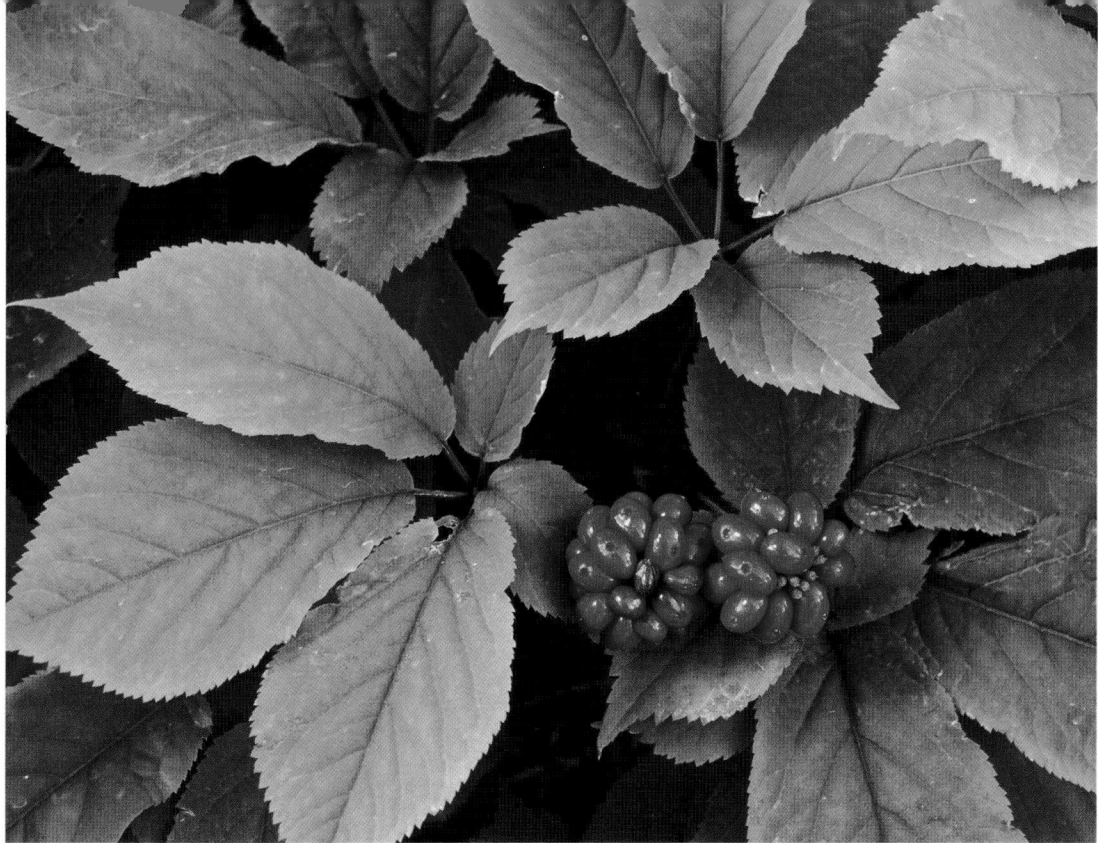

To make ginseng tea, simmer 1 teaspoon of the dried and sliced or powdered root in 1 cup of water for 10 minutes. Strain. Drink 1 or 2 cups per day.

Caution: Because wild American ginseng is an endangered species, you should purchase only roots that have been commercially cultivated. Use Asian ginseng if American ginseng is not available.

The Roots of Vitality

Ginseng root is a remarkable medicinal herb. Many years ago, I was nodding off at a scientific meeting—it was 2:30 in the afternoon, and the postprandial dip from eating a full lunch was kicking in. My friend, who also was feeling a bit tired, took out her small box of ginseng roots and began to chew on a piece the size of a pencil eraser. She suggested I try it, which I did. Within a few minutes this small root produced a newfound alertness and energy.

The two types of ginseng, American and Asian, have very useful properties that are similar in some ways. American ginseng reduces postprandial glycemia in people with type 2 diabetes, as well as in nondiabetics. It also benefits mental performance and enhances cardio-respiratory endurance, boosting athletic performance.

Asian ginseng is an excellent general tonic, known in herbal medicine as an adaptogen. It is used to improve the body's response to stress, anxiety, and fatigue. Human studies involving athletic performance have not always supported this benefit for this species, however. One clinical trial suggested that Asian ginseng helped ease menopausal symptoms. Herbalists also recommend ginseng as an aphrodisiac, to treat erectile dysfunction.—M. J. B.

Passiflora incarnata

PLANT PROFILE

Common Names: Maypop, Passionflower, Passion Vine, Purple Passionflower

Description: Vine, 25 to 30 feet tall, with alternate, lobed leaves; showy flowers have white petals, lavender sepals, and a bright pink or purple corona; 3-inch yellow or orange fruits

Hardiness: To Zone 7

Family: Passifloraceae

Flowering: Early to late summer

Parts Used: Flowers, fruit, and roots

Range/Habitat: Ranges from southeastern North America to northern South America, as well as the Caribbean and Madagascar; edges of wooded areas, thickets, and fence lines

This evergreen perennial vine grows naturally in fields and along roadsides from southeastern North America to northern South America. Sometimes called maypop, the plant produces egg-size, sweet, edible fruit that makes a popping sound when mashed. The filaments of the showy blossoms were thought to resemble the crown of thorns worn by Christ during his crucifixion, and the five anthers represented the five wounds he received. Because of this, the Spanish friars who saw the flowers of this genus in South America called it the "flower of passion," or as it is known today, passionflower. *Passiflora incarnata* is the most useful medicinal plant in this genus.

CULINARY USE

A sweet pulp covers the seeds of the maypop's ripe fruit. Native Americans boiled the fruits to make syrup and crushed and strained them to make juice. You can prepare the fruit in similar ways, using a sieve or strainer to remove the hard seeds. Also, try the pulp in jellies and frozen desserts.

MEDICINAL USE

Native Americans made preparations from the roots to treat wounds, ear infections, and liver problems; they also used the plant as a sedative to treat nervous conditions. Other medicinal uses for this herb include the treatment of colic, menstrual pain, dysentery, diarrhea, and muscle spasms.

Today, passionflower is best known for its sedative and tranquilizing properties, and it may be used to treat insomnia, anxiety, and nervousness. A recent clinical trial showed that drinking passionflower tea at night improved patients' sleep quality, as compared with a placebo. Another human clinical study showed that this herb could manage some of the symptoms of generalized anxiety disorder; after several weeks of comparison against patients using oxazepam—a member of the benzodiazepine class of drugs (which includes Valium)—the group using passionflower extract showed less "job performance impairment" as compared to the group using oxazepam.

Caution: Do not use this plant if you are pregnant.

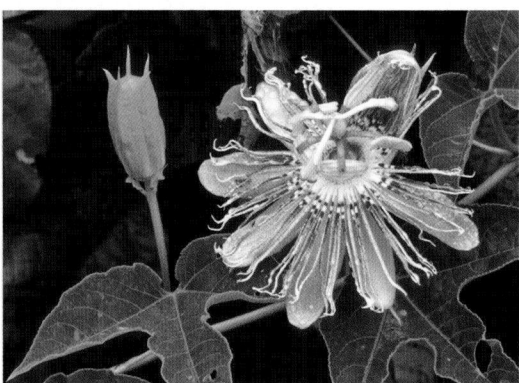

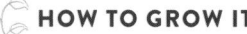

HOW TO GROW IT

Passionflower grows easily from seed or cuttings in deep, fertile, well-drained soil and full sun to partial shade. (If you live in Zone 6 or colder, you can grow the vine in a large container; bring it indoors in fall.) For best blooming, enrich the soil with compost, and fertilize two or three times during the growing season. Prune out weak or crowded stems in early spring each year. Passionflower is considered invasive in some areas; control its spread by removing suckers regularly. Harvest the fruit when it turns yellow-brown.

Paullinia cupana

Guarana is a climbing perennial vine indigenous to the Amazon basin, particularly northern Brazil on the Maués Açu River. The red-orange fruits of this species pop open to reveal shiny black seeds surrounded by a thin white pulp, giving the fruits an eyelike appearance. The common name, guarana, derives from a Tupi-Guarani reference to this resemblance.

Indigenous people used guarana as a stimulant and appetite suppressant as they traveled rainforest paths for days or weeks at a time. The plant contains three to five times the caffeine found in coffee beans—up to 5 percent by weight. The caffeine is thought to serve the plant as a kind of chemical defense, allowing it to repel pathogenic organisms that might otherwise attack the fruits and seeds.

CULINARY USE

The pulverized seeds of guarana are made into a thick, brown syrup used in carbonated beverages that are widely consumed by the people of Brazil, as well as other guarana aficionados around the world. Marketed by Brazilian, Peruvian, and multinational corporations, the soda can often be found in supermarkets and small stores that cater to South American shoppers. It is also used as a

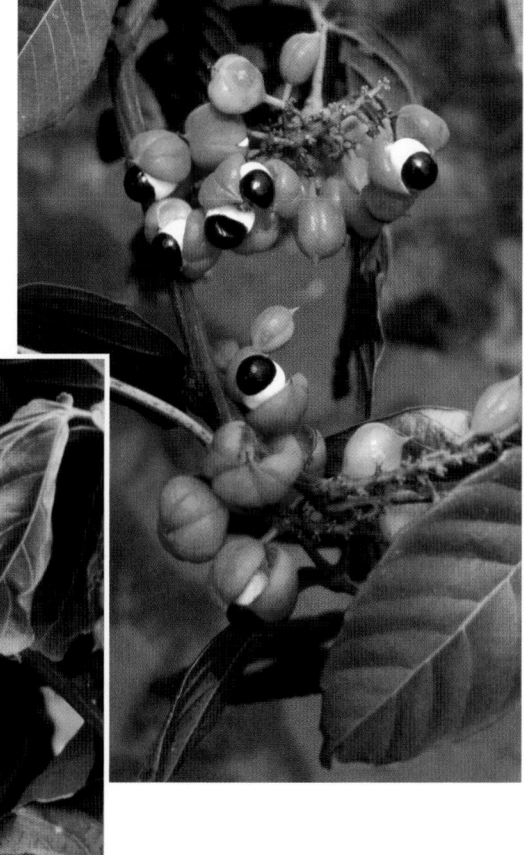

Guarana: Gift from the Amazon

In the early part of my career as a tropical botanist, I spent a great deal of time in the Amazon Valley, having been sent there by my mentor, Harvard professor Richard Evans Schultes, the most widely recognized Amazon plant explorer and ethnobotanist of his time. Much of my PhD dissertation research was spent in this region, with the indigenous people who used plants as part of their daily lives. One of these plants was guarana, a bright green vining herb found in the forest and cultivated near their houses.

I learned that its shiny black seeds are harvested, ground into powder, mixed with a local starch to give it a doughlike consistency, hand-rolled into 1-inch-wide cylinders, and heat dried. As needed, these are rasped against the dried, filelike tongue of the pirarucu fish to produce a brown powder, which is then added to hot or cold water and is often consumed with a bit of sugar.

I drank a lot of guarana in those days, and I found that it reduced my appetite and gave me an energizing lift. One of my favorite artifacts from the Harvard Botanical Museum was a beautifully sculpted bottle of ZIL, a guarana-based "champagne" introduced during the 1950s. It did not sell well, and I always presumed one reason was that partygoers found out that after drinking a few bottles, they were happier and livelier . . . but they probably could not go to sleep for a day or two.—M. J. B.

caffeine source in energy drinks. (See "Field Notes" for more about preparing the beverage.)

MEDICINAL USE

The seeds' high caffeine content speeds heart rate, relaxes blood vessels, and opens bronchial airways. Other potentially bioactive compounds in the seeds are tannins and saponins, which could be responsible for some of this herb's effects. Guarana is taken to treat fatigue, headache, and diarrhea, as well as to increase libido. A recent small clinical trial with healthy adults showed that guarana can improve cognitive performance as well as mood. The authors of this study noted that the result was most likely due not only to the caffeine in guarana, but also to other as yet undetermined substances. There are case reports of heart palpitations caused by taking large doses of guarana supplements, similar to the effects some people report after large doses of caffeine. Guarana also has diuretic activity. It is widely used in weight-loss formulas.

 HOW TO GROW IT

A tropical rainforest plant, guarana requires warm to hot conditions, high humidity, and acidic soil. Throughout most of North America, you'll need a greenhouse to grow this tall vine.

Start with the freshest seed possible. Soak the seed in water for 24 hours, then plant it in pots filled with a moist growing medium. Set the pots in a bright location, atop a germination mat; maintain a minimum temperature of 65°F. Transplant 3-inch-tall seedlings to 8- to 10-inch pots (with drainage holes) filled with an acidic medium (a pH of 3.5 to 4.5). Provide good air circulation, and keep the soil moist but not saturated. Mist daily in the morning, but do not fertilize, so the soil will remain acidic.

Continue to pot up the growing plants, and provide support for the growing vines. Beginning in the second year, prune out old or damaged branches and unwanted new growth. Wait until the orange fruits split open to reveal black seeds. Remove the seeds, rinse them, then let them air-dry in a warm place. Toast the seeds in a moderately hot oven, then grind into a fine powder and store in an airtight container. To use, mix with warm water.

Pausinystalia yohimbe

Yohimbe is a 100-foot-tall evergreen tree native to the forests of western Africa, particularly in Cameroon, Zaire, and Gabon. A relative of the coffee plant, yohimbe has red to yellow wood; glossy, dark green leaves; and clusters of tubular white or pink flowers.

In its native region, yohimbe is valued as a stimulant, male aphrodisiac, and mild hallucinogen; the gray-brown bark is taken as a tea, smoked, or sniffed. This plant is highly toxic when taken in large doses, however, due to the presence of a group of psychoactive indole alkaloids. Because of increased demand for this herb, yohimbe trees have been overharvested in the wild, and there is concern that the tree soon will become endangered.

MEDICINAL USE

A bitter, warming herb, the bark of the yohimbe tree has a reputation as an aphrodisiac in Africa, particularly among the Bantu people. One of the indole alkaloids in the bark is yohimbine, which has been made into the pharmaceutical drug yohimbine hydrochloride, used to treat impotence and erectile dysfunction. An extract of this plant also has been used to increase saliva flow in patients taking antidepressants who experience dry mouth as a side effect.

In herbal medicine, however, yohimbe is not widely used because of its potentially toxic effects, which include increased heart rate and elevated blood pressure. Other side effects associated with the use of this herb include dizziness, headache, shaking, anxiety, nausea, and vomiting.

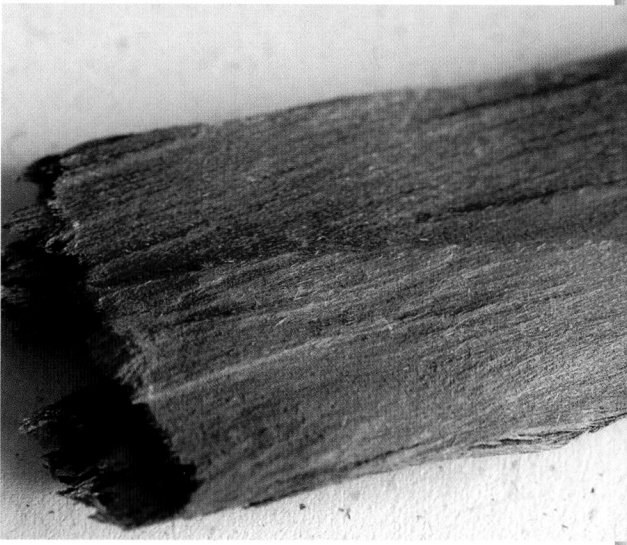

Caution: Yohimbe should not be used by those with high blood pressure or kidney or liver disease. Excess use can cause depression. Use this herb only under the supervision of an experienced medical professional.

 HOW TO GROW IT

Yohimbe grows in tropical conditions that include moist soil, high humidity, and minimum temperatures of 59° to 64°F. In North America, it will survive outdoors only in the warmest locations, such as Hawaii, southern Florida, or Puerto Rico. In colder areas, try growing this plant in a large, warm greenhouse. (Although it's difficult to find propagating material of this species in the commercial trade, sources of seeds can sometimes be found on the Web.) In Africa, the bark is collected throughout the year and dried in strips.

Pelargonium spp. and hybrids

The genus *Pelargonium* includes more than 200 species of annual, perennial, and subshrub plants commonly known as geraniums. The *Pelargonium* species and hybrids grown for their culinary, fragrant, and medicinal qualities are known as scented geraniums. Native to parts of Africa, Asia, Australia, and New Zealand, scented geraniums have been cultivated for centuries, but they gained their greatest popularity during the mid-1800s. The French discovered a way to substitute the oil from rose-scented geraniums for attar of roses in perfume making, introducing a popular commercial use for scented geraniums. Later, Victorian gardeners and herbalists used them in bouquets, potpourris, ointments, poultices, teas, desserts, and wines.

Popular species include rose-scented geranium (*Pelargonium capitatum* and other species, as well as hybrids), nutmeg-scented geranium (*P. × fragrans*), and lemon-scented geranium (*P. crispum*). The name of this genus comes from the Greek word *pelargos*, meaning stork, a reference to the beak-shaped fruits of scented geraniums.

CULINARY USE

Use scented geranium leaves to flavor teas, vinegars, breads, and desserts. Rose-scented geranium makes a flavorful jelly. To add subtle flavor to a cake, place scented geranium leaves flat on a buttered and floured pan just before pouring in the batter. Discard the leaves after removing the baked cake from the pan. To flavor sugar with geranium leaves, alternate layers of sugar and rose- or peppermint-scented geranium leaves in a jar, and set the jar in a sunny window. Remove the leaves after 2 weeks.

MEDICINAL USE

Scented geraniums contain complex volatile oils with more than 2,000 components. The oils are extracted by steam distillation of the leaves, stems, and flowers. Geraniol, an antiseptic compound found in geranium oil, is commercially used in the manufacture of many high-quality perfumes. In aromatherapy, essential oil of scented geranium, especially rose geranium, is used as an ingredient in facial creams and bath and massage oils. It is also used as an antidepressant and to help ensure restful sleep. It is particularly useful in skin care, for the treatment of conditions such as acne, burns, cuts, and wounds, and as a natural mosquito repellent. In South Africa, where many of the scented geraniums are native, the leaves have been used to treat diarrhea.

 HOW TO GROW IT

Scented geranium is a commonly grown aromatic garden plant that thrives in well-drained neutral to alkaline soil in full sun or partial shade. A tender perennial that requires minimum temperatures of 45° to 50°F, scented geranium can be grown year-round in a container moved indoors for the winter. Propagate by softwood cuttings. For maximum oil content, harvest the leaves just before the flowers begin to appear, preferably early on a dry, sunny day. Dry the leaves out of direct light to preserve their fragrance.

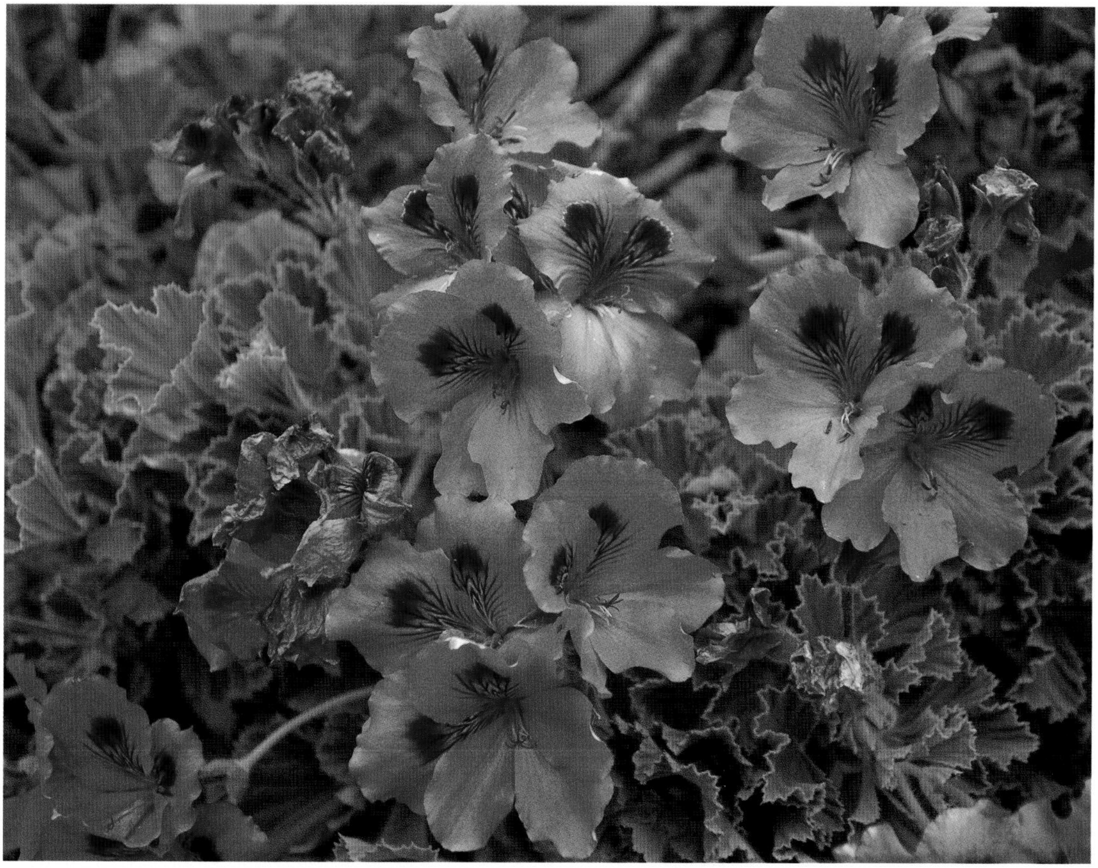

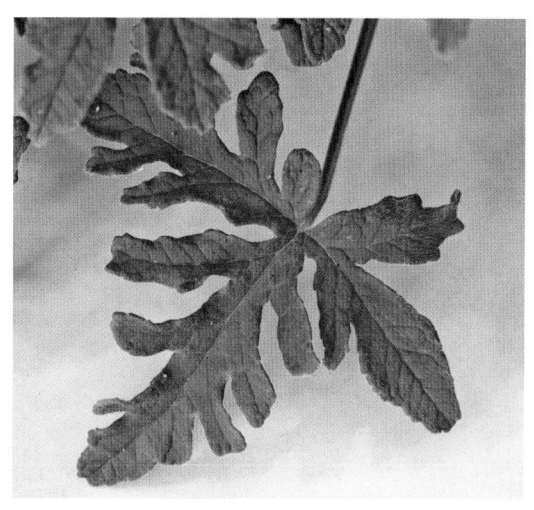

With bright blooms and fragrant foliage, pelargonium hybrids add charm to garden beds and containers.

Caution: Do not use geranium oil if you are pregnant.

ORNAMENTAL USE

Scented geraniums make lovely house and garden plants, filling the air with delightful scents when brushed. Many varieties also offer striking blossoms and foliage. Grow them where their aromatic leaves can be touched and enjoyed.

OTHER USES

As in the past, the dried leaves and flowers of scented geraniums make fragrant sachets and potpourris. Mildly astringent and stimulating, the leaves can be used for herbal facials and in baths. Certain scents are still used in the commercial perfume industry.

Petroselinum crispum

Although this aromatic biennial is best known as a garnish for other foods, parsley is much more than a frilly face. Native to the Mediterranean region and naturalized in Europe, parsley is cultivated throughout the world. The plant's curled leaves have a fresh, slightly peppery flavor. One of the first herbs to appear in early spring, parsley is used in the traditional Jewish Passover meal (known as the Seder) to represent new beginnings. Ancient Greeks planted parsley on graves and fed the herb to chariot horses. Ancient Romans ate parsley with soft cheese on bread. The ancients also used wreaths of parsley to ward off drunkenness.

CULINARY USE

Among the world's most popular culinary flavorings, parsley is used in sauces, fillings, and savory dishes. It pairs especially well with egg and chicken salads, tomatoes, cheeses, egg dishes, and peas. The herb makes a tasty addition to pasta dishes and is a crucial component of the Middle Eastern bulgur wheat salad called tabbouleh. In Burgundy, France, *persillade,* a fine mince of garlic and parsley, is added at the final moment of cooking to grilled meats, sautés, and poultry. Parsley is also one of the herbs in bouquet garni, a bundle of herbs used to flavor soups and stews.

MEDICINAL USE

Parsley is a good dietary source of iron, calcium, and vitamins A and C. Used since ancient times to freshen the breath, parsley contains high levels of chlorophyll, an ingredient in many commercially available breath fresheners. It is soothing to the

digestion and may be taken to relieve intestinal gas and bloating. The herb has a diuretic effect and has been used to treat urinary tract infections, edema, and kidney stones. Parsley also has traditionally been used to relieve menstrual pain.

Caution: Parsley leaf should not be used in medicinal amounts during pregnancy or by individuals with kidney disease. Photodermatitis, a rash caused by the sun, occurs in some people who harvest or handle parsley routinely.

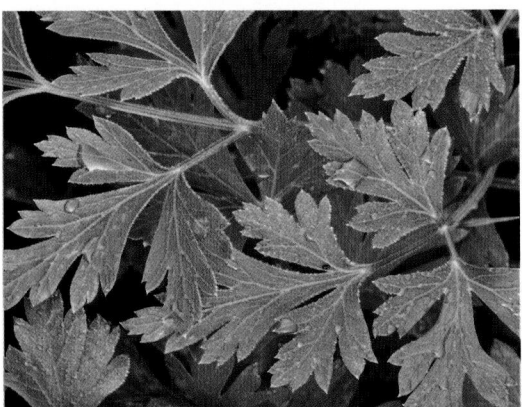

> **PLANT PROFILE**
>
> **Common Name:** Parsley
>
> **Description:** Plant, 10 to 18 inches tall, with flat or curly leaves divided pinnately into sections; umbels of tiny greenish yellow flowers form in the second year
>
> **Hardiness:** Biennial; hardy to Zone 3
>
> **Family:** Apiaceae
>
> **Flowering:** Spring or summer of second year
>
> **Parts Used:** Leaves
>
> **Range/Habitat:** Sardinia east to Lebanon; cultivated throughout temperate zones

 HOW TO GROW IT

Parsley grows in rich, well-drained, neutral soil in full sun or partial shade. Although parsley is a biennial, it is often planted as an annual because it develops a bitter flavor during its second year. Plant seeds or transplants in spring or early summer, after the soil temperature has warmed. Harvest leaves as needed throughout the growing season, removing the outer stems first. Crush the dried leaves and store them in an airtight container.

Phytolacca americana

Pokeweed is a perennial native to North America and naturalized around the Mediterranean and in northern Africa. It bears spikes of greenish white flowers, followed by juicy, deep purple berries that are a good source of food for birds. Native Americans used the berries to stain baskets a dark blue, and poke berries (called ink berries in some localities) provided one of the first natural inks used by settlers of the New World. The ink proved so lasting that it can still be seen on period documents preserved in museums. In the 19th century, tinctures made from the root were popular for joint pain, but poisonings were common due to the plant's toxicity. Pokeweed berries, roots, leaves, stems, and seeds are poisonous.

CULINARY USE

Eating pokeweed is *not* recommended, as it can cause nausea, vomiting, abdominal cramps, and diarrhea. Traditionally, the young shoots were cooked and eaten as a spring vegetable in parts of the southeastern United States, but foragers recommend against this practice unless you are *very* experienced in preparing this species.

MEDICINAL USE

Pokeweed has stimulant, purgative, and emetic properties. Native American people and traditional herbalists used the roots, berries, and leaves to treat conditions such as acne, arthritis and joint pain, fungal infections, scabies, folliculitis, and sore or infected nipples. A few modern herbalists recommend the herb to stimulate the thyroid or lymphatic system.

Caution: Pokeweed is highly toxic. When consumed, all parts of the plant can cause digestive irritation, vomiting, diarrhea, and decreased blood pressure. Overdoses can be fatal. Pokeweed should be used only under the guidance of a qualified health practitioner, if at all. Some authors recommend handling this plant with gloves, as toxins can be absorbed through cuts, scrapes, and other breaks in your skin.

OTHER USES

Poke berries can be used to create a red, brown, or pink natural dye. In a hedgerow or wild area of your landscape, pokeweed berries provide food for many wild birds.

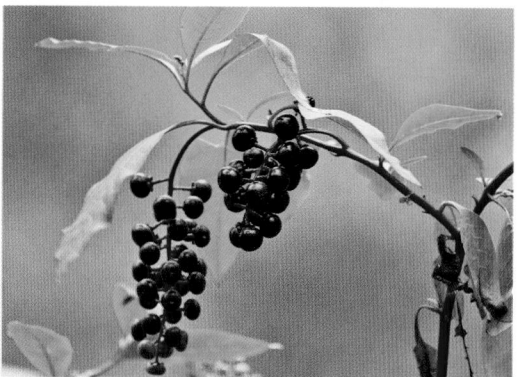

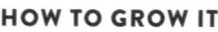

HOW TO GROW IT

Pokeweed thrives in woodland areas and open spaces in rich, moist, well-drained soil in full sun or partial shade. It is rarely grown in the garden and can become invasive. If you choose to grow pokeweed in a wild area as a wildlife food or ornamental, plant the seeds or root divisions in a location with moist but well-drained soil and full sun to partial shade. Harvesting the plant for medicinal use is not recommended. Pokeweed self-seeds readily throughout its native range.

Pimenta dioica

This evergreen tree is indigenous to South America and the West Indies, and it's grown extensively in Jamaica. Christopher Columbus found it growing on that island in 1494, during his second voyage to the Caribbean. Its wood was once in such demand for the making of walking sticks that the tree was nearly harvested to extinction. The dried berries are used to produce allspice, a common culinary flavoring. The botanical name *Pimenta* is derived from the Spanish word for pepper because the ripe fruits resemble peppercorns.

CULINARY USE

One of the most popular baking spices, ground allspice adds a sweet, warm flavor to pumpkin pie, banana bread, and cookies. Allspice also contributes a key flavor to barbecue sauce. The whole fruits are used to flavor soup, brine, mulled wine, and cider.

MEDICINAL USE

Allspice has been used to treat ailments such as indigestion, flatulence, and muscle pain. It contains the compound eugenol, an anesthetic and antiseptic. In Belize, the berries and leaves are made into a flavorful warming tea to treat upset stomach, gas, and infant colic. To prevent and cure fungal infections of the feet—a frequent consequence of living in tropical rainforest conditions—local people crushed allspice berries into a fine powder and mixed this with animal fat, rubbing the concoction liberally on the affected sites. Laboratory studies have confirmed that compounds in this plant have antifungal activity. For toothaches, indigenous people chew allspice leaves or berries into a paste and apply it to the sore tooth and surrounding gum. A similar preparation is used externally to ease joint pain: The crushed berries are boiled into a paste, applied to a cloth, and used as a plaster.

PLANT PROFILE

Common Names: Allspice, Jamaican Pepper

Description: Slow-growing evergreen tree, up to 40 feet tall; large, leathery leaves; grayish white peeling bark; clusters of small white flowers followed by purple berrylike fruits; aromatic

Hardiness: To Zone 10

Family: Myrtaceae

Flowering: Early summer

Parts Used: Fruits, seeds, and leaves

Range/Habitat: Native to tropical areas of South America and the West Indies

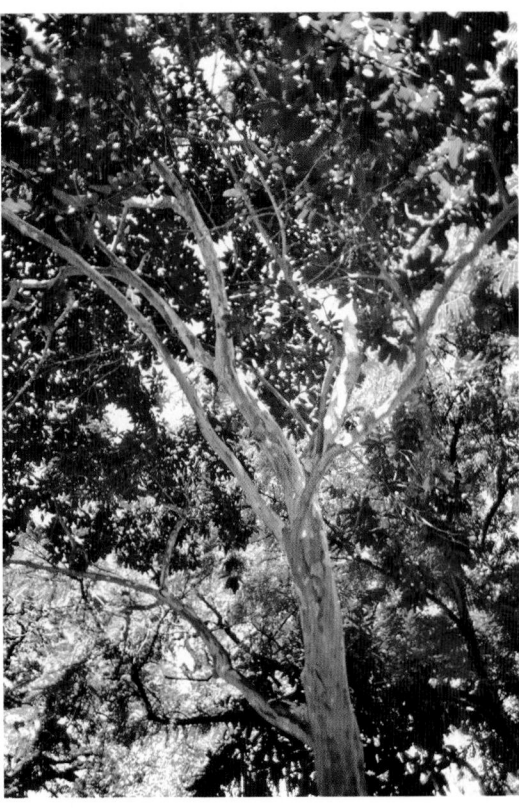

 HOW TO GROW IT

Jamaican allspice requires warm, frost-free growing conditions with rich, well-drained soil and full sun. In Zone 9 and colder, grow this small tree in a large container that can be moved indoors for the winter, or grow it in a warm greenhouse. Amend the soil or potting medium with compost. Feed with a tropical plant fertilizer every 3 to 5 weeks, and water during dry periods. The tree should begin fruiting during its third year; harvest berries about 4 months after they form, while they are still green and unripe. When sun-dried, they turn brown and can be used. Propagate by planting fully mature seed.

Pimpinella anisum

Anise, a member of the same family as parsley and carrots, is widely grown throughout North America, Europe, and Asia for its seeds, which are used medicinally and in cooking. The herb has been recommended for health problems since at least the 6th century BCE, when the mathematician and philosopher Pythagoras (ca. 580–ca. 500) suggested that holding it could prevent epileptic seizures. The 1st-century Roman herbalist Pliny the Elder (23–79 CE) stated that anise "removed all bad odors from the mouth, if chewed in the morning." The Romans mixed anise seed with other savory spices and meal to make a cake called *mustaceum*, a digestive aid and dessert served after heavy meals.

Dogs love the scent of anise: In greyhound racing, the artificial hare is scented with this herb.

CULINARY USE

Anise imparts a licorice flavor to foods. The seed can be used whole or ground with eggs, fruit, cheese, spinach, or carrots, as well as in bread or crackers. Anise seed intensifies the sweetness of desserts. Anise liqueurs, including the Greek ouzo, are made all over the world. To make anisette, combine equal parts anise, coriander, and fennel seed, and steep them in vodka; sweeten with simple syrup (one part sugar dissolved in one part boiling water).

MEDICINAL USE

John Gerard, in his *Herball, or Generall Historie of Plantes*, published in 1597, noted that anise seeds were good for the treatment of intestinal gas ("winde") and "belching and upbraidings of the stomacke." He counseled that the seeds could be chewed to make the breath "sweete," and when eaten with bitter almonds (a wild almond related to the cultivated species), anise would "helpe the old cough."

Anise seed is used today to relieve gas, bloating,

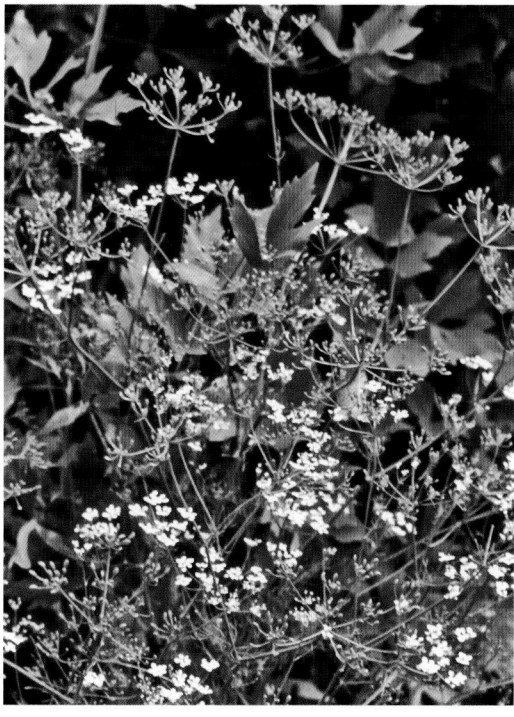

PLANT PROFILE

Common Names: Anise, Aniseed

Description: Stems, 2 feet tall, topped with yellowish white flower umbels; feathery, divided leaves; flattened oval gray-brown seeds up to ⅛ inch long

Hardiness: Annual

Family: Apiaceae

Flowering: Summer

Parts Used: Seeds and leaves

Range/Habitat: Native to the Mediterranean region and western Asia; widely cultivated

nausea, bad breath, and indigestion. It has antispasmodic and expectorant properties, which may make it helpful in the treatment of menstrual cramps and respiratory complaints such as asthma, coughs, and bronchitis.

HOW TO GROW IT

Sow anise seeds directly in your garden in light, well-drained soil and full sun. Harvest whole seed heads after the seeds have ripened, but before the heads open, clipping them directly into a bag so the seeds do not scatter. Dry the seeds in the sun or in a warm, dry area indoors. Store the dry seeds in airtight containers. Start new plants from the saved seeds.

Piper methysticum

People have grown kava for so many centuries that its original birthplace is unclear, although the highest diversity of cultivars (often an indicator of a plant's origin) is found in the Pacific Island nation of Vanuatu. Today, kava grows throughout the Pacific Islands from Hawaii (where it is called "awa") to New Guinea. A member of the pepper family, this tender, sprawling, perennial shrub has stout rhizomes and bears large, heart-shaped leaves and small green spikes containing tiny flowers. The plant roots are harvested only after the plants have grown for at least 3 years. The remaining long, thin stems are then cut into sections and replanted, to be harvested when mature. Traditionally, people macerate the roots and make them into a beverage consumed for ritual use and social interaction (see "Field Notes" below). Kava derives from a Greek word meaning "intoxicating."

PLANT PROFILE

Common Names: Awa, Kava, Kava Kava, Sakau, Yangona

Description: Sprawling, perennial shrub, up to 8 feet tall; bears large, heart-shaped leaves and small green spikes of tiny flowers; stout rhizomes

Hardiness: To Zone 10

Family: Piperaceae

Flowering: Summer

Parts Used: Roots and leaves

Range/Habitat: Believed to be native to the Pacific Island nation Vanuatu; sunny, moist highlands and tropical forests

MEDICINAL USE

Kava contains kavalactones, compounds that relieve pain and relax muscles. Kava root extracts in the form of tinctures, pills, or capsules are used to treat nervousness, anxiety, stress, and restlessness. Human clinical studies have shown that

FIELD NOTES
Sakau: The Sacred Root

On the remote tropical island of Pohnpei, in the Federated States of Micronesia, where I have studied plants and their cultural uses since 1997, the most powerful, sacred, and important plant is kava—known locally as Sakau. Bite on the root and it tastes somewhat peppery, with a numbing quality; people place the leaves of the plant on an area stung by a stingray to dull the pain.

Traditionally, the roots are pounded, releasing a bioactive liquid, then mixed with other substances and consumed. The bitter root extract is an acquired taste, but the effects are quite pleasant—mild euphoria, amicability, and greatly reduced anxiety. It is also a muscle relaxant, so drinking too much Sakau results in a lack of motor coordination (so moving around is not suggested) while your mind remains crystal clear.

On Pohnpei, people come together regularly to drink Sakau and to discuss the day's issues, exchange stories, and gossip. The beverage promotes social interaction, perhaps in the same way as that first glass of wine at a dinner party. In Germany, where physicians are trained to prescribe both pharmaceutical and herbal medications, Sakau (kava) is recommended for the treatment of anxiety, stress, and restlessness. Tinctures and teas of this plant can usually be found in your local health food store under various brand names. Note that the tea should not be made with extremely hot water, as the kavalactones—the bioactive compounds—are thought to degrade with high heat.—M. J. B.

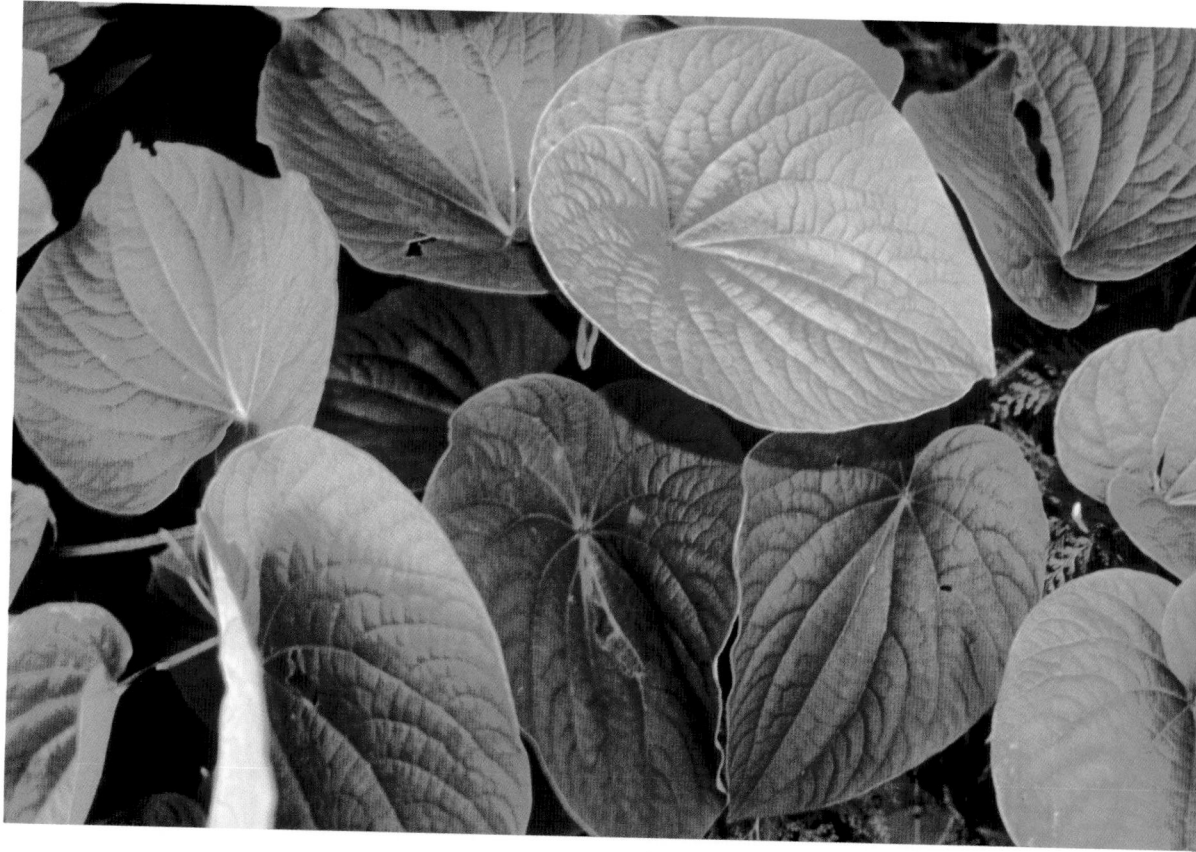

dosages containing 60 to 120 milligrams of kava-lactones can be very effective for treating anxiety disorder. Some studies have found kava to work as well as benzodiazepines (a class of drugs that includes Valium). One study showed that kava might help prevent the uptake of noradrenaline, a hormone that initiates a stress response.

In traditional use, people chew kava to relieve the pain of a sore throat or toothache; they also apply the leaves to wounds and stings. Kava's anes-thetic properties are about twice those of aspirin. Combined with pumpkin seed oil, kava has been used to treat irritable bladder and irritable bowel syndrome.

To make a kava tea, gently simmer 1 teaspoon of the dried and sliced root in 1 cup of water for 10 minutes. Strain. Drink 1 or 2 cups per day.

Caution: Kava should not be taken by pregnant or nursing women, and its long-term use should be monitored by a health-care professional.

HOW TO GROW IT

Kava grows in moist, sunny highlands or wet tropical forests at elevations to 1,000 feet above sea level. The plant cannot tolerate temperatures below 55°F, but you can grow it in a container in a warm greenhouse if you mist frequently to maintain a high humidity level. Amend the growing medium with coarse sand or grit to ensure good drainage and aeration. Gradually increase the pot size and replant as needed. Begin harvesting the roots when the plants are 3 years old. After harvesting the roots, propagate new plants from stems that contain two or three nodes.

Piper nigrum

The genus *Piper* includes about 2,000 species of climbing plants, shrubs, and small trees. *Piper nigrum* (black pepper) is native to Southwest India and is cultivated in tropical areas throughout the world. This woody-stemmed, pungent-smelling climber bears large, oval leaves; spikes of tiny white flowers; and clusters of small berries (called peppercorns) that turn red when mature.

Black peppercorns consist of the entire fruit, called a drupe, harvested from plants that are at least 3 years old, and then dried. Although black pepper is relatively inexpensive now, it was once so highly valued and so difficult to obtain that it was used as currency. In 408 CE, the Mongol warrior Attila the Hun is said to have requested 1½ tons of black pepper as a ransom during his siege of Rome. In the 15th century, European explorers searched for trade routes to the Far East, where they could obtain peppercorns. The wealth of some European ports, such as Venice, resulted from the quest for black pepper.

CULINARY USE

Black pepper, one of the world's oldest-known spices, is used in some form in nearly every regional cuisine. Before the invention of refrigeration, black pepper was used to preserve meat and to mask the taste of meat that was not fresh. Today, the spice is used to flavor savory dishes, including meats, dressings, and pickles. It is an ingredient in many commercially available food products, such as baked goods, condiments, and nonalcoholic beverages. Whole black peppercorns, ground immediately before use, provide more flavor than preground pepper. White pepper, which comes from the same plant but is prepared differently, has a slightly milder flavor because it lacks the fruit coating.

MEDICINAL USE

High in antioxidants, black pepper contains volatile oil and alkaloids that cause the herb to have a stimulating, warming effect on your digestive and circulatory systems. Used to relieve stomachache, nausea, constipation, bloating, and flatulence, black pepper is also taken to stimulate appetite by increasing gastric secretions. In China, where black pepper is known as *hu jiao*, the herb is popular for alleviating phlegm from a cold, stomach reflux, and diarrhea. Essential oil of black pepper, produced by steam distillation of the fruit, has antiseptic and antibacterial properties. It can be diluted in carrier oils and applied externally as a chest rub to warm your body and alleviate congestion from cold and flu. The oil is also added to liniments and creams to ease sore joints and relax tight muscles.

Caution: Essential oil of black pepper is for external use only.

PLANT PROFILE

Common Name: Black Pepper

Description: Woody vine, up to 12 feet tall; bears large, oval leaves and spikes of tiny white flowers; clusters of small berries turn red when mature; aromatic

Hardiness: To Zone 10

Family: Piperaceae

Flowering: Summer

Parts Used: Fruit

Range/Habitat: Native to India; cultivated in tropical regions worldwide

---

HOW TO GROW IT

Black pepper grows in rich, well-drained soil in full sun to light shade. It requires high humidity and moisture and will not tolerate temperatures below 60°F. In colder climates, black pepper can be grown as a houseplant in a warm spot that receives bright sunlight. Support the vine on a stake or trellis, and mist the plant to maintain humidity. Hand-pick the fruits when they are half-ripe (red-green in color). Propagate by stem cuttings.

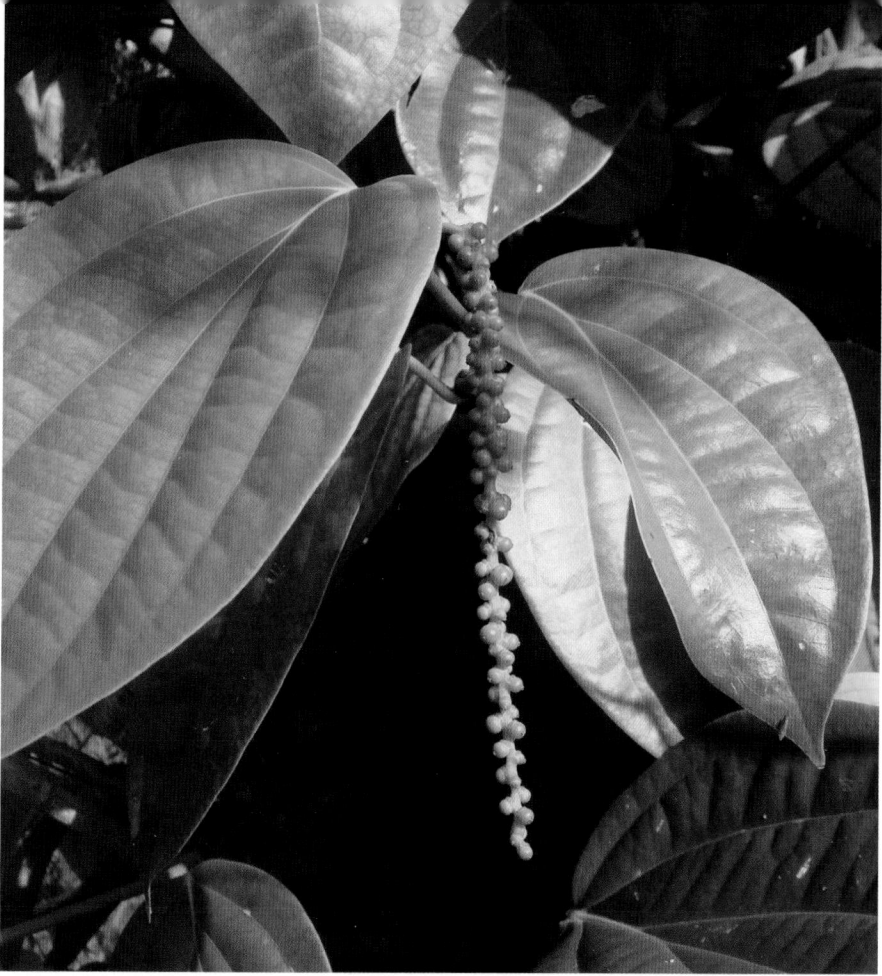

Pepper: The World's Most Important Spice

Cultivated in tropical regions throughout the world, pepper is produced on large plantations or in fields managed by small farmers. The low-growing evergreen vines are usually planted on poles, for easier harvest of the berries. If you walk through a pepper field, you'll see several crops growing together in layers—the pepper vines on their supports, annual crops (such as cucumbers or squash) at their bases, and, often, tree crops overhead.

Thousands of miles away, on our supermarket shelves, we can find different kinds of pepper: black, green, and white. All come from Piper nigrum but are handled differently. Immature berries are used to produce green pepper. Half-ripe, red-green berries are used to produce black pepper. And fully ripe, bright red berries become white pepper, after the fruit's outer layer is removed. Each type has a different flavor, but all contain the alkaloid piperine, one of

the compounds that give the seed of this species its pungent flavor. By the way, the "red pepper" seeds in some P. nigrum blends are not from a pepper at all—that's the seed of Schinus molle, an invasive tree native to the Peruvian Andes. That species, in the same family as poison ivy and poison oak, can provoke allergic reactions if handled by those sensitive to it and can be toxic when ingested.—M. J. B.

Plantago major

The wide green leaves and yellow-green flower spikes of broad-leaf plantain are a familiar (and, usually, unwelcome) sight in lawns and gardens throughout North America, where this weedy perennial has naturalized. The species is native to Eurasia; its common name, plantain, is the French version of the Latin *plantago*, which means "plant." Some Native American tribes called plantain "Englishman's foot" because it seemed to flourish in areas visited by British colonists—as a weedy species, it would spread to disturbed habitats, including the fields, pastures, and roads developed by the settlers. Despite its wild nature, broad-leaf plantain can be highly useful.

CULINARY USE

Young plantain leaves can be eaten in salads or steamed lightly and eaten as a vegetable. In recipes that include cooked spinach, try substituting cooked young plantain leaves. Noted forager

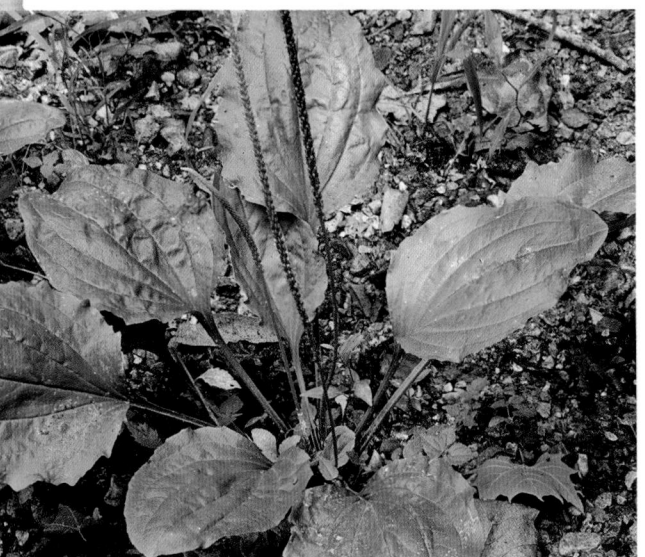

"Wildman" Steve Brill suggests using the older, fibrous leaves along with other herbs and vegetables to make a mineral-rich vegetable stock. (Remove the plantain leaves before eating.)

MEDICINAL USE

Plantain leaves have long been used as a folk medicine. In Shakespeare's 16th-century play *Romeo and Juliet*, Romeo tells Juliet that plantain leaf is excellent as a treatment for broken skin. Indeed, plantain leaves contain soothing, anti-inflammatory, antibiotic, and vulnerary (blood coagulant) compounds. The astringent, antibacterial leaves, bruised or crushed and rubbed against the affected area, are a traditional remedy for poison ivy, insect bites and stings, superficial wounds, and skin conditions such as eczema. Plantain leaf tea is also soothing to the respiratory system and the urinary tract, and it makes a good mouthwash, reputed to help heal sores. It has been used as a diuretic and to relieve dry cough.

Caution: Plantain may cause contact dermatitis in sensitive individuals. Avoid harvesting plantain from roadsides or other areas commonly treated with herbicides or otherwise exposed to toxic substances.

HOW TO GROW IT

Plantain grows in moist sandy or gravelly soil in full sun or partial shade. Considered an invasive weed throughout most of the United States, the plant self-seeds freely. Harvest the leaves before the plant flowers.

Podophyllum peltatum

Native to the moist woodland areas of eastern North America, the mayapple bears large, umbrella-like leaves that form a lush groundcover during spring. Its scientific name derives from the Greek words *podos* and *phyllon*, meaning "foot-shaped leaves," and *peltatum*, which means "shieldlike." After the leaves develop, a single, white, strong-smelling flower forms, followed by a fleshy yellow fruit known as the mayapple.

CULINARY USE

In some folk traditions, the ripe fruit is used to make jam. If you wish to try making mayapple jam, harvest only fully ripe fruit (the green, unripe fruit is poisonous). Ripe mayapples are soft, lemon yellow in color, and fragrant. Use only the pulp—not the rind or seeds—for jam. To do this, cook the fruit, mash it, and then squeeze the puree through a sieve to separate the pulp. Process the pulp the same way you would for other jams.

MEDICINAL USE

Native Americans used mayapple roots or rhizomes as a laxative and purgative, as well as a treatment for joint pain, cancers, and many other conditions. Several tribes employed the fruit to remove skin warts. By the late 18th century, American settlers were also using the resin from the roots of mayapple as a laxative and treatment for cholera, dysentery, genital warts, hepatitis, tumors, and other conditions and diseases. An antitumor agent identified in the plant's roots is the basis for modern drugs used against certain cancers. An extract is also used topically to treat genital herpes. (See "Field Notes" on page 238.)

Caution: Other than its ripe fruit, which can be eaten in small quantities, mayapple is extremely poisonous and should not be taken internally.

PLANT PROFILE

Common Names: American Mandrake, Duck's Food, Ground Lemon, Mayapple

Description: Perennial, 12 to 18 inches tall; stems each bear one or two large, deeply divided lobed leaves; nodding white flowers give way to 2-inch fleshy green fruits that ripen to yellow; long, creeping rhizomes

Hardiness: To Zone 4

Family: Berberidaceae

Flowering: April and May

Parts Used: Ripe fruit and rhizome

Range/Habitat: Eastern North America; damp, open woods and moist meadows

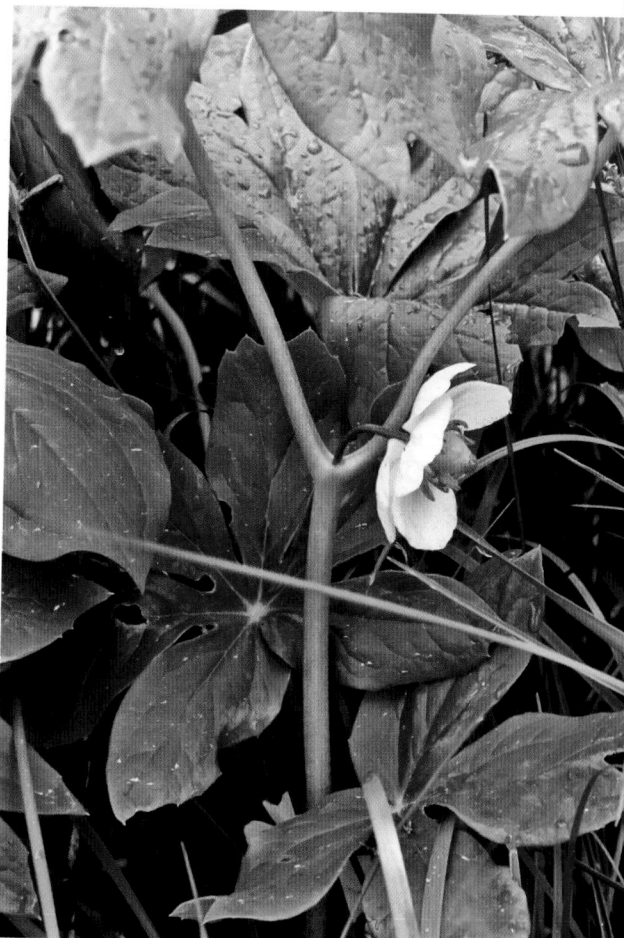

The Plant Kingdom's Untapped Potential

Throughout northeastern forests of the United States, it is easy to find large colonies of mayapples, which spread by their underground rhizomes. Native Americans, such as the Penobscot of Maine, used these rhizomes to treat warts and certain cancers. A century and a half ago, American medical practitioners also began using mayapple widely against various tumors, polyps, and other skin granulations. In the late 19th century, a resin derived from the root (which contains a compound known as podophyllin) was used to treat genital warts. Two modern derivatives of this compound, etoposide and teniposide, are now used as anticancer therapies for conditions including testicular cancer, small-cell lung cancer, Kaposi's sarcoma, and lymphomas. These drugs block the replication of rapidly dividing tumor cell DNA, leading to cell death.

The mayapple is just one example of the plant kingdom's potential. While many plants already have provided important pharmaceuticals used in modern medicine, only a very small percentage of the several hundred thousand plants known to exist on earth have been exhaustively studied for their chemical composition and healing potential. So much remains untapped.—M. J. B.

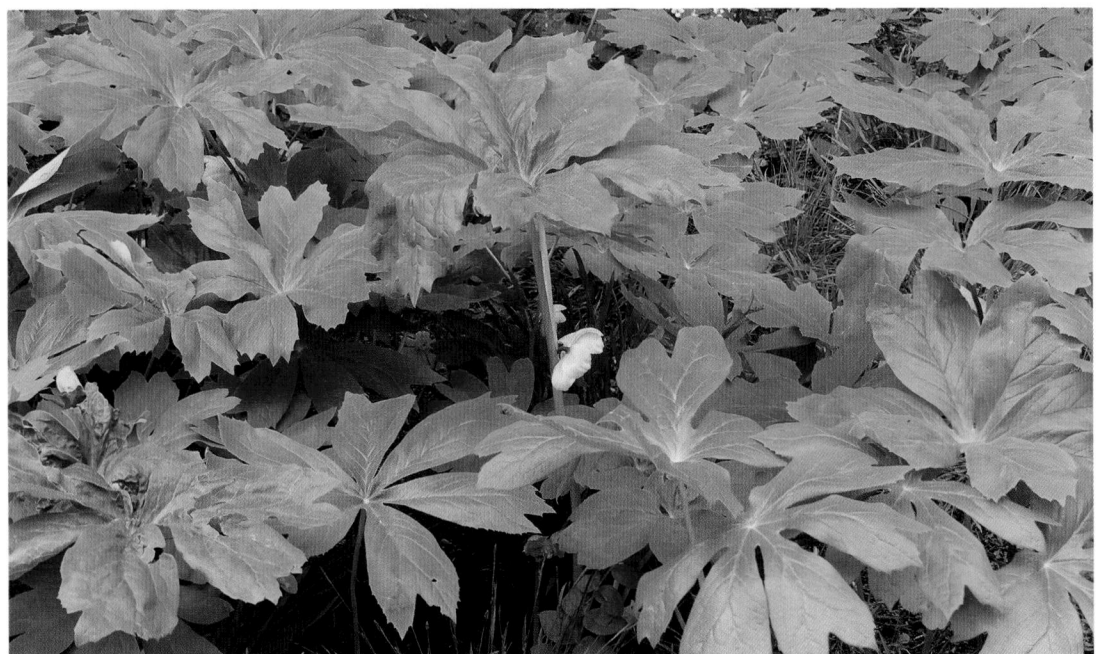

HOW TO GROW IT

Mayapple can form a handsome groundcover in woodland areas. If you wish to grow it as an ornamental, provide rich, moist, humusy soil and partial shade. Sow the seeds in spring, or divide the plant in early spring or fall and plant the root divisions immediately. The plants colonize by underground rhizomes and can take 5 years or more to become established. Harvest ripe yellow fruits when they are soft and fragrant, in late summer to fall.

Pogostemon cablin

Best known for its richly scented essential oil, patchouli is native to the tropical regions of India and Malaysia. The 2- to 3-foot-tall plant has soft, fragrant leaves and small, pale pink or white flowers that appear in fall to early winter. The name patchouli comes from the Tamil *pachchai* and *ilai*, meaning "green leaf." Most of the world's patchouli oil now comes from Indonesia, where the plant is often grown in rotation with other crops or as an understory plant. After the leaves are harvested, they are partially dried, stacked, and fermented, then sent to steam distilleries for extraction of the essential oil. The oil is highly valued as a perfume ingredient, as well as for healing.

MEDICINAL USE

Patchouli oil has antibacterial, antifungal, and anti-inflammatory properties. The oil is used externally—mixed with carrier oils, creams, or gels—to treat conditions such as dry, cracked, or oily skin and scalp; athlete's foot; acne; inflamed skin; and eczema. Alone or mixed with other oils, patchouli oil is also a good insect repellent. In aromatherapy, the oil is used to treat exhaustion, depression, and stress, and to enhance libido. Practitioners of traditional Chinese medicine use the whole plant to treat headache, stomach gas, vomiting, and diarrhea.

OTHER USES

Prized for making perfume, the fragrant oil of patchouli has a warm, spicy scent that improves with age. It is used to scent massage and bath oils, soaps, and cosmetic products. The leaves and oil can be added to potpourri or used in drawers and closets to scent linens and clothing and to repel moths.

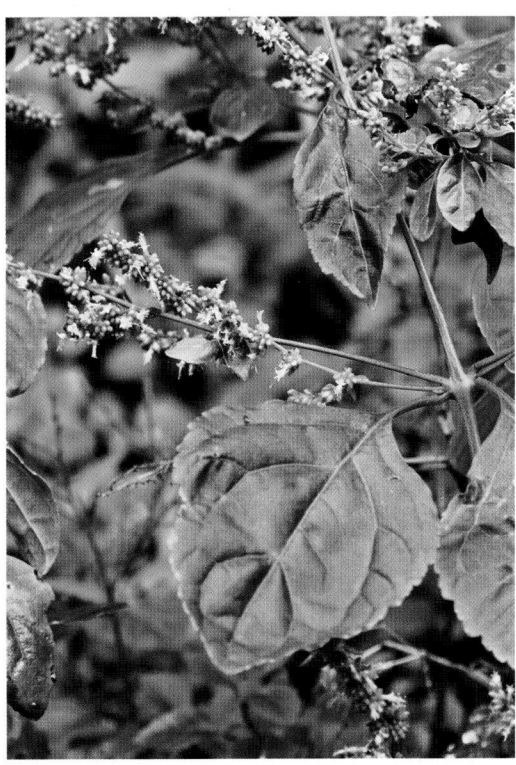

PLANT PROFILE

Common Names: Patchouli

Description: Perennial, 2 to 3 feet tall, with serrated leaves, hairy stems, and white or pale pink flowers; highly fragrant leaves

Hardiness: Tender perennial

Family: Lamiaceae

Flowering: Midautumn to early winter

Parts Used: Leaves and stems

Range/Habitat: Native to tropical regions of India and Malaysia

HOW TO GROW IT

A tropical understory plant, patchouli thrives in moist, warm, shady conditions and languishes in temperatures lower than 50°F. In cooler climates, it can be grown as an annual or as a potted indoor plant. Indoors or outdoors, provide bright, indirect light and rich, moist soil. Never allow the soil to dry out completely; mist frequently to increase humidity. Pinch back stem tips to keep the plant bushy. In late summer, harvest up to one-third of the plant by cutting back the stems along with their leaves and any flowers. Dry them in a warm, dark location for 7 to 10 days. To promote flowering in winter, keep the plant in total darkness after sunset, starting in fall. Patchouli is easy to propagate by cuttings.

Portulaca oleracea

An annual plant found wild and cultivated in many areas of the world, this low-growing succulent green is eaten fresh or cooked wherever it is found. In the United States, it grows in vacant lots, fields, and gardens, where it is often considered an invasive weed. Yet this common plant is uncommonly nutritious. Writing about his voyage to the South Seas, Englishman and adventurer Sir Richard Hawkins (1562–1622) observed that his crew, suffering from scurvy, was saved by eating "the hearbe purslane," which they found in abundance on an island they visited. Purslane is a very rich source of vitamin C, a deficiency of which is the cause of that terrible disease.

PLANT PROFILE

Common Names: Pigweed, Purslane

Description: Trailing, 6- to 8-inch-tall plant with clusters of flat, succulent, dark green leaves; smooth stems often have a reddish hue when mature; small, yellow flowers

Hardiness: Annual

Family: Portulacaceae

Flowering: Early summer to fall

Parts Used: Leaves and stems

Range/Habitat: Native to Eurasia, widely naturalized throughout the world

CULINARY USE

The tender young leaves of purslane can be pinched off of the young stems from summer to fall and added fresh to salads or cooked in the same way as spinach. Eaten raw, purslane has a tart, lemony flavor with peppery undertones. One Pennsylvania German folk recipe combines chopped fresh purslane, egg, bread crumbs, currants, and seasonings.

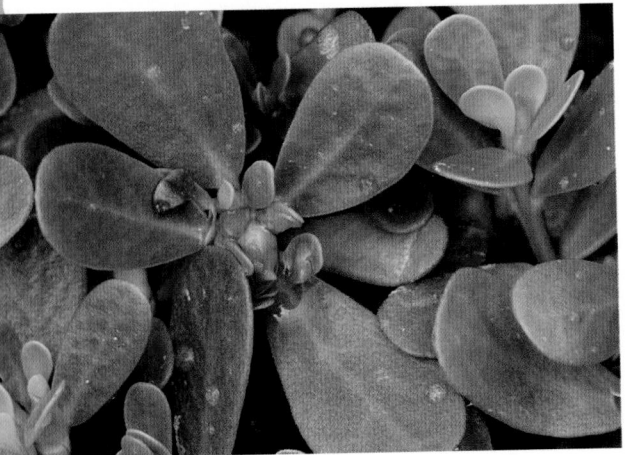

The mixture is formed into small cakes that are sautéed until light brown; the cakes make a very tasty and nutritious substitute for sausage. The stems can be pickled like cucumbers or blanched and frozen for use in winter.

MEDICINAL USE

Purslane is an important plant in traditional Chinese medicine (TCM) and is cultivated throughout China. The young leaves are ground and used as a wash for treating skin problems, such as sores. It is a cooling plant thought to relieve "fire toxicity" and is taken internally for urinary problems, as well as for dysentery. Human clinical trials have shown both purslane juice and tablets to be effective against intestinal parasites such as hookworm. The herb is also used topically to treat swellings and stings.

A nutritional powerhouse, purslane is high in omega-3 fatty acids, containing more than any other leafy vegetable, as well as vitamins A, B, C, and carotenoids. For those who don't eat enough omega-3 fatty acid–rich fish, purslane should be the herb of choice to maintain optimum health and prevent disease. The leaves also contain a great deal of oxalates, however, so people with a history of oxalate-based kidney stones should avoid eating too much of this plant.

HOW TO GROW IT

Purslane can often be found growing in garden beds or between paving stones. If you don't find it there, it's easy to grow in full sun and sandy, well-drained soil. Sow the seed on the surface of the soil after danger of frost has passed. Harvest young leaves and stems and use them fresh; remove flowers to prevent unwanted seedlings.

Primula veris

In country meadows throughout much of the world, the sweet-smelling, yellow, bell-shaped blooms of cowslip are nearly synonymous with spring. The attractive perennial—which bears clusters of nodding flowers atop long, thin stems—is native to Europe and western Asia and has naturalized in temperate areas of the world, including the northeastern United States and Canada. Cowslip is strongly associated with springtime. In Spain and Italy, this perennial herb is known as *primavera,* meaning "spring." The name "cowslip" is derived from the Anglo-Saxon *cu-sloppe,* a reference to the plant's tendency to bloom among herds of dairy cattle.

CULINARY USE

Cowslip flowers have a very distinctive fresh fragrance, and they make a nice addition to springtime salads. Also try candying them like you would violets to make a decorative garnish for desserts.

MEDICINAL USE

Shakespeare's play *A Midsummer Night's Dream* makes reference to a traditional belief that cowslip flowers are good for the complexion. Modern herbalists use cowslip flowers prepared as a lotion to treat skin blemishes, and for sunburn. The flowers have antioxidant, anti-inflammatory, antispasmodic, and diuretic properties. Taken as a tea, they are used to treat asthma and allergies. Cowslip tea is also a traditional treatment for anxiety and insomnia.

The roots, which contain triterpenoid saponins, have powerful expectorant properties. Decoctions of cowslip root have been used to loosen phlegm in people with chest colds.

Caution: Do not use cowslip if you are pregnant or taking aspirin or prescription anticoagulant drugs, such as warfarin.

ORNAMENTAL USE

Long-blooming, deer-resistant cowslip is a good choice for mixed borders, woodland plantings,

and cottage gardens. Its long-stemmed blooms make attractive springtime bouquets. Related *Primula* species have yielded many garden cultivars, including the pastel-colored mix drumstick primrose (*P. denticulata*), pink 'Quaker's Bonnet' (*P. vulgaris*), and purple 'Wanda' (*P. juliae*).

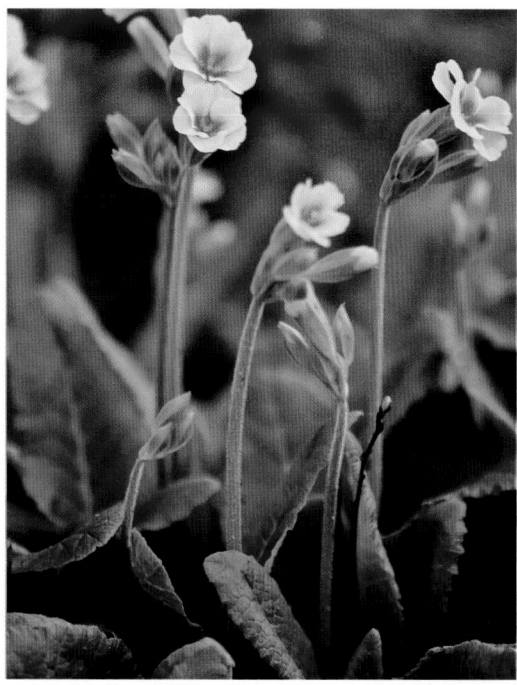

HOW TO GROW IT

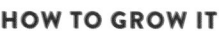

Cowslip grows wild in fields and pastures with chalky soil. It prefers dry, neutral to alkaline soil in full sun or partial shade. Plant seeds in summer; root divisions can be planted in late spring or early fall. Harvest the flowers and roots in spring.

Prunella vulgaris

Heal all, a low-growing mint relative, is native to Eurasia and can be found in temperate regions worldwide. Naturalized throughout North America, the plant spreads so readily that it's often considered an invasive weed. Its scientific name can be traced to a fever known as "the browns" (for the brown-colored tongue coating of infected patients), which spread through German armies during the 16th century. Because heal all was a common treatment for the browns, the herb became known as *Brunella*, and later *Prunella*.

CULINARY USE

The minty flavored leaves, stems, and flowers of heal all can be used in salads, soups, or stews or boiled as a potherb. To make a tasty, healthful tea, bring 2 cups of water to a boil, then pour the water over 1 ounce of fresh leaves or flowers. Steep for 5 minutes, then strain.

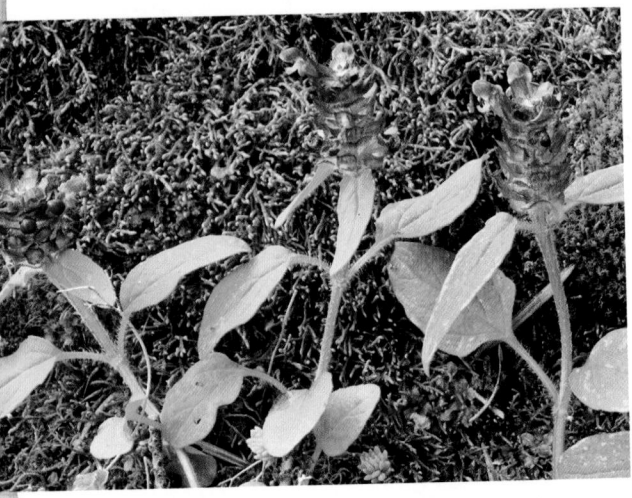

PLANT PROFILE

Common Names: Heal All, Self-Heal

Description: Low-growing perennial with creeping rhizomes; reddish stems bear small, oval leaves and spikes of violet-blue blooms

Hardiness: Hardy throughout most of North America

Family: Lamiaceae

Flowering: Midsummer to autumn

Parts Used: Flowers, leaves, and stems

Range/Habitat: Native to Eurasia, naturalized throughout temperate regions

MEDICINAL USE

As its name suggests, heal all has been used to alleviate a wide range of conditions. It can be taken as a tea, tincture, mouthwash, poultice, or salve. The plant is rich in rosmarinic acid, which regulates the production of thyroid hormone, making it useful in the treatment of overactive or underactive thyroid. As an immune-system stimulant with antiviral properties, it may be beneficial in the treatment of the herpes simplex virus. The herb also soothes inflamed mucous membranes and has been taken traditionally to relieve gingivitis, sore throat, and diarrhea. In lab studies, it has been found to lower LDL ("bad") cholesterol.

Practitioners of traditional Chinese medicine use an extract of the herb to treat hypertension. The great 17th-century English herbalist Nicholas Culpeper (1616–1654) recommended applying heal all externally as a plaster or unguent to treat skin wounds and other sores. Heal all is a key ingredient in many natural skin-care products.

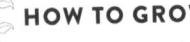

HOW TO GROW IT

Heal all commonly grows on sunny banks, in grassy areas, and in open woodlands. It can be propagated by seed or by division of the creeping rhizomes, although the plant spreads quickly and is considered weedy. For best germination, chill seeds for about 1 month before sowing them indoors in flats. Transplant 8-week-old seedlings outdoors in early spring, spacing plants about 1 foot apart in either full sun or partial shade. Keep the soil evenly moist for the first year. Harvest the flowering stems just before the blooms open.

Punica granatum

The pomegranate is a 15- to 20-foot-tall evergreen native to central Asia from Iran to the Himalayas. Mentioned in the Bible, Koran, and other ancient books, the tree has been cultivated since ancient times throughout the Mediterranean region of Asia, Africa, and Europe. Its red flowers develop into rounded, scarlet fruits up to 5 inches in diameter. The name comes from the Medieval Latin words *pomum* (apple) and *granatum* (seeded), and indeed the fruits are filled with crunchy seeds,

PLANT PROFILE

Common Name: Pomegranate

Description: Evergreen tree, 15 to 20 feet tall, with twisted, multiple trunks; red flowers are followed by scarlet fruits up to 5 inches in diameter; seeds are covered with a juicy red pulp

Hardiness: To Zone 8

Family: Lythraceae

Flowering: Early to midsummer

Parts Used: Fruit and root bark

Range/Habitat: Native to central Asia, from Iran to the Himalayas

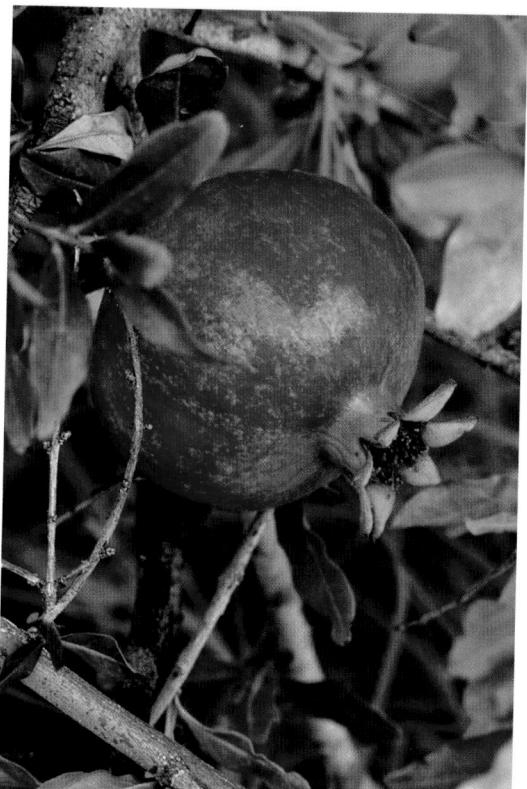

each of which is encased in the sweet or somewhat sour red pulp known botanically as an aril. Believed by some to be the forbidden fruit of the biblical Garden of Eden, the pomegranate has been regarded as a symbol of fertility, prosperity, and even immortality by ancient cultures. The Ebers Papyrus (ca. 1550 BCE), one of the world's oldest medical texts, discusses the plant's healing properties. The rind of the fruit has long been used as a dye. Depending on the preparation method and what the rind is mixed with, it can produce yellow to green tints.

CULINARY USE

Flavorful, crunchy pomegranate seeds and their juice are important ingredients in many traditional Middle Eastern sauces, salad dressings, marinades, soups, and desserts. The seeds can also be used in salads, ice creams, custards, breads, muffins, chutneys, and more.

To remove the seeds from the fruit, cut the fruit in half, then submerse the halves in water. (Be careful; the pulp-covered seeds can stain.) Gently scoop out the seeds with your fingers, letting them sink to the bottom of the bowl, then skim off any pith that floats to the surface. Pour

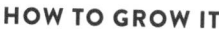

HOW TO GROW IT

Pomegranate thrives in subtropical climates with slightly alkaline, loamy soil, such as in the southwestern region of the United States. Provide full sun and well-drained soil. Feed in late winter and spring with a slow-release, balanced organic fertilizer. Pomegranate is self-fruitful, but potted indoor plants require hand pollination to set fruit. Or, for insect pollination, move the pots outdoors when the weather warms up in spring; bring them indoors when temperatures drop below 40°F in fall. Pomegranate can be propagated by hardwood cuttings taken in late winter, or by layering.

From Ancient Symbol to Modern Superfruit

The Old City of Jerusalem is honeycombed with narrow alleys that twist and turn, eventually opening into larger open spaces. Wandering through this area is like visiting an earlier culinary, cultural, and spiritual time. Here and there, vendors stand behind tables with small steel presses and large pyramids of pomegranates. They shout out a friendly invitation to sample the fruits' refreshing red juice.

According to archeological evidence, the pomegranate tree has been cultivated for at least 5,000 years. Native to the Middle East—most likely Persia—it is believed by some to be the biblical "tree of knowledge." Since ancient times, the fruit was considered a symbol of fertility because of its many seeds. The cultivation of this fascinating plant eventually spread to India,

northern Africa, Asia, Europe, and the New World. As modern research began to uncover the fruit's many health benefits, pomegranate has gained popularity. Known to relatively few Americans just a decade ago, the pomegranate is now considered a "superfood," widely consumed as a fresh fruit, juice, and in an array of commercially packaged products and supplements.—M. J. B.

the water through a mesh strainer to separate the seeds. To obtain the juice, wrap the seeds in cheesecloth and squeeze the liquid into a bowl.

The seeds from one pomegranate will yield about ⅓ cup of juice, which can be used to flavor sauces, vinaigrettes, marinades, or desserts. The original grenadine syrup, used in cocktails, was made with pomegranate juice.

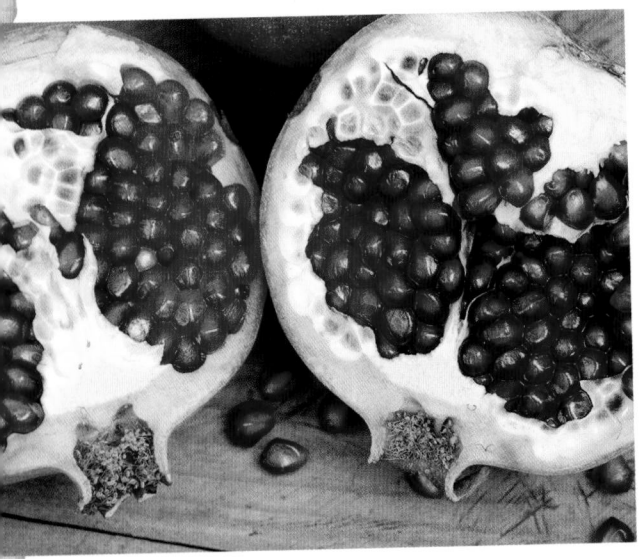

MEDICINAL USE

This fruit is both medicine and food, low in calories and rich in many important nutrients and compounds. Pomegranate juice is gaining popularity as an antiaging, free-radical-fighting antioxidant "superfood" that protects cells from oxidative stress and reduces inflammation. It could also prove helpful for treating or preventing many health conditions, including diseases of the heart and blood vessels. In Ayurvedic medicine, pomegranate's astringent root bark has been used to expel worms, especially tapeworms, from the body. Its astringent fruit rind is very rich in tannins and highly effective for treating diarrhea. To treat infants with that condition, the rind is powdered and mixed with buttermilk. In some studies, pomegranate rind has also inhibited the herpes simplex virus.

ORNAMENTAL USE

Older plants develop an appealing sculptural form with multiple twisted trunks. Ornamental cultivars have been developed with large double blooms and white or pink flowers and small, inedible fruit. Dwarf varieties make attractive potted ornamentals and can be used for bonsai.

Rauvolfia serpentina

Named in honor of the 16th-century German physician and explorer Leonhard Rauwolf, the genus *Rauvolfia* includes more than 100 species native to the moist tropical forests of the Pacific region, South America, Asia, and Africa. Serpentwood, *Rauvolfia serpentina*, is a small deciduous shrub that grows as an understory plant in India, Indonesia, Burma, Thailand, and Ceylon. According to legend, holy men in India, including Mahatma Gandhi, chewed the root of serpentwood to help achieve a state of philosophic detachment while meditating. The herb was first mentioned in the ancient Indian medical text *Charaka Samhita* (ca. 600 BCE) as useful for the treatment of mental illness. It also has a long history of use in India as a treatment for snake and insect bites, diarrhea, fever, and worms.

MEDICINAL USE

In traditional Indian medicine, this plant was valued as a sedative and tranquilizer. In 1952, serpentwood was found to contain an alkaloid called reserpine, which has powerful depressant and sedative properties. Reserpine—isolated from the dried, thick, snakelike roots of *Rauvolvia* that gave the plant its common name—was found to be useful as an antipsychotic and antihypertensive drug. At one time, reserpine was the only drug available to calm patients with serious psychological illnesses. Other tranquilizers have replaced reserpine in mental health therapy, but it is still used in some parts of the world, often in combination with other therapies, for the treatment of hypertension. Because of its numerous side effects and interactions with other medications, reserpine

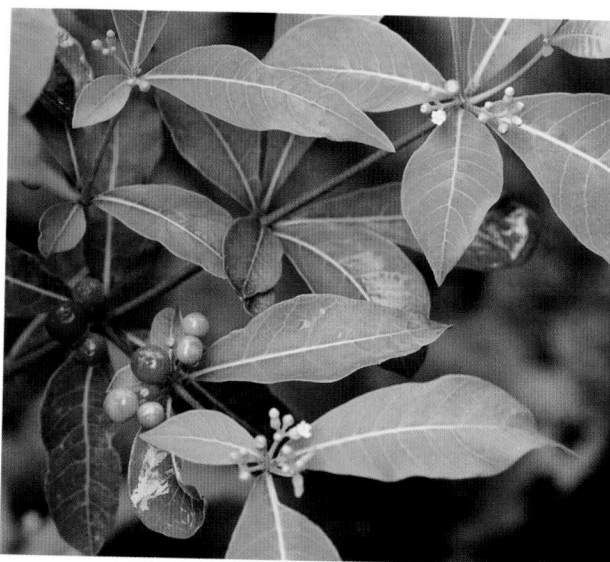

has been replaced in Western medicine by other antihypertensive drugs.

Caution: This plant should be administered only under the supervision of a health-care professional.

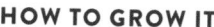

HOW TO GROW IT

Serpentwood thrives in tropical climates, where temperatures do not drop below 50° to 55°F. To grow serpentwood in a greenhouse, provide rich, acidic soil; high humidity; and full sun to partial shade. In winter, reduce watering. Propagate by taking stem cuttings in spring or summer, or take root cuttings in winter. For commercial preparations, roots of mature plants are harvested (leaving the taproot intact) in winter.

Ricinus communis

Although the castor bean plant is considered a weed in many of the world's tropical regions, the plant is cultivated in temperate regions, not only for its seed oil but also for its beauty as an accent plant in the garden. Castor bean is native to parts of Africa and India and has been used in these areas for cosmetic, healing, and household purposes since ancient times. Seeds of the plant have been found in 4,000-year-old Egyptian tombs. The Ebers Papyrus, an Egyptian medical text dating to ca. 1550 BCE, specified that the oil was useful as a laxative. In the Middle Ages, European herbalists used the herb as a liniment.

The seeds, commonly called beans, contain up to 5 percent of the protein ricin, which is one of the most toxic natural poisons. The extraction process used to produce oil from the beans removes the poisonous compound.

MEDICINAL USE

In addition to its use as a mild laxative, commercially produced castor bean oil can be applied topically as a skin moisturizer and to treat skin inflammations and warts.

Caution: Castor bean oil (also called castor oil) is not recommended for pregnant and nursing women and young children. The beans should never be taken internally in any form; the body can absorb the ricin in the seeds and the result can be severe poisoning and death.

ORNAMENTAL USE

Fast-growing castor bean is a popular foundation plant for new homes in southern regions. The plant's height and large, showy leaves also make a dramatic backdrop for lower-growing ornamentals in mixed borders. Planted in a large container, castor bean gives decks, porches, and verandas a lush, tropical look.

OTHER USES

Sometimes called "mole plant," castor bean reputedly deters rodents and rabbits, so some gardeners plant a castor bean hedge around their vegetable garden to repel animal pests. It is said that if you put a few seeds in a mole's hole, the little animals will move elsewhere. Certain eco-friendly mole repellents have castor oil as a major ingredient. Researchers at Michigan State University found that a commercial mole repellent containing 65 percent castor oil was effective for a period of 1 to 2 months. The bean's toxicity is probably a mechanism that evolved to ward off insect and pest attacks. It has been studied as a potential insecticide, but this would seem to be very toxic to humans and animals, as well.

HOW TO GROW IT

Plant castor bean seeds 1 inch deep in fertile, well-drained soil and full sun. In Zone 7 and colder, grow castor bean as an annual. Start the seeds indoors about 1 month before the last spring frost date, then transplant the seedlings outdoors after all danger of frost has passed. Keep plants well watered and away from young children and pets. Harvesting the plant for medicinal use is not recommended.

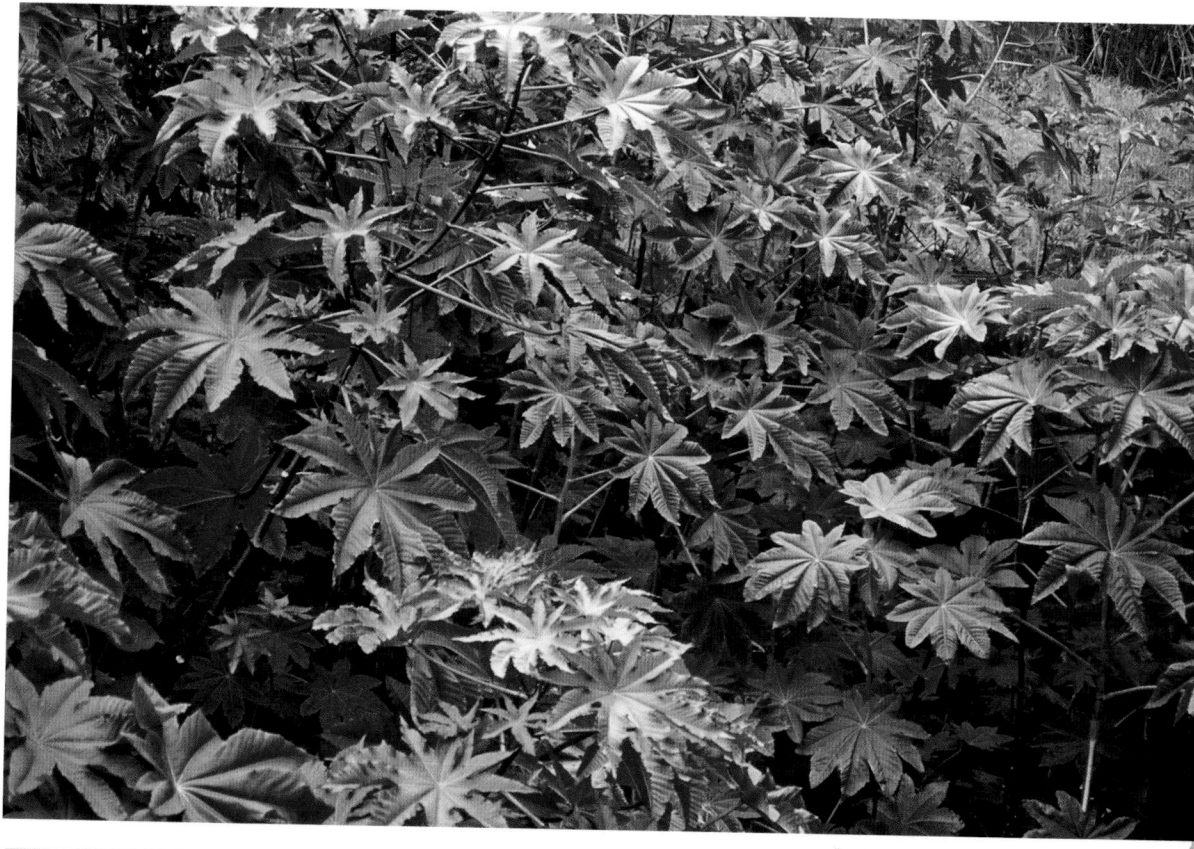

Castor Oil and Early Flying Machines

When I think of early aviators, the romantic image that immediately comes to mind is of the World War I pilot, sitting in an open cockpit wearing a leather jacket, goggles, and a white silk scarf that's wrapped around his face. Cutting through the clouds in acrobatic formations with the high winds whipping against his face, the smell of the rotary engine permeating the air—those early days of flying machines were indeed magnificent.

The goggles and scarf were not just a fashion statement; they were an essential part of flying. The design of the rotary engine that powered many of these planes—the fact that it spewed lubricating oil into the air during flight—caused the pilot's face and parts of his body to be covered with the spray. Castor oil was the best lubricant for this type of engine, which meant that pilots ingested a great deal of it during each hour of flight. And because castor oil is a purgative, this had an immediate effect on the pilot's intestinal system, resulting in the need to run to the facilities after every flight. Thus, the long, protective silk scarf wrapped in many layers around the pilot's nose and mouth became a mandatory part of flying gear. In later years, closed cockpits and other types of engines eliminated the need for the scarf, but the style was set. Today, there are still some high-performance motor lubricants that contain oil extracted from the castor bean.—M. J. B.

Rosa spp.

A member of the rose family (which also includes apple, strawberry, peach, and hawthorn), this familiar perennial is known by its fragrant flowers, serrated leaves, and thorny stems. The showy blooms—which range in color from pink and red to lavender, yellow, and white—give way to scarlet berries called rose hips. The genus *Rosa* includes more than 100 species, distributed throughout temperate regions in both hemispheres.

Roses were probably cultivated first in Iran, at least 3,000 years ago; from there, garden roses were introduced to ancient Greece and, later, Rome. Sappho, a 6th-century BCE Greek poet, called the rose "queen of flowers." Ancient Romans (not known for their restraint) also were enamored with the crimson blooms of *Rosa gallica*. They wore rose garlands and crowns, and they lavishly scattered the petals across banquet tables and floors and in the paths of victors.

In North America, Native Americans used wild roses ornamentally, as well as for food and medicine, long before Europeans introduced garden roses. Native American healing preparations included a mixture of rose petals and bear fat for mouth sores, rose petal powder for fever sores and blisters, and rainwater-soaked roses for soothing irritated eyes.

CULINARY USE

Rose hips and petals can be made into teas, fruit drinks, jellies, jams, candies (such as Turkish delight), and syrups. Also, try substituting the tart-flavored hips for cranberries in sauces, relishes, and muffins. Add rose petals to fruit or vegetable salads. Fill dessert crepes with rose jelly and garnish them with candied rose petals. Rosewater, a

distillation of rose petals in water, is a popular flavoring in Indian and Middle Eastern cuisines. *Lassi,* an Indian yogurt drink, is traditionally flavored with a few drops of rosewater.

MEDICINAL USE

The rose isn't used much in modern herbal medicine. Pure rose essential oil, known as rose attar or attar of rose, is used in aromatherapy and in perfumes. Rose oil has mild sedative, antidepressant, and anti-inflammatory effects. Rose hips, which usually come from *Rosa canina* (dog rose), are a good source of vitamin C. Studies using rose hip powder derived from a specific cultivar of *Rosa canina* grown in Denmark have shown promise for treating the symptoms of osteoarthritis.

ORNAMENTAL USE

The rose is beloved as a garden plant, and thousands of varieties have been developed. Many are disease resistant and bloom virtually nonstop from late spring through frost. Versatile roses can be used in

HOW TO GROW IT

Roses thrive in well-drained, moist, fertile, neutral to slightly acidic soil in full sun. Space the plants at least 30 inches apart to provide good air circulation. Prune them in late winter or early spring to remove old or dead canes, and thin them lightly to increase bloom size. In spring, top-dress beds with compost, then feed plants weekly with compost or manure tea through midsummer. Keep roses well watered and mulched during dry weather; remove all mulch in spring, when temperatures have warmed. To propagate roses, take hardwood cuttings in fall.

Harvest rose petals before the blossom opens completely. Pluck the petals from the bloom's center, and dry them in the sun until crisp. Harvest rose hips when they are fully mature, after the weather turns cold.

mixed borders, formal garden settings, and informal cottage gardens; as hedges and groundcovers; and as flowering covers for fences, pergolas, and trellises.

OTHER USES

The rose is a favorite source of fragrance for perfumes, bath oils, soaps, ointments, creams, and more. Varieties of *Rosa × damascena, R. gallica,* and *R. × centifolia* are the most fragrant. To obtain 1 ounce of essential oil of rose, 60,000 roses are needed, but you can make a less-potent rose oil at home simply by soaking rose petals in a light oil, such as grapeseed oil. Rosewater is sometimes used as a mild astringent in skin-care products. To make rosewater, place 6 cups of fresh rose petals in a medium-size saucepan; add 1 quart of water. Heat the mixture gently and then simmer for 15 minutes. Remove the pan from the heat, and steep for several hours. Strain out the petals. Store the rosewater in an airtight container in the refrigerator for up to 1 month. Rose petals also add fragrance and beauty to potpourris and sachets.

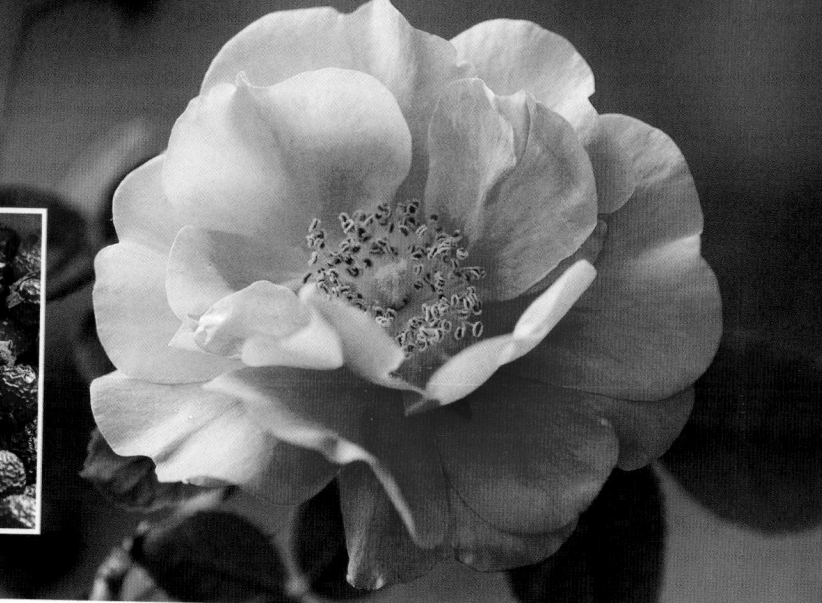

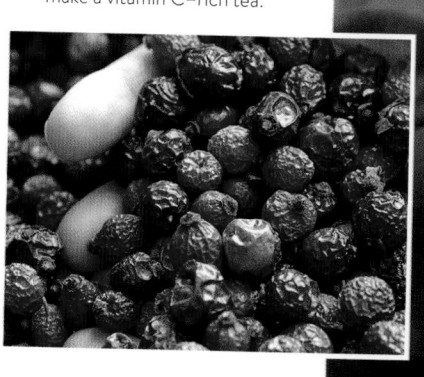

Fragrant *Rosa gallica,* sometimes called the apothecary rose, is valued for perfumes and cosmetics. The hips of dog rose (*R. canina*) make a vitamin C–rich tea.

The Apothecary Rose

Known botanically as Rosa gallica var. officinalis, the common name for this rose denotes its early use in medicine, as well as the fact that it was commonly grown outside of apothecary shops—a living sign that the establishment prepared and dispensed healing herbs. Its flowers have been used for herbal therapies since ancient times, when the Romans steeped the petals in wine to treat hangovers. Today this species is prized as a garden plant; its fragrant petals can be used for potpourri, and the essential oil, produced by steam distillation, is used in cosmetics. You can mix a few drops of the essential oil with several tablespoons of a carrier oil to make a rose-scented massage oil. During the War of the Roses in England (a civil war fought between 1455 and 1487), this red rose was the House of Lancaster's insignia.—M. J. B.

Rosmarinus officinalis

A bushy evergreen shrub with pale blue flowers and needle-shaped, aromatic leaves, rosemary belongs to the family Lamiaceae—also known as the mint family. The scientific name for the genus comes from the Latin *ros* ("dew" or "spray") and *marinus* ("sea"), a reference to the plant's tendency to grow on ocean cliffs in its native Mediterranean habitat. An old French name for this herb was *incensier* because it once was used as an inexpensive substitute for incense in religious ceremonies.

Rosemary has long been an emblem of fidelity and memory. Traditionally carried by brides, the herb appears in Shakespeare's *Hamlet,* when Hamlet's doomed lover, Ophelia, says, "There's rosemary, that's for remembrance." In the home, rosemary has long been valued for its antiseptic and antibacterial properties. At one time, it was rubbed on meat not only for flavor but also to help delay spoilage. Rosemary was also placed in sickrooms to fight illness and infection, and World War II nurses are said to have burned a mixture of rosemary leaves and juniper berries to disinfect hospitals.

CULINARY USE

Rosemary's flavor is pungent, somewhat piney, and mintlike. The fresh or dried leaves complement soups, breads, roasted meats (especially lamb, poultry, and pork), eggs, cheese, pasta dishes, marinades, sauces, and dressings. Rosemary also enhances tomatoes, spinach, peas, mushrooms, squash, and lentils, and it combines well with other herbs, such as chives, thyme, parsley, chervil, and bay. Finely chop the rough-textured leaves before you add them to fresh or cooked foods.

Fresh sprigs of rosemary and rosemary flowers can be steeped in vinegar, wine, or olive oil to add a subtle flavor. Use rosemary branches as skewers for grilling meat and vegetable kebabs.

MEDICINAL USE

Rosemary leaves have antispasmodic, carminative (gas-relieving), antioxidant, and anti-inflammatory properties. The herb is used primarily to treat poor digestion and appetite, joint pain, and sluggish circulation. It may help increase the flow of blood to your heart, and it has been recommended for elderly individuals with impaired circulation and for young adults who lack physical stamina. The herb also has been shown to have some liver-protective and antitumor properties.

 HOW TO GROW IT

A drought-tolerant plant, rosemary requires well-drained, fairly dry, rocky to sandy soil in full sun. Rosemary does not tolerate cold temperatures well, although several named cultivars—including 'Arp' and 'Hill Hardy'—are reported to tolerate temperatures as low as -10°F. In general, varieties with lighter colored flowers and thin leaves are most hardy; prostrate varieties are least hardy. In areas where temperatures drop below freezing, mulch rosemary during the winter. To overwinter rosemary indoors, lightly prune back the top, and then pot the plant before the first hard freeze. Rosemary is susceptible to root rot, so use a porous container and a medium that drains well. Keep potted rosemary in a cool, bright location indoors. Do not overwater, but mist regularly. Rosemary can be propagated by seed, cuttings, or layering. Harvest sprigs as needed throughout the growing season. To dry rosemary, hang small bundles upside down in a warm, dark location for 1 to 2 weeks. Strip the needles from the stems, then store them in an airtight container.

Oil of rosemary, made by steam distillation of the herb's fresh flowering tops, is used to ease irritation by increasing the blood supply to your skin. The oil is also useful as a steam inhalant, helping relieve nasal and chest congestion from colds, flus, and allergies. Rosemary oil contains natural camphor, which has an affinity for the nervous system. Applied externally, the oil has been used to relieve muscle and nerve pain, such as sciatica. In aromatherapy, rosemary oil is believed to have stimulating properties.

OTHER USES

Rosemary's pleasant fragrance and antioxidant properties make it a beneficial addition to cosmetics, skin creams, soaps, and lotions. Diluted rosemary oil can be rubbed into the scalp or added to shampoo to stimulate hair growth and prevent dandruff. A rosemary bath or facial, made by adding a strong rosemary infusion to water, is stimulating and refreshing. You can also add antiseptic rosemary oil to your homemade cleaning products.

ORNAMENTAL USE

Shrubby rosemary varieties make handsome landscape plants, especially in warm, dry climates. Use them near foundations, in rock gardens, or in containers on porches or decks, where their blue blooms and aromatic leaves will be within sight and touch. Plant trailing forms where they can cascade over the edge of a stone wall, hanging basket, window box, or pot.

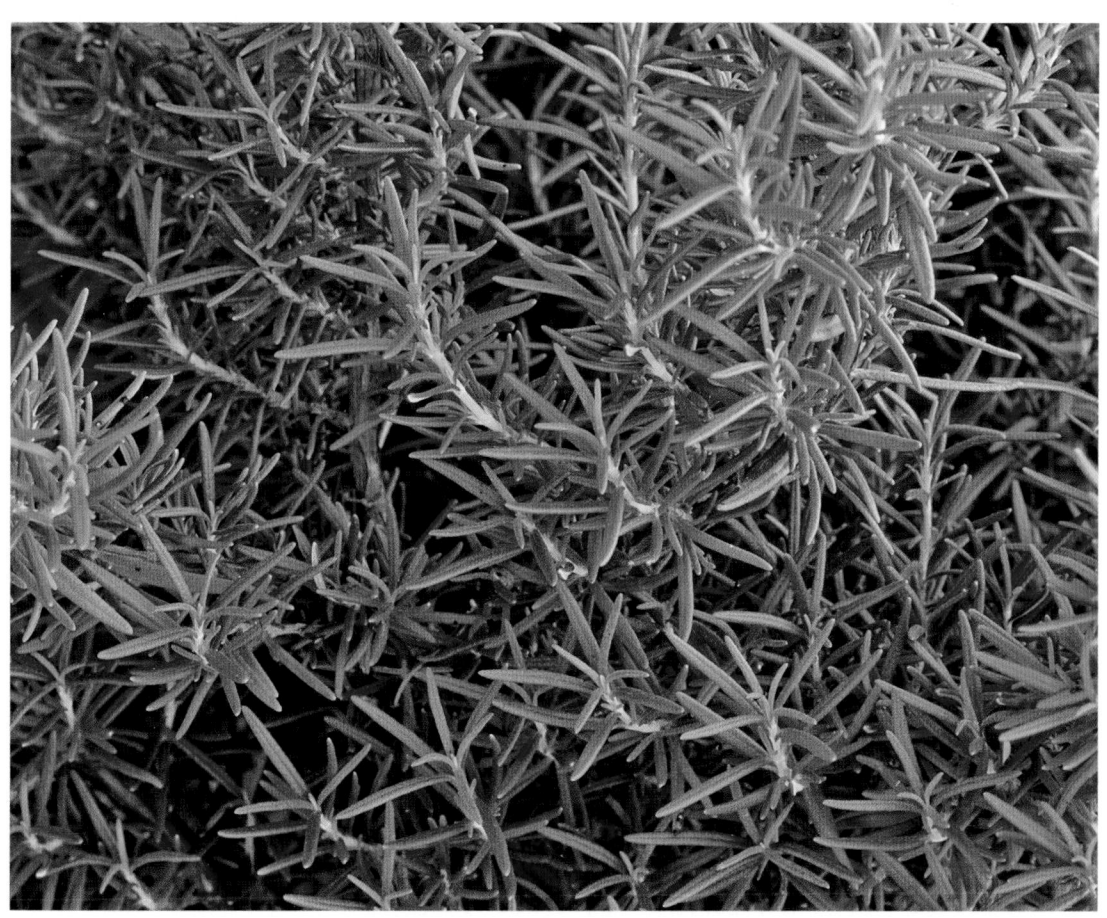

Rubia tinctorum

A relative of coffee (*Coffea arabica*), this southwestern Asian perennial has been valued since ancient times as a source of red dye for fabrics and leather. The species name in Latin refers to its use for dyeing. A piece of fabric dyed with madder root was found in the tomb of the Egyptian King Tutankhamen (ca. 1370–1352 BCE), and there is very early evidence of its use to dye clothing in India, as well. Even the "red coats" of 18th-century British soldiers were colored with madder dye. Madder began to fall out of favor as a dye in 1869, when scientists were able to synthesize alizarin, one of the pigments found in madder root.

MEDICINAL USE

Madder roots and stems were once used medicinally, especially by the ancient Greeks. The herb was believed to stimulate menstruation and to promote the flow of urine. At various times, it also was said to cure jaundice, inflammations, kidney stones, dysentery, diarrhea, and more.

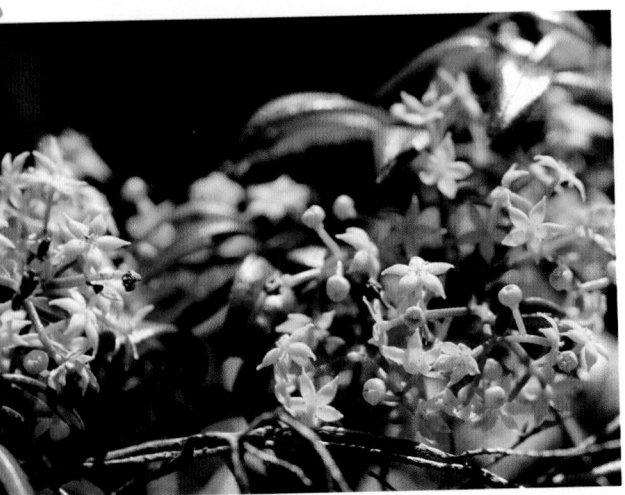

Although some lab experiments have shown that madder can stimulate uterine contractions, there is little clinical data on the efficacy of madder when used internally. Due to its possible risks and side effects, madder was not recommended by the German Commission E monographs for internal medicinal use. Applied externally, however, it can be used to treat wounds.

The compound alizarin is used in medical testing to color bone tissue, cells, and fluids for study.

OTHER USES

Artisans still use madder as a natural red or orange dye for wool, cotton, and silk.

To prepare madder for making dye, the roots are dried and then peeled. (Removing the root's outer layer of bark makes a better-quality dye.) Dyers recommend grinding the roots and then putting the powder in a cheesecloth bag before adding it to the dye bath. To make the dye colorfast, a mordant blend of alum and cream of tartar is often used.

Ancient Egyptian artists are believed to have made the world's first two red pigments, using madder root and cinnabar. The best reds were said to come from madder that had grown in alkaline soil.

HOW TO GROW IT

Madder thrives in deep, well-drained soil and full sun. The herb takes a long time to establish from seed, so start with nursery-grown plants, if possible. Space madder plants at least 1 foot apart. After 3 years, you can harvest the roots after the plant's top growth dies back in fall. Medium-size roots are best for making dye.

Rumex crispus

The scientific name of this green-yellow native European perennial refers to the shape of the plant's leaves: *Rumex* means "lance" and *crispus* means "curly." The genus consists of cultivated species (the sorrels) used mainly in cooking and wild species (the docks) used mainly as medicinal plants. Dock roots have been used throughout history as a laxative, a remedy for anemia, and a blood "purifier."

Native Americans applied the crushed roots and leaves to cuts, swellings, itchy areas, and boils.

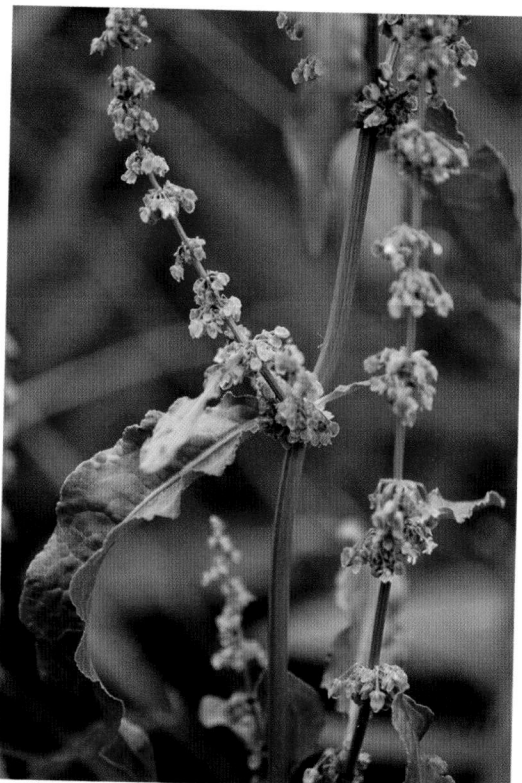

They also cooked and ate the leaves, often together with other greens. Eating yellow dock as a vegetable isn't recommended, however: Although the leaves are nutritious, they're also high in oxalic acid, which can damage your kidneys and liver if eaten in large amounts. Eating the leaves can also irritate your mouth.

MEDICINAL USE

Yellow dock root has been taken internally as a laxative and to strengthen blood and used externally to provide relief from inflammatory skin conditions, boils, rashes, and burns. A poultice of the leaves can be used to treat ringworm and other skin fungi. When applied to an area touched by stinging nettle, it is said to relieve the irritation and pain. In the mid-1800s, practitioners of Eclectic medicine—a branch of medicine based on botanicals and natural healing that developed in the United States—prepared an ointment from the roots to treat irritated skin sores and swellings. The plant's roots contain iron, calcium, and tannins that are astringent and antibacterial.

HOW TO GROW IT

Considered an invasive weed throughout North America, yellow dock thrives in rich, heavy soil in full sun. Buried seed can remain viable for 50 years or more. Wild plants can be found in disturbed sites, such as ditches and roadsides, as well as in moist clearings, along stream banks, and in meadows. If you harvest wild dock, be sure it has not been treated with herbicides.

Ruta graveolens

The namesake of the rue family and kin to citrus, rue is native to southeastern Europe and is cultivated worldwide. This evergreen shrub bears grayish blue, spade-shaped leaves and bright yellow flowers. It has a repellent odor. Its genus name, *Ruta,* is thought to come from the Greek word *reuo,* meaning "to set free," referring to the plant's reputed ability to free people from disease. The herb once was used as an antidote to poisons and

PLANT PROFILE

Common Names: Common Rue, Herb-of-Grace, Rue

Description: Semiwoody evergreen shrub, 2 to 3 feet tall; grayish blue, spade-shaped leaves; bright yellow flowers

Hardiness: To Zone 4

Family: Rutaceae

Flowering: June through August

Parts Used: Leaves

Range/Habitat: Native to southeastern Europe and northern Africa; locally naturalized in old fields, and waste areas and along roadsides

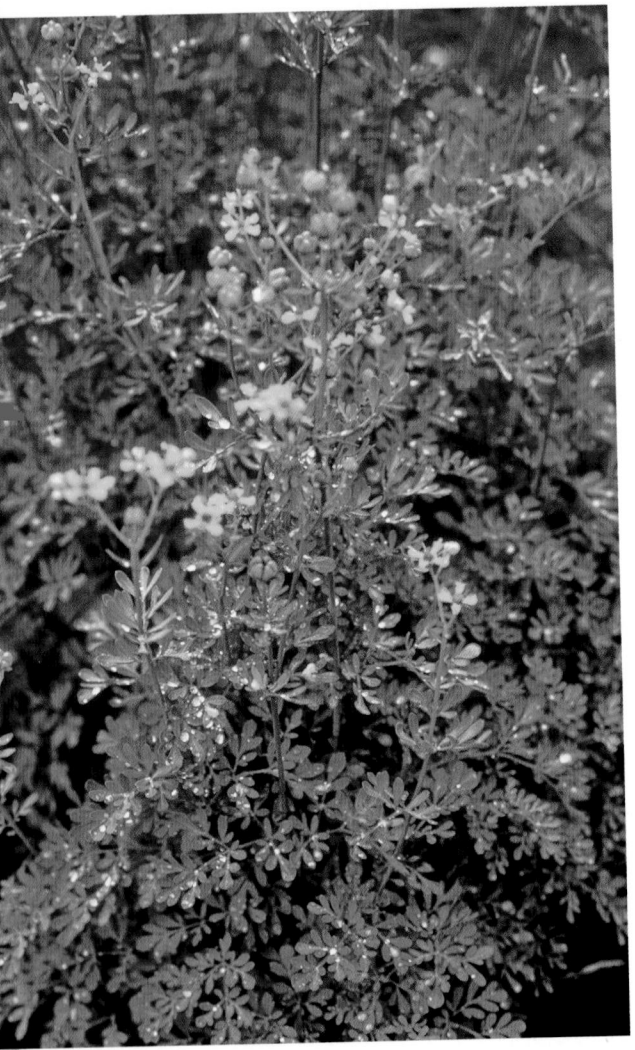

as a protection against witches and the bubonic plague. In ancient Rome, artists ate rue to preserve their eyesight. The common name herb-of-grace comes from the Catholic tradition of using a rue brush to sprinkle holy water during mass.

CULINARY USE

Add rue leaves to cream cheese, salads, and egg dishes; use the herb sparingly, however—it has an acrid flavor. Rue is very popular in Ethiopia, where the fresh leaves are used as a flavoring for coffee. It is also an essential ingredient in the Ethiopian spice mix berbere. Rue leaves are used to flavor some varieties of the Italian grape liqueur grappa, as well.

MEDICINAL USE

Once considered an important herb for treating hypertension, diabetes, and allergic reactions, rue is no longer widely used in medicine. Rue leaves contain volatile oil, bitters, astringent and antiseptic tannins, and the flavonoid rutin, which helps strengthen capillaries (explaining the herb's traditional use as a treatment for failing eyesight). Today, rue is primarily used to regulate the menstrual cycle. It contains alkaloids that have antispasmodic effects, making it useful not only for treating menstrual cramps, but also digestive upset, bowel tension, and spasmodic cough.

Caution: Do not use rue if you are pregnant or breastfeeding. It is a very powerful plant that contains toxic compounds. Exposure to sun following contact with this plant, such as handling it in your garden, can cause severe photodermatitis.

Powerful Protector

Rue is an extremely important plant in the traditional medical systems of Belize. Working with my colleagues and friends Dr. Rosita Arvigo and Dr. Gregory Shropshire, we developed an understanding of the variety of uses of this plant during more than a decade of fieldwork with dozens of traditional healers who collaborated with us on a project to inventory the useful plants of that nation.

In Belize, rue is used internally for certain conditions, but only under the watchful eye of an experienced healer. A few drops of juice are carefully squeezed out of nine small branchlets and into a glass of water; this is strained and consumed twice daily for stomach cramps or to rid the body of intestinal worms, reduce nausea, and calm a nervous person. More commonly, the leaves are soaked in alcohol and used externally as a liniment for sore muscles, backache, and muscle spasms.

The most common use of rue in Belize is as a charm that protects a person from evil and from the envy of others who wish to do them harm. People carry a few sprigs of leaves with them for this purpose, or they form the sprigs into the shape of a cross and place it over the entrance of their home, thus cleansing anyone who may enter with harmful intentions. Does it work? Local people swear by its protective powers, and it has been a prominent protective amulet for centuries in the area.—M. J. B.

ORNAMENTAL USE

With its mounded form, beautiful yellow blooms, and finely textured leaves, rue makes an attractive garden plant. Butterflies love it, while dogs and cats seem to avoid it. Rue's blue-green leaves are a nice foil for roses in informal beds and borders. Tolerant of hot, dry conditions, rue also shines in rock gardens. Or grow the plants to form a low hedge or edging, such as for a knot garden. The flowers are good for cutting and drying, too.

OTHER USES

Rue may have antibacterial and antifungal properties. The essential oil, extracted from a steam distillation of the fresh flowering plant, is sometimes used in soaps, detergents, creams, and lotions. But because it is an oral toxin and skin irritant, the oil must be used at *extremely* low concentrations.

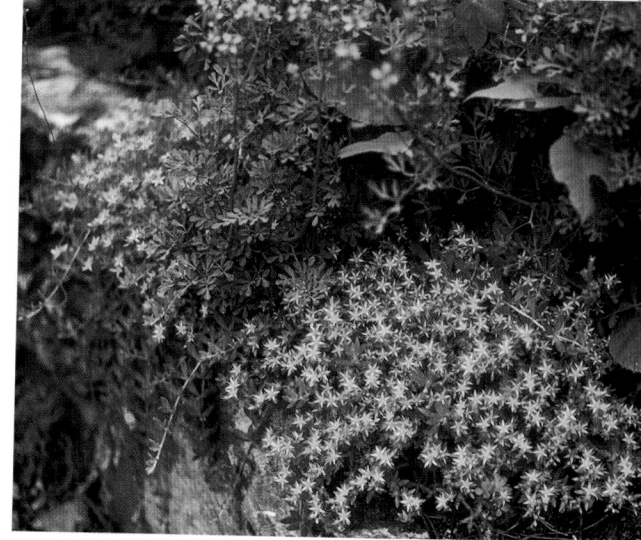

 HOW TO GROW IT

Rue thrives in well-drained, neutral to alkaline soil in full sun. Start seeds indoors under lights in late February, and transplant seedlings to your garden in spring, when the soil and air have warmed. To propagate, take semiripe cuttings in summer, root them in the shade, and plant them in a sunny location. Rue can also be grown in a pot on a sunny windowsill.

Harvest rue leaves before flowers form. Dry them in the shade, then store them in an airtight container.

Salix alba

Willow, one of 400 *Salix* species, is a large tree native to Europe and western and central Asia. *Salix*, derived from a Celtic word that means "near water," refers to the plant's tendency to grow in damp soil or near waterways. Willows have slender, supple branches and large fibrous root systems. The lance-shaped leaves of the white willow (*Salix alba*) are covered with fine hairs, which give the foliage a silvery sheen. In the folklore of many cultures, the willow is associated with death and the afterlife. The tree was sacred to several ancient Greek goddesses of the underworld and was linked to the mythological Orpheus. According to legend, he received his gift of poetry and music after touching a willow.

PLANT PROFILE

Common Names: White Willow, Willow

Description: Deciduous tree up to 75 feet tall; gray-brown bark; narrow, alternate, lance-shaped leaves; flowers in cylindrical catkins

Hardiness: To Zone 3

Family: Salicaceae

Flowering: Midspring

Parts Used: Bark

Range/Habitat: Native to temperate climates in Europe and western and central Asia; usually found near water

MEDICINAL USE

Commonly called "herbal aspirin," the bark of the willow tree has been used for more than 2,000 years to reduce fever and relieve pain. In the first century CE, the Greek physician Dioscorides wrote that willow "mashed with a little pepper and drunk with wine" could relieve lower backache. Native American healers used the bark of white willow and related North American species as a poultice to treat

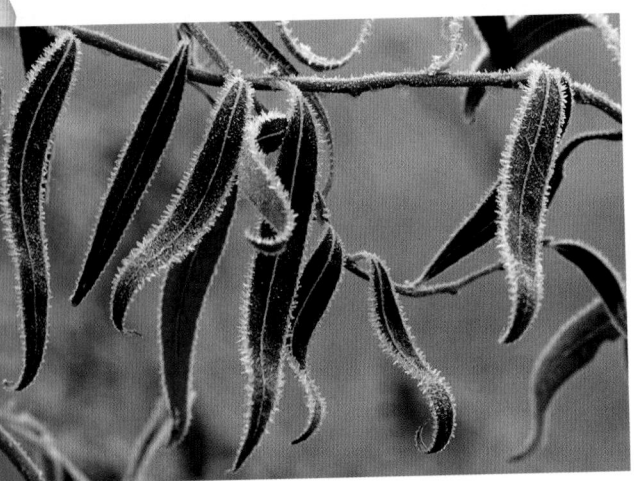

sores and stop bleeding and as an infusion to treat diarrhea, fever, and head and body aches.

Willow contains salicylic acid, which was synthesized by the Bayer company from the herb meadowsweet as the basis of pharmaceutical aspirin. Bayer was looking for a substitute for its popular pain formula, which included as ingredients toxic wintergreen and black birch oil. Willow has a weaker action than aspirin, but it also provokes fewer side effects. The tree does not share aspirin's blood-thinning effects, nor does it irritate the lining of the stomach.

Caution: Willow should not be used by pregnant or nursing women, by people who are sensitive to aspirin or have stomach ulcers, or by children younger than age 16 who have a fever related to cold, flu, or chickenpox.

ORNAMENTAL USE

The soft, graceful form and foliage of the willow adds a tranquil look to the landscape. It is a favorite for planting near pools and water gardens, and it can help control erosion on stream banks.

OTHER USES

Astringent decoctions of willow bark can be used in facial preparations and herbal baths. Though not easily worked, willow wood has been used to make tool handles and fencing. The pliant young stems are prized for basket weaving.

HOW TO GROW IT

Willow trees grow in heavy, moist to wet soil in full sun. The trees are difficult to transplant, but cuttings root easily in summer. Harvest bark from 2- to 5-year-old trees in spring or summer.

Salvia officinalis

An evergreen shrub native to the Mediterranean region, *Salvia officinalis* bears oval-shaped silvery green leaves with a velvety texture and white, pink, or violet flowers. The botanical name *Salvia* derives from the Latin *salvere*, meaning "to save," a reference to the herb's reputation as a powerful healer. In medieval England, people added sage to ale as a toast to good health. The Chinese held sage in such high esteem that they traded it for black tea (*Camellia sinensis*).

The genus *Salvia* includes many other interesting and useful species, including blue sage (*S. clevelandii*), an evergreen shrub that bears wrinkled aromatic leaves and spikes of blue-violet flowers; diviner's sage (*S. divinorum*), which has large green leaves, white flowers, and psychoactive properties; Greek sage (*S. fruticosa*), which bears lavender-scented leaves with downy undersides and mauve to pink flowers; narrow-leaved sage or Spanish sage (*S. lavandulifolia*), an evergreen perennial with hairy stems bearing wrinkled gray lavender-scented leaves; Chinese sage, or red sage (*S. miltiorrhiza*), a popular Chinese medicinal herb that has red roots and bears purple flowers; and painted sage (*S. viridis*), which has erect stems and bears soft leaves and small pink or purple flowers. Many of these species and their cultivars are beautiful and useful garden plants.

CULINARY USE

Sage tastes lemony, camphorlike, and pleasantly bitter. Add the young leaves to salads, omelets, fritters, soups, breads, pasta dishes, cheeses, and meats (especially pork and poultry). Sage also partners well with beans, artichokes, tomatoes, eggplant, potatoes, carrots, squash, corn, Brussels sprouts, and cabbage. For a unique and tasty appetizer or accompaniment for potatoes, dust larger sage leaves with flour, then fry them in ¼ inch of hot oil for about 30 seconds, until crispy. Sage leaves and flowers can also be candied.

Because sage has strong antioxidant and antibacterial properties, people traditionally added it to sausage and other meats as a preservative and flavoring. Commercial beverage-makers add sage oil to both nonalcoholic and alcoholic beverages, including vermouth and bitters.

MEDICINAL USE

Salvia officinalis has antimicrobial properties and contains volatile oils that help soothe mucous membranes. The herb is a classic remedy for sore throats, coughs, and colds. Herbal practitioners suggest drinking sage leaf tea or using it as a gargle to treat laryngitis, pharyngitis, tonsillitis, gingivitis, and mouth sores. Sage also seems to relax the stomach and may ease indigestion and flatulence.

One of the traditional uses of this plant is to enhance memory, and a recent small pilot study using *Salvia officinalis* extract confirmed that it could help in the early stages of illnesses involving

HOW TO GROW IT

Sage grows best in fairly rich, well-drained loam in full sun. Mulch the plants to retain moisture during extended hot, dry periods. Where temperatures drop below 0°F, apply winter mulch.

Harvest the leaves as needed for fresh use. To dry sage leaves, snip them from their stems and spread them on cloth or paper in the shade. Store the dried leaves in an airtight container.

Replace or divide the plants every 3 years to encourage vigorous, productive growth. Propagate sage by seed, cuttings (taken in fall and planted in spring), or root division. When dividing sage, replant only the outer, newer root sections.

cognition. Other studies have shown that sage can help reduce hot flashes and night sweats during menopause. German health authorities recognize the herb as a treatment for excessive perspiration.

To make sage leaf tea, pour 1 cup of hot water over 1 teaspoon of dried (or 2 teaspoons of fresh) sage leaves. Steep for 10 minutes, then strain. Drink, or use the tea as a gargle.

Caution: Do not use sage in therapeutic amounts if you are pregnant or nursing. (Culinary use is safe.)

ORNAMENTAL USE

The silvery green leaves of garden sage add a restful accent to the ornamental border and can serve as a beautiful backdrop for orange lilies and daylilies or red roses. The varieties 'Aurea' (compact with gold and green variegated leaves), 'Purpurea' (aromatic purple foliage), and 'Tricolor' (variegated cream, purple, and green leaves) offer added garden interest.

OTHER USES

Traditionally used to control excess perspiration, sage is an ingredient in some present-day antiperspirant formulas. Sage also stimulates the skin when used in lotions or bathwater. A sage leaf and lavender infusion makes a soothing, astringent aftershave. Traditionally, women darkened their hair by rinsing it with sage leaf tea.

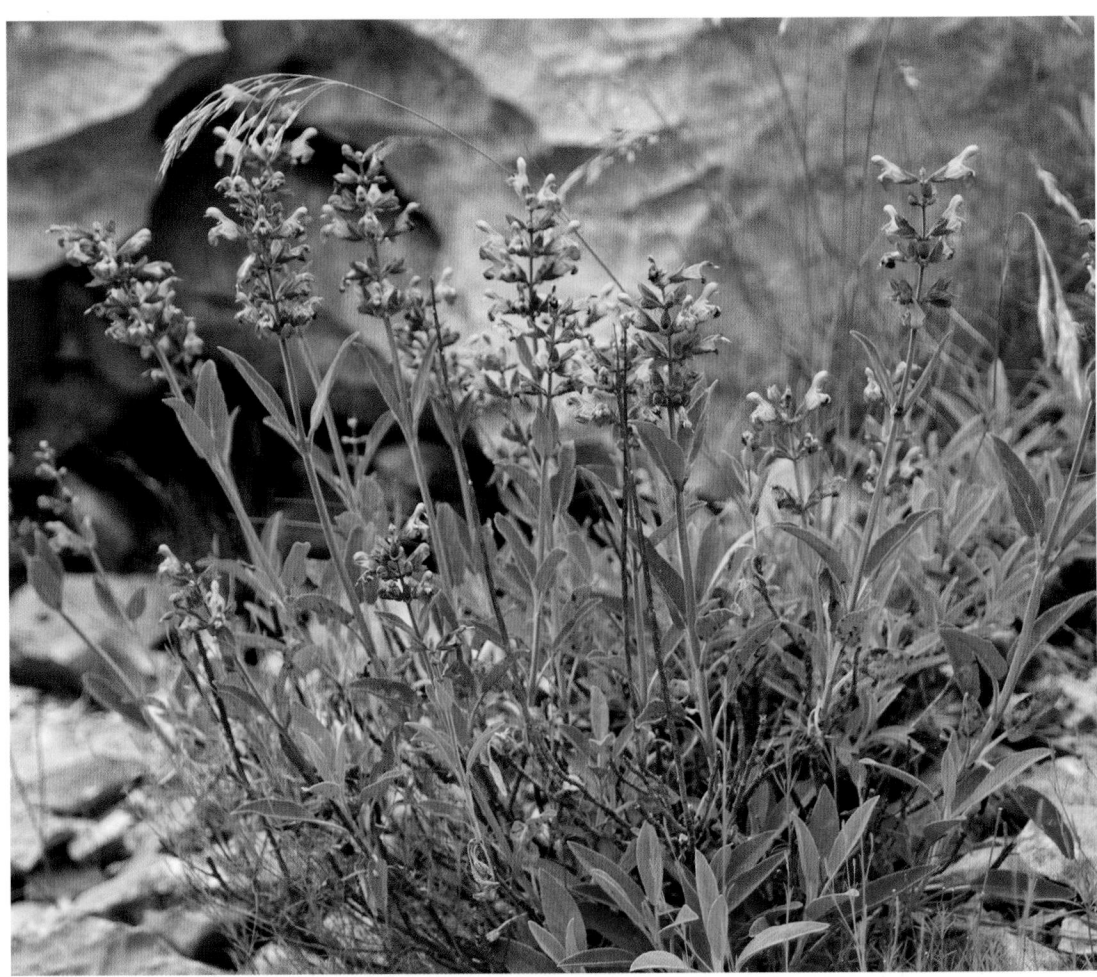

Salvia sclarea

An erect biennial in the mint family, clary sage is native to southern Europe and the Mediterranean region. The herb is best known as a traditional treatment for eye afflictions; in fact, its species name, *sclarea*, is derived from the Latin word *clarus*, meaning "clear."

Clary sage was also once used as an ingredient in wine and beer. During the 16th century, German wine merchants made an infusion with clary sage and elder flowers, and then added the liquid to Rhine wines to make them taste more like expensive muscatel wines. In England, the herb was sometimes substituted for hops when making beer.

CULINARY USE

Use the fresh or dried leaves of clary sage as you would use garden sage (*Salvia officinalis*). The chopped fresh or dried leaves add an earthy flavor to beans, eggs, pasta dishes, pork, potatoes, poultry, salads, and soups.

MEDICINAL USE

In the Middle Ages, clary sage was a very important medicinal herb used as a treatment for eye problems, digestive disorders, menstrual and uterine conditions, and kidney disease. Because a decoction of the seeds is mucilaginous, traditional herbalists believed that its use as an eyewash would clear foreign matter from the eyes.

Today the herb is not used widely for these conditions, although some herbalists still recommend clary sage seed eyewash for removing foreign particles. An infusion, or tea, made from the herb's leaves can help soothe digestive discomfort.

Essential oil of clary sage, obtained by steam distillation, is commonly used in aromatherapy because it is less toxic than the oil of *Salvia*

PLANT PROFILE

Common Names: Clary, Clary Sage, Muscatel Sage

Description: Erect biennial (or short-lived perennial), 3 to 4 feet tall; broad; opposite, heart-shaped leaves 6 to 9 inches long; spikes of purple or pale pink flowers; aromatic

Hardiness: To Zone 5

Family: Lamiaceae

Flowering: Early summer

Parts Used: Leaves and seeds

Range/Habitat: Native to southern Europe and the Mediterranean region

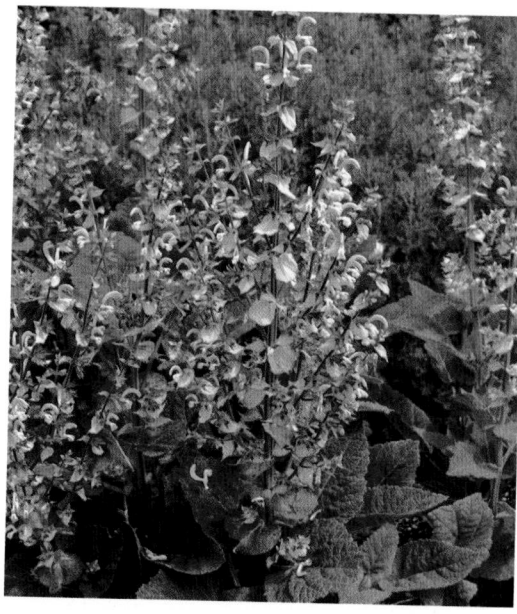

officinalis. The oil is considered effective for treating muscle tension and pain, menopausal hot flashes, acne, skin inflammation, and dandruff.

HOW TO GROW IT

Clary sage thrives in average, well-drained soil and full sun. The herb is easy to grow from seed sown in spring, but the plants will not flower until their second year. Harvest the leaves as needed for fresh use. To dry clary sage leaves, snip them from their stems and spread them on cloth or paper in the shade. Store the dried leaves in an airtight container. In areas with harsh winters, mulch the ground around the plants with straw or evergreen boughs when the soil has frozen to about 1 inch deep.

Sambucus nigra,
S. canadensis

PLANT PROFILE

Common Names: Black Elder, Elderberry

Description: Shrub or small tree, up to 12 feet tall; compound, opposite leaves; flat-topped clusters of creamy white flowers followed by small, seedy berries ripening to a deep purple-black

Hardiness: To Zone 3

Family: Adoxaceae

Flowering: Early summer

Parts Used: Bark, flowers, and fruit

Range/Habitat: European elder is native to Europe, American elder is native to eastern and central North America; found in moist or wooded areas

Both the European elder (*Sambucus nigra*) and North American elder (*S. canadensis*) grow naturally along riverbanks and in moist woodland thickets. A shrub or small tree, the elder bears flat-topped masses of sweetly scented, cream-colored flowers that are followed by purplish blue edible berries. In many of the folk tales of northern Europe, the elder held supernatural powers and was believed to ward off evil. The name *Sambucus* is similar to the name of an ancient musical instrument and could refer to the traditional use of the plant's hollow stems as a whistle or flute.

CULINARY USE

You can use fully ripe elderberries to make delicious juice, wine, and preserves. Mix the flowers into pancake batter; coat them with milk and eggs

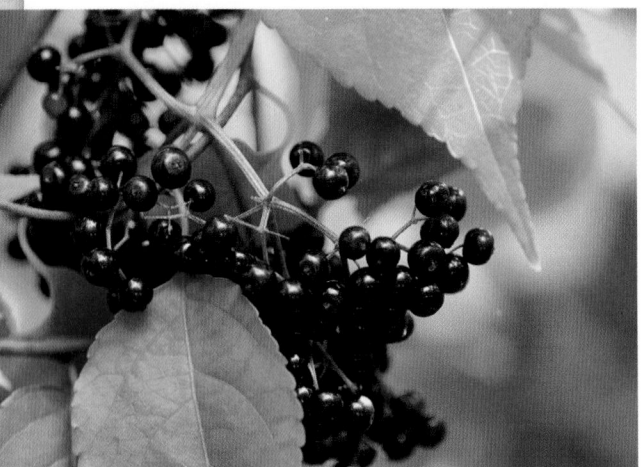

and then cook them to make fritters; or use them to make tea, wine, or vinegar.

Caution: Unripe fruits of *Sambucus* can be mildly toxic.

MEDICINAL USE

Elderberry has been called "the medicine chest of the people" because of the plant's many therapeutic uses. The herb has anti-inflammatory and antiviral properties, and the flowers have a long history of use for relieving the symptoms of sinusitis, colds, fever, and flu. Commercial syrups and extracts made from elderberry fruit are widely available in health food stores. Studies have shown that elderberry syrup and extracts can reduce flu symptoms and duration, as compared to a placebo. Elderberry is also believed to have diuretic and diaphoretic (sweat-promoting) activity; herbalists recommend warm elder flower tea to promote sweating and reduce fever.

OTHER USES

The berries produce a deep blue dye. The leaves can be used to make a green dye.

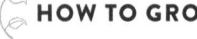

HOW TO GROW IT

Grow elder in rich, moist soil and full sun or partial shade. Amend the site with compost or aged manure before planting, and water the plants regularly until they're established. Harvest the flowers in spring and early summer; harvest fully ripe berries in late summer. To propagate elderberry shrubs, take softwood cuttings in summer or hardwood cuttings in winter.

Caution: Be careful when harvesting elderberry. While reports of poisoning are rare, the leaves, stems, roots, and unripe fruit of European and American elderberry can be toxic. Also be careful if you're harvesting berries from wild plants; similar-looking species have highly toxic berries.

Sanguinaria canadensis

Bloodroot, native to the deciduous woods and woodland slopes of eastern North America, is a relative of the poppy (*Papaver* spp.). This low-growing perennial bears white flowers and a single, rounded, gray-green leaf that wraps around the flower. The genus name *Sanguinaria* comes from the Latin *sanguis,* or "blood," which refers to the red sap found in the plant's rhizomes and roots. Native Americans once used the red-orange liquid as a fabric dye and body paint. They also made a tea from the plant's roots to treat colds, sore throats, fevers, joint problems, and many other conditions. Tribes in the Lake Superior region applied the sap to cancerous growths on the skin.

PLANT PROFILE

Common Names: Bloodroot, Red Paint Root, Red Puccoon

Description: Herbaceous perennial, 4 to 6 inches tall; naked stems rise from thick, horizontal rhizomes; 1- to 2-inch white flowers; deeply lobed palmate leaves up to 8 inches across at maturity

Hardiness: To Zone 3

Family: Papaveraceae

Flowering: April

Parts Used: Rhizomes

Range/Habitat: Native to eastern North America; cool, moist woodland slopes

MEDICINAL USE

The rhizomes of bloodroot contain many types of alkaloids; one of the most important is sanguinarine, which has antifungal, expectorant, antispasmodic, cathartic, and cardiovascular actions. The herb has a relaxing effect on the bronchial muscles and has proven useful in the treatment of bronchitis. In extremely small doses administered under the supervision of a medical professional, bloodroot has been used to treat asthma, croup, and laryngitis.

Bloodroot is sometimes used externally to treat conditions such as skin sores, eczema, warts, nasal polyps, and benign skin tumors. Bloodroot extracts are used in dental hygiene products, such as mouthwash, to fight plaque formation and gum disease, although it is known to induce mutations in DNA, and some sources suggest that long-term use of these products should be avoided.

Caution: Bloodroot is considered a toxic plant and shouldn't be ingested or used during pregnancy. It should only be used under the supervision of a qualified medical professional. Bloodroot has been overharvested in the wild and is at risk of becoming endangered. If you buy this herb, check the source to be sure that the herb has been cultivated, not harvested from the wild.

ORNAMENTAL USE

The pure white blossoms and uniquely shaped foliage of bloodroot are a lovely addition to informal shade gardens and woodland plantings. The cultivar 'Multiplex' has full, long-lasting blooms.

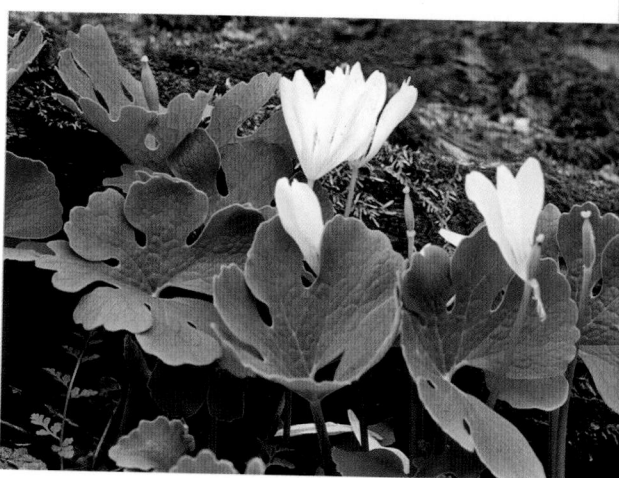

HOW TO GROW IT

Plant nursery-grown plants or sow seeds in partial shade and moist, well-drained soil amended with compost. Space plants 6 to 8 inches apart. To harvest the rhizomes, dig up mature plants (5 years or older) in early fall. Reserve some of the rhizomes and replant them at their original spacing.

Sanguisorba minor

PLANT PROFILE

Common Names: Burnet, Salad Burnet

Description: Perennial, up to 3 feet tall, in bloom; basal rosette of toothed, parsleylike leaves; small, thimble-shaped, purplish to pinkish flowers

Hardiness: To Zone 3

Family: Rosaceae

Flowering: May to June

Parts Used: Leaves and roots

Range/Habitat: Native to western Asia and Europe, naturalized in North America

A relative of the rose (*Rosa* spp.), salad burnet is one of 15 to 20 species in the genus *Sanguisorba*— a name that refers to the herb's traditional use to staunch wounds. *Sanguisorba* comes from the Latin *sanguis*, meaning "blood," and *sorere*, meaning "to soak up." Native to Europe and western Asia, this perennial herb was once a common addition to salads and wines and was extensively cultivated as fodder for sheep and cattle. The dried leaves of salad burnet are popular for making pressed flower arrangements.

CULINARY USE

When bruised, salad burnet leaves smell and taste like cucumber. Use the tender, young leaves in salads, dressings, herb vinegars, herb butters, and iced beverages. Add the seeds to vinegars, marinades, and cheese spreads. Toss the edible pink flowers into salads or use them as garnishes.

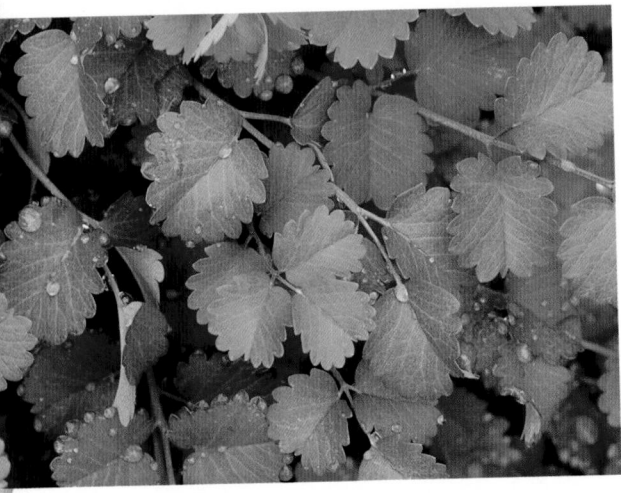

MEDICINAL USE

Salad burnet contains astringent and antiseptic tannins and has been used throughout history to staunch the bleeding of wounds. Herbalists still sometimes suggest applying a leaf poultice of this herb to stop external bleeding. A tea made from the herb's roots and leaves has been used to stop internal bleeding and to treat diarrhea and fevers. A salad burnet leaf infusion can be applied as a wash to soothe sunburn and other skin irritations.

ORNAMENTAL USE

In spring, salad burnet's flowering stems grow to 3 feet tall, bearing rounded heads of tiny pink flowers. Consider using it as an edging plant for your herb or kitchen garden.

HOW TO GROW IT

Salad burnet prefers full sun to partial shade and average, well-drained soil. It is not drought tolerant, so provide water during dry periods. Remove flower stems to encourage new foliage growth. Although it's easily grown from seed sown directly in the garden, the herb can also be propagated by root division in spring or fall. Once established, burnet needs little attention. Harvest the leaves for fresh use as needed throughout the growing season. (The leaves do not hold their flavor well when dried.) A few of the roots of established plants can be harvested in fall.

Saponaria officinalis

This pink-flowered, leafy-stemmed perennial is native to Europe and Asia and is naturalized throughout sunny, open areas of North America. Long ago, native peoples learned that rubbing this plant's roots in water would produce foamy suds. This is due to the presence of compounds known as saponins, a term derived from the Latin word for soap. Soapwort contains 15 to 20 percent saponins by weight. Before soap was invented in the early 1800s, soapwort and other saponin-rich plants were used to cleanse both the body and clothing. At one time, soapwort was also added to

beer to create a frothy head. In the Middle Ages, the herb was called *Herba fullonis*, referring to its use to "full" or clean and thicken woolen cloth.

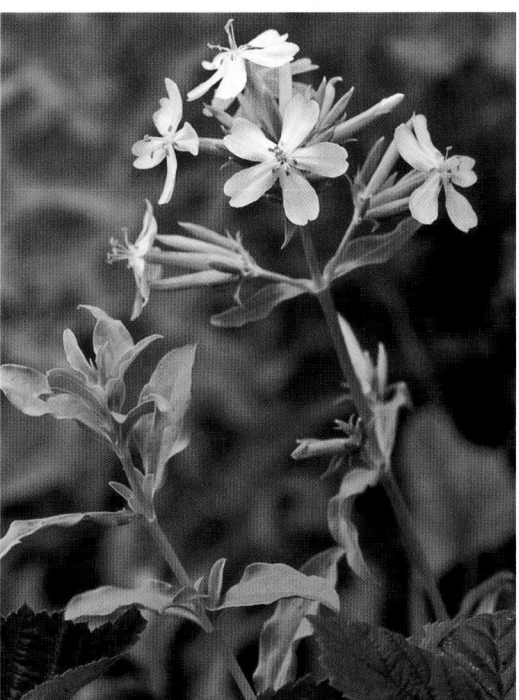

MEDICINAL USE

The root may have antibacterial and expectorant properties. In folk medicine, it has been taken internally to treat upper respiratory conditions, such as coughs and bronchitis, and applied externally to treat skin problems, such as eczema, psoriasis, acne, and poison ivy. Soapwort and other plants that contain saponins are not widely used in herbal medicine today, however, as these compounds are very irritating to the intestinal tract and can cause nausea, vomiting, and diarrhea.

ORNAMENTAL USE

A familiar wildflower, soapwort is lovely when naturalized along the edge of a woodland garden or hedgerow. The blooms draw butterflies and hummingbirds. The double-flowered variety 'Rosea Plena' and others have been bred for garden use.

OTHER USES

When mixed with water, the viscous saponin in soapwort forms a lather that can be used to cleanse delicate fabric or skin. Soapwort can cause eye irritation, so be cautious if you use it as a body cleanser.

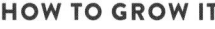 **HOW TO GROW IT**

Soapwort is very easy to grow in average soil and full sun to partial shade. Plant seed outdoors in either spring or fall or, for earlier bloom, start seed indoors under lights in late winter. The plants will self-sow, and propagation is rarely necessary. To prevent soapwort from becoming invasive, cut back the plants immediately after the flowers have faded. Use the cut tops to make natural cleaning products. Dig up roots for the same purpose in fall.

Sassafras albidum

The root of this handsome native North American tree was one of the first exports to Europe—and possibly the first medicinal herb—from the North American colonies. Sassafras bears clusters of aromatic yellow-green flowers, followed by distinctive "mitten-shaped" leaves that turn bright yellow or orange in fall. Native American tribes of the eastern woodlands and colonial settlers used the tree's root bark to make a soothing tea taken as a spring tonic and as a remedy for circulatory, digestive, and respiratory disorders, as well as skin conditions. The leaves were also used to flavor food.

CULINARY USE

Sassafras oil was used to flavor foods, root beer, and chewing gum until the FDA banned its use in commercially prepared foods after studies showed that safrole, a major ingredient in sassafras oil, is a carcinogen. Today, safrole is removed from sassafras extracts to make them safe for use in foods.

When mixed with water, the finely ground leaves of sassafras (known as filé) make a flavorful thickener for soups and stews, such as the Cajun dish gumbo. Sassafras leaves contain relatively little safrole; using a pinch of filé powder in cooking is generally considered harmless.

MEDICINAL USE

This plant has a long tradition of use in Native American medicine as a general tonic and as a healing poultice and wash for treating skin conditions such as bee stings, burns, and measles. Although the herb should not be taken internally unless the safrole has been removed, sassafras preparations are still used externally to treat skin irritations such as insect bites, eczema, psoriasis, and poison oak and ivy.

ORNAMENTAL USE

Sassafras adds spectacular foliage color—shades of yellow, orange, and red—to the fall landscape,

and the tree's young leaves have a pleasant citrus fragrance. Sassafras is ideal for naturalizing in poor, rocky soils or damp locations.

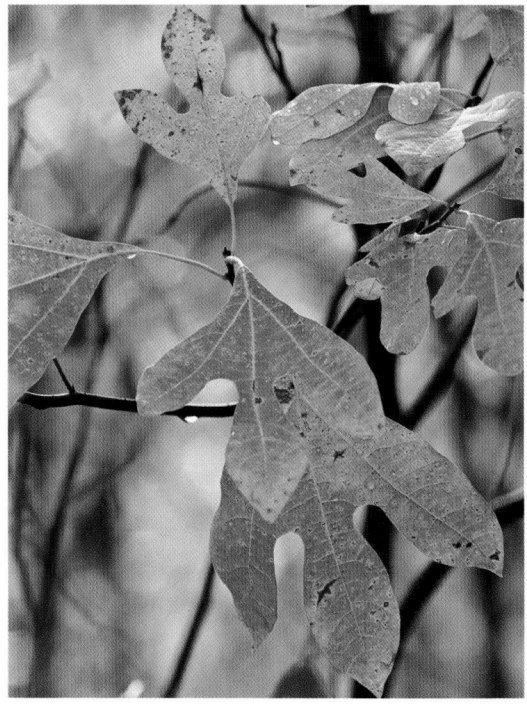

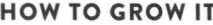

HOW TO GROW IT

Plant sassafras in moist, well-drained, acidic soil in full sun or partial shade. The trees have long taproots, and only the smallest trees transplant successfully. For commercial use, the roots are harvested in spring before the leaves appear or in autumn after the leaves have fallen. Propagate sassafras from root cuttings or suckers taken from mature trees.

Satureja hortensis

Native to the Mediterranean region, summer savory is naturalized in southwest Africa, Asia, and North America and is a popular garden plant in temperate and warm areas throughout the world. The plant is a small annual that has widely branched stems and bears whorls of white or pale pink flowers. Used as a food flavoring for more than 2,000 years, summer savory tastes like a cross between thyme and mint. The genus *Satureja*, which includes 30 species of annuals, perennials, and subshrubs, is so often included in pea and bean dishes that Germans call the herb *bohnenkraut*, which means "bean herb." Its genus name is derived from the Latin word *satyrus*, meaning "satyr," because summer savory is reputed to be the food plant that gave these mythical creatures their sexual powers.

CULINARY USE

Summer savory is milder in flavor than its perennial relative, winter savory (*Satureja montana*). In recipes, summer savory is a heavier substitute for mint and a lighter substitute for sage. It adds a piquant flavor to soups, meat and fish dishes, beans, eggs, and pâtés. It also complements tomato sauce, potatoes, eggplant, asparagus, squash, cabbage, and Brussels sprouts. Use the herb sparingly, though—a small amount goes a long way.

MEDICINAL USE

Like many culinary herbs, summer savory helps improve digestion and relieve intestinal gas. This is one reason it is so often added to bean dishes, which can cause this problem. It is also used in herbal medicine to treat nausea, colic, menstrual disorders, and to ease muscle spasms and alleviate lung congestion. Summer savory contains astrin-

gent and antibacterial properties, making it a useful remedy for diarrhea.

Caution: Summer savory should not be used in medicinal doses during pregnancy. Small amounts used in cooking do not pose a problem.

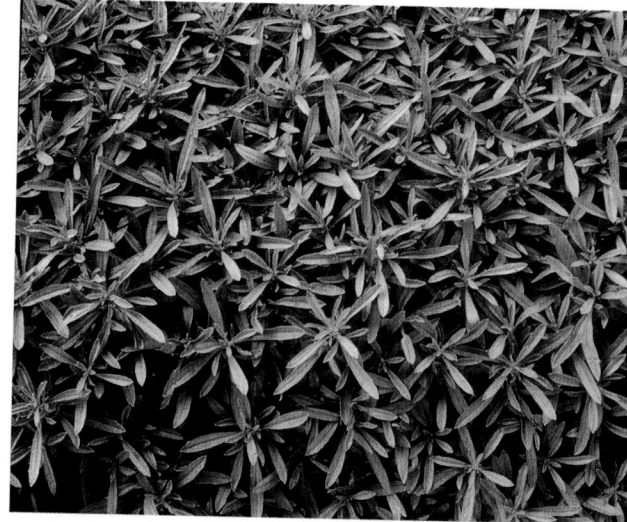

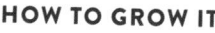 **HOW TO GROW IT**

Summer savory is easy to grow from seed sown in neutral to alkaline soil and full sun. Use only fresh seed, however—viability decreases quickly after the first year. Begin harvesting leaves when the plants are about 6 inches tall; snip often to prevent flowering and extend leafy growth. When flowering begins, cut the whole plants and dry them on a screen or piece of paper in a warm, shaded location. Strip the dried leaves from the stems, and store them in an airtight container.

Senna alexandrina

(= Cassia senna)

A member of the pea family, Alexandrian senna is native to Egypt and Sudan and is cultivated in the warm regions of the world, particularly India and Somalia. Used for centuries as a tea to treat constipation, Alexandrian senna now is an ingredient in many commercially prepared, over-the-counter laxatives. It has a very strong effect and is generally recommended for use only when other remedies—such as lifestyle and dietary changes, as well as more gentle laxatives—have not been effective.

MEDICINAL USE

Alexandrian senna has a long history of use as a laxative in both Eastern and Western herbalism. Arab physicians first wrote of the herb's bowel-stimulating effects in the 9th century, but it was probably used for centuries before that. The herb contains compounds called anthraquinones, which stimulate the colon. Most modern commercial products are made from the plant's leaflets or fruits, but some authorities say products made from the seedpods have a more gentle laxative effect than those made from the leaves. When digested, the herb provokes intestinal muscle contractions (peristalsis), thereby speeding the body's elimination of waste. It's often taken with carminative (gas-dispelling) herbs, such as ginger (*Zingiber officinale*), both to reduce intestinal cramping and to mask senna's bitter and unpleasant—even nauseating—taste. This plant has been well studied in clinical settings.

Caution: Alexandrian senna may cause intestinal discomfort and cramping. To reduce the risk of laxative dependency, the herb should not be used for more than 1 week unless directed by a healthcare provider. It should not be taken by women who are pregnant or nursing, by children younger than 10 years old, or by anyone suffering from chronic gastrointestinal conditions, such as colitis or ulcers.

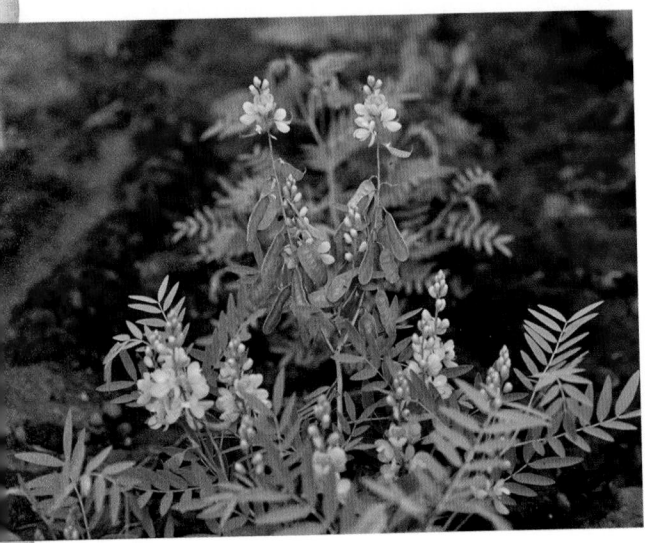

HOW TO GROW IT

Alexandrian senna grows in moist but well-drained soil in full sun. In Zone 9 and colder, grow this herb in a large container and move the plant indoors when temperatures drop below 45°F. Plant seeds in spring, when temperatures have warmed. Harvest the leaves in summer and the pods in autumn. Propagate the herb from seed or take cuttings in early summer.

Serenoa repens

This evergreen palm is the only species in its genus; its natural habitat includes pinelands, coastal dunes, and sand hills. Saw palmetto was named in honor of Sereno Watson (1826–1892), the American botanist who undertook many collection expeditions while a curator of the herbarium at Harvard University. Native Americans ate saw palmetto seeds as one of their staple foods and used the leaves for making medicine baskets. This species was first commercialized as a therapeutic medicine by Eli Lilly and Company in the early 1900s.

MEDICINAL USE

Once called "the old man's friend," saw palmetto has long been recommended as a treatment for enlarged prostate, and preparations of this fruit are now widely prescribed by health-care practitioners for the treatment of prostate conditions. Saw palmetto berries contain fatty acids and steroids, which help strengthen the male reproductive system, supporting healthy prostate and urinary function. The herb appears to inhibit the production of dihydrotestosterone (DHT), the compound that causes the multiplication of prostate cells, resulting in prostate enlargement. It also may relieve symptoms related to enlarged prostate, including trouble with urination. In addition, saw palmetto has

PLANT PROFILE

Common Names: Sabal Palm, Saw Palmetto

Description: Clumping evergreen palm, 6 to 12 feet tall; fan-shaped, sharply toothed leaves; tiny, fragrant flowers in dense clusters followed by small, blue-black fruits

Hardiness: To Zone 7

Family: Arecaceae

Flowering: Spring

Parts Used: Fruit

Range/Habitat: Native to southeastern United States; pinelands and coastal dunes

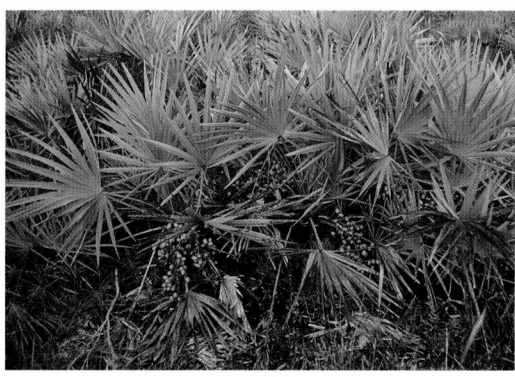

been used as a sleep aid and a treatment for cystitis, chronic bronchial coughs, and laryngitis.

 HOW TO GROW IT

Saw palmetto thrives in well-drained, moist soil in full sun or light shade. It does best with a minimum temperature of 50° to 55°F, but it can survive temperatures as low as 0°F. If given adequate light, saw palmetto can be grown as a houseplant.

FIELD NOTES

A Most Useful Palm

The Seminole Tribe of Florida has used the saw palmetto for many purposes, including construction, handicrafts, food, and medicine. My friend and colleague Bradley Bennett, PhD, who studied this species, noted that, "for humans, saw palmetto is one of Florida's most versatile plants, providing food, fiber, oil, medicine, wax, and roof thatch." He and his coworkers estimated that nearly 7 million kilograms of fruits are harvested annually in Florida to be processed into preparations for the treatment of enlarged prostate and other conditions. To date, 17 human clinical trials have shown that "the old man's friend" has value in contemporary medicine.—M. J. B.

Silybum marianum

European settlers carried milk thistle with them to North America. An annual or biennial native to the Mediterranean, the herb bears oblong, spiny, variegated leaves and purple flowers, followed by black seeds. The common name milk thistle comes from the milky sap that exudes from the plant's leaves, as well as its traditional use of stimulating milk flow in nursing mothers. The name St. Mary's thistle derives from a Biblical story. According to legend, Mary, mother of Jesus, was resting beneath a thistle plant while nursing the baby Jesus when a drop of her milk fell on the plant, producing the leaves' characteristic white markings.

CULINARY USE

Remove the prickly outside edges of young thistle leaves, then lightly steam the leaves and eat them as a spring vegetable. The seeds are high in antioxidants, protein, and healthy fat. To prepare the fresh seeds, soak them overnight, and then drain them. Use a mortar and pestle or spice mill to grind them into a powder, and sprinkle it on cereal or add it to smoothies. You can also lightly roast the seeds, grind them, and then brew them with water (like coffee) to make a hot beverage. Store whole seeds in your freezer for future use.

MEDICINAL USE

For more than 2,000 years, people have used milk thistle to treat liver conditions such as hepatitis, cirrhosis, and drug-induced damage. The seeds contain silymarin, a complex of flavonoid compounds that are powerful antioxidants that reduce inflammation. Herbalists value standardized milk thistle products for their ability to protect the liver from damage by environmental toxins, medications, and alcohol. More recent studies suggest that the extract

may also protect the kidneys in a similar way.

Herbal practitioners also believe that milk thistle can help the liver repair damaged cells and generate new ones. In Europe, milk thistle extract is used along with standard medical interventions to treat poisoning from mushrooms in the genus *Amanita*, a deadly group of fungi.

Milk thistle has been used to treat poor digestion, female hormone imbalance, constipation, mood disorders, hemorrhoids, varicose veins, atherosclerosis, and skin conditions including psoriasis and acne. Milk thistle seeds are high in protein and linoleic acid, a healthy fat that might help balance the menstrual cycle and improve cardiovascular health.

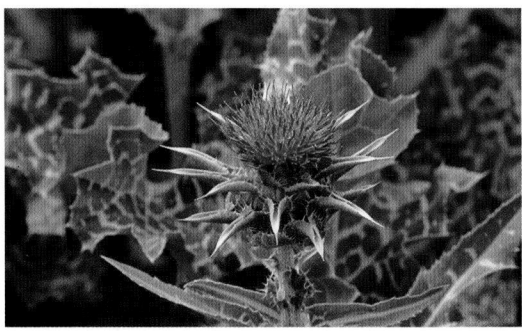

HOW TO GROW IT

Considered an invasive (and in some states "noxious") weed, milk thistle self-seeds readily and is not recommended for the garden. To harvest wild milk thistle, look for the plants in dry, stony soil in fields or ditches. (Be sure the plants have not been treated with an herbicide.) Cut off the seed head after it has dried, remove the seeds, and then remove the hairlike fringe from the seeds.

Solidago spp.

There are more than 100 species of goldenrod, a fast-growing perennial with yellow flowers, found throughout North and South America, Europe, northern Africa, and some parts of Asia. This late summer–blooming plant is often unfairly blamed for causing "hay fever" because it flowers at the same time, and often in the same locations, as the truly allergenic ragweed.

Traditionally associated with wound healing, goldenrod's genus name, *Solidago*, derives from the Latin *solida*, meaning "whole," and *ago*, meaning "to make." Native Americans are reported to have used nearly two dozen different *Solidago* species for a variety of conditions, ranging from external applications as a hair rinse and a wash for burns, sores, and boils, to internal use to treat diarrhea, fevers, and sore throat. Because of its pleasant smell and aniselike taste, goldenrod tea was once used to disguise the unpleasant flavors of other ingredients—an early herbal equivalent to sugar coating on a pill.

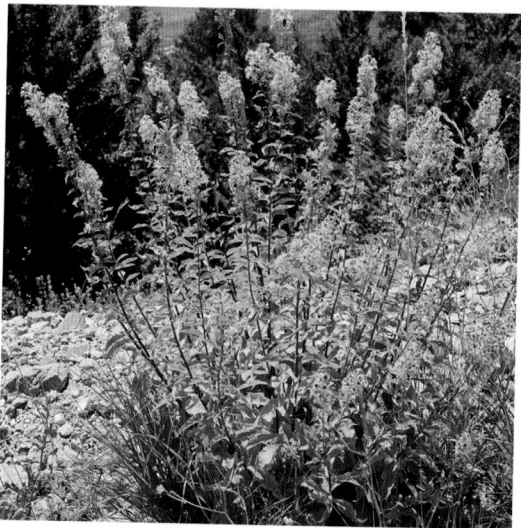

PLANT PROFILE

Common Name: Goldenrod

Description: Perennial, 3 to 7 feet tall, with showy yellow flower spikes and simple, alternate leaves; woody stems seldom branch

Hardiness: To Zone 4

Family: Asteraceae

Flowering: Late summer

Parts Used: Flowers and leaves

Range/Habitat: Native to North and South America, Europe, and Asia; found in open fields and along roadsides

MEDICINAL USE

Three species in particular, *Solidago nemoralis* (gray goldenrod), *S. odora* (sweet goldenrod), and *S. virgaurea* (European goldenrod), have been used as astringents, diuretics, and diaphoretics (sweat inducers). A tea made from the flowers of sweet goldenrod has been used to treat urinary obstructions, while goldenrod leaf tea has been used for flatulence and vomiting. European goldenrod has been administered for gum disease, arthritis, and kidney inflammation, as well as for wounds and skin conditions such as eczema, sores, and insect bites. In traditional Chinese medicine, European goldenrod is prepared as a headache remedy and for treating flu, sore throat, malaria, and measles.

ORNAMENTAL USE

Several horticultural varieties have been developed with larger flower heads and a more compact form. These dwarf varieties add bright color to ornamental borders in late summer.

OTHER USES

The flower heads dry to a nice golden color that looks lovely in everlasting herb and flower arrangements. Goldenrod blooms can also be used to make a yellow dye.

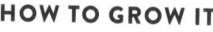

HOW TO GROW IT

Goldenrod species, as well as named cultivars, are sold as plants or seeds. If you aren't able to find the herb at a retail garden center, check mail-order suppliers that sell native plants. Don't bother to enrich the soil—goldenrod thrives in average to poor soil and full sun. Harvest goldenrod when it is in full bloom, cutting the top third of the plants. Hang bunches of two or three stems upside down to dry in a warm, airy location.

Stachys officinalis

A member of the family that includes the mints (*Mentha* spp.), wood betony is native to Europe and naturalized in many parts of the world. This soft-textured plant bears stiff, slightly hairy pointed leaves and lavender-pink flowers arranged in whorls on top of the spikes. Its genus name, *Stachys,* is Greek for "spike." Once known as woundwort, betony was traditionally applied to stop the bleeding of wounds, draw out splinters, and drain boils. The herb's healing powers were esteemed by the ancient Greeks, Romans, and Anglo-Saxons. Antonius Musa, the physician to the Roman emperor Augustus (ca. 63 BCE–14 CE), listed 47 diseases treatable with wood betony. The common name "betony" is said to derive from the ancient Celtic words for "good head," a reference to the herb's early use as a treatment for headaches.

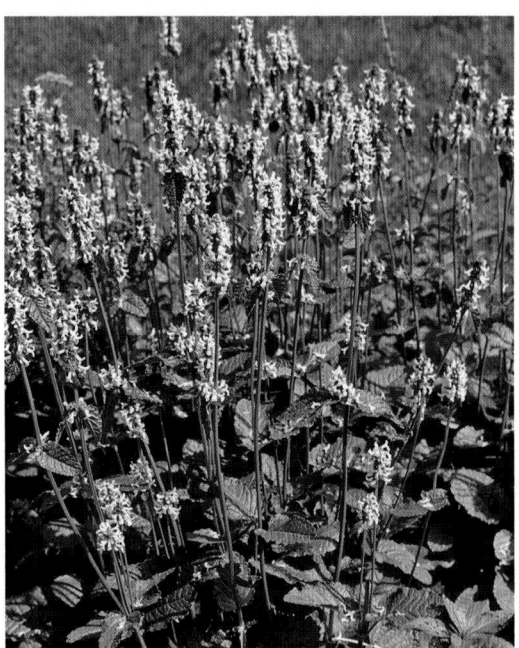

CULINARY USE

Wood betony has a refreshing, astringent flavor. Although it is not usually used in cooking, the leaves can be a pleasant-tasting substitute for black tea (*Camellia sinensis*).

MEDICINAL USE

Wood betony leaves contain the alkaloid betonicine, which has the ability to reduce inflammation and is used to strengthen the nervous system and treat nerve pain. Wood betony also has sedative properties and has long been used to treat headaches, particularly those due to tension and anxiety. The herb's astringent and antiseptic tannins account for its early use to staunch wounds and for digestive conditions. Once considered a cure-all, wood betony is not widely used for healing today.

Caution: Do not use wood betony if you are pregnant.

ORNAMENTAL USE

The lavender bloom spikes of wood betony are attractive in mixed flower borders, cottage gardens, and woodland plantings, as well as in cut flower arrangements. Shorter varieties are also suited to rock gardens. The plants are drought tolerant and deer resistant.

HOW TO GROW IT

Found in meadows and open woodlands, wood betony prefers a well-drained, dry, neutral to acidic soil in full sun or partial shade. Plant seeds in spring or fall; root divisions can be planted when the herb is dormant. Harvest the flowering plants in summer.

Stellaria media

Native to southern Europe and a member of the family that includes garden pinks (*Dianthus* spp.), chickweed now grows throughout the world as a common weed. A hardy, low-growing, spreading annual, chickweed often overwinters, meaning that it does not completely die back during the winter months. It bears oval leaves and small, white, star-shaped flowers. The genus *Stellaria* takes its name from the Latin word *stella*, meaning "star," a reference to the shape of the species' flowers. Chickweed has been a popular healing herb for centuries. In many countries, it was also used as a food for birds and domestic fowl.

CULINARY USE

Fresh chickweed leaves, harvested in early spring, taste like spinach and are a nutritious addition to salads, soups, or stews. Cook the delicate leaves for no more than 5 minutes.

MEDICINAL USE

Although chickweed has been used medicinally in the past, there has been very little research conducted on the herb. Chickweed leaves have been applied externally as a juice, ointment, or poultice to treat irritated skin, eczema, psoriasis, ulcers, and boils. The leaves contain steroid saponins, which may help soothe rashes and relieve itching. Native Americans used a chickweed leaf decoction to treat sore eyes. In homeopathy, it is used in minute amounts to treat psoriasis and rheumatic pain. Chickweed has also been used as a digestive aid. The root of a related species is used in Chinese medicine to treat fevers.

Caution: Do not use chickweed if you are pregnant. Excessive amounts of the herb may cause vomiting and diarrhea.

PLANT PROFILE

Common Names: Chickweed

Description: Spreading annual forms mats 4 to 8 inches tall, 16 inches across; small, oval, opposite leaves; white, star-shaped flowers with five clefted petals

Hardiness: Annual

Family: Caryophyllaceae

Flowering: Spring through fall

Parts Used: Leaves

Range/Habitat: Native to southern Europe, naturalized in temperate climates worldwide

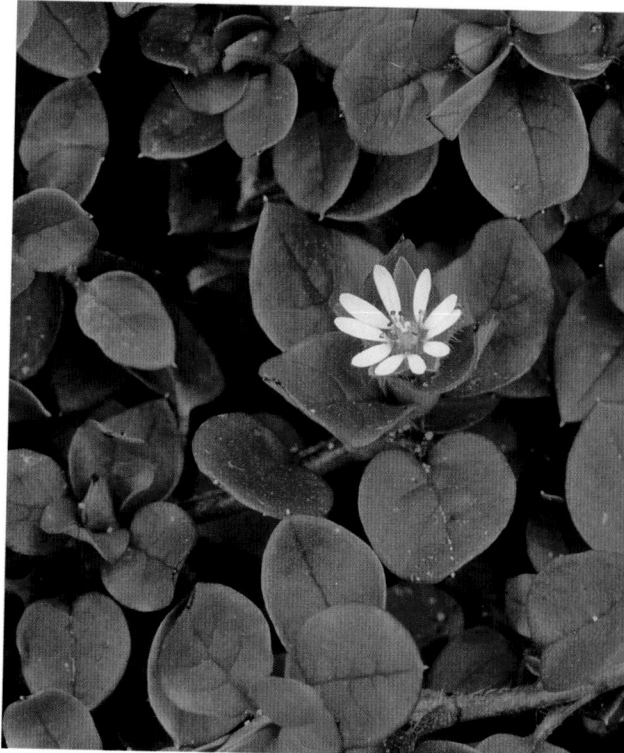

 HOW TO GROW IT

Considered an invasive weed in some states, chickweed is not recommended for the garden. Look for wild plants growing in moist soil in sun or partial shade. For culinary use, harvest the leaves of untreated plants in early spring. For medicinal use, harvest the leaves as needed.

Stevia rebaudiana

This low-growing bushy perennial bears dark green, serrated leaves that are intensely sweet. In recent years, stevia has grown in popularity as a healthful sugar substitute; it's sold in leaf, liquid, and powdered forms. Stevia extracts are said to be 200 to 300 times sweeter than granulated sugar, but with no calories and apparently none of sugar's negative side effects, such as causing tooth decay. The plant has been used commercially in various parts of the world for more than 3 decades. It is especially popular in Japan, where it is used to sweeten many products, including soft drinks, chewing gum, and pickles. In Paraguay, where this species grows wild, stevia leaf has been used for centuries to sweeten the herbal beverage maté. The sweetness in this plant comes from compounds known as steviol glycosides, initially identified in 1931. The first commercial use of these compounds took place in Japan, in 1971, in response to concerns over the possible toxicity of other artificial sweetener products in use at that time. Crystals of stevia extract are produced by drying the plants and processing them in water to collect the steviol glycosides, then treating the extract with alcohol, causing the glycosides to crystallize.

CULINARY USE

Intensely sweet, stevia can be used as a healthful substitute for sugar and artificial sweeteners. It has a mild, aniselike aftertaste that most people enjoy. Powdered commercial products that contain crystallized leaf extracts are available for use in baking and for sweetening beverages. Because they are, by weight, so much sweeter than cane or beet sugar, use them sparingly; depending on the product, 1 to 4 teaspoons of stevia extract equals the sweetness of 1 cup of sugar. Stevia will not brown or caramelize the way sugar does when heated, so it cannot be substituted in certain desserts.

MEDICINAL USE

Although stevia's principal value is as a noncaloric natural sweetener, it could benefit people with hypertension or type 2 diabetes, as well. The plant contains rebaudioside and stevioside, glycosides responsible for its sweet flavor. A clinical study published in 2003 showed that patients with mild hypertension taking a capsule of stevioside powder over a 2-year period had significantly lower systolic and diastolic blood pressure and no adverse effects. A small-scale human clinical trial also supported stevia's effectiveness for lowering blood sugar in type 2 diabetics, a traditional use for the plant. Stevia has also been used traditionally as a contraceptive in Paraguay.

Caution: Because of limited data showing that stevia may prevent conception, the herb should not be used by pregnant women or by those trying to conceive.

> **PLANT PROFILE**
>
> **Common Names:** Stevia, Sweetleaf
>
> **Description:** Small perennial, 1 to 3 feet tall; hairy stems with opposite, serrated, dark green leaves; white, tubular flowers
>
> **Hardiness:** To Zone 11
>
> **Family:** Asteraceae
>
> **Flowering:** Mature plants bloom constantly
>
> **Parts Used:** Leaves
>
> **Range/Habitat:** Native to subtropical highlands of Paraguay and Brazil

HOW TO GROW IT

Grow stevia in full sun and well-drained soil. It will not survive freezing temperatures, but it is easy to grow in a 10- or 12-inch pot filled with a lightweight growing mix. The potted plant can be kept outdoors when temperatures are above 50°F and there is no danger of frost. Stevia is difficult to grow from seed, so start with young, nursery-grown plants (available from several mail-order suppliers). Water lightly but often during the summer; a thin mulch of compost will help keep the plant's shallow feeder roots from drying out. During the growing season, feed plants with a slow-release, low-nitrogen organic fertilizer. Harvest the leaves in fall, when shorter days and cooler temperatures have intensified their sweetness. Dry the leaves on a screen in full sun for about 12 hours, then crush them by hand or with a coffee grinder and store them in an airtight container. Stevia can be propagated by root division or cuttings.

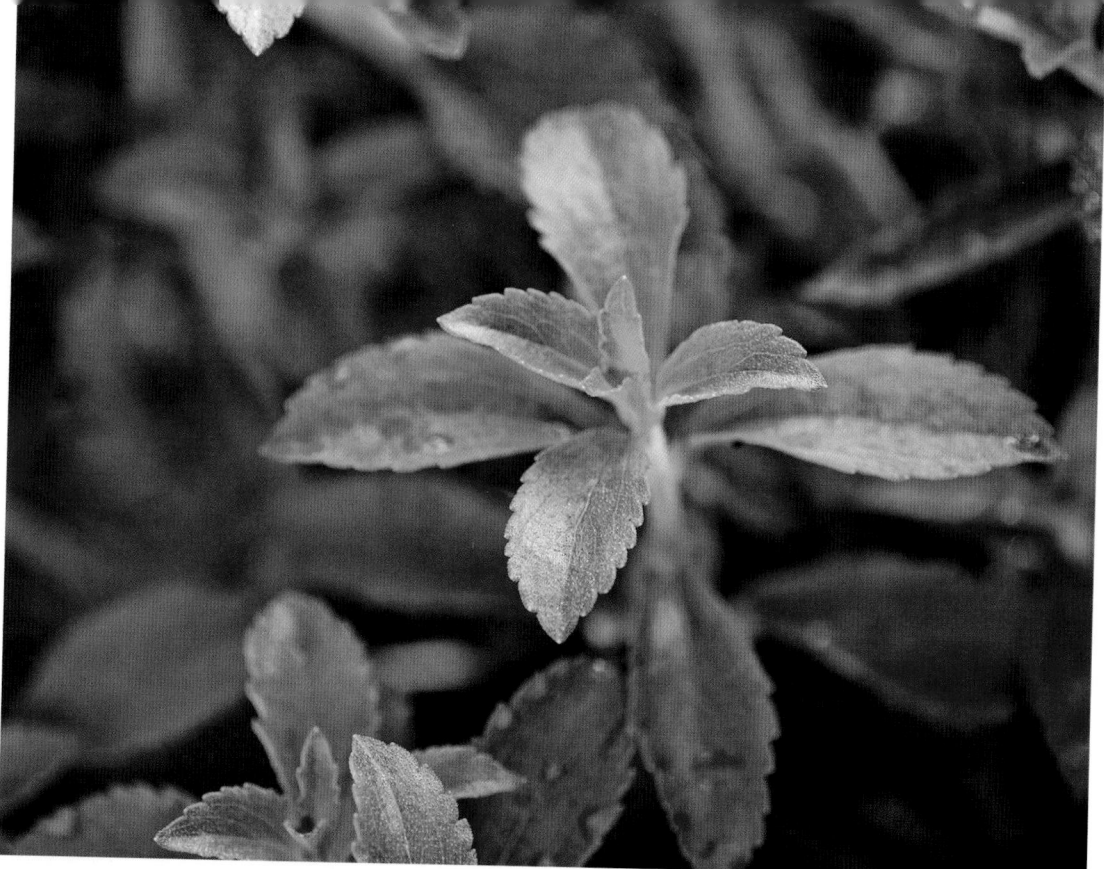

Searching for Sweetness

In the early 1980s, plant explorer D. D. Soejarto, a student of Professor Richard Evans Schultes and my classmate, investigated native Stevia populations in Paraguay, Peru, Colombia, and Mexico. During a period of 3 months, he and his team collected more than 30 species in this genus. Each time he collected a plant, he tasted the fresh leaves, noting their taste and degree of sweetness. He also gathered information from people in each area, recording the traditional uses of these species. In Paraguay, a root decoction of Stevia balansae is used to treat diarrhea; in Peru, the whole plant of S. macbridei is made into a decoction and used for a bath for women; in Mexico, the leaves and stems of S. salicifolia are treated with water and used as a rub for people with joint problems. Carefully gathering data, Soejarto and his colleagues reported in the Journal of Economic Botany that S. rebaudiana, the commercial source of stevia sweetener, was the only member of this genus that had sweetening properties. He also warned that the species' genetic diversity was being diminished by the destruction of native habitats for farming, logging, and other uses.

Tragically, this story is being repeated around the world with many species—wild populations of plants critical to our future are being destroyed for short-sighted and unsustainable resource extraction. Their genetic diversity could someday help plant breeders create varieties more tolerant of warming, drought, floods, and other challenges posed by global change.—M. J. B.

Symphytum officinale

Comfrey is a stout, vigorous perennial plant that bears large, tapered, prickly leaves and purple, pink, blue, or white bell-shaped flowers. It has been used as a medicinal plant since ancient times, and its botanical name refers to the plant's traditional use to repair broken bones: *Symphytum* is from the Greek *symphytos,* which means "to unite." "Comfrey" comes from the Latin *con firma,* meaning "with strength." Women whose virginity was in doubt were once encouraged to bathe before marriage in water infused with comfrey. The herb was believed to repair a woman's hymen, and in some places it is still used for this purpose, considered to be able to repair tears in the vagina. Although the leaves were at one time added to soups, stews, and salads, this use is no longer recommended due to the plant's toxicity.

MEDICINAL USE

Comfrey root and leaves contain allantoin, a chemical that promotes cell proliferation and may contribute to the healing properties of the plant. The herb has been used to heal burns and insect stings, as well as broken bones, strains, and sprains. A paste of the root, spread on cloth, will stiffen into a cast. A compress of comfrey tea, applied immediately after a sprain, may help reduce the sprain's severity. Comfrey is a common ingredient in herbal ointments and salves. A synthesized form of comfrey is used in pharmaceutical hemorrhoid preparations.

Caution: Comfrey contains pyrrolizidine alkaloids, which may cause liver damage and are considered toxic. Comfrey leaves should not be used internally, except under the advice of a qualified medical professional. Comfrey root preparations should not be used internally under any circumstances, nor should they be applied to broken skin.

The herb should not be used in any form by pregnant or nursing women. Poisonings have occurred when people have collected the highly toxic foxglove (*Digitalis purpurea*), mistaking it for comfrey.

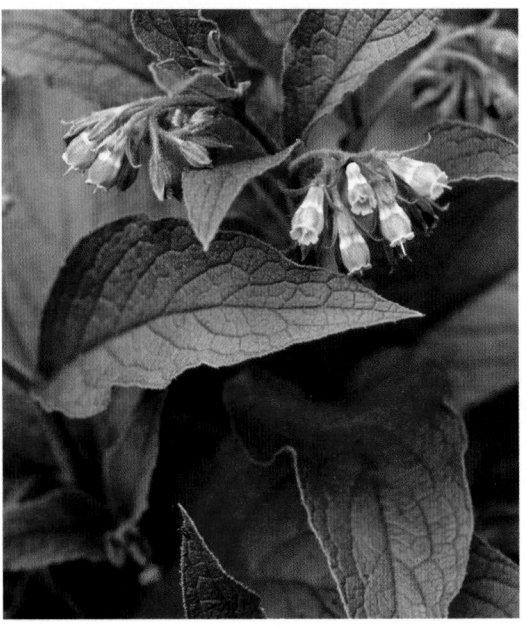

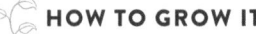

HOW TO GROW IT

Comfrey grows wild in marshy areas, meadows, and ditches, but it will thrive in any good garden soil in sun or partial shade. The plant can be invasive. To keep it contained, many gardeners plant it in a submerged pot with drainage holes. Plant seeds or root divisions in spring or fall. Harvest leaves in summer; lift the roots in fall.

Syzygium aromaticum

A highly aromatic evergreen, the clove tree grows up to 35 feet tall in tropical southeastern Asia, where it is native. The dried, unopened flower buds are commonly used in cooking. Clove buds also yield a pale yellow essential oil used in dental products, soaps, creams, lotions, and insect repellents. It's said that in China, during the Han Dynasty, subjects who addressed the emperor were made to hold cloves in their mouths as a breath freshener.

CULINARY USE

Clove buds are a distinctive spice, commonly used whole or in powdered form as an ingredient in curries, pies (particularly pumpkin pie), pickles, tea blends, and mulled wine and cider. The sharp, strong flavor complements beets, carrots, squash, fruit dishes, and desserts.

MEDICINAL USE

Clove oil contains a high concentration of eugenol, which has pain-relieving and mildly antiseptic properties (but can be toxic to the liver if used in large amounts). The oil is an ingredient in liniments used to relieve muscle and arthritic pain. It's also used to alleviate toothache and is included in dental cements, fillings, and other preparations. Because of eugenol's antiseptic properties, clove has the potential to fight bacteria, viruses, and fungi, such as *Staphylococcus aureus* and *Candida albicans*. Clove oil is also thought to have carminative (gas-relieving) activity and is used to treat stomachache and flatulent colic. In aromatherapy, clove oil is used to reduce drowsiness and alleviate the pain of headaches.

To treat a toothache, stomach discomfort, or indigestion at home, make a soothing infusion by steeping cloves in hot water for 10 minutes. Clove oil can also be applied to cotton and used to alleviate toothache by pressing it against the affected site.

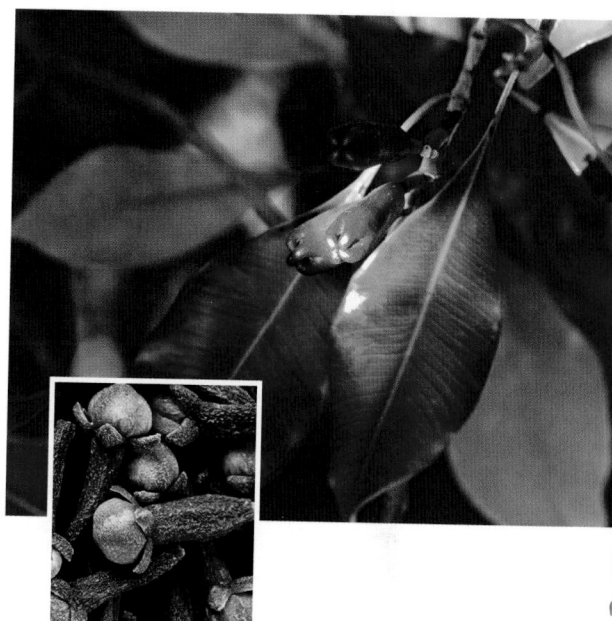

HOW TO GROW IT

Clove trees thrive in humid, tropical conditions with well-drained, fertile soil and full sun or partial shade. In Zone 9 and colder, grow your clove tree in a heated greenhouse. Be sure the growing medium includes compost or other organic matter to ensure good drainage, and protect the young plants from direct sun. Provide 1 inch of water per week to keep the soil consistently moist, and mist frequently. Feed in spring and early summer with a slow-release organic fertilizer. Commercial growers harvest the flower buds when the lower parts of the flowers turn purple. They are then sun dried until they are a deep reddish brown.

Tanacetum balsamita

(= *Chrysanthemum balsamita*)

(= *Balsamita vulgaris*)

The genus *Tanacetum* is named for the Greek *athanasia*, meaning "immortality"—a reference to the plants' long-lasting flowers. Costmary, a 3-foot-tall perennial, bears clusters of yellow, daisylike blooms in late summer. It was once known as Bible-leaf because early American settlers used its long, balsam-scented leaves as bookmarks. Legend has it that this bookmark served double duty on Sunday mornings. If a person had difficulty staying awake during a sermon, they simply had to scratch the dried leaf or chew a bit of it and the invigorating scent revived them—at least temporarily! A native of Europe and Asia, costmary was introduced to England in the 16th century, and it quickly became a widely cultivated and popular garden plant. Today, it's rarely seen in herb gardens; you're more likely to find it in an old family Bible, marking a page for later reference.

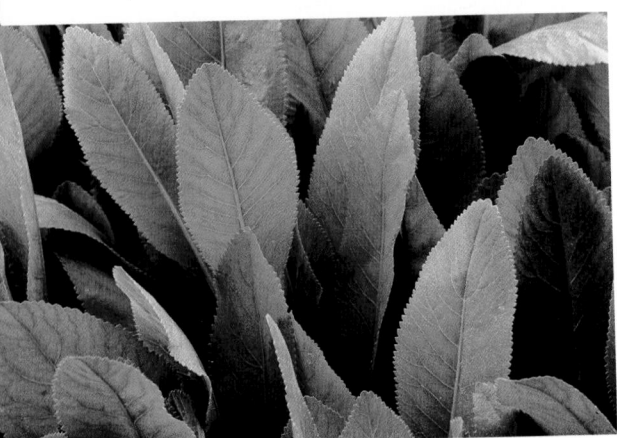

CULINARY USE

Costmary's tender leaves have a refreshing, minty flavor that complements iced tea, lemonade, iced soups, and fruit salads. Also try adding the minced leaves to tuna, egg, or shrimp salads. Steep fresh or dried costmary leaves to make a hot tea.

MEDICINAL USE

In 17th- and 18th-century Europe, costmary was widely used as a diuretic, gentle laxative, and remedy for acute fever. Today, the leaves are used externally to treat wounds, burns, and bee stings. Its properties are thought to be similar to those of its botanical relative, tansy (*Tanacetum vulgare*).

ORNAMENTAL USE

Costmary's appealing yellow blooms attract butterflies. Plant groups of three or five plants at the back of a perennial border or in a cottage garden.

OTHER USES

The herb's astringent and antiseptic qualities are soothing to the skin. Use an infusion of the leaves as a facial toner, or add it to bathwater. The balsam-like fragrance of the leaves is pleasant in potpourris and sachets, too.

 HOW TO GROW IT

Costmary grows best in a site with well-drained loam and full sun. Plant it in spring, spacing the plants about 2 feet apart. Costmary spreads easily and requires division every few years. Harvest a few leaves at a time throughout the growing season; most of this herb's leaves grow from the base of the plant. To preserve the leaves, dry them at a temperature of about 100°F, then store them in an airtight container in a cool, dark location.

Tanacetum parthenium

Feverfew's common English name refers to its earliest use to treat fevers, along with headaches. The ancient Greek physician Dioscorides (ca. 40–90 CE) valued the herb for its effect on the uterus. It was often used in childbirth to help with the delivery of the afterbirth, if contractions were not regular. In more recent times, it has been taken as a tonic, and a Cuban variety has been used as an ingredient in confectionaries and wines, as an aromatic to ward off disease, and as an insect repellent.

CULINARY USE

Feverfew has an extremely bitter taste. In Italy, it is sometimes used as a seasoning (in small amounts) to stimulate the appetite.

MEDICINAL USE

Feverfew has long been used to treat fevers and headaches. In the 1970s, it was discovered that consuming the fresh leaves could ward off migraines along with the nausea, vomiting, and sensitivity to light that accompany them. This discovery, made by a Welsh physician's wife, spawned a great deal of clinical research on the bioactivity and clinical efficacy of this plant. The herb contains the compound parthenolide, a sesquiterpene lactone that inhibits the release of prostaglandins and histamine, preventing the blood vessel spasms in the head that cause migraine attacks. For best effect, the herb, often in pill form, is taken regularly and at the onset of a migraine. Feverfew also has antispasmodic activity, making it useful in the treatment of indigestion and menstrual problems such as cramps and amenorrhea. Feverfew leaves can be applied externally to soothe the pain and itching of insect bites.

Caution: Feverfew should not be used during pregnancy. Those who take blood-thinning medications should consult with their health-care pro-

PLANT PROFILE

Common Name: Feverfew

Description: Vigorous, hardy biennial or perennial, 2 to 3 feet tall; small, white, daisylike flowers in tight, flat-topped clusters; strongly scented alternate leaves up to 4 inches long

Hardiness: To Zone 6

Family: Asteraceae

Flowering: Midsummer to late summer

Parts Used: Flowers and leaves

Range/Habitat: Native to Europe, naturalized in temperate regions, including North America

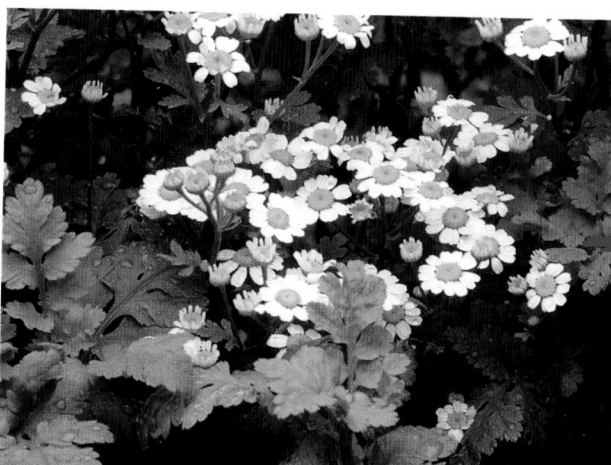

vider before using this herb. Some people are allergic to feverfew and other members of this plant family.

ORNAMENTAL USE

The herb has many outstanding cultivars. Plant low-growing varieties as annuals in rock gardens, window boxes, or containers for summer and fall blooming.

OTHER USES

The pulverized flowers can be used to make an insect repellent spray or dust.

HOW TO GROW IT

Feverfew grows in well-drained, dry soil in full sun or partial shade. Plant seeds or root divisions in spring or fall. Deadhead the flowers to prevent self-seeding. Harvest leaves and flowers as needed throughout the growing season.

Tanacetum vulgare

Like its cousin, feverfew, tansy is native to Europe and naturalized throughout North America. According to Greek mythology, the plant gave immortality to Ganymede, the cup-bearer of the gods. Both its common and genus names come from the Greek word for immortality, *athanasia*. Because of its strong odor, tansy is a natural insect repellent. In the Middle Ages, dried tansy was strewn on floors, hung from rafters, and packed between bed sheets and mattresses to discourage lice, flies, and other vermin from attacking people as they slept. It has also been used in embalming, packed in coffins, and wrapped in funereal garments to keep away insects, as well as rubbed on meats as a preservative.

MEDICINAL USE

In the past, tansy was used to relieve indigestion, rid the body of intestinal worms, and induce abortion; however, the plant contains varying levels of toxic thujone, a compound also found in wormwood and used to make absinthe.

Caution: Even in small amounts, tansy is highly poisonous and not recommended for medicinal use.

ORNAMENTAL USE

Tansy's lush foliage and golden, buttonlike blooms add interest to garden beds and everlasting arrangements. Try fernleaf tansy (*Tanacetum vulgare* 'Crispum')—a shorter form with more delicate foliage—in a container or along a pathway, where passersby will brush against the leaves to release their fragrance.

OTHER USES

As a dye, the young leaves and flowering tops produce yellows and greens in wool. Tansy was also

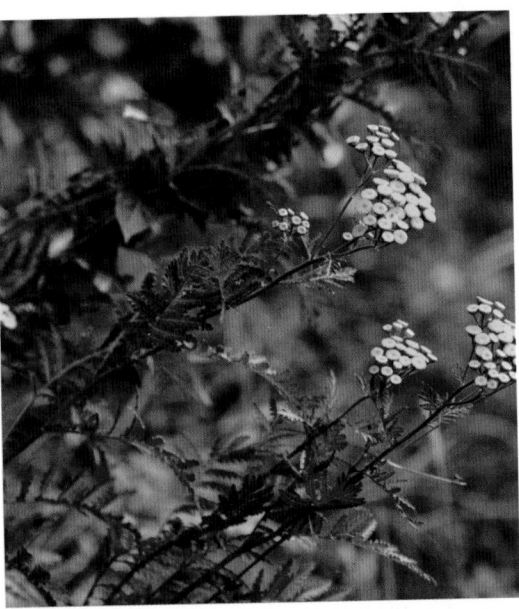

traditionally used as an insect repellent, although modern housekeepers and gardeners report mixed results. Consider experimenting with the old-time practices of planting tansy near a doorway to deter flies, or tucking sprigs into kitchen cabinets to repel ants.

PLANT PROFILE

Common Name: Tansy

Description: Vigorous perennial, up to 4 feet tall; spreads by underground rhizomes; dark green, fernlike foliage; loose clusters of yellow flower heads, ⅓ to ½ inch across

Hardiness: To Zone 4

Family: Asteraceae

Flowering: Midsummer to late summer

Parts Used: Leaves and flowers

Range/Habitat: Native to Europe, naturalized throughout North America; found along roadsides

---

HOW TO GROW IT

Considered a weedy plant, tansy is extremely easy to grow and can become invasive if not contained. If you wish to grow it in a border or garden bed, plant it in a pot with drainage holes, and sink the pot into the ground. Plant tansy in spring or fall in average soil and full sun to partial shade. Harvest the leaves and flowering stems as needed throughout the growing season.

Taraxacum officinale

PLANT PROFILE

Common Names: Dandelion, Lion's Tooth

Description: Herbaceous perennial, up to 18 inches tall; dark green leaves with toothed margins grow in rosettes close to the ground; golden yellow flower heads open in the daylight

Hardiness: To Zone 3

Family: Asteraceae

Flowering: Late spring

Parts Used: Entire plant

Range/Habitat: Native to Europe and Asia, naturalized throughout temperate regions of the world; lawns, fields, and roadsides

This seemingly ubiquitous perennial, with its characteristic thick taproot, is both a stubbornly pervasive weed and a useful medicinal and culinary plant. Dandelion bears toothed leaves, a single bright yellow flower that opens with the morning sun and closes in the evening, and ribbed fruits with fine white hairs. The name "dandelion" comes from the Latin *dens leonis,* which means "lion's teeth," in reference to the plant's toothed leaves. The French name *pissenlit* ("wet the bed") refers to the plant's potent diuretic effects. Its medicinal use was recorded in the 10th-century medical journals of Arabian physicians. By the 16th century, British apothecaries considered dandelion a valuable drug and referred to it as Herba Taraxacon or Herba Urinaria, for its diuretic effect. By the 19th century, dandelion had become a valuable potherb in Europe and America. Native to Europe and Asia, dandelion is grown commercially in North America and Europe, especially in France.

CULINARY USE

Young dandelion leaves are a tasty green vegetable, rich in antioxidant carotenoids, potassium, and vitamins A, B, C, and D. The slightly bitter-tasting

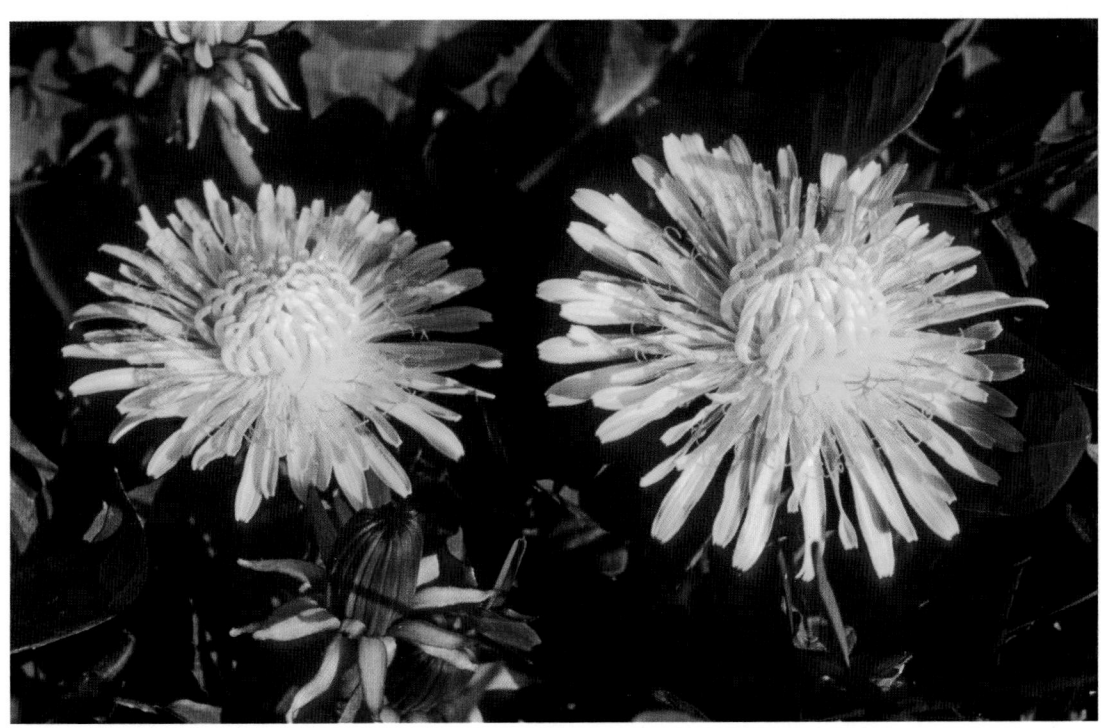

When Is a Plant a Weed?

It was Ralph Waldo Emerson who asserted that a weed is "a plant whose virtues have never been discovered." Growing up in the Northeast, I was trained to consider dandelions weeds—their brilliant yellow spring blossoms exploding into seeds, quickly spread by the wind to the four corners of the yard, producing hundreds more of these plants each year. We pulled them out of the ground and we poured herbicides on them—mostly to no avail. It was not until I began to study ethnobotany in Belize that I realized how useful this plant actually was. One of the traditional healers I worked with, the late Mr. Percival Reynolds, had an herb garden where he carefully tended the remedies his patients needed. All were species that could survive the hot, humid environment of the tropics.

One day he told me his dream was to grow dandelions and use them to treat his patients, particularly people with urinary problems. While dandelions grew quite abundantly around my home garden up North, I never brought him any viable seeds as I didn't want to introduce what to me was an invasive weed. Actually, we both were correct in our perceptions of dandelion—a weed to some, a food to others, and to healers, a remedy.—M. J. B.

---

leaves can be added to salads or cooked like spinach. Dandelion flowers can be minced and added to butters or herbal vinegars for color, or they can be used to make wine. The roots of the plant can be roasted, ground, and used as a coffee substitute.

MEDICINAL USE

Dandelion has powerful diuretic effects. Unlike conventional diuretics, which deplete the body of potassium, this herb is a good source of potassium, leaving the body with a net gain of the mineral after the herb is taken. As a result, there is less chance of a problem from electrolyte imbalance, compared to pharmaceutical diuretics. Dandelion root is believed to increase the body's flow of bile, which helps digest fats and may help prevent gallstones. The herb has been used to detoxify the liver, gallbladder, and kidneys, and it is often taken to treat skin conditions such as acne, eczema, and psoriasis. Dandelion root has mild laxative effects and moderate anti-inflammatory properties. It has traditionally been used to treat joint pain and stiffness.

Caution: Dandelion should not be taken by people who have gallstones or bile duct obstruction.

OTHER USES

Dandelion is reported to be a tonic herb externally, as well as internally. Use the leaves in herbal baths and facial steams. Dandelion flowers can be used to make yellow dyes for wool; using the whole plant produces a magenta dye.

HOW TO GROW IT

Dandelion, a very easy-to-grow plant, prefers moist to dry, neutral to alkaline soil in full sun. For cooking and healing, you can dig up "weedy" dandelions from your lawn or another location that hasn't been treated with herbicides. Or you can plant a dandelion variety specifically developed for the garden. Horticultural strains are available with longer leaves and a milder flavor. Plant the seeds in spring, summer, or fall, and thin seedlings to 6 inches apart. Deadhead the plants to prevent excessive spreading. For culinary use, harvest very young leaves.

Teucrium chamaedrys

PLANT PROFILE

Common Names: Germander, Wall Germander

Description: Slender herbaceous perennial, up to 18 inches tall; opposite, oval, bright green leaves with serrated edges; rose to purple blooms on small stalks in groups of two or three or in whorls of six or more

Hardiness: To Zone 5

Family: Lamiaceae

Flowering: Midsummer to late summer

Parts Used: Ornamental

Range/Habitat: Native to Europe, naturalized in North America and Europe

Germander was once known as "poor man's box" because the plant could be substituted for the more expensive boxwood in gardens. Its glossy, dark green foliage can be clipped to form a miniature hedge, such as those that edge Elizabethan knot gardens.

MEDICINAL USE

In earlier times, germander was also used to treat gout, and Dioscorides (ca. 40–90 CE) recommended it for the treatment of coughs and asthma. Herbalists also once recommended this plant for gallbladder conditions, fever, stomachache, and diarrhea. Some people have used it as a mouthwash to help kill germs and freshen breath. In the early 1990s wall germander, alone and mixed with other plants, was sold as a weight-loss product in Europe and caused several dozen cases of toxicity, including one fatality. *Caution:* Germander is no longer recommended for medicinal use due to significant safety concerns including possible liver toxicity and even death. The United States still allows small quantities of the herb to be used as a flavoring in alcoholic beverages.

ORNAMENTAL USE

Compact in form and drought tolerant, germander is an ideal edging for pathways and borders. Try it also in the crevices of a rock wall, allowing the stems to cascade downward, as the plant's common name suggests. Several cultivated forms have been developed, including a compact variety that grows to only 5 inches tall. With glossy, dark green leaves and long-lasting, lavender flowers, it makes an excellent groundcover, low edging, or rock garden plant. However, if growing it in your garden, remember that it is a toxic species.

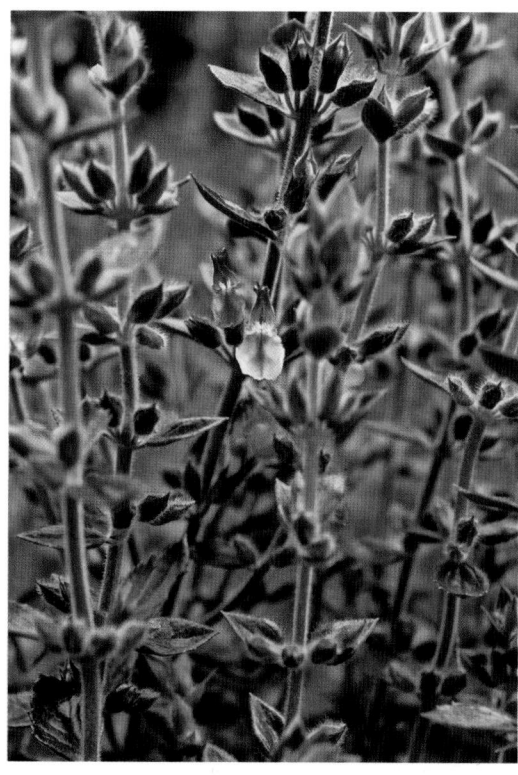

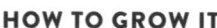

HOW TO GROW IT

Germander thrives in full sun and a well-drained, slightly acidic soil; its ideal growing medium consists of peat, sand, and organic matter. Seeds can take up to 1 month to germinate. For a faster start, buy young plants or use cuttings. Space established plants 1 foot apart. To create a formal edging, clip the plants in spring to encourage branching.

Theobroma cacao

The genus *Theobroma*, which translates to "food of the gods," includes *T. cacao*—the source of our beloved chocolate. Native to lowland tropical forests in Central and South America, cacao is a small evergreen tree that bears long, thin leaves and small yellow flowers formed directly on the plant's stems. The flowers develop into small, football-shape seedpods that contain the valuable beans. Cacao has been cultivated in Africa since the 19th century, and today, much of the world's cocoa bean supply comes from that region.

In Central and South America, cocoa beans formed the basis of the traditional Aztec drink *chocolatl* (also known as *xocoatl*, meaning "bitter water"), which was enjoyed by the ancient Inca, Maya, and Aztec peoples. Because the drink was made of pounded cocoa beans and spices, without sweeteners, it had an extremely bitter taste. Most people could afford the expensive drink only on special occasions, but members of royalty consumed this beverage frequently as a sign of their elevated position. The ancient Aztec king Montezuma believed the plant had powerful aphrodisiac effects. According to the Spanish conquistador Hernando Cortés, Montezuma consumed large quantities of chocolatl daily—drinking it from golden goblets—and freely shared it with Cortés. Cortés sent cocoa beans to the king of Spain, where it became popular in Europe in the mid-17th century. Today, the tree's seeds are dried and roasted to produce cocoa powder, cocoa butter, chocolate, and a skin-softening ingredient used in cosmetics.

CULINARY USE

Cocoa is best known as the base ingredient of chocolate. There are several types of chocolate: dark chocolate, which has the lowest sugar content; milk chocolate, which contains dried or condensed milk; and white chocolate, which is made from cocoa butter with added milk and sugar—but no cocoa solids. Chocolate can be used in candy, baked goods, and beverages, as well as in savory meat dishes and sauces, including Mexican mole sauce. It is also used to flavor liqueurs.

MEDICINAL USE

Chocolate is a rich source of the antioxidant compounds flavonoids and catechins. Studies show that chocolate may have an effect similar to that of red wine; daily consumption of dark chocolate—the variety highest in flavonoids and lowest in sugar—may help prevent cardiac problems, including reducing the risk of stroke. While chocolate does contain saturated fat, it does not raise cholesterol levels when enjoyed in moderation. Because chocolate contains a small amount of caffeine, it provides a mildly stimulating effect without the jitteriness that coffee can cause.

PLANT PROFILE

Common Names: Cacao, Chocolate, Cocoa

Description: Small evergreen tree, 20 to 50 feet tall (smaller when cultivated); long, thin leaves; small, yellow flowers develop into oblong seedpods that contain cocoa beans

Hardiness: To Zone 11

Family: Malvaceae

Flowering: Periodically

Parts Used: Seed

Range/Habitat: Native to tropical rainforests of Central and South America; cultivated in Africa, Indonesia, Hawaii, and elsewhere

---

HOW TO GROW IT

Cacao trees grow in fertile, moist, well-drained soil in shade. The trees require a minimum temperature of 61°F and high humidity, and they must be sheltered from the wind. In temperate North America, the cacao tree can be grown in a large pot in a warm greenhouse, exposed to bright but indirect light. After 2 or 3 years, flowers may form, and a few of these may in turn form seedpods. The pods contain edible white pulp and 20 to 60 seeds, which can be used to make cocoa. Commercial growers dry the seeds in the sun for 2 to 8 days, then roast and process them for use as cocoa. Plants are propagated by seed.

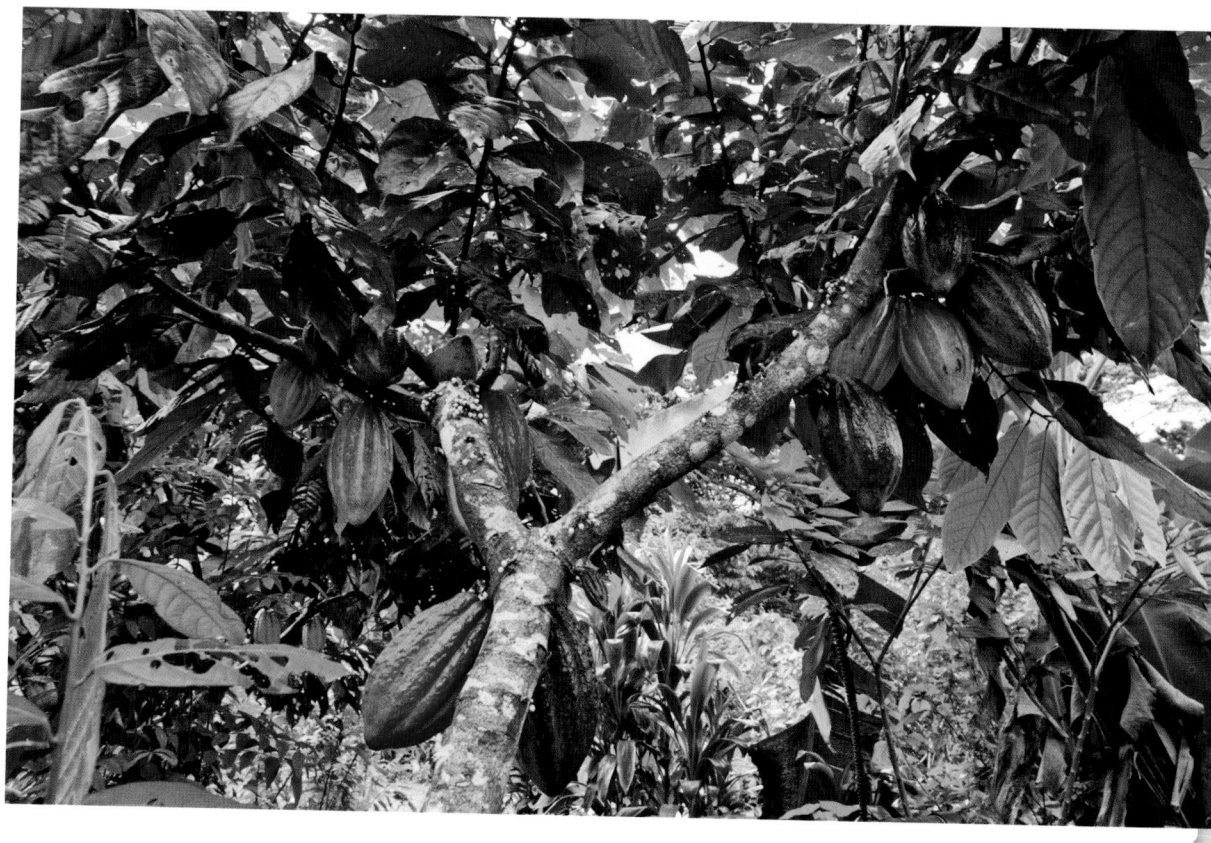

Rx Chocolate

The Maya people of Mexico and Central America make a chocolate beverage that is quite different from the sugary hot chocolate we know and love. They toast fresh cocoa beans on an open griddle and then pound them into a powder that they put in boiling water over a cooking fire. A piece of fresh vanilla pod, bursting with seeds, is tossed into the pot along with some very spicy chile pepper. As the water continues to boil, other ingredients—such as black pepper, cornmeal, and sometimes plantains—are added.

This fragrant brew tastes piquant, with no sugar or sweetness added to help the drink go down. After awakening in a hammock in the moist, cool forest, sipping this beverage is a most pleasant way to start the day. Its ingredients have helped indigenous people, such as Panama's Kuna Indians (who drink several cups daily), avoid hypertension and other conditions associated with aging. Interestingly, those Kuna who have migrated to the capital city and have begun to drink processed cocoa drinks have high rates of hypertension.

I believe we can learn to adapt to new foods and preparations, particularly if they offer a better quality of life and health. Try purchasing ground cocoa seeds, add a few spices (such as vanilla and chile pepper) to the boiling water, and see if this brew can become your new morning drink—it's certainly much healthier than what we call "hot chocolate."—M. J. B.

Thymus vulgaris

Thyme, a member of the mint (*Mentha* spp.) family, is among the most popular garden and kitchen herbs. Its tiny, gray-green leaves have a pungent, slightly lemony flavor and minty aroma. Native to the Mediterranean and southeastern Italy, thyme has naturalized in temperate regions throughout the world. The genus includes about 350 species of aromatic woody perennial shrubs and subshrubs that vary in flavor and aroma, but most can be used in cooking. Scientists believe that thyme was cultivated in Sumer in ancient Mesopotamia as long ago as 3000 BCE.

The plant's name is thought to come from the Greek word *thumus*, meaning "courage." In ancient times, people believed that thyme promoted bravery, and medieval knights carried sprigs of the plant as a symbol of their valor. At one time, thyme also symbolized death, and the souls of the dead were believed to rest in the herb's flowers. Ancient Romans burned the herb in the hope that the scented smoke would repel scorpions; they also strewed the sweet-smelling herb on floors and used it to flavor cheese. The emperor Charlemagne ordered the planting of thyme in all of his gardens for its culinary and medicinal attributes.

The herb's antibacterial properties—correctly ascribed in the 1700s to the presence of the compound thymol—helped preserve meats before refrigeration was available. The ancient Egyptians also used thyme as a preservative; the essential oil was used for embalming the dead.

CULINARY USE

Thyme is a popular and widely used flavoring in poultry, seafood, and vegetable dishes. The herb pairs particularly well with carrots, tomatoes, potatoes, summer squash, and mushrooms. It retains its flavor in slow-cooked dishes and can be bundled together with bay and sage to make a bouquet garni for soups, stocks, and stews. For hundreds of years, bees on Mount Hymettus near Athens, Greece, have produced a beloved wild thyme honey. Benedictine monks added thyme to their famous liqueur.

MEDICINAL USE

Thyme was used by the ancient Romans to treat coughs, improve digestion, and expel worms—much as the herb is used today. Thyme is rich in volatile oils that have powerful antimicrobial, antifungal, and antispasmodic properties, but it is best known for its expectorant effects. Thyme tea eases coughs and bronchial spasms and helps clear the congestion and mucus of a cold.

Like most culinary herbs, thyme benefits digestion by relaxing the smooth muscle tissue of your gastrointestinal tract. Thyme is also rich in disease-fighting antioxidants. Extracts of the herb can be used as an antibacterial against *Helicobacter pylori,* the bacteria thought to cause stomach ulcers. Thyme's antibacterial properties can be used externally, too. Placing crushed thyme leaves on a minor cut, scrape, or other wound can prevent bacteria from entering.

HOW TO GROW IT

Thyme thrives in well-drained soil and full sun. Plant nursery-grown transplants in spring. Or, about 8 weeks before your last frost date, start seeds indoors in flats under lights; transplant the seedlings to your garden when the weather warms. Space plants 12 to 18 inches apart. Mulch seedlings to prevent weed competition until the plants are established. Harvest sprigs of established plants just prior to flowering, in early summer. (Harvesting sprigs after flowering can make the plants more susceptible to winter kill.) Propagate thyme by root division in spring or fall, or by cuttings taken in summer.

Used in massage oil, essential oil of thyme helps warm and relax tired and sore muscles. Thymol, an extract of the herb's volatile oil, is an ingredient in many commercially available products, including cough drops, mouthwashes, dental-care products, chest rubs, and cosmetics.

Caution: Thyme should not be consumed in large amounts by pregnant women; small amounts used in cooking should not be a problem. Thyme essential oil is for external use only; always dilute it and do not give it to children or use it during pregnancy. The oil can irritate skin and mucous membranes.

ORNAMENTAL USE

Thyme makes an attractive edging or groundcover in garden borders, beds, and containers. Creeping varieties, such as 'Bressingham Pink' and 'Coconut', are excellent for planting between stepping stones in a pathway; the plants will grow to form a dense, carpetlike filler and will not be harmed by foot traffic. Thyme also adapts well to rock gardens, rock wall plantings, and raised terraces, where it can sprawl and cascade. The flowers attract butterflies and bees.

OTHER USES

Dried thyme leaves add a pleasant scent to sachets and potpourris. Some gardeners plant thyme near members of the cabbage family to discourage flea beetles, cabbageworms, whiteflies, and other pests. People have also used thyme indoors to repel moths.

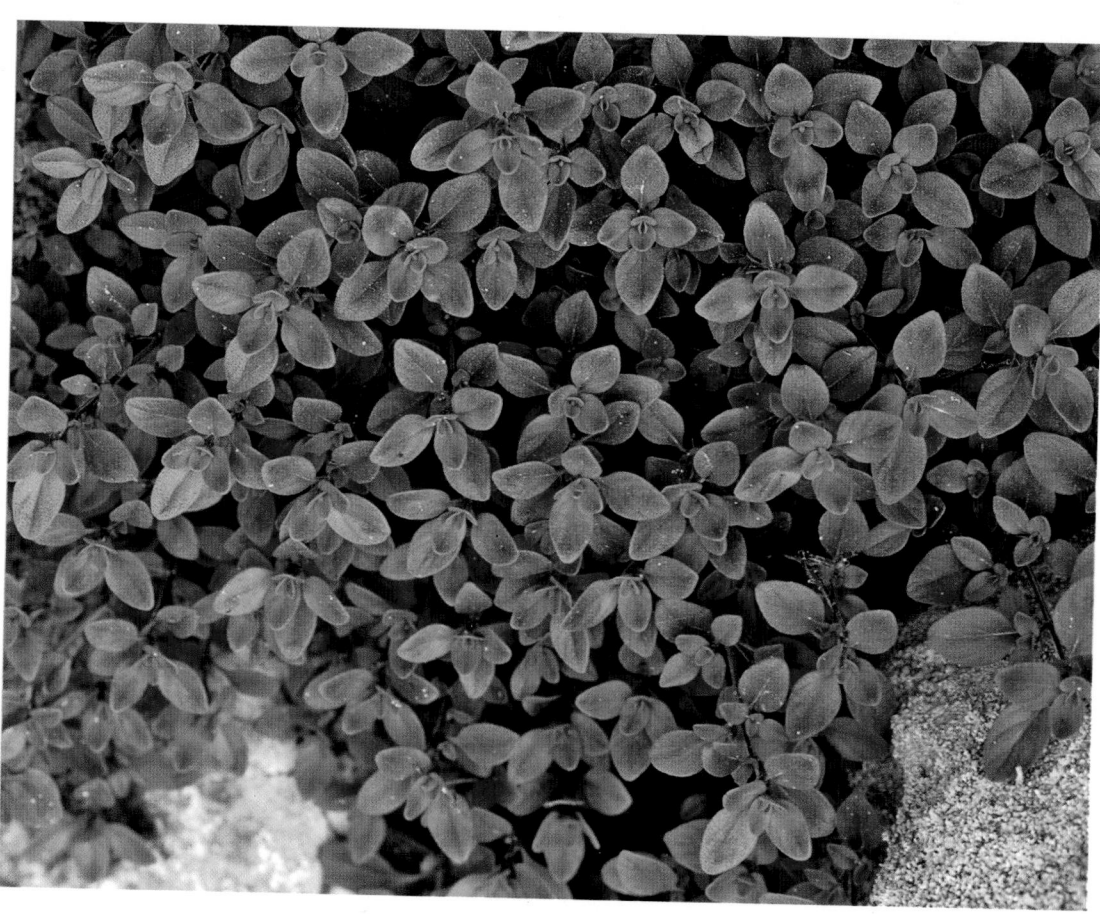

Trifolium pratense

A member of the pea family, red clover is native to Europe, Western Asia, and Northwest Africa, but it grows throughout North America. The herb bears pink flower heads on upright hairy stems; the flowers are highly attractive to bees and are an important source of wildflower honey. Clover's leaves grow in groups of three oval leaflets with pale crescent markings: The genus name *Trifolium* means "three leaves." To the ancient Druids, these three leaves symbolized earth, heaven, and ocean. And of course mutations of this plant that have four leaves are considered to bring good luck.

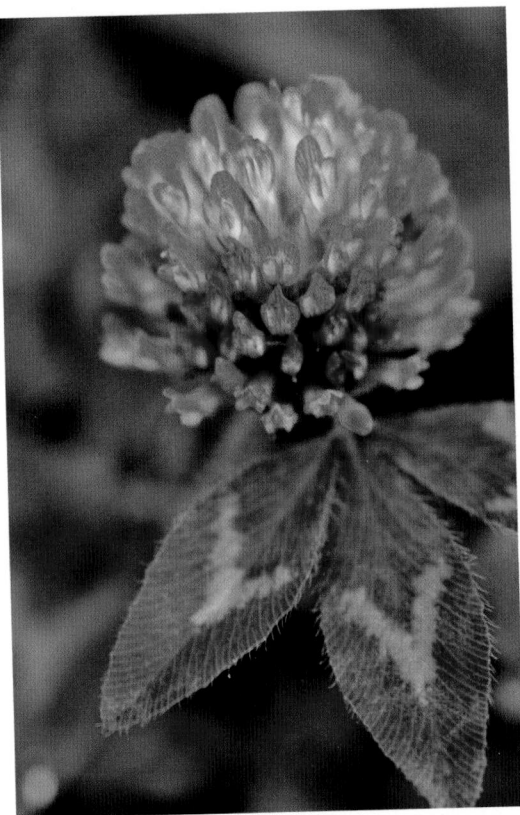

PLANT PROFILE

Common Name: Red Clover

Description: Fast-growing, up to 24 inches tall; three oval leaflets with pale, crescent-shaped markings; mauve-pink flowers on upright stems

Hardiness: To Zone 3

Family: Fabaceae

Flowering: Late spring to midsummer

Parts Used: Flowers, leaves, and sprouts

Range/Habitat: Native to Europe, western Asia, and northwest Africa; grows widely throughout North America

CULINARY USE

Red clover is abundant in vitamins and minerals, including calcium, phosphorus, and vitamins A, D, E, and K. Add red clover sprouts, flowers, and leaves to salads. The flowers can also be added to soup stocks or steeped to make tea.

MEDICINAL USE

The round, flowering tops of red clover contain estrogenlike compounds known as isoflavones, making the herb useful for treating menopausal symptoms such as hot flashes and night sweats. Red clover contains the compounds daidzein and genistein (also found in soy), which may help prevent cancer. Considered an expectorant, the herb is a traditional treatment for coughs, bronchitis, and chest congestion; a soothing tea can be made by steeping the dried flowers in hot water for 10 minutes.

Red clover has diuretic and liver-cleansing properties, and it can help rid your body of toxins. Herbalists recommend it to purify blood. A small-scale human trial has shown that ingesting red clover increases elasticity of the arteries, as compared to a placebo, and could reduce your risk of heart disease, although much more work is needed to confirm this. Externally, the herb has traditionally been applied as a poultice to cancerous growths and to treat skin conditions such as eczema and psoriasis, especially in children.

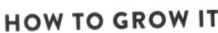 HOW TO GROW IT

Red clover grows in moist, well-drained, neutral soil in sunny areas such as meadows and along paths. It can tolerate shady habitats. The herb is easy to grow from seeds planted in spring, summer, or fall. Harvest leaves for salads before the plant blooms; harvest flowers just as they come into bloom. Dry the flowers in a warm, airy location.

Trigonella foenum-graecum

PLANT PROFILE

Common Name: Fenugreek

Description: Plant with three-lobed leaves, grows 12 to 24 inches tall; white flowers are followed by curved 2-inch seedpods containing up to 20 aromatic brown seeds

Hardiness: Annual

Family: Fabaceae

Flowering: Early to midsummer

Parts Used: Seeds

Range/Habitat: Native to western Asia and the Mediterranean, naturalized in North America, India, and northern Africa

Fenugreek, an annual native to southeastern Europe and western Asia, has been a source of flavoring, medicine, food, and fodder for thousands of years. Archeological remains of fenugreek seeds dating to 4000 BCE have been found in Iraq.

Bearing three-lobed leaves and white flowers on slender stems, the plant resembles wild clover. Its species name, *foenum-graecum*, in Latin means "Greek hay," referring to its use as a livestock food—valued for its ability to stimulate appetite and promote health. Because of the herb's unique scent (often compared to maple syrup), it also was used to disguise the smell of moldy fodder. Benedictine monks brought fenugreek to Western Europe during the 9th century. Today it is cultivated all over the world, with India being the largest commercial producer.

CULINARY USE

The ripe, dried seeds are commonly used as a spice in Asian and African cuisines. Their nutty flavor, which combines the taste of celery and maple, enhances meats, poultry, marinated vegetables, curry blends, and condiments, such as chutney. Use the whole seeds in pickling brine, or sprout them and add them to salads.

MEDICINAL USE

Fenugreek has been used to treat digestive disorders and ulcers, respiratory conditions such as bronchitis, and sore throats, fevers, and diabetes. It has also been used to promote lactation. Studies have shown that fenugreek might help lower cholesterol levels and, for those with type 2 diabetes, could help regulate blood sugar levels.

This herb also has a long tradition of use for soothing skin. It has been used externally to treat conditions such as boils, ulcers, hives, and eczema.

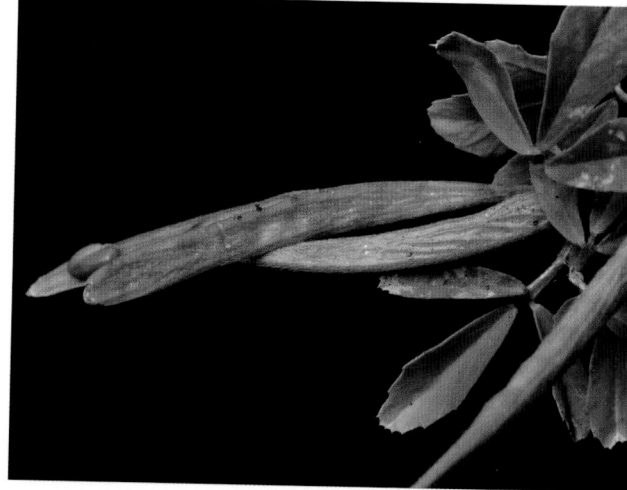

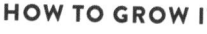

HOW TO GROW IT

Fenugreek thrives in full sun and rich soil that has been deeply cultivated. Broadcast the seed thickly when the soil has reached a minimum temperature of 55°F; in cold, wet soil, root rot can occur. Harvest seedpods when they are ripe but before they begin to shatter. Remove the seeds and dry them in the sun.

Tropaeolum majus

A popular garden flower, the nasturtium bears large, boldly colored blooms and rounded leaves on trailing stems. Its common name comes from the Latin for "twisted nose," a reference to the herb's pungent scent. Originating in the Andes Mountains of South America, nasturtiums were brought from Peru to Spain by the Spanish conquistadors during the 16th century, and their reputation as a culinary herb gradually spread across the continent. The plant was not grown in North America until the 18th century, when it was introduced by European settlers.

CULINARY USE

Nasturtium leaves and flowers have a peppery flavor, reminiscent of radish. Add them to salads, sandwiches, or butters, or float the flowers in soup

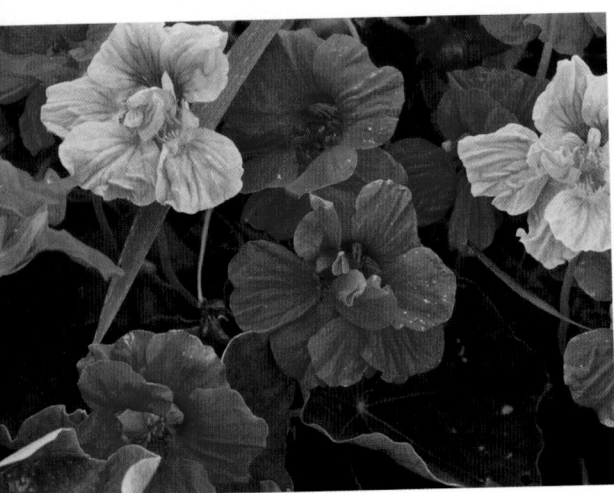

or punch. The young seedpods can be pickled and substituted for imported capers.

MEDICINAL USE

Nasturtium has disinfectant and antibacterial properties due to the presence of mustard oil compounds. The seeds were traditionally used as a poultice to treat sores and boils, and a drink made from the whole plant was taken to help rid the body of toxins and to treat urinary conditions. Some herbalists recommend a hair tonic of nasturtium leaf and rosemary extract to slow hair loss.

Caution: While nasturtium flowers and leaves are rich sources of vitamin C, there have been reports of toxicity associated with overconsumption of this species.

ORNAMENTAL USE

These brightly colored, long-blooming annuals are a favorite of gardeners, hummingbirds, and butterflies. Use the compact varieties in mixed borders and rock gardens. The trailing types are perfect for containers, window boxes, hanging baskets, walls, or banks—anywhere the stems can spill casually over the sides.

HOW TO GROW IT

Nasturtiums grow best in full sun and well-drained, moist soil. They are easy to grow from seed, either sown directly in the garden in spring or started indoors in late winter and then transplanted to the garden when the soil warms. Space the seedlings 6 to 9 inches apart. To grow nasturtiums in a container, use a coarse, porous medium that is not overly rich. Keep the container in full sun and water when the soil feels dry beneath the surface. Harvest the young leaves and flowers as needed. Propagate by gathering the ripe seeds late in the season.

Ulmus rubra

Named for its slick inner bark, slippery elm is native to eastern and central North America. The 50- to 60-foot deciduous tree has thick, reddish brown bark and bears red-brown winged fruits.

Native Americans traditionally used the tree to make canoes and baskets, as well as for food and healing; slippery elm teas and poultices were used to treat wounds, coughs, colds, sore throats, and many other conditions. By the 18th century, European settlers had learned to use the plant in similar ways. Soldiers applied slippery elm poultices to gunshot wounds during the American War of Independence. In the 19th century, the herb became a popular treatment for gastrointestinal problems.

CULINARY USE

The bark powder of slippery elm makes a restorative hot breakfast cereal. Mix 1 teaspoon of the powder with cold water to form a thin, smooth paste. Then add 2 cups of boiling water and cook the mixture for 10 to 15 minutes, stirring constantly. If desired, flavor the cereal with cinnamon, nutmeg, or lemon peel.

MEDICINAL USE

The inner bark of slippery elm contains soothing mucilage, making it a gentle treatment for cough, gastrointestinal conditions, including diarrhea, heartburn, and ulcers; and sore throat. It can also be applied topically to treat superficial skin wounds, inflammatory skin conditions, boils, abscesses, and burns. Slippery elm is available commercially in powder, tea, syrup, lozenge, and pill forms—although there is concern about the long-term viability of this popular herbal remedy due to the overharvesting of wild trees. To make

slippery elm tea, pour 1 cup of boiling water over 1 to 2 teaspoons of the powdered bark and steep for 5 minutes. Sweeten with honey, molasses, or stevia, if you like. You can also add cinnamon, ginger, or nutmeg for additional flavoring. Drink the tea two or three times per day.

Caution: Take other drugs 1 hour before or several hours after consuming slippery elm, as it could slow the absorption of oral medications.

> ## PLANT PROFILE
>
> **Common Names:** Slippery Elm
>
> **Description:** Broad tree up to 60 feet tall; rough, hairy, toothed leaves; small, light green flowers; thick, brown bark; winged seeds
>
> **Hardiness:** To Zone 3
>
> **Family:** Ulmaceae
>
> **Flowering:** Spring
>
> **Parts Used:** Bark
>
> **Habitat/Range:** Eastern and central North America

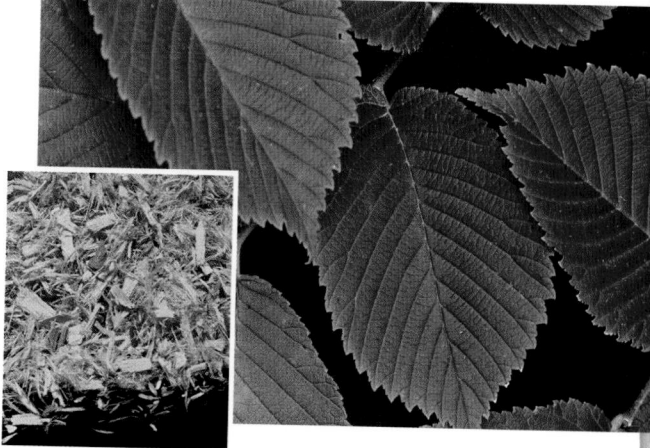

HOW TO GROW IT

Slippery elm grows best in moist, rich soil and full sun, but it will tolerate average soil. If you're planting this tree from seed, use only freshly harvested seeds collected in spring, and plant them immediately with the "wings" intact. (Removing them can damage the seeds.) Plant the seeds directly in prepared garden soil. Most of the seeds will germinate the following spring, after a cold period. The bark of established trees (10 years old and older) can be harvested in spring or fall. Harvest only from larger branches, never the trunk. If possible, use pruned branches because stripping the bark of existing branches increases the tree's susceptibility to Dutch elm disease. After the coarse outer bark is removed, remove the inner bark in strips or chunks, and dry it in a warm, well-ventilated area. Store the bark in a cool, dry location.

Uncaria tomentosa, Uncaria guianensis

PLANT PROFILE

Common Names: Cat's Claw, Uña-de-Gato

Description: Twining, woody vine to 100 feet long; large, glossy leaves; thorny spines curved like cats' claws grow at stem leaf junctions; tiny, yellowish white or red-orange flowers

Hardiness: Zone 11

Family: Rubiaceae

Flowering: Periodically

Parts Used: Bark

Range/Habitat: Native to the tropical rainforests of the Amazon Valley and surrounding regions

A relative of the coffee plant (*Coffea arabica*), cat's claw grows wild in the tropical rainforests of Central and South America. Two species are of medicinal interest, *Uncaria tomentosa* and *U. guianensis*; both are found in the Amazon Valley. The plant's twining woody stem, which can grow to 100 feet, bears large, glossy leaves and thorny spines curved like a cat's claws. In its native region, indigenous people have traditionally used cat's claw as a contraceptive and as a treatment for a wide range of health conditions. Much of the supply of this herb used for commercial purposes

FIELD NOTES

Sacred Seeds

The world's first Sacred Seeds Sanctuary—for the conservation of medicinal plants and the promotion of indigenous knowledge of healing traditions—was founded at Finca Luna Nueva in Costa Rica. Semillas Sagradas, as it is known in Spanish, is dedicated to "preserving both medicinal plant species and cultural memory." Gardens with this purpose are now found in more than 1,000 places as part of an international network. Located in a magnificent Costa Rican rainforest preserve and organic biodynamic farm and ecotourism lodge, Sacred Seeds Sanctuary is home to hundreds of medicinal plant species from Central America, as well as from many other regions.

I've had the chance to walk through the sanctuary with several of the preserve's founders (and my good friends), Rafael Ocampo, Steven Farrell, and Tom Newmark. We stopped along a rainforest trail, and Don Rafael began to tell the story of the uña-de-gato plant, which climbs up into the forest canopy. We learned of its medicinal properties, as well as its indigenous uses against inflammation, diarrhea, dysentery, rheumatism, and arthritis. We also learned how it is grown, harvested, and prepared—and that more than 1.5 million pounds of the plant's bark was collected from the Peruvian Amazon and exported to two dozen countries around the world in a single year, reducing the wild populations dramatically.

Don Rafael then explained why this important commercial herb must be sustainably harvested and cultivated—so that its extraordinary healing properties will be available to anyone who needs them. It was clear why Sacred Seeds Sanctuaries and places like them are so essential: They can help improve the health of millions of people around the world today, and they serve as a "Noah's Ark" to preserve these precious plants and the knowledge of their healing properties for future generations.—M. J. B.

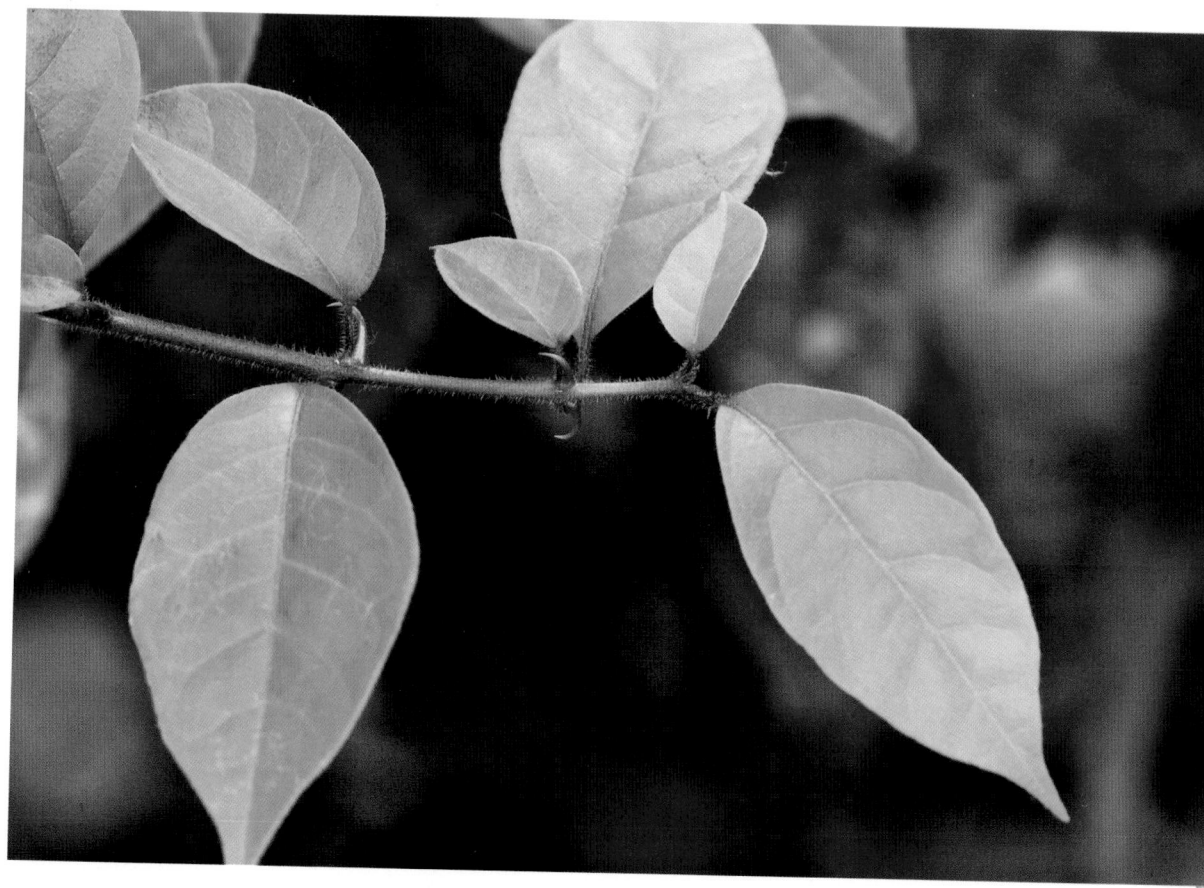

is wild-harvested from plants in South America, although cat's claw is increasingly being harvested from cultivated sources or managed plantings in secondary forests.

MEDICINAL USE

Cat's claw is a known anti-inflammatory agent. It has been used to treat osteoarthritis of the knee and rheumatoid arthritis (in conjunction with conventional therapy), as well as Crohn's disease, chronic prostatitis, canker sores, gastric ulcers and other stomach problems, sinus infections, and flu. The plant's roots and stem bark are believed to contain compounds that can stimulate the immune system. Cat's claw could be useful in the treatment of viral infections and for lowering cholesterol and blood pressure levels.

Caution: This herb should not be used during pregnancy, by those taking ulcer medications, or by transplant patients. The plant has been overharvested in the wild; choose products made from sustainably harvested stem bark.

HOW TO GROW IT

Cat's claw thrives in rich, moist soil; ample rain; and heat—typical conditions of a tropical rainforest. You can try growing it in a warm greenhouse where it will receive ample light—in the wild, its long vine helps bring this plant into the canopy of the rainforest. Harvesting begins when the plant is at least 8 years old; the vine is cut from the top to within a foot of the ground, and the bark is stripped and dried for use. Basal parts of the stem and roots are left in the ground to ensure that the rapidly growing vine continues to flourish. Propagate the vine from stem cuttings.

Urtica dioica

Native to North America and Eurasia, nettle is a
5-foot-tall perennial widely naturalized in fields
and woodland edges of temperate areas worldwide. The genus name comes from the Latin *urere*,
which means "to burn." Like other plants in its
family, nettle is well known for the burning sensation that occurs if you come in contact with the
plant's hairy, toothed leaves. Interestingly, you can
relieve the stinging by rubbing the affected area
with the leaves of yellow dock (*Rumex crispus*) or
jewelweed (*Impatiens capensis*), which often grow
near nettle.

Ancient Greeks used nettle juice medicinally to
treat many conditions, ranging from snakebites to
coughs, and Roman soldiers rubbed nettle on their
skin—a practice known as urtication—to improve
their tolerance of cold temperatures. From the
Bronze Age through the early 20th century, people
used the strong fibers of nettle stems to make cloth
and paper.

CULINARY USE

Nettle leaves are a favorite spring green. Cooking
(and drying, for use in winter) destroys the plant's
sting. To prepare the leaves, you can steam, sauté,
or stir-fry them; puree them and add them to
soups; or substitute them for spinach in recipes. In
Scotland, people make a traditional pudding with
nettle, leeks, broccoli, and rice. The herb is also
used in Russian and Italian dishes, such as Russian
nettle soup and risotto with wild greens.

MEDICINAL USE

Nettle leaves—which contain vitamins A and C, as
well as the mineral iron—have antihistamine, anti-
inflammatory, astringent, and diuretic properties.
Practitioners use nettle to treat anemia and poor
circulation; to relieve arthritis, seasonal allergies,

PLANT PROFILE

Common Names: Nettle, Stinging Nettle

Description: Single-stemmed perennial up to
5 feet tall; clusters of tiny, greenish flowers;
heart-shaped leaves with toothed edges, covered
with tiny, bristly hairs

Hardiness: To Zone 3

Family: Urticaceae

Flowering: Summer

Parts Used: Leaves, stems, and root

Range/Habitat: Native to North America and
Eurasia, widely naturalized in temperate areas

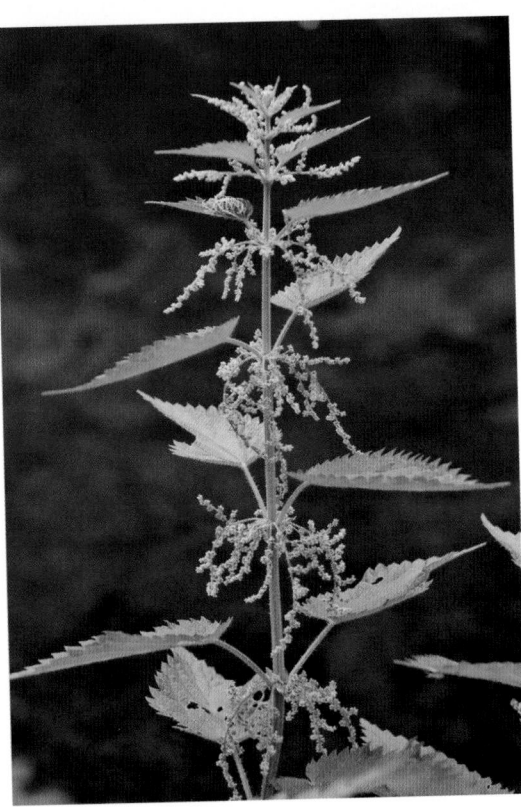

 HOW TO GROW IT

Nettle grows easily in moist, nitrogen-rich soil in full sun or partial shade. Plant seeds or root divisions in spring; to prevent unwanted spread, grow nettle in a large container. For medicinal use, wear gloves and harvest the whole plants in late
spring or summer, just before the plants flower. For culinary use, pick young leaf tips from plants less than 4 inches tall.

heavy menstrual bleeding, and inflammatory skin conditions; and to ease and prevent urinary tract infections and kidney stones.

Impressive research supports the ability of nettle root to ease the symptoms of enlarged prostate, including frequent and nighttime urination. The condition, known as benign prostatic hyperplasia, affects many men older than 50.

Herbalists frequently recommend nettle tea for its nutritive value and as a general tonic and "blood builder." To make nettle leaf tea, steep 2 teaspoons of the herb in 1 cup of hot water for 10 minutes. Strain, then sweeten the tea, if desired. Drink up to 3 cups per day. Wear gloves when handling the fresh herb; heat deactivates the plant's sting.

Other nettle preparations include extracts, tinctures, and fresh juice. The fresh leaves can be applied externally as a poultice to relieve joint pain and inflammation.

OTHER USES

Shampoos and other commercial hair-care products often contain nettle. The herb is thought to thicken hair and make it shiny. You can use a nettle infusion as a hair rinse or facial steam. Some gardeners use nettle tea as a fertilizer for garden plants.

IN THE KITCHEN: THE SOFTER SIDE OF NETTLE

Nettle can be a wonderfully nutritious and tasty spring green—*if* you learn to handle this prickly plant with care. To protect yourself from the herb's notorious sting, be sure to wear gloves when harvesting and preparing nettle.

For cooking, choose young plants, ideally no more than 4 to 6 inches tall. If the plants are older, use only the younger (top) leaves and discard the stems. While wearing rubber gloves, gently rinse the nettle and then chop it. Cooking nettle deactivates the sting. Steam it alone or with other vegetables, cooking the greens just until they wilt—3 or 4 minutes. Serve cooked nettle as a side dish, or add it to risotto, pasta sauces, or quiches. Here's another way to make the most of this springtime tonic and treat.

Spring Nettle Soup

1–2 tablespoons olive oil

2 shallots, chopped

1 stalk celery, diced

2 cloves garlic, minced

3 cups young nettle leaves, finely chopped

1 cup arugula, coarsely chopped

2 cups milk

2 cups vegetable stock

2 medium potatoes, peeled and diced

Salt (optional)

Pepper (optional)

2–3 tablespoons grated Parmesan cheese

2 teaspoons chopped parsley

In a 3- or 4-quart pot, heat the olive oil over medium heat. Cook the shallots and celery in the oil for about 5 minutes or until soft. Add the garlic and cook for 1 minute, then add the nettle leaves and arugula. Reduce the heat to low, cover the pot, and cook the greens just until they wilt, about 3 minutes. Add the milk and stock, then raise the heat just until the liquid comes to a boil. Add the potatoes. Reduce the heat to a gentle simmer, and cook for 30 minutes. Remove the pot from the heat. In a blender or food processor, puree the soup in batches to thicken it. (When pureeing hot soup, take care to avoid splashing yourself.) Return the soup to the pot and reheat over low heat. Season with salt and pepper, if using; add the grated cheese and garnish with the parsley just before serving. **Serves 4.**

Vaccinium spp.
including
V. angustifolium,
V. corymbosum

PLANT PROFILE

Common Name: Blueberry

Description: Shrubs (varying in height from trailing to 12 feet tall); dark green, oval leaves; bell-shaped white or light pink flowers; light blue to black fruits

Hardiness: To Zone 2, depending on species

Family: Ericaceae

Flowering: Spring to early summer

Parts Used: Fruit and leaves

Range/Habitat: Most are native to eastern and central North America; woodlands and bogs

The oak and pine forests of eastern and central North America are home to more than a dozen *Vaccinium* species commonly known as blueberry. Depending on the species, the shrubs range in height from ground-hugging to 12 feet tall. All bear dark green leaves, white or pink bell-shaped flowers, and sweet, round fruits that range in color from light blue to black. Selections of *Vaccinium corymbosum* (northern highbush blueberry) have produced a wide range of cultivars grown commercially in North America and throughout the world.

Blueberries were a staple food of Native Americans, who ate the fruit fresh, dried, or cooked into desserts, relishes, cakes, and sauces.

CULINARY USE

Fresh or dried, blueberry fruits are delicious in baked goods, such as muffins, cakes, and pies. They also make tasty jellies, jams, and syrups and can be added to many foods.

MEDICINAL USE

Blueberry fruits contain relatively large amounts of vitamins B_6 and C and the mineral manganese. They are also rich in antioxidants and flavonoids, which could inhibit the production of LDL (bad) cholesterol, improve heart health, and help prevent or reverse memory loss due to aging. One study with a small group of older men and women who had mild age-related memory decline showed that drinking three glasses of wild lowbush blueberry juice each day increased memory test scores compared to a group that drank a placebo. Other research suggests that eating blueberries may help prevent urinary tract infections.

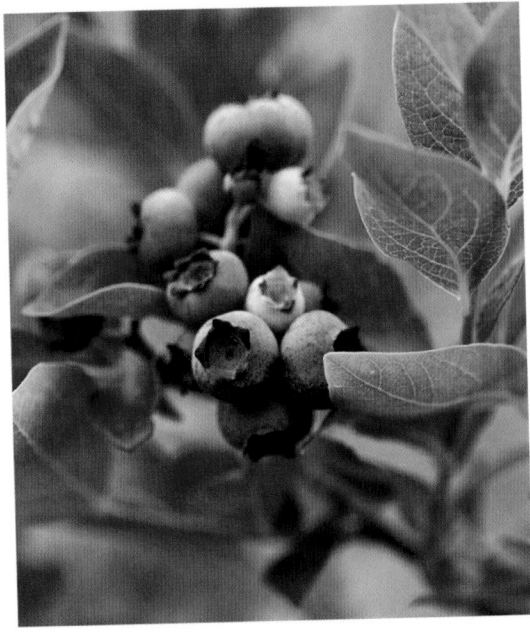

HOW TO GROW IT

Grow blueberries in full sun and moist, acidic (4.0 to 5.0 pH) loam. Blueberries won't thrive in soil that has a neutral or alkaline pH. Lower the soil pH before planting by amending with peat moss or elemental sulfur and composted leaves. After planting, mulch with a 4- to 5-inch layer of composted leaf litter or pine needles, and replenish it annually. Fertilize each spring with composted manure, cottonseed meal, or another high-nitrogen fertilizer. Plants begin bearing fruit during their third year. Cover the ripening fruits with netting to protect them from wildlife. Propagate by hardwood cuttings.

Vaccinium macrocarpon

The cranberry is a low evergreen shrub native to the coastal areas, bogs, and swamps of northeastern and western North America. The creeping plant bears dark pink flowers with curved petals, followed by white berries that turn deep red when ripe. European settlers in eastern North America called the plant craneberry because they thought its curved flower petals and anthers resembled the head of a crane. Native Americans used the fruit as food, often making it into cakes or mixing it with meat to make pemmican, which they used throughout the winter.

CULINARY USE

Because of their tartness, cranberries are generally cooked with sugar when they're made into sauces, jellies, jams, and baked goods. The fruits can also be dried and eaten like raisins or added to salads and desserts.

MEDICINAL USE

Cranberry fruits, which are high in vitamin C, were at one time eaten to prevent scurvy, a disease caused by vitamin C deficiency. The berries contain anthocyanins and flavonol glycosides, which have antibacterial properties. Studies have shown that drinking cranberry juice or taking cranberry extract tablets reduces your risk of a bladder infection—although there is little evidence that cranberry can cure an infection once it's begun. Active compounds in the fruit inhibit microorganisms from adhering to the cells lining your urinary tract, making a less hospitable environment for infection-causing bacteria such as *E. coli*. The same compounds are said to help prevent various types of bacteria from forming dental plaque, and some preliminary research suggests cranberry could inhibit the growth of *Helicobacter pylori,* a bacteria that can cause stomach ulcers. Cranberry also might benefit men with chronic prostatitis.

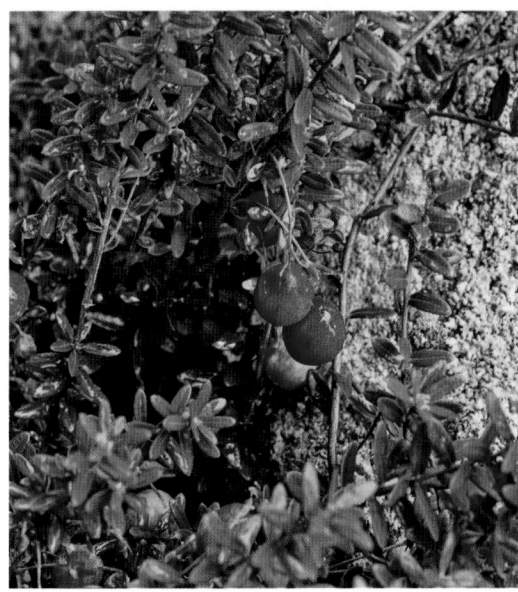

HOW TO GROW IT

Cranberry requires a unique combination of growing conditions to thrive: moist to wet acidic soil, cool temperatures, and a long growing season (April to November). The plant's creeping roots must remain cool and wet; commercial growers cultivate cranberries in bog soil composed of alternate layers of sand, gravel, and organic matter, adding new layers of sand every 2 to 5 years. If you do not have a natural wetland area, try growing cranberries in a sunken bed and flood it periodically, or use drip irrigation to keep the soil constantly moist. Cranberry fruit matures about 80 days after bloom, usually by late October; the ripe fruit is bright red and firm. The plants can be propagated by softwood cuttings taken in spring.

Vaccinium myrtillus

PLANT PROFILE

Common Names: Bilberry, Whortleberry

Description: Small, deciduous shrub, up to 2 feet tall; pink or yellow-green flowers; small, aromatic, dark blue to black fruits

Hardiness: Zone 2

Family: Ericaceae

Flowering: Midsummer

Parts Used: Fruit and leaves

Range/Habitat: Native to Europe and western North America; woodlands and meadows

Bilberry grows primarily in pine forests and meadows in Europe and western North America. The shrubs bear small, round, bluish fruits that can be distinguished from blueberries (*Vaccinium corymbosum* and others) by their dark blue, aromatic flesh. (Blueberry fruits are white or pale green when cut open and are not as aromatic.) Another difference is that bilberry fruits usually form singly or in pairs, while blueberries appear in clusters.

Bilberries are rarely cultivated; the fruits are generally harvested from the wild for food or medicinal use. Several related species, including *Vaccinium membranaceum* (big huckleberry) and *V. deliciosum* (Cascade bilberry), are also native to western North America and can be used in similar ways. Native Americans ate the fruit of the big huckleberry fresh, cooked, or dried, and they used an infusion of the plant's roots and stems to treat heart disease and arthritis.

CULINARY USE

The fruits of the bilberry and its relatives are more acidic and seedy than blueberries. But when cooked with sugar, they make delicious pies, syrups, and jams. You can also use them to make breads, muffins, compotes, and wine.

MEDICINAL USE

Bilberry has been used medicinally in Europe for more than 1,000 years. The fruits are rich in vitamin C and were eaten to prevent scurvy, a disease caused by vitamin C deficiency. In 17th-century England, people mixed bilberries with honey to form a mixture called "rob," which was used to treat diarrhea. During World War II, British pilots ate bilberry jam before night missions, claiming it improved night vision.

Bilberry fruits contain antioxidant pigments called anthocyanosides, which help improve blood flow by maintaining strong, flexible cell walls. Bilberries are especially beneficial for vision, because they increase blood flow to and oxygen levels in the eyes. Scientists believe that eye conditions such as cataracts and macular degeneration are promoted by free radical or oxidative damage.

Bilberry also might benefit the cardiovascular system by helping to reduce the buildup of calcium plaque deposits in arteries, inhibiting blood clot formation, and increasing heartbeat strength. Besides taking bilberry in its fresh form, you can also take the herb as a commercially prepared tea (made from the dried ripe fruit or leaves) or extract.

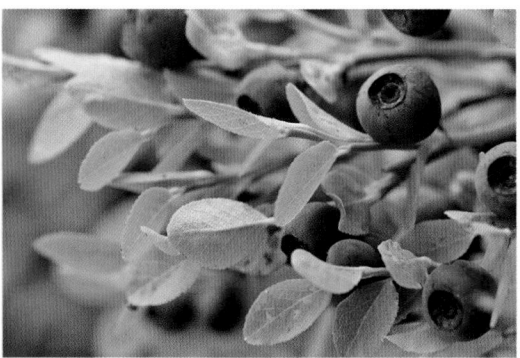

HOW TO GROW IT

Although this plant is rarely cultivated, it is possible to find commercial suppliers of seed. Sow the seed on the surface of the soil in fall. Bilberries thrive in moist, acidic soil in sun or partial shade; to propagate, take semiripe cuttings in summer. Harvest the berries when they turn blue-black.

Valeriana officinalis

According to folklore, the Pied Piper led rats out of the city of Hamelin, Germany, not with music, but because he carried valerian in his pockets. This tall perennial herb contains compounds similar to those in catnip (*Nepeta cataria*), and cats—as well as rats and mice—tend to find the unique scent of valerian appealing. Although the plant's pink or white flowers are sweetly fragrant, its leaves and roots have a strongly pungent odor that most people consider highly unpleasant. Like catnip, valerian has a calming effect on people, and the herb's common name is believed to derive from the Latin *valere*, which means, "to be well." Valerian is native to Europe and western Asia and is naturalized in North America.

CULINARY USE

Despite its strong scent and flavor, valerian was once eaten in salads and used as a pot herb. Today, extracts of valerian are used commercially as an apple flavoring in baked goods, soft drinks, beer, and tobacco.

MEDICINAL USE

Valerian root—taken in tea, extract, or capsule form—contains more than 100 physiologically

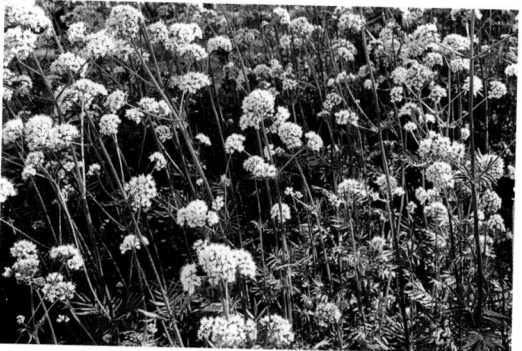

PLANT PROFILE

Common Names: Garden Heliotrope, Valerian

Description: Stems, 3 to 6 feet tall; dark green, lance-shaped serrated leaves; clusters of small white or pink flowers; large, pungent-smelling rhizomes

Hardiness: To Zone 3

Family: Valerianaceae

Flowering: Midsummer

Parts Used: Roots and leaves

Range/Habitat: Native to Europe and western Asia, naturalized in North America; damp meadows and wooded areas

---

active chemical compounds. Used as a mild sedative since ancient Roman times, this natural sleep aid is nonaddictive and has no known side effects, such as the hangover feeling associated with prescription sleep aids.

Valerian also dilates coronary arteries and helps normalize heart rhythm. It is used to relieve excitability, exhaustion, and anxiety-related symptoms such as heart palpitations, sweating, and feelings of panic. During World War I, it was used to treat soldiers with "shell shock" (a short-term condition now referred to as combat stress reaction), which can include memory loss. Valerian has antispasmodic properties and is a central nervous system (CNS) depressant. Clinical trials have shown it to be as effective (and sometimes more effective) at treating anxiety as some conventional pharmaceuticals.

To make valerian root tea, cover 1 teaspoon of the dried root with 1 cup of boiling water. Steep for 10 minutes and sweeten if desired.

Caution: Valerian can cause stomach upset in sensitive individuals, and in a small percentage of people it can be stimulating rather than calming. The herb should not be used together with a prescription or over-the-counter sleep aid, particularly a CNS depressant, or with alcohol. Pregnant women should avoid this herb.

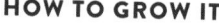 HOW TO GROW IT

Valerian thrives in moist, fertile soil and full sun or partial shade. Plant root divisions or seeds in spring or fall. Mulch with composted manure and remove flowers to increase root size. Harvest roots starting in fall of the plant's second year. Dry the roots in a 170°F oven until brittle. Harvest leaves for salads or soups as needed.

Vanilla planifolia

PLANT PROFILE

Common Names: Vanilla

Description: Climbing evergreen vine, up to 50 feet long; thick, succulent stem; bright green, pointed leaves; clusters of pale greenish yellow flowers; fruit contains hundreds of tiny seeds

Hardiness: To Zone 11

Family: Orchidaceae

Flowering: Periodically

Parts Used: Pod

Range/Habitat: Native to Mexico, Central and South America, and the West Indies

The only orchid that bears an edible fruit, *Vanilla planifolia* is a climbing evergreen perennial vine native to Mexico, Central and South America, and the West Indies. Vanilla has a thick, succulent stem and bears bright green, pointed leaves and clusters of showy, pale greenish yellow flowers. Its fruit, commonly called the vanilla bean, is a pendant pod that contains hundreds of tiny seeds. Vanilla beans have been highly prized for hundreds of years for use in sweets and perfumery.

CULINARY USE

A much-loved food flavoring around the world, vanilla was introduced to Europe in the 16th century by the Spanish, who learned of its use in

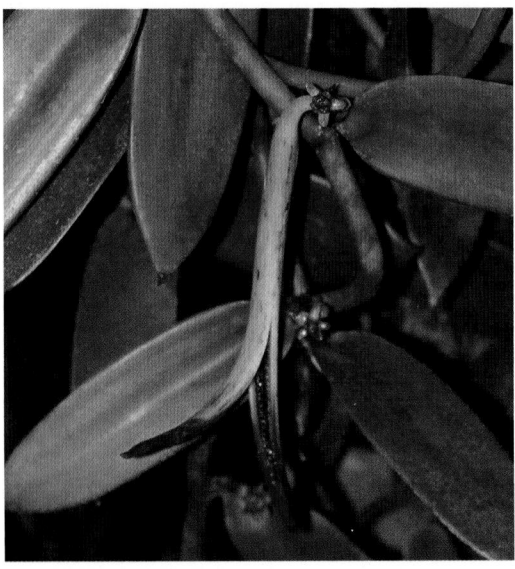

Mexico. Its enchanting flavor and aroma are due to a substance called vanillin, which develops during the curing process. To impart a delicate flavor to sugar, add a vanilla bean to your sugar bowl; use the sugar to flavor desserts and teas. Vanilla extract is used commercially to flavor ice creams, baked goods, syrups, soft drinks, and liqueurs, such as Kahlúa.

MEDICINAL USE

In folk medicine, vanilla has been used to stimulate the brain, prevent sleep, increase energy, and improve digestion. In aromatherapy, the scent of vanilla is believed to promote feelings of confidence and calmness. Massage oils that contain vanilla are said to have aphrodisiac properties.

OTHER USES

Vanilla is often included as a fragrance in hand and body lotions, soaps, cosmetics, deodorants, scented candles, and potpourris. In some places, the pods are woven into aromatic handicrafts.

HOW TO GROW IT

Vanilla is cultivated in plantations in many parts of the tropics, and it can be grown in a warm greenhouse if given a soil mix formulated for orchids, plenty of moisture, shade, humidity, and an average daytime temperature of 80°F with slightly cooler nights. Plant cuttings that are several feet long. Hand-pollinate the flowers to ensure that the plant will set fruits, or beans. Vanilla beans ripen in 5 to 7 months; harvest them when they're fully ripe but before they split open. In commercial production, the 10-inch-long beans are allowed to "sweat"—either by heating them in the sun or scalding them with boiling water—to produce an enzymatic reaction, then are stored for 3 to 6 months to develop their flavor. The pods can be stored whole in an airtight container.

Caution: Handling this plant can cause an allergic reaction in some individuals.

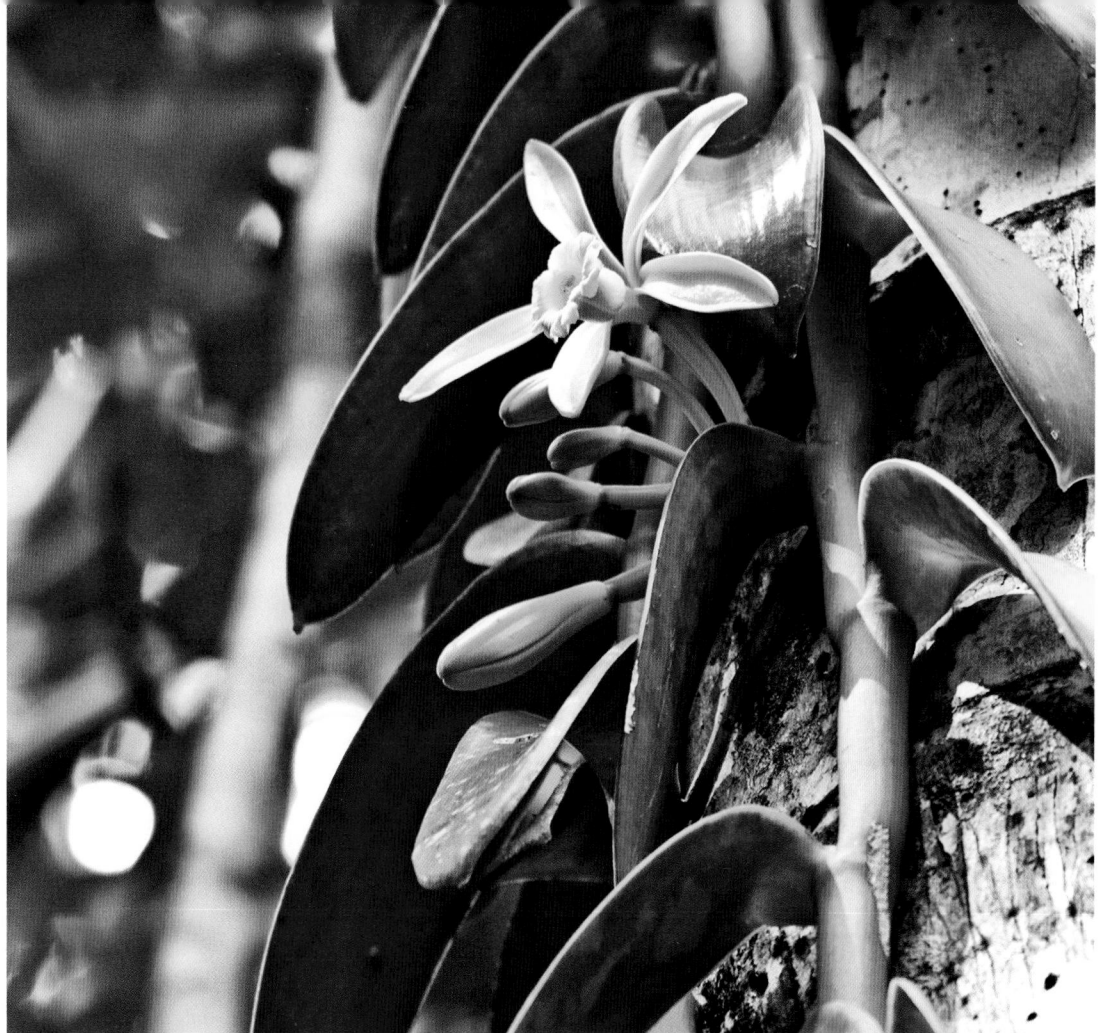

The Orchid and the Bee

The forests of Mexico and Central America are home to a very special vine—the vanilla plant, which is the only orchid used as a spice or food. Vanilla vines grow pressed against trees, creeping up to the canopy, and hanging down from branches. When their beautiful, large yellow flowers open, they are pollinated by a single type of insect, known in Mexico as the "mountain bee." Shortly after the bee does its work, the pod starts to grow and eventually opens, spreading its seeds.

In nature, the chances of this bee pollinating the vanilla flower are very small. So when people began transplanting the vanilla orchid to other places in the world, it was clear that an artificial method of fertilization was needed. In the 1840s, a system was developed that involved using a sliver of wood to open the flower and a finger to move the pollen from the anther to the tip of the stigma—ultimately putting the bee out of work. Today, this hand-pollination method is more or less equivalent to what was used 150 years ago, and it is employed in vanilla orchid plantations around the world.—M. J. B.

Verbascum thapsus

PLANT PROFILE

Common Names: Common Mullein, Torch Weed

Description: Rigid stems up to 6 feet tall; silvery green, velvety leaves up to 18 inches long; dense spikes of bright yellow blooms, followed by seed capsules with numerous small brown seeds

Hardiness: Biennial; to Zone 1

Family: Scrophulariaceae

Flowering: Midsummer to late summer

Parts Used: Leaves and flowers

Range/Habitat: Native to Europe and Asia; naturalized throughout North America; found along disturbed sites, such as ditches and roadsides

At 6 feet tall with dense spikes of golden blooms, common mullein makes an impressive display in fields, ditches, and other disturbed sites throughout North America. Mullein is also called torch weed because people used to soak its tall, rigid stems in oil and then used them for lighting. The hardy biennial self-seeds readily and is considered a pest in many areas, but healers long ago recognized the plant's virtues.

The Greek physician Dioscorides (ca. 40–90 CE) prescribed mullein for lung conditions 2,000 years ago. In North America, where the plant has naturalized, Native Americans found a multitude of uses for the velvety leaves and golden flowers. Many groups smoked the leaves or made them into a tea to treat coughs and colds, asthma, sore throat, and sore joints. Externally, they applied a poultice of the fresh, pounded leaves to cuts, swellings, abscesses, sores, bruises, sprains, earaches, and toothaches.

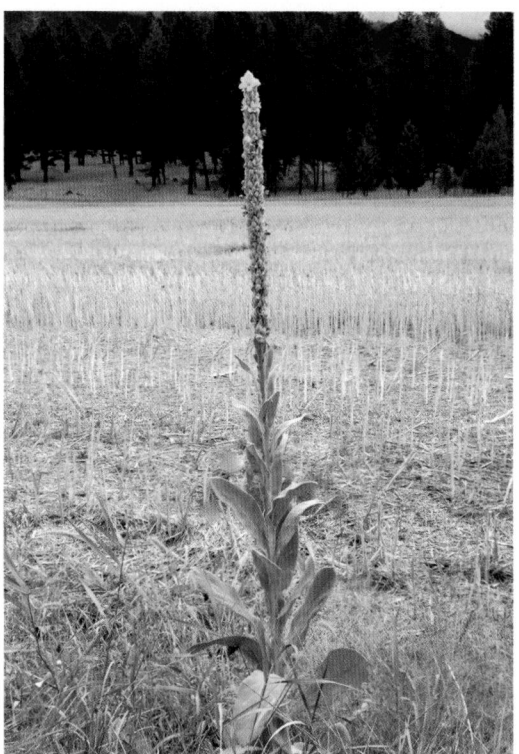

MEDICINAL USE

The plant's leaves and flowers contain antibacterial and astringent tannins and soothing emollient mucilage. Although little research has been conducted to support mullein's effectiveness, the herb has a long tradition of use, especially for treating respiratory problems. Modern practitioners recommend mullein leaf tea or decoction for respiratory conditions, as well as for sore throats, digestive discomforts, and urinary tract problems.

The fresh or dried flowers can be used to make an oil infusion for external use, such as for skin conditions, earaches, and joint pain. To make mullein tea, pour 1 cup of boiling water over 1 to 2 teaspoons of the fresh leaves. Steep for 10 minutes. Strain, then sweeten and drink as desired. Filter out any irritating plant hairs by pouring the liquid through cheesecloth or a coffee filter.

HOW TO GROW IT

Considered an invasive weed in many areas of the United States, common mullein can be difficult to eradicate and is rarely grown in the garden. The plant thrives in full sun and open, somewhat dry locations. Harvest the leaves and flowers in summer.

Verbena officinalis

Vervain was revered as a sacred herb by many ancient peoples, including the Romans, Persians, and Druids. The Egyptians believed the plant originated from the tears of the goddess Isis as she wept for the dead god Osiris. Vervain was also associated with the crucifixion: According to legend, the herb was pressed onto Christ's wounds to staunch the bleeding.

The genus name derives from the Latin for "sacred boughs," while the common name is believed to come from the ancient Celtic words *fer* ("to drive away") and *faen* ("stone"), reflecting a belief in the herb's ability to treat kidney stones. Native Americans prepared a decoction of the roots for the treatment of liver and kidney problems.

MEDICINAL USE

Vervain has been reported to have astringent, antispasmodic, diaphoretic (sweat-promoting), diuretic, and other healing properties, but there is virtually no scientific evaluation of its efficacy. The herb could have the ability to clear bronchial passages, stimulate the digestive system, promote lactation, flush excess water from the body, reduce inflammation, and relieve anxiety.

Vervain tea or tincture is sometimes recommended for the treatment of coughs, bronchitis, and sore throats, as well as for bladder infections, nervous tension, and joint pain. Herbalists recommend a vervain leaf poultice for headaches, nerve and joint pain, sores, abscesses, and burns. In Spain, vervain is mixed with other herbs to make a poultice used to heal wounds on cattle.

Caution: Do not use vervain during pregnancy. Also, a glycoside in vervain may cause vomiting.

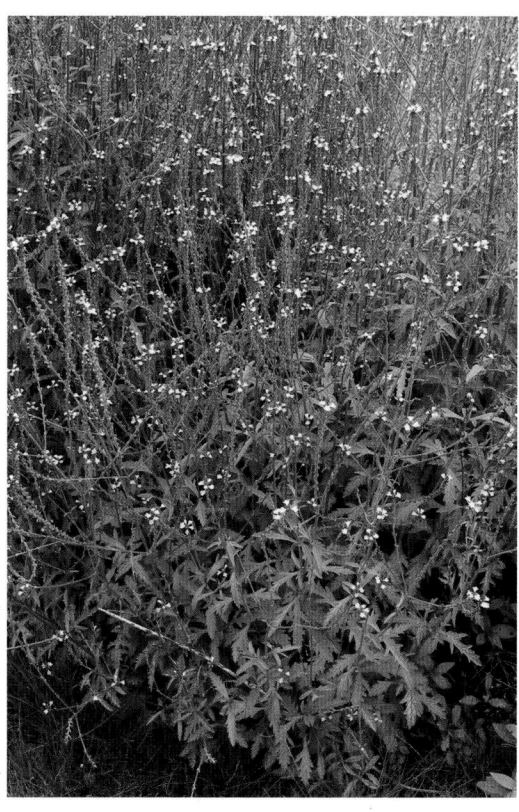

HOW TO GROW IT

Vervain is easy to grow in full sun or partial shade and rich, moist soil. Amend the soil with compost prior to planting the seeds after the last frost in spring. Or start seeds indoors in late winter to early spring, and transplant the seedlings to your garden after the weather has warmed. For medicinal use, harvest the leaves and stems before the plant flowers, and use them fresh or dried. To propagate, divide the roots in fall or allow the seed heads to dry on the plants, then remove and collect the seeds.

Viola odorata

The delicate, dark purple or white flowers of violet have a wonderful, sweet fragrance, but due to the plant's chemical composition, the scent fades quickly. Native to Europe and Asia and naturalized throughout the temperate regions of the world, violet has had a place in the kitchen, medicine cabinet, and garden for centuries. The ancient Romans infused wine with violets, then sweetened the drink with honey. The 1st-century herbalist Pliny the Elder wrote of the violet's medicinal virtues, recommending it for gout and disorders of the spleen. The flowers were the favorite of French emperor Napoléon Bonaparte (1769–1821) and his first wife, Josephine. When she died in 1814, Napoléon planted violets on her grave. Before he was exiled in 1815, he picked some of the violets and put them in a locket, which he wore around his neck until the end of his life.

PLANT PROFILE

Common Names: Sweet Violet, Violet

Description: Creeping perennial, up to 6 inches tall; oval to heart-shaped leaves and sweet-scented, dark purple or white, five-petaled flowers

Hardiness: To Zone 5

Family: Violaceae

Flowering: Spring

Parts Used: Flowers, leaves, and roots

Range/Habitat: Native to Europe and Asia, naturalized in North America; found along roadsides and in woodland areas

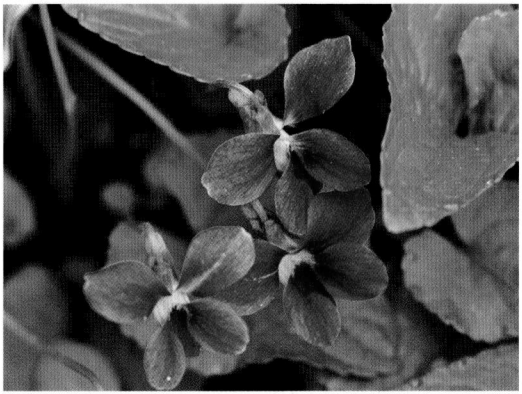

CULINARY USE

Violet flowers add color to salads and can be used fresh or candied as a dessert garnish. The fresh flowers can also be floated on cold soups.

MEDICINAL USE

Violet leaves and flowers have a mild expectorant action, and a tea or syrup made from them can be taken to treat coughs, colds, and congestion. Herbalists have used violet tea to alleviate headaches, lower fevers (by inducing sweating), and relieve gastritis and bladder inflammation. Externally, this species is used as a poultice or to make an ointment for treating skin conditions. A decoction of the roots can be applied as a dressing to sore and swollen joints. The plant contains salicylic acid, the primary chemical compound found in aspirin.

The tea of a related species, *Viola adunca,* is sometimes given to children to treat stomach pain and asthma.

Caution: This plant contains saponins. Consuming large amounts of violet leaves can cause diarrhea and vomiting.

ORNAMENTAL USE

Violets add welcome spring color to window boxes and other containers, rock gardens, and informal borders. In the garden, plant violets in large groups or masses for best effect.

OTHER USES

Violet leaf oil is used in various perfume and cosmetic products. Because it's made from the plant's leaves, the fragrance is described as "green" and fresh, rather than sweet or floral.

HOW TO GROW IT

Plant violets in well-drained, moist soil in full sun or partial shade. Sow the seeds outdoors in fall, and mulch with leaf litter for winter. Or plant divisions in early spring, spacing the plants about 1 foot apart. Harvest violet leaves and flowers as needed throughout the plant's flowering season. Use them fresh or dried.

Viscum album, Phoradendron spp., Arceuthobium spp.

PLANT PROFILE

Common Name: Mistletoe

Description: Semiparasitic plant, 20 to 60 inches tall; thick, evergreen leaves; small flowers followed by dense clusters of waxy white or yellow-green berries; sticky seeds

Hardiness: Varies with species

Family: Santalaceae

Flowering: Midspring to early summer

Parts Used: Leaves, fruit, and stems

Range/Habitat: *Viscum album* is native to Europe and Asia; *Phoradendron* spp. are native to the warm parts of North, Central, and South America; and *Arceuthobium* spp. are native to North and Central America, Asia, and Africa

Mistletoe is a semiparasitic plant that lives on trees, tapping water and nutrients from its host. European mistletoe (*Viscum album*), native to northern Europe and Asia, bears oval evergreen leaves and dense clusters of waxy white berries. More than 40 related mistletoe species (including those of *Phoradendron* and *Arceuthobium*, the latter known as dwarf mistletoe) grow in North America. Mistletoe seeds are usually spread by birds, which feed on the juicy berries. This mode of propagation could explain the plant's common name, which is said to derive from the Anglo-Saxon *mistel*, meaning "dung," and *tan*, meaning "twig."

Mistletoe figures prominently in folklore and mythology. In pre-Christian Europe, the plant was associated with romance and male vitality, and the Celtic Druids believed it possessed magical powers to protect and heal. Perhaps because of its pagan associations, mistletoe is also said to have been used for the cross of Jesus and for that reason was doomed to depend on other plants for its survival.

MEDICINAL USE

Although highly toxic, mistletoe species have a long history of use in traditional medicine. European mistletoe (*Viscum album*) has been used externally to treat varicose veins and leg ulcers.

Native Americans used *Phoradendron leucarpum* externally in steam baths and in infusions rubbed on the body to treat numbness and painful limbs and joints. An infusion of *P. californicum* was rubbed on sores, and crushed *P. juniperinum* plants were used for arthritis. Traditionally, species of *Arceuthobium* have been used to treat joint pain, lung disorders, stomachaches, and coughs.

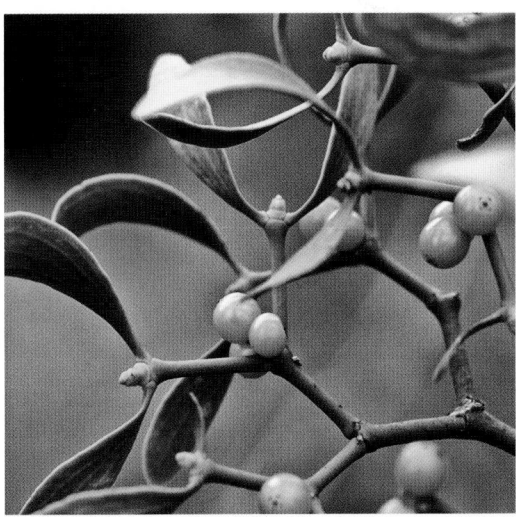

Standardized extracts of *Viscum album* are used to treat certain cancers.

Caution: All forms of mistletoe and mistletoe extracts must be used only under the direction of a qualified health practitioner. Mistletoe plants are highly toxic and the ingestion of any part—including the berries—warrants an immediate call to your local poison control center.

 HOW TO GROW IT

A parasitic plant, mistletoe is not usually cultivated. Plants used for medicinal preparations and decorations are harvested from the wild.

Vitex agnus-castus

This fragrant deciduous shrub bears showy purple flowers followed by dark, fleshy, peppercornlike fruits that are sometimes known as chasteberries. Native to the Mediterranean region and western Asia, this species has long been associated with chastity. According to the Roman scholar Pliny the Elder (23–79 CE), the fruits were placed, as a symbol of faithfulness, on the beds of the wives of soldiers going off to war. In the Middle Ages, branches of the herb were strewn on the ground as women entered convents, and monks are said to have consumed the ground dried berries to suppress their sexual urges. Even today, the flowers are used in Italian monasteries as a symbol of chastity.

MEDICINAL USE

Vitex has been used to treat female reproductive ailments for at least 2,500 years. The Greek physician Hippocrates (ca. 460–370 BCE) recommended using the herb after childbirth. About 500 years later, the Greek physician Dioscorides (ca. 40–90 CE) suggested consuming a beverage made from the plant's fruits to lower libido.

While there are no scientific studies of vitex's effect on libido, studies have confirmed the benefit of this plant for alleviating the symptoms of premenstrual syndrome, including breast tenderness, edema, tension, and constipation. Its long history of use to stimulate the production of breast milk in nursing mothers has also been confirmed by clinical studies.

Vitex has been used to regulate the menstrual cycle when there is excessive or too-frequent bleeding and to treat uterine fibroids, infertility caused by low progesterone levels, and problems associated with menopause. While vitex does not contain hormones, it does affect the pituitary gland, which has a regulating effect on hormone levels. It could be helpful in reducing hormone-related teenage acne in both genders.

Caution: Do not use vitex if you are pregnant, taking birth control pills, or receiving hormone replacement therapy.

ORNAMENTAL USE

This large, showy shrub produces a profusion of fragrant purple blooms that attract hummingbirds and butterflies. Use it as a landscape specimen, in a mixed border, or in a large container. The flowers can be harvested and dried for arrangements or crafts.

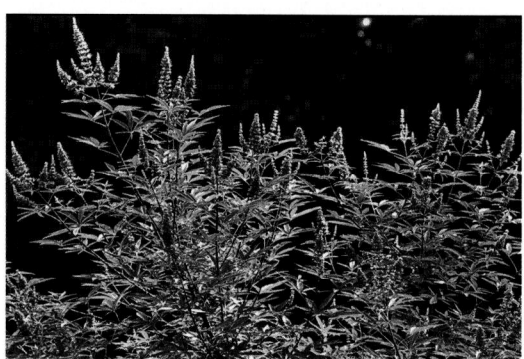

HOW TO GROW IT

Vitex is easy to grow in most any well-drained soil and full sun or partial shade. Once established, it is drought tolerant. Feed it lightly with fertilizer in spring and early summer. Prune back all bloom spikes immediately after flowering to encourage a second flush of bloom. For commercial extracts and tinctures, the ripe berries are harvested in fall and dried. Propagate by cuttings or seed; before sowing, chill the seeds for 3 months to improve germination.

Vitis vinifera

Grapes are cultivated in warm, temperate regions throughout the world. The deciduous climbing vine has a twisted trunk and bears clusters of oval to round, green to black fruits long used for food and drink.

Wine made from grapes has been tremendously important to many of the world's cultures. The earliest-known wine making is recorded through archeological findings from the Caucasus region in Europe around 8,000 years ago and in Iran around 7,000 years ago. Wine produced from grapes was a staple beverage and very important to ceremonial life in ancient Egypt at least 4,500 years ago. Grapes and wine are mentioned frequently throughout the Bible.

A recent study of important grape cultivars, using genetic mapping techniques, pinpointed the origin of *Vitis vinifera* as Georgia, in Eurasia. Most of the familiar varieties used to make modern wines originated with this species, although native North American grape species, such as *V. labrusca*,

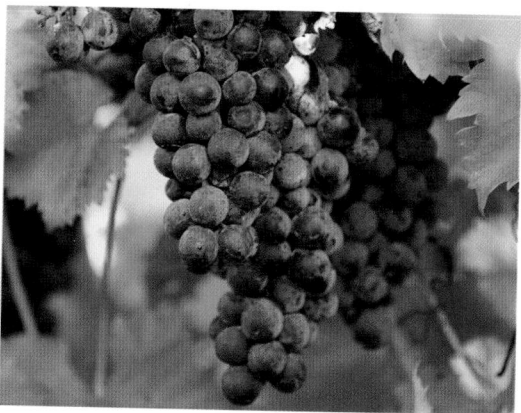

PLANT PROFILE

Common Names: Grape, Wine Grape

Description: Deciduous, woody vine, up to 12 feet long; alternate palmate leaves; inconspicuous greenish flowers

Hardiness: To Zone 7; modern crosses and varieties hardy to Zone 3

Family: Vitaceae

Flowering: Spring

Parts Used: Fruit, seeds, and leaves

Range/Habitat: Native to southern Europe and southwestern Asia

have been crossed with the European grape to make flavorful hybrids that are more cold hardy and disease resistant than the European varieties.

MEDICINAL USE

Grapes are rich in flavonoids that appear to lower the risk of heart disease. The fruits are mildly laxative, and the dried fruits (raisins) have mild expectorant properties. The skin of red grapes contains resveratrol, a strong antioxidant; both red wine and red grape juice are believed to offer antioxidant and heart-protective benefits. Grape leaves have astringent properties and may be used to treat diarrhea and varicose veins.

Grape seed contains the strong antioxidants oligomeric procyanidins (also known as procyanidolic oligomers, or PCOs). The antioxidant effects, along with the ability to bond with collagen, help promote skin health, elasticity, and flexibility, providing a more youthful appearance and possibly slowing your skin's aging. Extract of grape seed has been used to treat circulatory problems such as capillary fragility and varicose veins, and to reduce inflammation.

HOW TO GROW IT

Grape vines thrive in full sun and fertile, slightly acidic soil. The site should be well drained; the plants will not tolerate standing water. Planting on a southern slope or near the south side of a building will help ensure the plants get the warm temperatures and sunlight necessary for ripening. Each vine will require 8 feet of sturdy trellis to support the fruiting canes. Plant 1-year-old bareroot plants in spring as soon as the soil can be worked. Remove all but the most vigorous cane, then shorten the cane to two strong buds. After planting, apply balanced slow-release fertilizer on the surface of the soil around each vine; repeat monthly until early July. Proper pruning and thinning are essential, and many good books are available on the topic. Protect ripening fruits from birds with netting.

Withania somnifera

PLANT PROFILE

Common Names: Ashwagandha, Indian Ginseng, Winter Cherry

Description: Semiwoody, evergreen shrub, up to 6 feet tall; thick, grayish stems bear oval leaves and small green to yellow flowers; red berries

Hardiness: To Zone 9; grown as an annual in colder climates

Family: Solanaceae

Flowering: Summer

Parts Used: Roots, berries, and leaves

Range/Habitat: Native to India; widely naturalized and cultivated in Africa, the Middle East, and the Mediterranean region

Ashwagandha grows in the dry, stony soil of the mountains of India and countries around the Mediterranean and Africa. A small evergreen shrub, the plant bears oval leaves and inconspicuous green to yellow flowers. Its name is Sanskrit for "horse's smell," a reference to the root's strong aroma, which many say is reminiscent of a sweaty horse! The plant has tiny red berries that contain yellow seeds enclosed in a paper-thin calyx.

A very popular and important herb in India, ashwagandha is mentioned in 3,000-year-old Ayurvedic texts on health care. It is often used as a tonic, much like ginseng, although its effects are calming rather than stimulating. The species name *somnifera* refers to the herb's traditional use as a sedative.

CULINARY USE

The long, tuberous roots of ashwagandha have a bitter, sharp flavor. In India, they are used to make a tonic wine or are combined with milk, sugar, or rice to make a restorative food given to the elderly and the weak. The berries have been used as a thickener, much like rennet, for making cheese.

MEDICINAL USE

Ashwagandha is considered an adaptogen—a substance that increases immune function and helps your body cope with stress. The roots are widely used in Ayurvedic medicine to prevent premature aging and to treat age-related physical debility and impotence. Bittersweet and astringent, ashwagandha acts primarily on your reproductive and nervous systems and is believed to have sedative, anti-inflammatory, analgesic, and immune-strengthening properties. It is also considered a libido enhancer and aphrodisiac.

Animal studies have shown that ashwagandha protects the lining of your stomach and acts as an analgesic. A study with mice showed that one of its constituents significantly improved memory deficits. In other lab studies, the herb showed promise as an anticancer medicine.

Externally, ashwagandha leaves have been used to treat superficial skin wounds, sores, and inflammation. Rubbed on the skin, the leaves also reportedly repel insects.

To make ashwagandha tea, simmer 1 teaspoon of the chopped root in 8 ounces of water or milk for 10 minutes. Strain, then drink the tea once or twice per day.

Caution: Do not take this herb if you are pregnant; it can cause miscarriage when taken in large quantities. Also avoid taking it if you are taking a pharmaceutical sedative.

HOW TO GROW IT

Start the plants in a warm indoor location 10 to 12 weeks before your last frost date. Sow the seeds in flats, covering them with a thin layer of growing medium. Keep the medium moist but not saturated; germination usually occurs in 2 weeks.

When the weather is warm, transplant the seedlings to your garden or to a large outdoor container. Ashwagandha thrives in a slightly alkaline, sandy loam and full sun or partial shade. Allow the soil to dry completely before watering. In fall to early winter, when the berries turn bright red and the leaves begin to dry out, cut the stems to the ground and gently dig up the roots. Dry the roots for later use. Propagate by seed.

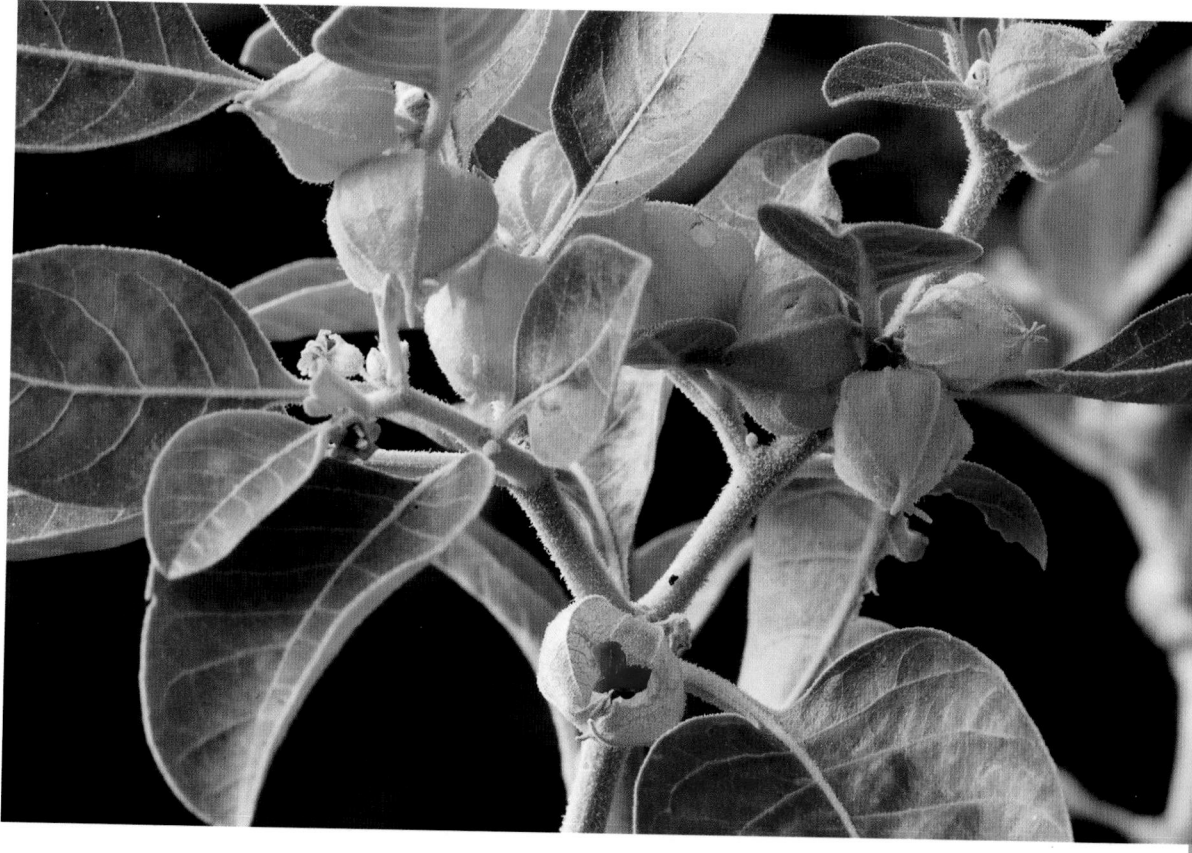

Ashwagandha for the Ages

One common name of this plant, "Indian ginseng," is quite misleading. Ashwagandha is not related to ginseng—it is not in the same plant family—nor are its adaptogenic properties entirely similar to those of ginseng. Although both ginseng (Panax ginseng) and Withania somnifera have antistress activity, the former is more of a stimulant, while the latter has sedative properties.

In my travels to India to study Ayurvedic medicine, I learned how this plant's thick root can be ground to make medicinal preparations for treating bronchitis, asthma, ulcers, insomnia, and senile dementia. Local research hospitals and clinics have conducted many animal and human trials using this herb and have obtained promising results. One year-long human study with healthy, middle-aged men showed that ingesting this root did have antiaging effects.

In Egypt, where this plant also grows, ashwagandha fruits were part of the floral collar found in the great King Tutankhamen's embalming cache—materials used in the mummification process and then buried with the body. According to the beliefs of the time, people were buried with the possessions they thought were necessary in the next world. Did King Tut consider ashwagandha so essential that he ordered its seeds to remain very close to his body so they could be planted and used for their important properties in the life to come?—M. J. B.

Zingiber officinale

The thick, pungent rhizomes of this tropical plant have been a favorite of cooks and healers for millennia. Greek bakers reportedly imported ginger from the Orient more than 4,000 years ago, and the plant has been used medicinally in Asia for at least 5,000 years. A relative of cardamom and turmeric, ginger bears long, pointed, lanceolate leaves and yellowish green flowers with deep purple lips. Botanists believe that the species is native to India. In the 1500s, the Spanish introduced ginger to the Caribbean and Central America, where it was developed as an export crop for Europe. Today, China and India are the leading commercial producers of ginger.

CULINARY USE

Ginger is essential to Asian cuisine. Fresh or dried, it flavors curries, chutneys, pickles, meat and fish

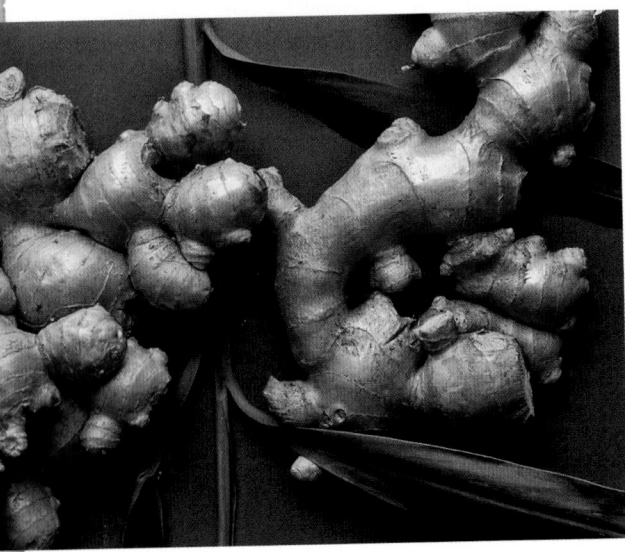

PLANT PROFILE

Common Names: Ginger

Description: Herbaceous perennial, up to 2 feet tall; grasslike leaves; 6- to 12-inch stems topped with conelike spikes of yellow-green flowers occurring between overlapping green bracts

Hardiness: To Zone 9

Family: Zingiberaceae

Flowering: Rare when cultivated

Parts Used: Rhizome and leaves

Range/Habitat: Believed native to India; cultivated throughout the tropics and subtropics

dishes, soups, and marinades. The people of India and China also combine ginger root with cinnamon to make a warming tea.

Powdered dry ginger is a popular ingredient in pies, cakes, cookies, and muffins. The grated root can be added to salads, dressings, and smoothies, as well as to cooked carrots, squash, and tomatoes. It adds a warm, spicy flavor to custard and ice cream when the milk is infused with sliced fresh ginger root. Ginger leaves impart a similar but more subtle flavor. Use them to stuff chicken, or wrap fish with them before poaching in water. Remove the fibrous leaves before eating.

Ginger oil—extracted from the freshly ground, dried rhizome—is used commercially to flavor ice cream, candy, and soft drinks (including ginger ale).

MEDICINAL USE

Ginger—a premiere remedy for easing nausea, vomiting, and upset stomach—is an important herb in many ancient traditional medicines. Ayurvedic medicine recommends eating the root daily, before afternoon and evening meals, to

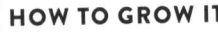

HOW TO GROW IT

Ginger thrives in well-drained, humus-rich soil in sun or partial shade. It will not tolerate freezing temperatures, but it is easy to grow indoors. Plant the rhizome in a container filled with equal parts loam, sand, and compost. Keep the pot in a warm, humid location and provide even moisture. When the weather is warm, move the potted plant outdoors to a semi-shaded location. To harvest the rhizome, remove the plant from its pot 8 to 12 months after planting. Cut off the leaves and remove the fibrous roots. Save a piece of the rhizome for replanting.

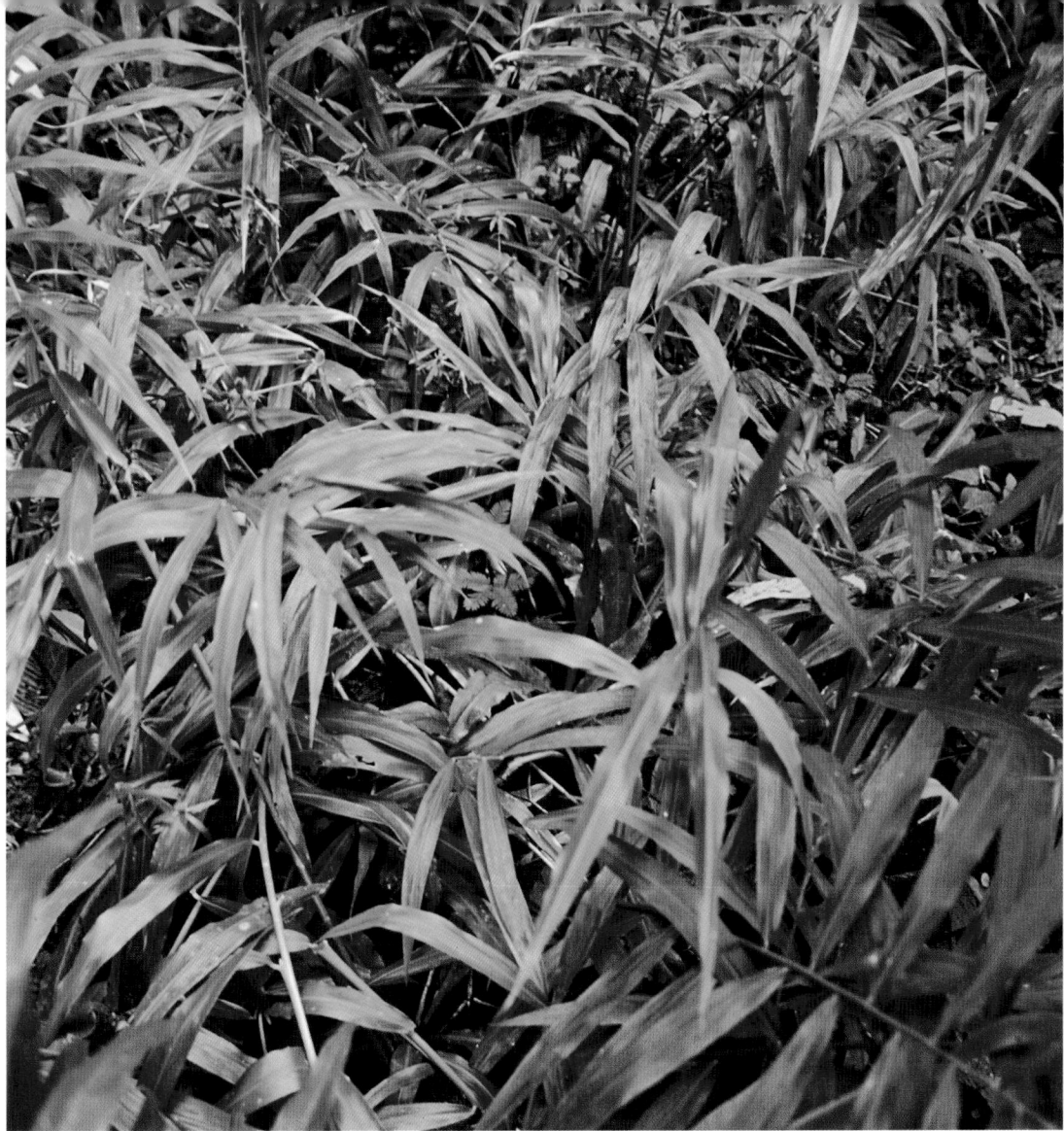

promote digestion. Traditional Chinese medicine formulas use ginger to treat stomach ulcers, stomachaches, diarrhea, and nausea.

Ginger's thick rhizomes, which contain anti-inflammatory and antiseptic compounds, can be added to soups or used to make a tea for relieving cold and flu symptoms, joint pain, and poor circulation. To make ginger tea, simmer 1 teaspoon of the chopped fresh root in 1 cup of water for 10 minutes, then strain. Or, pour 1 cup of boiling water over ½ teaspoon of powdered ginger, and steep for 10 minutes. Pour off the liquid and discard the powder. Drink 1 or 2 cups of the tea per day, or use it as a gargle to ease a sore throat.

Ginger tea is used externally, too. Hot ginger tea compresses are applied to painful or stiff joints, strains, and sprains. Cool ginger tea compresses are used to ease the pain of minor burns and rashes.

Caution: Although safe when used as a spice, ginger should not be taken medicinally during pregnancy or by those who have gallstones.

OTHER USES

Ginger oil is used as an antiseptic and fragrance in soaps, body creams, and perfumes.

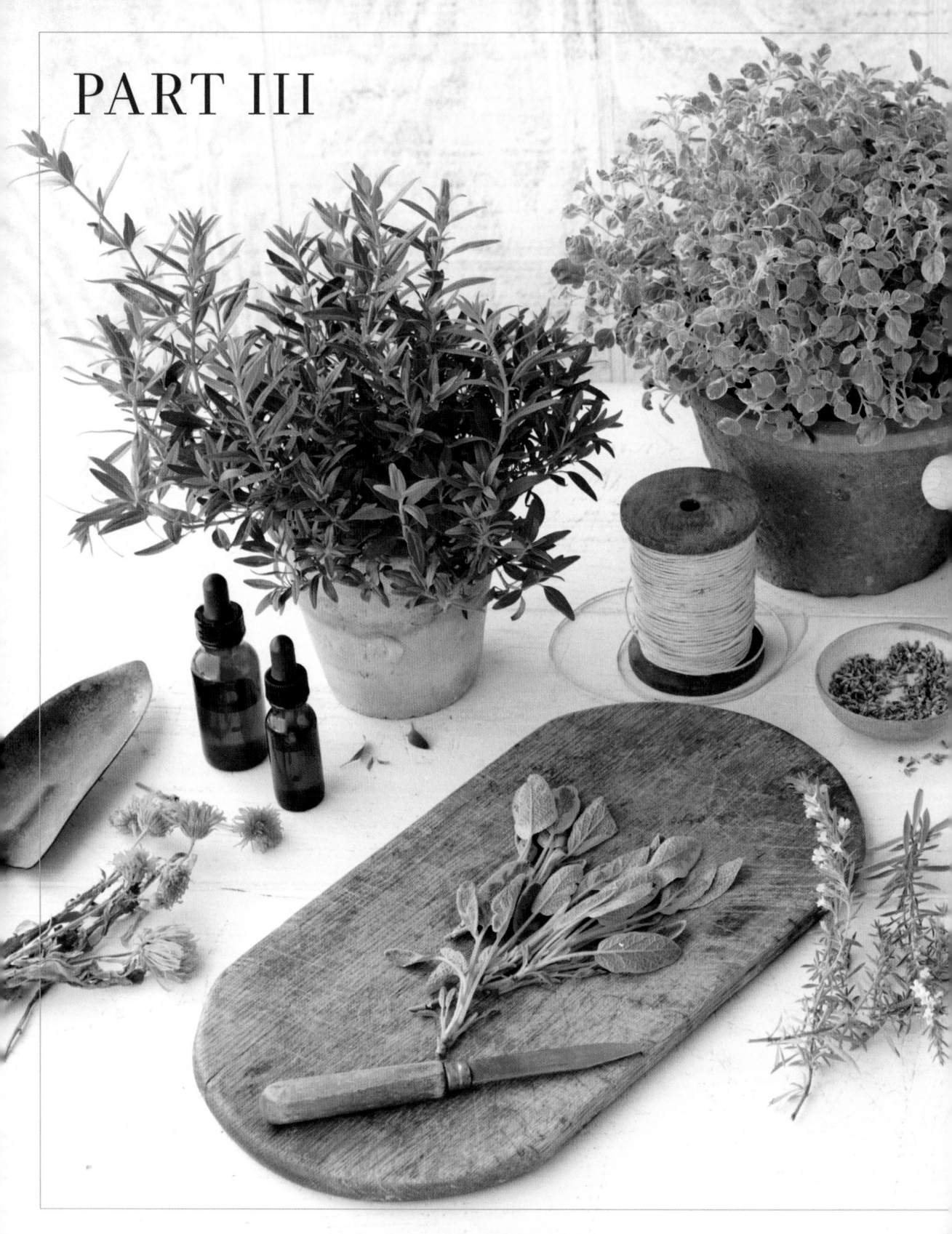

PART III

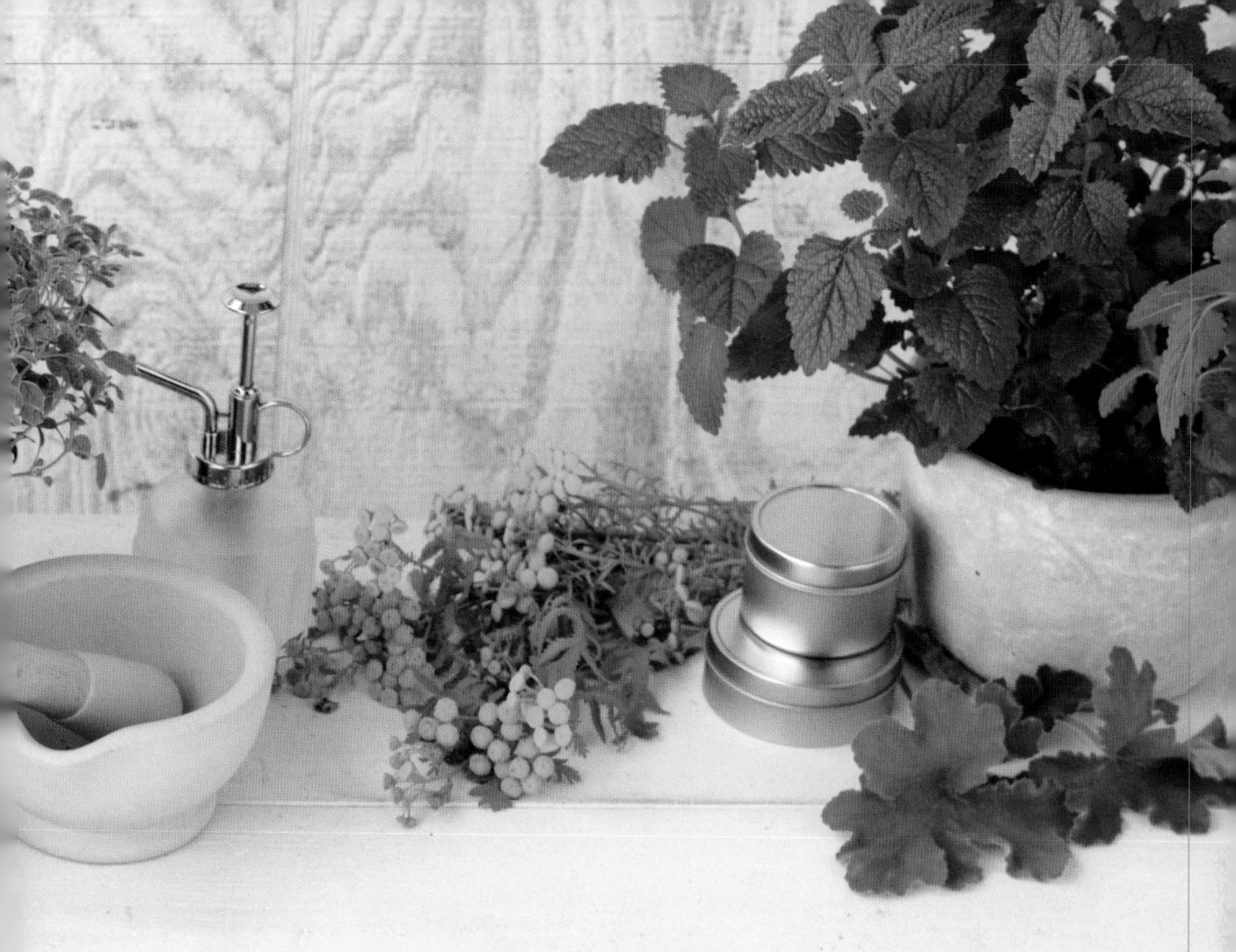

HERBS
for LIFE

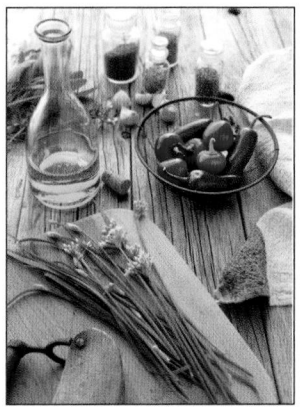

CHAPTER 4

COOKING
with HERBS

S ince the beginning of recorded history, people have added herbs and spices to their meals. Whether used to preserve food, to mask the taste of spoiled meats before the days of refrigeration, or simply to enhance the flavor of a dish, herbs and spices have always played an important role in cuisine. Although spices are technically herbs, the two terms are applied separately in cooking, according to their usage. In culinary terms, an herb generally is the leaf of a plant, and it is often used fresh. Spices, on the other hand—the seeds, roots, bark, buds, or fruits of a plant—are usually used in their dried forms.

For most of the Middle Ages, Arab traders brought exotic spices such as peppercorns, cloves, and nutmeg from Asia to Europe. Spices were so valued in medieval times that they were often used as currency. In fact, the demand for spices and the search for a shorter trade route to Asia for spices took Christopher Columbus and others across the Atlantic and led to the discovery of the New World—and its own rich array of herbs and spices. Today, it is nearly impossible to imagine certain dishes without the flavors of the herbs and spices introduced so many years ago.

HERBS AND SPICES IN THE CULINARY WORLD

Most, if not all, of the world's cultures have incorporated herbs and spices into a unique culinary signature. In Japan, for example, a seven-spice powder—which may include sesame seeds, poppy seeds, and dried chiles—is sprinkled over udon noodles and grilled chicken yakitori. In India, garam masala, an intricate blend that varies regionally, adds nuance to grilled meats. In Italy, basil and garlic mingle with olive oil, pine nuts, and Parmesan or pecorino cheese to make a delicious pesto sauce. The Middle East's signature spice, za'atar, is a blend of ingredients that includes thyme, sumac, sesame, and salt. It is used in cooking and put on hummus, as well as mixed with olive oil and sprinkled on flat bread. In Hungary, mild and piquant varieties of paprika add color and taste to goulash and other foods. On the following pages are just a few examples of the ways herbs and spices have influenced food customs around the world.

NORTH AMERICA AND THE CARIBBEAN ISLANDS

The cuisines of North America and the islands of the Caribbean are largely shaped by the tastes of Europeans, who imported the spices of Asia, combining these with local herbs. Each wave of immigration to the New World brought along the unique dishes, herbs, and spices of the immigrants' native land. As a result, the cuisine of North America and the Caribbean region blends together the flavors of the world. In the United States, the melting pot of flavors includes the spices cinnamon and paprika, as well as the herbs basil, oregano, and parsley. In Cuban cuisine, the salsalike *mojo* is made with garlic, orange juice, dried oregano, cumin, and cilantro. In the Caribbean islands, the spices nutmeg, allspice, and ginger commonly flavor stews, while the sultry spice of jerk seasoning—made with dried chiles, thyme, garlic, pepper, and allspice—infuses grilled meats.

CENTRAL AND SOUTH AMERICA

The cuisines of Central and South America were greatly influenced by European explorers of the 16th century. In Mexico, Chile, and Argentina, herbs and spices introduced by Spanish conquistadors were integrated with native dishes based on corn, beans, chiles, and cassava. Mexico's magical mole sauces commonly include chiles, cinnamon, chocolate, nuts and seeds. *Recado* spice pastes—used as rubs for pork, chicken, and fish—are made with annatto, peppercorns, cloves, cumin, oregano, and cinnamon. In Chile, *pebre* sauce, used to flavor casseroles, combines garlic, chiles, and cilantro. In Argentina, *chimichurri* sauce, made with oregano, parsley, garlic, and paprika, adds a flavorful edge to soups, vegetables, and grilled meats. Portuguese colonists and African slaves contributed much to the cuisine of Brazil. The Portuguese influence is evident in the use of herbs such as garlic and parsley along with ingredients such as

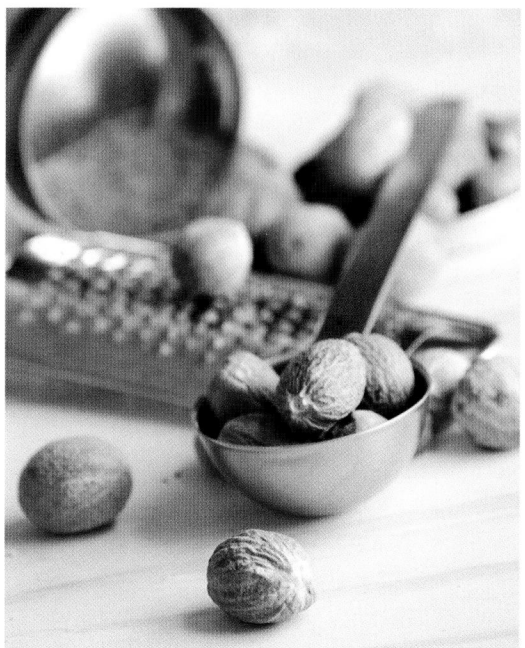

Freshly grated nutmeg—the seed of the evergreen nutmeg tree (*Myristica fragrans*)—adds a warm flavor and fragrance to beverages, sauces, stews, and desserts.

dried and salted cod, olives, wine, garlic, and onions; the African influence is evident in the extensive use of coconut, plantain, and palm oil.

NORTHERN AND EASTERN EUROPE

In the cool climates of Northern and Eastern Europe, cooks have traditionally favored the use of strongly flavored spices and warming herbs. Nutmeg, mustard seed, and cloves are frequently added to hearty soups and casseroles, stews, meat pies, dumplings, and pickled and cured fish. In warmer months, fresh herbs such as dill, stinging nettle, and tarragon help lighten the flavor of heavy fare. In Scandinavia, fresh dill and juniper berries are key additions to pickled herring. In Ukraine, the classic relish *hrin* combines grated horseradish, red beets, vinegar, and sugar. In Ger-

many, caraway is used in sauerkraut, breads, and cheeses, and in Poland, bay leaf is used to flavor *bigos*, a traditional hunter's stew.

THE MEDITERRANEAN REGION

Mediterranean cooking is best known for its use of fresh herbs, such as sage and tarragon. The cuisines of southern Italy and France draw heavily upon fresh basil, oregano, and rosemary, while Portuguese dishes feature the use of garlic, coriander, and parsley. In Greece, dried oregano and thyme find their way into dishes ranging from fish and stuffed vegetables to the layered moussaka, while in Spain, saffron elevates paella from a humble rice and seafood dish to a culinary tour de force. *Herbes de Provence*, a common Mediterranean blend often used to flavor roasted meats, features basil, fennel seed, marjoram, thyme, rosemary, and savory.

THE MIDDLE EAST, NORTH AFRICA, AND EAST AFRICA

Middle Eastern, northern African, and eastern African cuisine tends to draw upon spices that passed through the region while being transported to Europe and the West from the Far East. Iranian dishes often call for the addition of luxurious aromatics, such as rose and saffron. Cinnamon is a key ingredient in Moroccan harina, a lentil and tomato soup. Ethiopia's currylike stews echo the flavors of the Middle East and India and often feature a spice mix called *berbere*, which includes cloves, dried chiles, and fenugreek.

EAST AND SOUTHEAST ASIA

The cuisines of China, Japan, and Korea have three spices in common—garlic, ginger, and sesame seed—yet each remains distinctive. Korean cuisine, the spiciest of the three, is characterized by the use of chiles, garlic, and ginger, such as in kimchi, a pickled cabbage condiment. China's cuisine varies in flavor by region, from the intense pungency of Sichuan preparations (which typically use dried chiles and garlic) to the subtle flavors of the lower Yangtze Plain (which incorporate ginger). The cooking of Japan is the most austere, with sesame seed, ginger, or wasabi root used to add dimension and decoration to pristine presentations of singular items such as raw fish or grilled beef.

INDIA AND SOUTH ASIA

This region is home to many of the world's most beloved spices, such as peppercorn, star anise, garlic, and ginger. Blends such as curry powder, which combine many of these spices, are an integral part of the region's cuisine. Recipes for curry powder vary widely, not only by locale, but also from family to family. In northern India, two spice blends are quite common: garam masala and *chaat masala,* which include cumin, fennel seed, and cardamom. In southern India, another common blend consists of as many as 20 ingredients, including coconut and tamarind. Indonesian cuisine draws heavily from galangal and lemongrass. The foods of Malaysia are often flavored by *sambal bajak,* a condiment comprised of chiles, tamarind, galangal, garlic, and kaffir lime leaves. Vietnamese *pho,* a traditional noodle dish, is flavored with cilantro, Thai basil, lemon or lime, and chiles. In Thailand, the most important flavoring agents include cilantro, basil, garlic, and ginger.

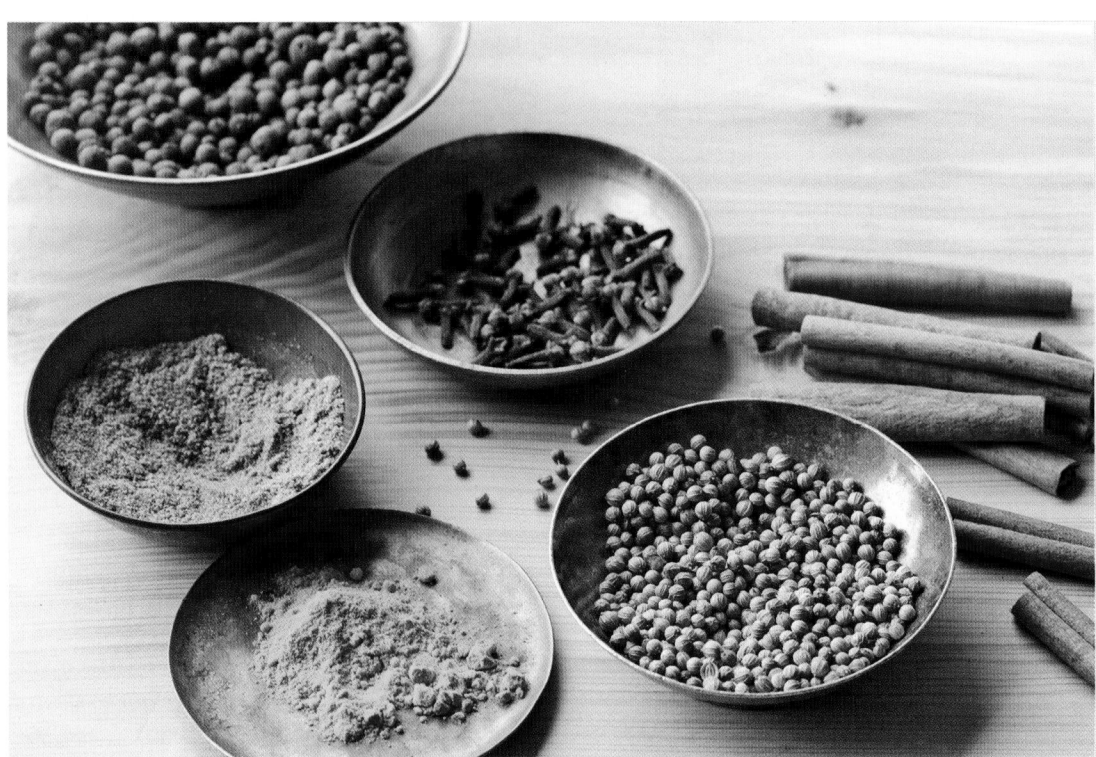

Richly flavored spices, such as (clockwise from top right) cinnamon, coriander, turmeric, cardamom, black pepper, and cloves, are at the heart of many Asian cuisines.

AUSTRALIA AND THE SOUTH PACIFIC

In Australia and New Zealand, influences from British colonists and Southeast Asian immigrants combine with Mediterranean flavors. Ingredients traditionally used by native Aborigines, including Tasmanian pepper leaf, hibiscus flowers, and purslane, are also beginning to find their way onto restaurant menus. In the South Pacific, the cuisine of the islands of French Polynesia has been influenced by the flavors of Asia and North and South America, as well as by colonial Europe. Popular dishes range from French-inspired foie gras with vanilla bean to ginger-laden chow mein to fish salad with cilantro.

HERBS AND SPICES IN THE KITCHEN

At one time, because they came from so far away, were often carried at risk of life and limb, or were very hard to grow or collect, many spices and herbs were too expensive and precious to use on a daily basis. Today they are affordable and are an integral element of contemporary cooking. Incorporating these flavors into marinades, main dishes, desserts, and even beverages allows the cook to utilize some of the finest tastes that the world has to offer and to create meals that allow us to travel around the globe simply by opening a kitchen cupboard or stepping into a garden.

As with any culinary ingredient, knowing a few basics will allow you to make the best use of herbs and spices. Here's how to select, store, and preserve them.

SELECTING HERBS AND SPICES

Herbs and spices get their aromas and flavors from essential oils and oleoresins, present in the plant's fresh and dried states. These oils are fragile and dissipate over time, making it critical to purchase the freshest herbs and spices available from grocers whose herbs and spices sell quickly and are replaced often. You can test the properties of essential oils by leaving a teaspoon of cinnamon out on a plate for a week and then comparing its aroma and flavor to that of the spice still in the bottle it came from.

When purchasing fresh herbs, look for healthy, unblemished leaves that are vibrant in color and not bruised, yellowed, or browning. They should be fragrant, especially when rubbed between your fingers. If you are purchasing dried herbs from a bulk bin, evaluate them for both color and aroma before buying. Their perfume should be deep and heady, not musty.

When purchasing dried spices, check for an aroma that is vivid and rich. To test whole spices, break off a piece of the stick or scrape off some of the nut and examine its color and fragrance. For ground spices, check the packaging date on the bottle or jar. It is generally best to buy dried herbs and spices in tightly sealed bottles. Self-serve bulk bins or packaging made of cardboard and cellophane allow oxygen to reach the herb, causing its fragrance and flavorful essential oils to deteriorate.

STORING HERBS AND SPICES

Fresh herbs have a limited shelf life—some last only a few days before wilting and losing their potency. To maintain their flavor and fragrance for as long as possible, store them in a plastic bag in the crisper section of your refrigerator. Tender leafy herbs such as basil, chervil, and cilantro can be wrapped in a damp—but not wet—paper towel and then placed in a plastic bag to prevent wilting.

Keep them in a moderately cool area of your refrigerator, such as in the door or on a top shelf. Herbs that have been packaged with their roots, such as basil, can be kept in a glass on the kitchen counter. Add just enough water to cover the roots and be sure to change the water every day or two to keep the herbs as fresh as possible.

Store dried herbs in a cool, dark, dry place such as a pantry or cupboard rather than in a kitchen spice rack, where they could be exposed to heat or sunlight. Check dried herbs and spices every 6 months, and discard any that are dull in color and fragrance or that do not release essential oils when they're crushed between your fingers, grated, or broken in half.

PRESERVING HERBS AND SPICES

Modern cooks can incorporate some of the world's finest flavors when preparing marinades, main dishes, desserts, and even beverages to create delicious and healthful meals. Simply by opening a kitchen cabinet or stepping into your garden you can gather the flavors of far-away places to prepare authentic dishes from around the globe.

Drying Herbs

Drying is one of the easiest ways to preserve herbs for future use in cooking. Several techniques can be used. (For drying whole flowers or stems, see page 394.)

Air Drying

Hanging: For centuries, people have dried herbs by tying them in bunches and hanging them upside down. Over time, the herbs gradually lose their moisture and become brittle. They remain flavorful, however, because the plants' essential oils remain in their leaves.

The best herbs to air-dry are sturdy, low-moisture plants, such as bay, lavender, oregano,

rosemary, sage, thyme, and winter savory. Always work with newly harvested plants. Use a rubber band, string, or twine to tightly fasten together several stems at their ends. (Keep in mind that as the stems shrink during drying, the rubber bands will tighten around them, while string may need to be retied periodically.) Bundle large-leafed, tender herbs loosely to speed drying and retain color.

To shield the drying herbs from light and dust, fasten a paper bag around the bunched herbs; puncture the bag with small slits for air circulation. Hang the bunches upside down in a dark, dry place where air can flow freely around them: from a rafter, ceiling hook, or on a rack. Do not hang them near a stove or furnace, as heat will speed the breakdown of the herbs' essential oils, affecting

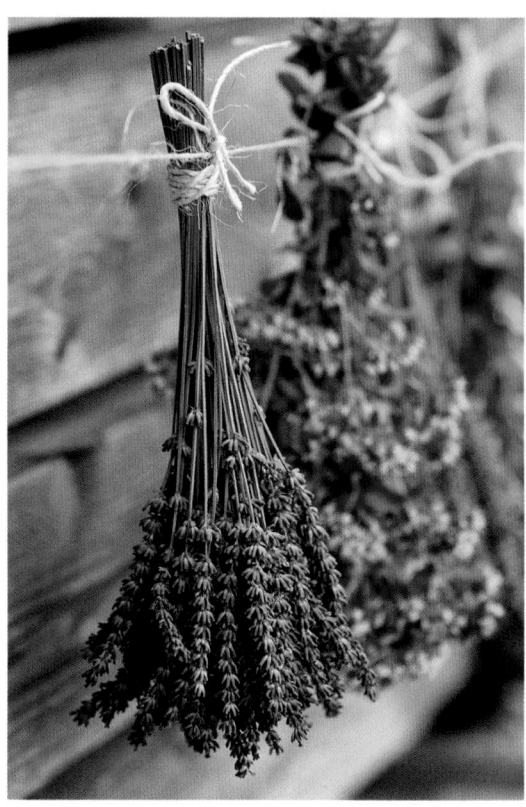

When air-drying herbs such as lavender, choose a well-ventilated and shady spot so they will dry thoroughly.

their flavor. Try not to dry your herbs in a garage where chemicals or engine exhaust will affect their flavor or add toxic elements.

To dry herb seeds (caraway, coriander, dill, and fennel, for example), put the almost-ripe seed heads into paper bags, keeping different varieties in separate bags. Handle the heads carefully, as seeds fall out easily when ripe. Hang the open bags in a well-ventilated spot for 2 or 3 weeks, until the seed heads are dry and papery. Then spread the heads on paper or a tray covered with very fine mesh screening (available at hardware stores), and rub or shake them to separate the seeds from the chaff. Label and store the seeds in airtight jars.

Trays: Herbs can also be air-dried on trays. This approach works especially well for drying tender leaves, such as those of basil and lemon balm, and for drying herb roots, bark, and stems. Spread short-stemmed herbs or individual leaves in a single layer on racks or screens. An old window screen can be used, or make a drying tray by stretching steel screening or cheesecloth over a wooden framework. (Do not use galvanized metal screens; some plant acids can react with them to form toxic compounds.) You can stack the trays, placing a wooden block or other spacer at each corner to allow air to circulate between them. Keep the trays in a warm (not hot), dry, dark place until the leaves become brittle.

To dry the roots, bark, and sturdy stems of plants such as ginger, ginseng, horseradish, licorice, and marshmallow, first clean the plant parts; do not peel the roots. Chop, slice, or shred the roots and stems into small pieces; they can become extremely hard once dried, making them difficult to cut or grind later. Lay the plant parts on racks and turn them periodically until they are dry; this can take 2 to 3 weeks. When thoroughly dried, roots and stems become light and brittle. Store them in airtight tins or in opaque or amber glass jars.

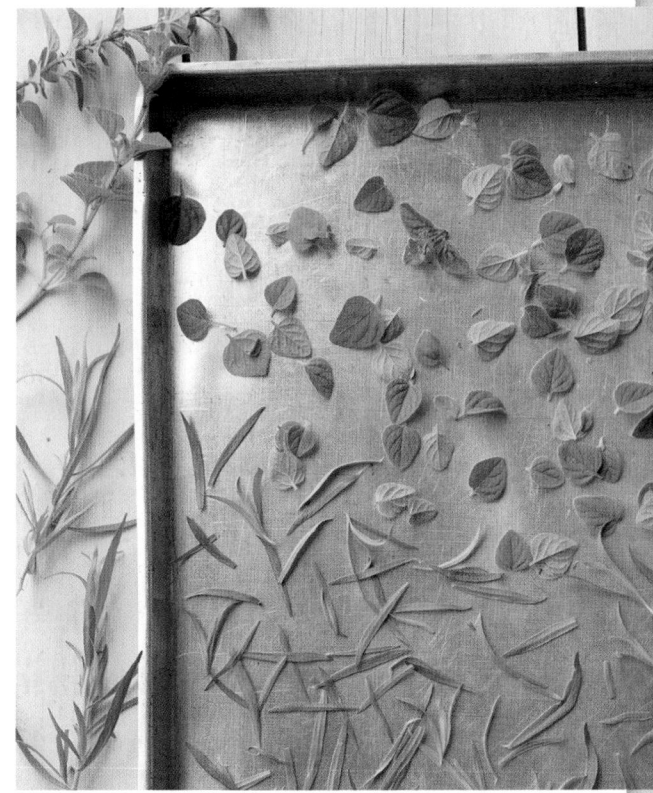

When drying herbs such as tarragon and oregano in a warm (90°F) oven, check them after 2 hours. If they are not completely dry, return them to the oven.

Oven Drying

To accelerate the herb-drying process, add heat. But proceed carefully; heating herbs too much or too quickly can cause the loss of essential oils, aromatic compounds, and flavor. Oven drying works great for lavender, oregano, rosemary, sage, thyme, basil, summer savory, parsley, lemon balm, mints, and tarragon. To speed-dry herbs using an oven, first clean the herbs and spread them on a cookie sheet or drying rack. Remove larger-leaved herbs (like basil, lemon balm, sage, and mints) from their stems and dry only the leaves.

Place the sheet in the oven, set at its lowest possible temperature, for up to several hours. Check the herbs every half hour and remove them when

To test the dryness of herbs, bend a leaf in half. If it cracks and crumbles, it is completely dry. If it bends, folds, or has a leathery feel, it still contains moisture and should be dried further.

Herbs can also be tested for moisture by sealing a small quantity of dried herbs in an airtight jar. After a day or two, check the contents. If condensation has formed inside the jar, the herbs are still moist and need to be dried for a longer period. It's important to dry herbs completely because those stored with even a small amount of moisture will develop mold and spoil. If mold is visible at any point, discard the entire batch of herbs.

---

they are dry. It may not be possible to set older gas ovens to a low enough temperature, so try drying herbs in these ovens using the heat from the pilot light. Roots and tough stems can be dried at 120°F. Check the herbs regularly to make sure they do not blacken and shrivel.

Microwave Oven Drying

Another way to speed-dry herbs is by putting them in a microwave oven. First, remove the leaves from the stems. Spread a single layer of the leaves on a paper towel–covered plate, so that the leaves are not touching, then transfer the towels to a microwave oven. Microwave the leaves for 1 minute, using a low power setting, and then check them. If they are still fairly moist, microwave again for 20 seconds. If necessary, continue heating the leaves for 20-second intervals until they are crisp but not burnt. It might take a few trials to get this process right. Cool the leaves on a baking rack, then store them in airtight containers.

Dehydrators

Dehydrators are appliances that blow warm air over foods, removing their moisture. Arrange herbs in a single layer on each tray of the dehydrator, and set the device to 90° to 100°F. Do not set the temperature higher, as the oils in the herbs may dissipate. The herbs will dry within several hours.

Freezing Herbs

One of the simplest and quickest ways to retain the flavors of herbs and spices for culinary use is to freeze them. The herbs best suited for freezing are tender-leaved plants with fleeting flavors: basil, chervil, chives, cilantro, dill, lemon balm, lovage,

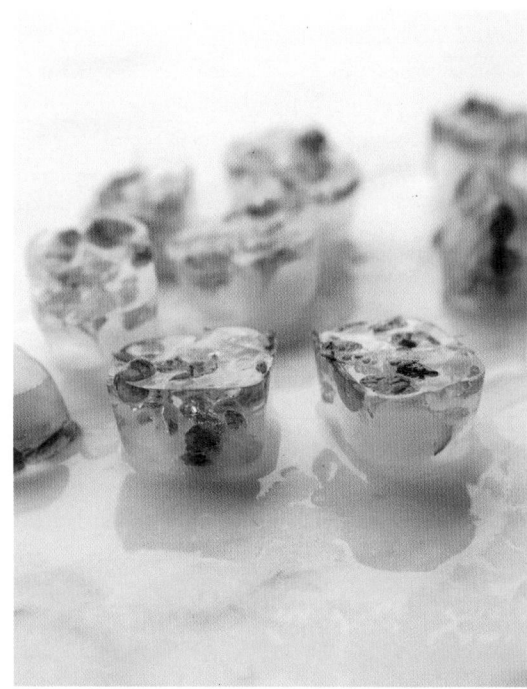

Add frozen herb cubes made with fresh herbs such as parsley, chives, or basil to winter sauces and soups for fresh summertime flavor.

marjoram, most mints, parsley, savory, sorrel, sweet cicely, sweet fennel, tarragon, and some thymes.

Freezing Herb Cubes

Frozen herb ice cubes are easy to make and useful to have on hand in your kitchen. They work well as flavorings in soups, stews, sauces, and braised dishes. To make herb cubes, chop fresh herb leaves to the desired texture, and then divide them among the sections of an ice cube tray. Add just enough water to cover the chopped leaves, then place the tray in the freezer. When the cubes are frozen solid, remove them from the tray and store them in the freezer in zipper-lock bags labeled with the herb type and date. Use them within 3 months for the freshest flavor.

You can use the same method to freeze edible herb flowers (from plants such as anise hyssop, basil, borage, lavender, mint, scented geraniums, and violets). These herbal ice cubes make spectacular additions to drinks.

Freezing Herbs in Oil

Herbs and spices are commonly used in dishes that also contain oils: dressings, marinades, dips, and spreads. An excellent way to retain the powerful flavors of fresh herbs is to mix them with oil and freeze them, creating a sort of frozen pesto. In a blender or food processor, puree 1 cup of loosely packed clean herb leaves (basil, dill, lovage, marjoram, oregano, or tarragon, for example) with ¼ cup of olive oil or another mild oil, such as canola. Freeze the puree in labeled containers or zipper-lock bags.

Herb Salts and Herb Sugars

Both salt and sugar are age-old herbal preservatives, as they inhibit the growth of bacteria. A traditional method of preserving herbs for cooking is to salt cure them. In a container, place alternating layers of chopped or whole herbs and noniodized coarse-grade or regular table salt. Make sure each herb layer is completely covered with salt. Seal the mixture in an airtight container such as a glass jar or plastic tub. After a week or so, sift out the herbs.

The salt will have drawn the moisture from the leaves and absorbed some of their essential oils, creating both a seasoning salt and crisp, dried herb leaves for cooking. Thin-leaved herbs such as dill, marjoram, rosemary, savory, tarragon, and thyme dry well with salt.

Herb-flavored sugars make a perfect addition to teas, icings, or other sweet foods that will showcase but not overwhelm their subtle fragrance and flavor. Herbs that combine well with sugar include lavender, lemon or bee balm, lemon verbena, mint, orange or lemon zest, and rose- or lemon-scented geraniums. Tightly wrap 3 tablespoons of chopped fresh herbs in a piece of cheesecloth. Bury this bundle in a jar filled with ¾ pound of granulated sugar. Or, you can simply layer herb leaves in a jar of sugar, covering each layer completely with sugar. Leave the mixture for 2 weeks to let the flavor permeate the sugar. Stir occasionally to prevent clumping and distribute the flavor. Remove the cheesecloth bundle or sift out the loose herbs. Seal the jar tightly to retain the herbs' fragrance and flavor.

Candied Herbs

The process that captures the beauty and flavor of fresh herb flowers and leaves, creating ethereal additions to cakes and other sweets, is referred to as candying. Be sure to candy only organically grown edible flowers and leaves. Good choices for candying include lemon verbena, mint, and scented geranium leaves, as well as borage, violet, and rose blooms.

To make these garnishes, select and then set aside several unblemished blossoms or leaves. Lightly whisk an egg white and strain it through a sieve. Hold one blossom or leaf with a pair of tweezers, and use a fine-bristled watercolor paintbrush to apply a coating of egg white. Next, dip the blossom or leaf into superfine (not confectioners') sugar. Lightly sprinkle more sugar on top. Gently shake off the excess sugar and let the herb dry for 4 to 8 hours on a tray lined with parchment paper. Candied herbs will last around 3 months if they're stored in an airtight container at room temperature.

USING HERBS IN COOKING

From pastes to rubs, herbs contribute fresh flavors and aromas to a wide variety of dishes, including grilled meats and seafood, soups, salads, and baked goods.

COOKING WITH FRESH HERBS

Herbs can be used fresh or dried, chopped, whole, pureed, or ground. Using whole herbs is perhaps the easiest way to put them to work. By simply adding a sprig or whole leaf to a sauce, soup, or pan of meat or vegetables, you can impart a delicate flavor into the dish. This method of using fresh herbs in cooking is called "infusion." Whole herbs are generally removed prior to serving.

If more intensity is needed from herbs, they can be torn, chopped, minced, or ground into a paste. Of these forms, a paste contributes the most powerful flavor to a dish. Torn, leafy, tender herbs, such as fresh basil or cilantro, will supply a soft, nuanced flavor that is more intense than an infusion (since the herbs are being consumed) yet less concentrated than chopped herbs. Torn herbs can be tossed in salads or sprinkled on vegetables and meats as an edible garnish. Chopping and mincing herbs completely integrates them into a dish, imparting a fuller, richer flavor with each bite. Chopped herbs can also add color and texture to food.

When using fresh herbs as an ingredient, be sure to add hardy, slower-cooking herbs, such as ginger, thyme, rosemary, and bay leaves, at the beginning of the cooking process. This allows time for their flavors to be released. More tender herbs, such as basil, tarragon, and parsley, should be added at the end of cooking to preserve their delicate flavors. To prepare tender herbs for cooking,

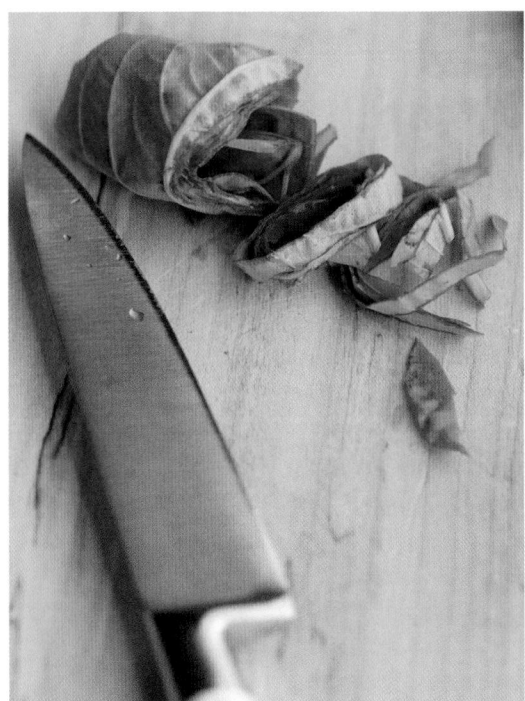

To chiffonade fresh basil or other fresh, leafy herbs, rinse the leaves and pat them dry. Stack six to eight of the leaves, then gently roll them into a tight cylinder. Hold them firmly and, using a sharp knife, cut the cylinder into thin strips, each about ½ inch wide. When the leaves are sliced and separated, you can keep them fresh for 30 minutes by placing them in a bowl of ice water.

pluck the leaves from the stems and chop them. (Basil leaves can be stacked and rolled lengthwise and then sliced into thin ribbons; see page 322.) The easiest way to remove hardy herbs, such as lavender, thyme, or rosemary, from their woody stems is to pull the needles or buds in the opposite direction of their growth.

COOKING WITH DRIED HERBS AND SPICES

Dried herbs and spices can be convenient for cooking with because they can be stored for up to 12 months in a cool, dark, dry place. When dried, fresh herbs lose water (this loss can constitute as much as 90 percent of their weight), which evaporates during the drying process. The herb's essential oils become more concentrated, which means that a more intense (but not as fresh) flavor is imparted. When substituting dried herbs for fresh, use about half the amount required for fresh herbs. If the dried herbs are finely ground or pulverized, further reduce the substitution to one-third as much as fresh.

Hardy herbs such as rosemary, lavender, thyme, and oregano are fine to use dried. It is best to add them to a dish during the early stages of cooking or during initial preparation; for example, sprinkle lamb with dried oregano prior to roasting, or add dried thyme to onions as they cook in a skillet. With the exception of dried sage, most leafy, tender herbs are best used in their fresh state, rather than dried. Tender herbs, such as basil, tarragon, and parsley, lose much of their distinctive flavor when dried.

Dried herbs and spices can be used whole or ground. As with whole fresh herbs, whole spices infuse flavor into a dish. They can be placed in a tea ball, wrapped in cheesecloth (see page 331), or added whole to a dish. Saltwater brines (salt dissolved in a large quantity of water), used to tenderize pork or poultry prior to cooking, can benefit from the addi-

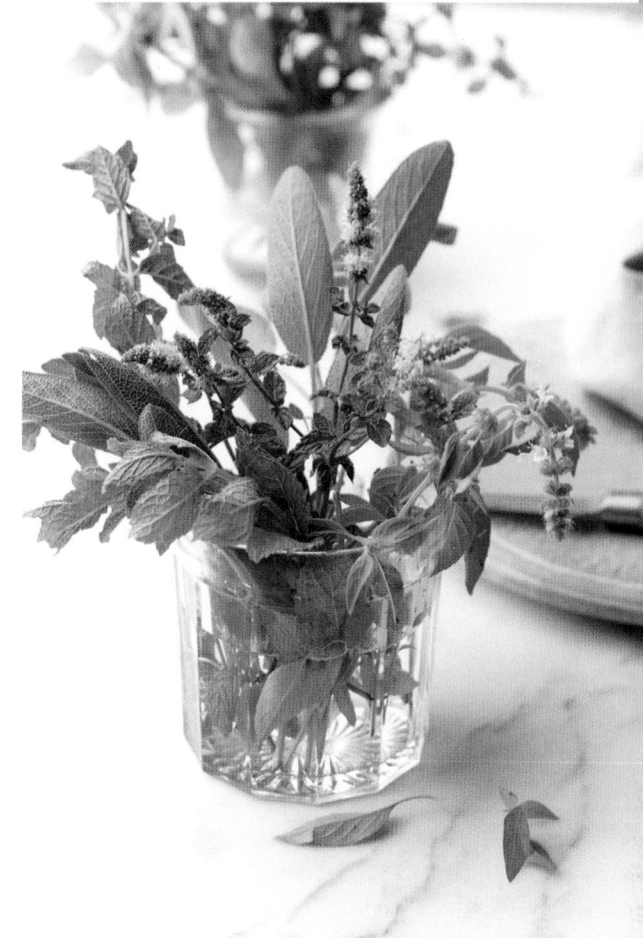

To store fresh herbs that will be used within a day or two, such as sage or mint, stand them up in a glass of cool water on your kitchen counter or windowsill, or in your refrigerator.

tion of whole spices such as allspice, clove, and peppercorn. Whole spices can also be sautéed with butter or oil to add flavor and crunch to puddings, pilafs, and stir-fried vegetables.

Ground spices are used to add an extra layer of intensity to a food's flavor. To grind spices, a coffee mill comes in handy. (Many cooks have one mill specifically for grinding spices, in addition to one for grinding coffee.) Other options for grinding large, whole spices, such as nutmeg and

CREATING HERB *and* SPICE BLENDS

Many types of cuisine use traditional herb or spice blends, which are generally prepared ahead of time and stored for future use. Curry powder, used in many of India's stews and braises, can contain more than 20 different spices. The French-inspired blend *herbes de Provence*, which can contain basil, fennel seed, marjoram, thyme, summer savory, sage, rosemary, and lavender, is used to flavor roasted meats, soups, and sauces. Italian food so frequently uses a combination of basil, marjoram, oregano, and thyme that creating a ready-to-use custom blend can be a real time-saver.

To create your own ready-to-use herb and spice blends, simply mix together the selected crushed spices and dried herbs. Experiment with different proportions to suit your taste. Store your blends in labeled, dated spice jars or resealable plastic bags. Here are eight classic combinations to get you started.

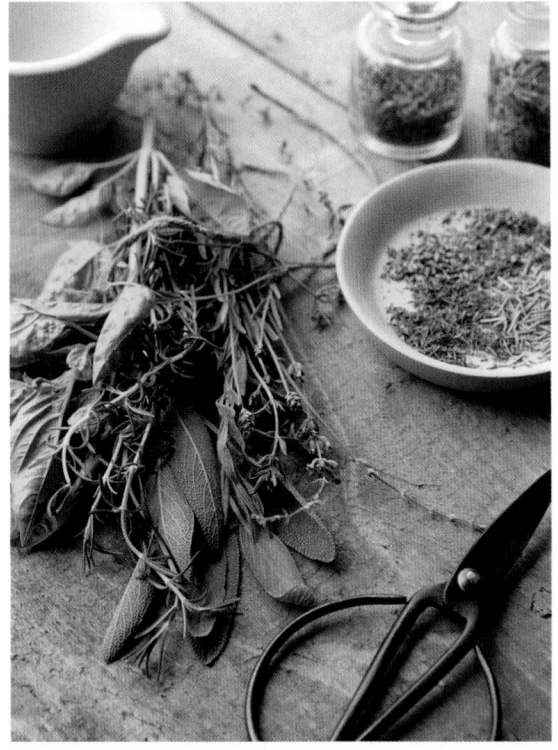

BLEND	ORIGIN	HERBS AND SPICES
Alino	Chile	Lemon balm, marjoram, oregano, rosemary, sage, spearmint, tarragon, and thyme
Berbere	Ethiopia	Ajowan, allspice, black peppercorns, cardamom, cinnamon, cloves, coriander, cumin, dried chiles, fenugreek, ginger, and nutmeg
Chili powder	North and Central America	Cloves, coriander, cumin, dried chiles, garlic, oregano, and paprika
Five-spice powder	China	Cinnamon, cloves, fennel seed, Sichuan peppercorns, and star anise
Garam masala	India	Black pepper, caraway, cardamom, cinnamon, cloves, coriander, cumin, dried chiles, fennel seed, mace, and nutmeg
Herbes de Provence	France	Basil, fennel seed, lavender, marjoram, rosemary, sage, summer savory, and thyme
Italian herb blend	Italy	Basil, marjoram, oregano, and thyme
Za'atar	Middle East	Marjoram, oregano, sesame seed, sumac, thyme

cinnamon, are a mortar and pestle, spice mill, or a microplane grater.

To coax more flavor from herbs and spices, toast them prior to grinding them. Dry-toast herbs and spices such as cumin seeds, mustard seeds, chiles, peppercorns, poppy seeds, and sesame seeds by placing them in a dry skillet (do not add fat) over low to medium heat. Shake the skillet occasionally until the spices become fragrant. In some instances, they may even crackle and pop. Immediately remove the spices from the skillet once they are toasted. Toasted spices can be used whole or, after cooling for 5 to 10 minutes, ground and used as a powder.

When it is desirable to have more flavor than whole spices can provide but less intensity than ground spices, crushed spices are an option. They can be used in infusions or to coat food prior to cooking, as in the classic French dish steak au poivre. To smash spices, place whole spices in a heavy-duty plastic bag. Use a heavy-bottomed skillet or rolling pin to crush the spices inside the bag.

COOKING WITH HERB-INFUSED OILS

One of the best ways to make use of herbs in cooking is by infusing them in oil. The aromatic compounds (essential oils) of herbs are fat soluble, so oil is an excellent medium for holding their intense essences. Herb-flavored oils have many uses in cooking: in salad dressings, as marinades, as dips for bread, to stir-fry or sauté meats and vegetables, or to drizzle on fresh tomatoes, meats, seafood, and vegetables headed for the grill.

There are three basic methods for infusing oils with herbs. In the traditional method, whole herbs are submerged in oil to flavor the oil over time. In a warm infusion, herbs are heated with oil so they rapidly release their essential oils. In a cold infusion, herbs are blanched, and then pureed with oil and later strained out.

Making herb-infused oils is not an exact science, and the quality of the infusion depends on the strength and freshness of the herbs used. Start by making small batches. When making oils for cooking, experiment to see which method and which combination of oil and herbs results in the best flavor.

If not stored properly, herb-flavored oils can become dangerous to consume because of the potential growth of food-poisoning bacteria—particularly the type that cause botulism. Be sure to label these infusions with the date they were made, store them in your refrigerator, and use them within 1 week of preparation. Refrigerated oils will thicken, but they'll liquefy again at room temperature. (You can speed the process by running the jar under hot water.)

When making herb-flavored oil, use either a high-quality olive oil that does not have an assertive, fruity taste that can overwhelm the flavor of the herbs, or use a mild-flavored oil such as grapeseed, canola, or sunflower. Herbs can also be paired with more flavorful oils, such as nut oils.

Traditional oil infusion: To use the traditional method of herb infusion to make a cooking oil, combine the desired herbs and oil in a one-to-one proportion: 1 cup (1½ ounces) of fresh herbs to 1 cup of oil. If the flavor is too weak or too strong, it can be adjusted later with the addition of oil to dilute the infusion or more herbs to strengthen the flavor of the final product.

To begin, wash a glass jar with hot, soapy water, then fill it with boiling water and set it aside for 10 minutes. Discard the water and thoroughly dry the jar, then fill it with the herb and oil mixture. To discourage the growth of bacteria, avoid overpacking the jar with herbs; be sure the herbs are submerged in the oil and that there are no air pockets. Cover the jar with plastic wrap, seal it tightly, and place it in your refrigerator. Taste the oil daily for up to 2 weeks. When the flavor is to your liking, strain out and discard the herbs. The

HERBS *for* OIL INFUSIONS

Add fresh herbal flavor to veggies and meats by stir-frying them in herb-infused oil. Or drizzle the oil over salads, breads, risotto, or other grain dishes for a delicious finishing touch. Store your prepared oils in your refrigerator for up to 1 week. Caution: Do not use garlic in herb-oil infusions; cases of botulism (caused by the neurotoxin *Clostridium botulinum*) have been linked to garlic oil. These herbs make flavorful cooking oils:

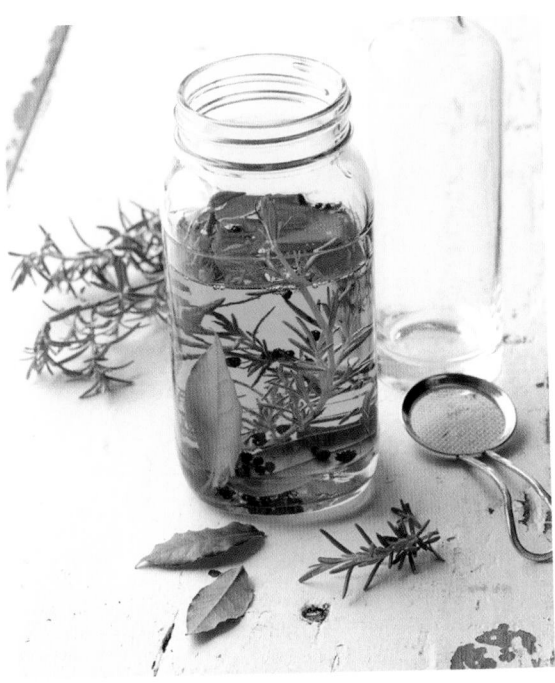

Anise seed

Basils, especially sweet, lemon, and 'Dark Opal'

Bay leaf

Chervil

Chiles

Chives

Cilantro

Dill (leaves and seeds)

Fennel (leaves and seeds)

Ginger

Lemon balm

Lemongrass

Marjoram

Mint

Oregano

Parsley

Peppercorns

Rosemary

Savory

Tarragon

Thyme

COMBINATIONS INCLUDE: Bay, peppercorn, rosemary, and thyme; bay, dill, and peppercorn; and tarragon and chiles

resulting oil will be flavorful, but it will lack the more vibrant color achieved through warm infusion.

Warm oil infusion: This method works particularly well with strong-flavored, resinous herbs such as thyme, sage, marjoram, rosemary, and savory. Prepare a jar as directed for the traditional infusion, and then heat a one-to-one mixture of herbs and oil in a heavy-bottomed saucepan over medium heat. Stir constantly until the oil starts to bubble. Lower the heat and cook for another minute, or until the oil is very aromatic. Remove the

pan from the heat and let the oil and flavorings cool. Taste the oil to make sure the herb flavor has reached the desired strength. If it's too weak, add more herbs and reheat the mixture. If it's too strong, dilute the mixture with additional oil. Strain the infused oil through cheesecloth, pour it into the prepared jar, and seal it tightly. Store the oil in your refrigerator.

Cold oil infusion: The cold-infusion method results in intensely colored and flavored oils. Quickly blanch leafy herbs by dunking them in boiling water for 5 seconds, or pour boiling water over herbs in a sieve, then immediately submerge the herbs in icy water to halt the cooking process. Blanching helps preserve the color of the herbs and gives the finished oil a lovely hue.

Thoroughly dry the blanched herbs with a paper towel, then combine a one-to-one mixture of herbs and oil in a blender or food processor. Blend or process until smooth. Pour the mixture into a wide-mouth container with a tight lid and store this mixture in your refrigerator.

Taste the oil after a week or so, and if the flavor is to your liking, run the jar under hot water to liquefy the oil. Strain the oil through a very fine sieve or a funnel lined with a double layer of cheesecloth. (You can also use a paper coffee filter that has been moistened and squeezed dry.) After straining, the oil will be ready to use.

COOKING WITH HERB PASTES

Chopped fresh herbs and ground spices are often blended with oil to create a paste that can be served as a condiment, sauce, spread, or dip. Italian pesto (basil pulverized with olive oil, Parmesan or pecorino cheese, garlic, and pine nuts) and Argentinean *chimichurri* (parsley, oregano, onion, and garlic blended with olive oil, vinegar, and cayenne pepper) are two examples. Herb pastes also can be used as a seasoning rub before cooking. Try rubbing a ham roast or lamb chops with a mixture of sage, garlic, salt, and pepper prior to cooking.

═══ PESTO'S ORIGINS ═══

Pesto alla genovese, or pesto sauce, is commonly believed to have originated in Genoa in northern Italy. But pesto (a shortened form of the Italian word *pestato*, meaning pounded) has been known in various forms since ancient Roman times, most likely originating in North Africa. A German variety uses ramson leaves (*Allium ursinum*) instead of basil.

Other simple blends such as minced garlic with basil and hot pepper flakes will have a profound effect on the flavor of shrimp or kebab-size pieces of chicken or fish. Store herb pastes, including pesto, for up to 1 week in your refrigerator. Or store meal-size quantities in zipper-lock bags in your freezer for up to 2 months.

Cooking with Herb Butter

Like oil and herbs, butter marries well with herbs including basil, chervil, chives, dill, fennel, and thyme. Float disks of herb butter on soups just before serving, or use herb butter as a spread for bread, melted on fish or vegetables, or whisked into sauces. Brightly colored flecks of chopped nasturtium or calendula petals will add a splash of color and intriguing flavor to an herbal butter.

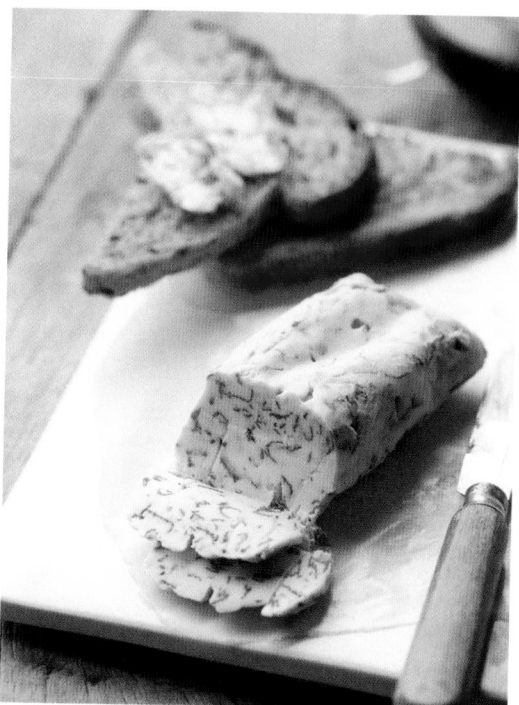

Herb butters are easy to prepare and make an elegant and flavorful addition to any table.

HERB BUTTER PAIRINGS

Just a bit of herbal butter can heighten the flavor of an ordinary dish to make it something truly special.

HERB BUTTER MIXTURES	COMPLEMENTS
Chives and garlic	Eggs, seafood, and vegetables
Cilantro, garlic, and lime zest	Beef, seafood
Mint and lemon zest	Lamb, seafood, and vegetables
Sage and orange zest	Pork
Tarragon and shallots	Beef, eggs, seafood, and vegetables

To make herb butter, finely chop dry, clean herbs. Depending on how intensely flavored and colored you want the butter to be, you'll want to use between ½ cup and 4 cups of herbs per pound of unsalted butter.

Soften the butter to room temperature and thoroughly combine the herbs and butter by hand or in a food processor. If desired, add 1 teaspoon of citrus zest or juice for each ¼ pound of butter. Minced shallots and garlic can also be added to herb butter. Store herb butter in your refrigerator, sealed in an airtight container or molded into your desired shape and tightly covered in plastic wrap. For the best flavor, use within 12 weeks.

If you shape your herb butter into a log before you chill it, you'll be able to create uniform "coins" of sliced butter. This makes for a more attractive presentation when serving. To make a ¼-pound herb butter log, place a 10-inch piece of plastic wrap or waxed paper on your kitchen counter. Beginning near the bottom center of the wrap or paper, spread the soft butter horizontally in both directions to form a 1-inch-wide band, allowing several inches to remain butter-free on each end. Next, use the wrap or paper to help you roll the butter into a tight cylinder. Twist the excess on the ends in opposite directions to seal the cylinder. Refrigerate the log until it is firm. Before serving, unwrap the cold butter and use a sharp knife to slice it into coins. At the table,

serve the butter garnished with an herb sprig or nasturtium blooms.

COOKING WITH HERB-FLAVORED VINEGARS

Herbs preserved in vinegar make a versatile, flavor-packed addition to your condiment shelf. Flavored vinegars bring piquancy and nuance to any recipe that calls for plain vinegar. Add them to marinades for meats and fish or to dressings for salads and pastas. Drizzle them on raw tomatoes or cucumbers or on cooked greens or beans.

When preparing herbal vinegars, don't use kitchen tools made of metal such as aluminum, stainless steel, or copper, because they could react with the vinegar's acids and impart an unpleasant flavor. Use glass or enamel pots for heating, wooden spoons for stirring, plastic funnels for bottling, and glass containers for storage.

A wide variety of culinary herbs can be used to flavor vinegars: For example, you could try basil, bay, chervil, chives, dill (seeds and leaves), fennel, garlic, ginger, lavender, marjoram, mint, rosemary, savory, tarragon, and thyme. For variety, add herb flowers, including borage (which will impart a blue tint to vinegar), chives, and nasturtium (include a little of the stem and leaves as well as the flowers for a more intense flavor). Combine herb flavors or pair them with fruits, such as raspberries and orange, lemon, or lime zest, or with spicy or hot elements, such as chiles, onions, and peppercorns.

Almost any variety of cooking vinegar will work as a base. However, for reasons of safety, only commercially produced vinegars, which are free of sediment and contain at least 5 percent acetic acid, which retards spoilage almost indefinitely, should be used. Distilled white vinegar is sometimes recommended for making herb vinegars, but keep in mind that its flavor is sharp and acidic and can overpower the flavors of some herbs. Wine and champagne vinegars, on the other hand, have more delicate flavors that work well with lemony herbs such as lemon thyme, lemon verbena, and lemongrass. Red wine vinegars pair well with stronger herbs, such as rosemary. Pair hearty herbs, such as garlic and chives, with robust vinegars, such as those made from apple cider and malt. Experiment with flavors, too: Combine herbs with sherry, rice, and fruit vinegars, for instance.

Other classic vinegar and herb combinations include tarragon and white wine vinegar, with or without garlic; bay, garlic, rosemary, and thyme in red wine vinegar; raspberry and thyme in white wine vinegar; chive flowers with lemon balm in white wine vinegar; and basil, chiles, and garlic in red or white wine vinegar.

To make an herb-infused vinegar, first clean the herbs and pat them dry, then place them in a clean, wide-mouth glass jar or plastic container. Most recipes call for three or four sprigs or ½ cup (¾ ounce) of coarsely chopped fresh herbs for every 2 cups (16 ounces) of vinegar. More or less vinegar can be used according to taste. In a nonreactive saucepan set over medium heat, warm the vinegar to just below boiling. Pour it over the herbs, and then stir.

To prevent the vinegar from reacting with metal lids, cover the mouth of the jar with waxed paper or plastic wrap before sealing. Place the

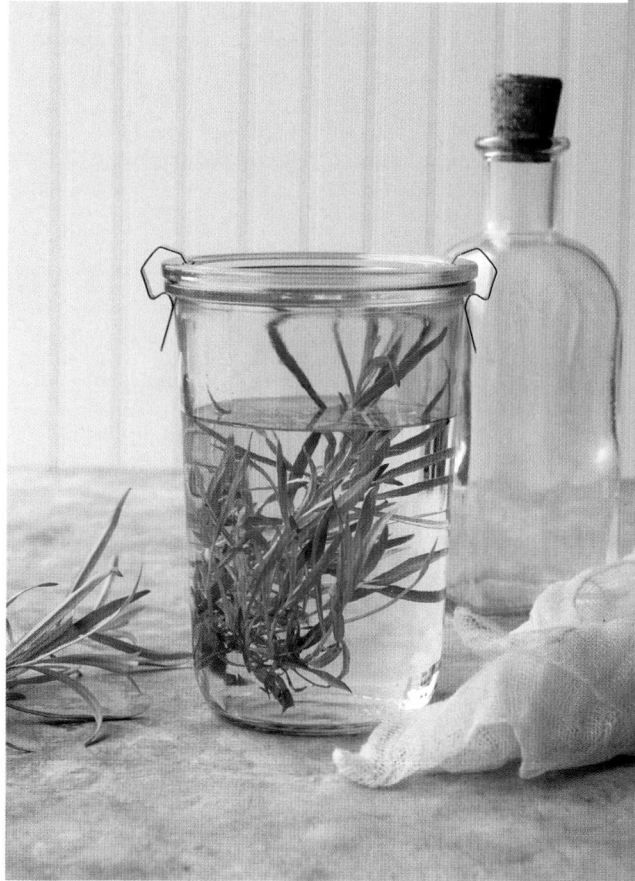

Tarragon-infused vinegar can be ready to use or give as a gift in just 1 week.

mixture in a cool, dark place for a week, then taste. If the flavor is too weak, allow it to infuse for another week or so. When the vinegar tastes right, prepare your storage jars: Wash with hot, soapy water and rinse well. Fill the jars with boiling water and let them stand for 10 minutes before discarding the water.

Next, strain the vinegar through a cheesecloth-lined funnel or moistened coffee filter into a decorative bottle or jar that has a tight-fitting, nonreactive lid. Add a decorative sprig of the herb to the mixture, if desired.

Remember to store the flavored vinegar in a cool, dark place. It will keep for about 6 months.

Do not store flavored vinegars in sunny or very hot areas; sunlight leaches flavor and makes the infusions more prone to spoiling. Bacterial growth is less of a concern with herb-infused vinegars than it is with herb-infused oils because vinegar's high acidity can retard or eliminate it. However, homemade flavored vinegars can develop mold or yeast, so immediately discard any flavored vinegars that show signs of fermentation, such as bubbling, cloudiness, or sliminess.

PAIRING FOODS WITH HERBS AND SPICES

There are many ways to pair foods with herbs. Regional cuisines tend to feature their own unique pairings. In Greece, for example, lamb is often roasted with rosemary; in India, it may be coated with a spice blend—or a masala—that includes chiles and cinnamon; in England, lamb is roasted and served with mint sauce. The chart on pages 332 to 333 shows some of the most common matches of herbs and spices with foods. Use these pairings as guidelines, or experiment to discover favorite new combinations.

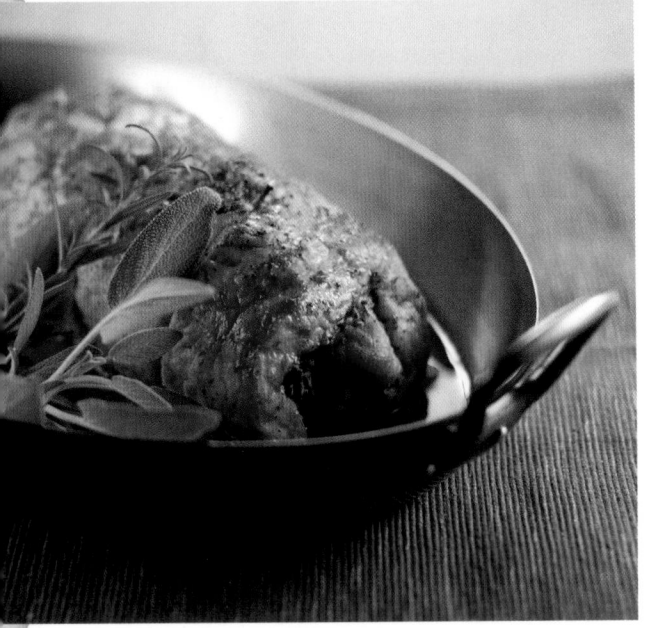

A sage-rubbed pork loin roast surrounded by sprigs of fresh sage is the basis for a tasty and festive holiday meal.

MEAT AND POULTRY

When meat and poultry are roasted or grilled with whole herbs, the heat of cooking transfers flavor from the herbs to the meat. You can impart flavor by stuffing whole herbs and spices into a chicken's cavity, tucking them into small slivers made on the surface of meat or fish, or adding them to saltwater brines used for tenderizing meat or poultry. Herbs and spices can also be blended to form a rub that's added before roasting, grilling, or broiling meat or poultry. Dry rubs often include coarse-grained sea salt, while wet rubs combine oil with herbs to make a paste.

SEAFOOD

Though seafood is often perceived as having a delicate flavor, many varieties actually have very bold flavors that are complemented by strongly flavored herbs and spices. Whole herbs can be stuffed into a deboned fish. And herbs with sturdy or woody stems—such as rosemary and lemongrass—can act as skewers when grilling or broiling shrimp or mussels. Be sure to select woody sections stiff enough to pierce the seafood, and strip the lower leaves from the stems, but leave the tops intact. And while wooden skewers need to be soaked for around 20 minutes before using them on a grill, it is not necessary to soak herb stems.

Another excellent use for herbs is for "smoking" fish and shellfish on a grill. To do this, loosely wrap robustly flavored herbs, such as rosemary, vanilla beans, black tea, or basil stems, in a sheet of heavy-duty aluminum foil, and then poke ventilation holes in the top layer of the foil to allow steam to escape. Place the herb packet on the grill rack, along with the food being prepared, and cover during cooking.

You can also transform minced herbs and ground spices into wet or dry rubs for fish that has a steaklike consistency, such as salmon, swordfish, and tuna. The flavor of the herbs and spices will permeate the fish as it cooks on the grill, in the oven, or on the stove top.

VEGETABLES AND GRAINS

Herb and spice flavors—from subtle and delicate to bold and piquant—team up beautifully with vegetables, from eggplant to turnips, and grains, including amaranth, quinoa, and rice. Vegetables can be drizzled with olive oil and roasted with whole herbs or sautéed with dried herbs at the beginning of the cooking process. (Fresh herbs should be added at the end of cooking because their flavor is more delicate and can become bitter if overcooked.)

Rosemary stems, lemongrass, and other sturdy herbs can act as skewers when grilling or broiling vegetables. When choosing herbs for this purpose, select woody sections stiff enough to pierce the vegetables. Strip the lower leaves from the stems, but leave the tops intact.

Herbs such as basil, dill, garlic, oregano, and thyme blend well with rice and other grains to make a flavorful pilaf. Or toss couscous or cooked chickpeas with chopped fresh herbs such as bay, garlic, parsley, or spearmint just before serving.

SOUPS AND SAUCES

Herbs and spices are great natural additives to soups and sauces. A liquid can be infused with herbal flavor from either fresh whole herbs or dry

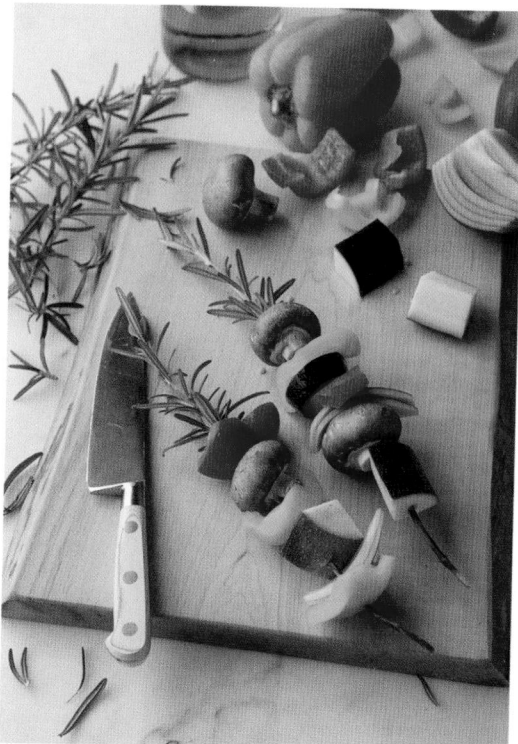

To grill vegetables on a rosemary skewer, use the stem's pointy end to pierce pieces of squash, bell peppers, mushrooms, onions, tomatoes, or other vegetables. Move each piece down toward the tip of the skewer and continue adding vegetables.

herbs in a tea ball or wrapped in a square of cheesecloth tied into a bag with twine (also known as a bouquet garni). Leave one end of the twine long and tie it to the soup pot or saucepan handle for easy removal. Let the herbs steep for a few minutes at the end of the cooking process, and remove them before serving. Sprinkle fresh herbs over the finished soup or sauce as an accent.

Also try using herb-infused oil to enhance the flavors of soups and sauces. In a skillet over medium-low heat, gently cook herbs and spices such as basil, garlic, ginger, and dried chiles in hot olive or vegetable oil. Drizzle the oil over each bowl of soup before serving, or add the oil to a sauce for an extra hit of flavor. This method works

DELICIOUS WAYS *to* PAIR FOODS *with* HERBS *and* SPICES

Generations of cooks from many cultures throughout the world have discovered that certain herbs and spices make especially good partners for different foods. Try these classic combinations, then experiment on your own.

VEGETABLES AND GRAINS

Food	Herbs	Spices
Artichokes	Basil, chives, garlic, oregano, rosemary, thyme	Cardamom, chiles
Asparagus	Chives, sage, savory, tarragon, thyme	Chiles, saffron, sesame seeds
Broccoli	Basil, curry leaves, garlic, marjoram, oregano, tarragon	Cayenne pepper, chiles, fenugreek, mustard seed
Brussels sprouts	Dill, garlic, parsley, rosemary, tamarind, tarragon	Anise, caraway, chiles, mustard seed, turmeric
Cabbage	Curry leaves, dill, marjoram, savory, tarragon	Caraway, cayenne pepper, cumin, paprika, turmeric
Carrots	Basil, chervil, chives, ginger, lemon balm, marjoram, parsley	Anise, cardamom, cinnamon, clove, coriander, cumin
Cauliflower	Basil, chives, cilantro, dill, rosemary	Caraway, coriander, cumin, turmeric
Corn	Basil, chervil, chives, cilantro, thyme	Chiles, paprika, saffron, turmeric
Couscous	Bay, garlic, parsley, spearmint	Anise, chiles, cinnamon, saffron
Eggplant	Basil, ginger, mint, oregano, parsley	Chiles, cinnamon, coriander, paprika
Green beans	Basil, dill, garlic, marjoram, savory, spearmint, thyme	Caraway, cloves, coconut, cumin, tamarind
Legumes, dried	Basil, bay, garlic, mint, oregano, parsley, rosemary, sage, thyme	Chiles, cinnamon, coriander, cumin, mustard seed, turmeric
Mushrooms	Chives, garlic, parsley, rosemary, tarragon, thyme	Coriander, cumin, nutmeg
Peas	Basil, chervil, chives, garlic, lemon balm, spearmint	Caraway, chiles, coconut, fenugreek, turmeric
Potatoes	Basil, chives, garlic, lovage, rosemary, tarragon, thyme	Caraway, chiles, cumin, mustard seed, turmeric
Rice	Basil, dill, garlic, lemon balm, oregano, parsley, thyme	Cardamom, cinnamon, clove, nutmeg, saffron
Spinach	Basil, chervil, dill, garlic, lovage, marjoram, parsley	Anise, caraway, cinnamon, nutmeg, sesame seeds
Squash	Basil, ginger, marjoram, rosemary, sage, thyme	Caraway, cardamom, cinnamon, nutmeg, star anise
Tomatoes	Basil, cilantro, lemongrass, oregano, spearmint, thyme	Chiles, coriander, mustard seeds, saffron, turmeric

MEAT, POULTRY, AND SEAFOOD		
Food	Herbs	Spices
Beef	Basil, bay, ginger, hyssop, oregano, parsley, thyme	Caraway, cumin, fenugreek, juniper, paprika
Lamb	Bay, fennel, garlic, ginger, oregano, spearmint, tarragon	Allspice, cayenne, cinnamon, cumin, saffron
Pork	Cilantro, fennel, garlic, rosemary, sage, thyme	Allspice, chiles, cinnamon, cloves, paprika, turmeric
Poultry	Basil, garlic, ginger, lovage, rosemary, tea	Allspice, cumin, fenugreek, paprika, poppy seed
Flaky freshwater fish *(catfish, perch, trout)*	Chervil, fennel, ginger, lemon balm, lemongrass, thyme	Chiles, cloves, cumin, saffron, tamarind
Firm deep-sea fish *(halibut, swordfish, tuna)*	Garlic, ginger, lemongrass, rosemary, thyme	Chili powder, cinnamon, cloves, cumin, juniper, paprika
Oily saltwater fish *(anchovies, bluefish, mullet)*	Basil, garlic, ginger, oregano, rosemary, sage, thyme	Cayenne, chiles, horseradish
Shellfish *(lobster, mussels, shrimp)*	Basil, chervil, garlic, ginger, marjoram, mint, tarragon	Chiles, coconut, mustard seed, saffron, turmeric

especially well with paprika and saffron, since they add color as well as flavor to the oil.

BAKED GOODS AND FRUIT

Both sweet and savory baked goods can benefit from the addition of herbs and spices. Rye bread with caraway seeds, gingerbread, anise biscotti, and semolina pudding with saffron and cardamom are but a few examples. When you're preparing biscuits, cakes, breads, and cookies, fresh or dried herbs (such as lavender, grated ginger, and thyme) and spices (like cinnamon, nutmeg, poppy seeds, and allspice) can be added to the dry ingredients before you mix in the wet ingredients. Spices—including cinnamon, nutmeg, and ground cloves—can also be tossed with sliced fresh fruit such as apples or peaches before you bake, roast, or grill them. Herbs and spices easily transform a simple bowl of fruit into something special. Use anise hyssop with peaches, melons, and berries; try thyme with dried fruits and pears; and accent apples and berries with rose-scented geranium.

ICE CREAMS AND CUSTARDS

Infuse milk- or cream-based desserts, such as ice cream or custard, with fresh herbal scents and flavors. To do this, bring milk or cream just to a boil, then add herb sprigs or leaves. Use four to six herb sprigs for each 2 cups of milk or cream. Cover the pan and remove it from the heat. Steep for 30 minutes, then strain out the herbs. Cool the liquid, if necessary, before using it in your recipe. Try anise hyssop–infused cream in desserts that feature apricots, currants, or peaches. Mint complements chocolate and berry-flavored custards and ice creams. English thyme makes an interesting accent for fig, pear, and cranberry flavored milk-based desserts.

HERBAL AND SPICED BEVERAGES

Teas, cocktails, fruit and vegetable juices—almost any beverage can be made even more flavorful with the addition of herbs and spices. In Spain and Mexico, cinnamon is added to rice milk to make a popular drink called *horchata*. Fresh mint- or sage-steeped tea is a trademark drink throughout the Middle East. Ground cinnamon, clove, and nutmeg are used in North America to spice apple cider. And in Central America, cinnamon gives a spicy kick to hot chocolate.

HERB-FLAVORED COCKTAILS

From Kentucky mint juleps, made with fresh mint, sugar, and bourbon, to Cuban mojitos made with rum, mint, and sugar, herb-flavored cocktails are becoming increasingly popular in restaurants and bars around the world. A Bloody Mary can be made with fresh wasabi, horseradish, or hot pepper flakes and cumin. Martinis can be flavored with herbs such as basil or lemongrass. A spice mixture applied to the rim of a glass adds a kick to a cocktail. To do this, run a damp napkin around the rim of a glass, and then dip the rim in a mix that's savory (such as celery salt) or sweet (such as ground anise mixed with granulated sugar).

HERB-INFUSED VODKAS

When herb leaves, flowers, roots, or bark are immersed in alcohol, their aromatic elements are drawn out and preserved in the liquid. Vodka—a pure alcohol and water blend that has usually been filtered through charcoal to remove flavors and

Fresh herbs can also be used for decorative purposes. Serve a cocktail garnished with sprigs of mint or lemongrass, or make a beautiful centerpiece with lavender, mint, and fresh bay leaves.

impurities—is the base for medicinal remedies called tinctures, as well as traditional beverages enjoyed throughout the Slavic and Nordic regions of Europe and Asia. Slavs combine flavorings such as cayenne pepper, ginger, various fruits, vanilla, unsweetened chocolate, and cinnamon with vodka. Ukrainians produce a commercial vodka using St. John's wort. In the Nordic region, vodka is seasoned with herbs, fruits, and spices to make drinks for traditional midsummer festivities. Sweden alone makes 40 common varieties of herb-flavored vodka, which are called *kryddat brännvin*. Russia produces vodkas that have been flavored with herbs such as aralia, which is related to ginseng, and magnolia vine, which is more commonly known as schisandra.

To make an herb-infused vodka, use a good-quality vodka that has no added color or flavor—an alcohol content of 35 to 45 percent is optimal. Place clean, chopped herbs in a jar. Pour vodka over the herbs, and store the jar in a dark place at room temperature.

Steep for 1 to 7 days, tasting every day or so to determine when the flavor has reached its peak. If the infusion is too strong, dilute it with additional vodka. If it's too weak, add more fresh herbs and allow the mixture to infuse for a few more days, or enhance the flavor by adding a bit of sugar syrup or honey.

Pour the finished vodka through a steel strainer, fine-mesh sieve, or steel funnel lined with cheesecloth. Store the liquid in a clean glass bottle or jar. To prevent oxidation, seal with a tight-fitting lid or screw cap. Store it in the freezer to preserve the flavor.

You can even combine several different infusions to create a tasty blend. Steep each herb individually, then mix the resulting infusions. For example, dill blends well with coriander, rosemary blends with peppermint, and lemon balm blends with tarragon.

Or make your own herbal liqueur starting with

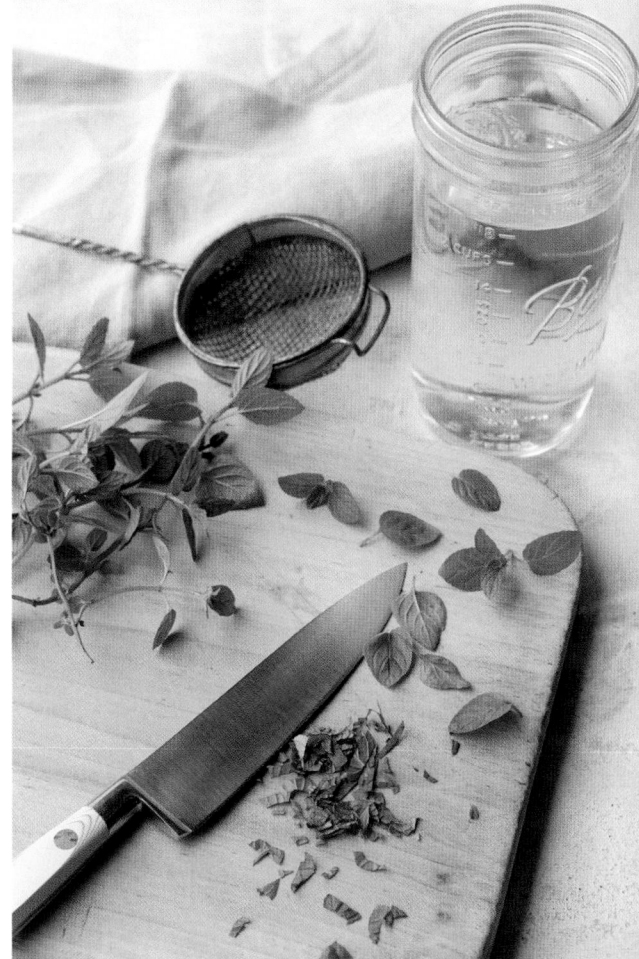

Vodka is an ideal base for tasty herbal cocktails.

your infused vodka as a base and then adding a simple syrup solution. For 1 quart of vodka, make a simple syrup from 2 cups of sugar and 1 cup of water. In a medium saucepan over medium-high heat, combine the sugar and water. Bring the mixture to a boil, then lower the heat and simmer uncovered for 5 minutes. When the syrup has cooled, add it to the infused vodka. Cover the bottle with a nonmetallic lid and allow the liqueur to mellow for about 4 weeks. Mints, lemon verbena, and lemon balm make great liqueurs.

ICED HERBAL TEAS AND LEMONADES

Iced herbal teas are refreshing summertime drinks. You can use fresh herbs, herbal tea bags, or loose dried herbs in a tea ball. Mints, chamomile, and lemon verbena are great choices. To make your tea, bring the water to a boil, then remove the pot from the heat. Add the herbs, allow them to steep until the mixture is heady and intense, and then strain out the herbs. Let the tea cool, and pour it over ice to serve. Garnish with a sprig of mint or lavender.

Lemonades can be made more complex and interesting with the addition of finely chopped ginger or mint. Sweeten both iced tea and lemonade with an herbal simple syrup. In a medium saucepan, combine 2 cups of water with 1 cup of sugar. Place the pan over high heat and bring the mixture to a boil as you stir to dissolve the sugar. Reduce the heat to a gentle simmer and add a handful of chopped herbs, such as basil. Turn off the heat and allow the mixture to steep for 5 to 10 minutes, then strain before use.

MASALA CHAI: SPICY TEA BLEND

Derived from the Chinese *chá*, "chai" means tea in much of the world, including Asia, Eastern Europe, parts of Africa, and Brazil. Masala chai is an aromatic blend of green or black tea with warming spices. Sugar and milk are often included, too.

In India, Nepal, and Tibet, where masala chai originated, vendors often peddle the tasty brew on

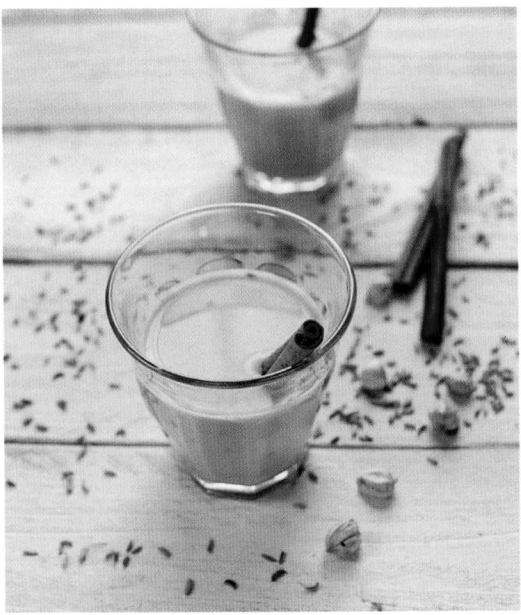

An herb garnish in iced tea serves as a visual reminder of the natural quality of the beverage's ingredients.

Masala chai, a soothing blend of tea and spices, often includes cinnamon, cardamom, and cloves, along with milk and honey.

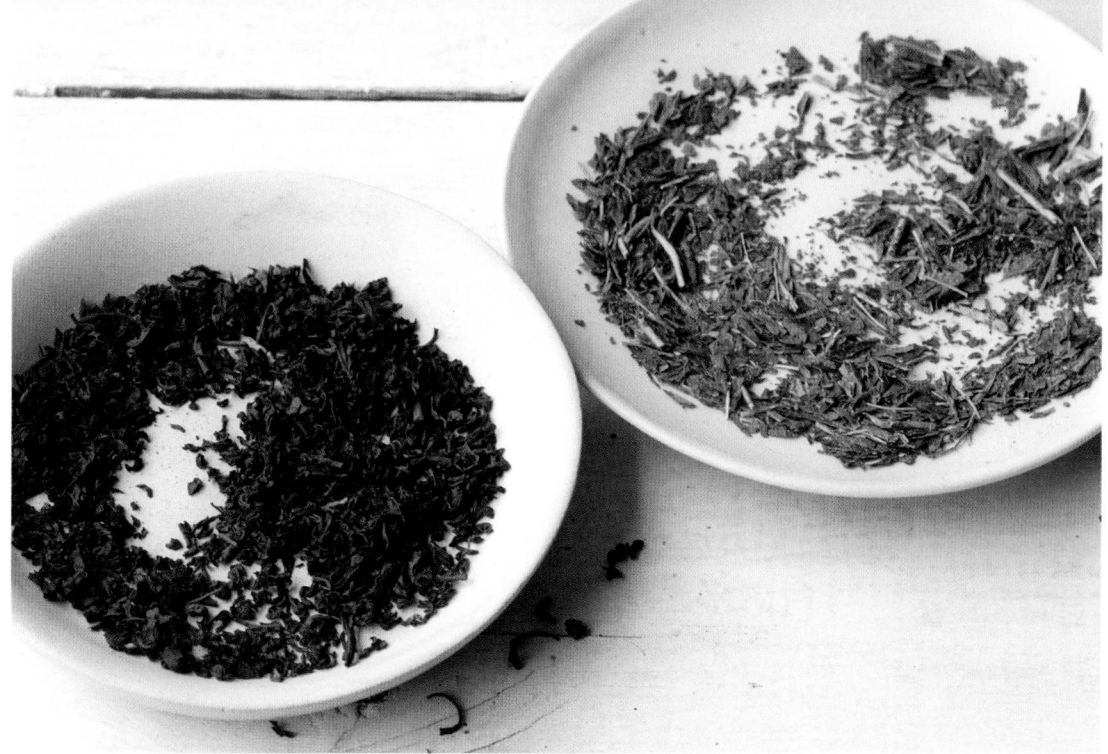

Unfermented green teas, such as sencha (right), give desserts and vegetables a grassy, herbal flavor; oxidized black teas, like Darjeeling (left), add full-bodied flavor to meat marinades, poaching liquids, and dry rubs.

street corners and at train stations. According to Ayurvedic tradition, masala chai boosts the immune system, enhances metabolism, relieves stress, aids digestion, and sharpens the mind.

There are hundreds of chai recipes associated with different locales and even families. Spices commonly used include cinnamon sticks, cardamom seeds, fresh ginger, black peppercorns, and whole cloves. Preparation methods vary, too—some boil the tea, spices, and milk together, while others briefly steep the tea leaves and spices in hot water, strain them out, and then add hot milk and sweetener last. To create your own favorite blend, experiment by adding fennel seeds, coriander seeds, nutmeg, star anise, and lemon or orange peel.

COOKING WITH TEA

After water, tea is the most-consumed beverage in the world. There are also many culinary uses for this versatile herb. In the Asian countries of China, Japan, and Vietnam, tea leaves are traditionally used to flavor, tenderize, and color food. In the West, many chefs have begun to experiment with tea, adding it to everything from ice cream to poaching liquids for fish and fruit.

Loose-leaf tea may be simmered with rice or stuffed into fish or chicken before roasting. Tea leaves can be finely ground in a coffee or spice mill and combined with other herbs to make a dry rub for meat and poultry, or they can be added to the dry ingredients for sweet shortbread or tea cakes. Tea oil, which is made from cold-pressed tea seeds, is a sweet, herbaceous addition to vinaigrettes that can be drizzled over salads, steamed vegetables, or delicate seafood.

Black and green teas are the most commonly used varieties in cooking. Unfermented green tea contributes a grassy, herbal, astringent flavor; fermented black tea adds full-bodied dimension to soups and spice rubs. To make tea for cooking, brew 2 teaspoons of loose-leaf tea per 1 cup of liquid (water, stock, or milk). Steep the tea in below-boiling water for 20 to 30 minutes. Strain the mixture before using it in any recipe.

Tea is so versatile a culinary ingredient that you can enjoy its flavor and health benefits from breakfast through dinner. Begin your day with a green tea smoothie: Blend chilled green tea, plain yogurt, cubed mango, banana, and a few ice cubes until smooth. Top with a dash of freshly grated nutmeg. For lunch, top a spinach, cucumber, and flank steak salad with a dressing made from peanut butter, cooled black tea, soy sauce, lime juice, and mint.

For dinner, make a flavorful rub for grilled salmon steaks using loose green tea leaves, green and black peppercorns, and cardamom. Use a mortar and pestle to grind the spices into a powder, lightly coat the salmon with oil, and then apply the rub. Tea leaves are the secret ingredient in many fabulous desserts, too. Add a teaspoon of smoky lapsang souchong leaves to a chocolate glaze for an out-of-this-world chocolate mousse cake. Or finish the evening with chocolate ice cream made with green tea–infused cream.

TEAS USED *in* COOKING

The flavorful world of tea goes well beyond the familiar black blends and varieties. Explore different teas to add subtle smoky, fruity, or spicy flavors to foods, including vegetables and grains, meats and fish, and desserts.

BLACK TEAS	FLAVOR	USES
Assam	Medium-bodied	Dessert infusions and sauces
Darjeeling	Full-bodied	Dessert and savory infusions; dry rubs; marinades; smoking poultry
Earl Grey	Astringent, fruity	Dessert infusions; chocolate desserts; marinades
Keemun	Smooth, spicy	Dessert bases, poaching liquids and sauces; savory infusions for poultry and shellfish
Lapsang souchong	Smoky, strong	Chocolate desserts; dry rubs; smoking poultry
Yunnan	Astringent, peppery	Savory infusions; poultry sauces
GREEN TEAS	FLAVOR	USES
Genmaicha	Smoky	Fish and rice infusions; smoking poultry, fish, and shellfish
Gunpowder	Fresh, grassy	Dessert bases and infusions; shellfish sauces, infusions, and broths
Matcha	Light, sweet	Dessert bases; vegetable infusions and sauces
Sencha	Astringent, sweet	Dessert bases; vegetable infusions and sauces

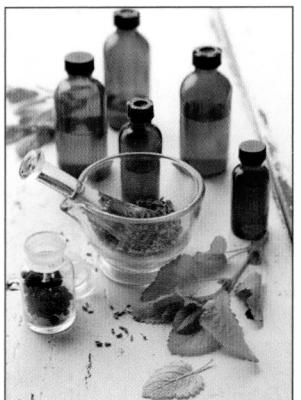

CHAPTER 5

HERBAL HEALTH
and HEALING

As early as 2500 BCE, physicians in Sumer (modern-day Iraq) recorded their use of herbal medicines and preparations on clay tablets using one of the earliest known forms of writing—cuneiform. Plants—including thyme, mustard, and willow—were prescribed for a wide range of conditions, administered as poultices or internal therapies.

Today, plants continue to play a vital role in everyday health care around the world. Several billion people use herbs for conditions ranging from bites, stings, and skin irritations to life-threatening illnesses such as malaria. Some 30 to 40 percent of people in the United States use herbal remedies in some form, either directly or processed into supplements, tinctures, extracts, or creams. And interest in herbs as preventive medicines, self-care for minor health conditions, and low-cost, nontoxic alternatives to standard treatments for common health problems continues to grow. Plants also play a critical role in the mainstream pharmaceutical industry. An estimated 25 percent of our prescription pharmaceuticals derive their molecules directly from plants, and many more drugs are based on compounds inspired by or derived from nature.

HERBS AS MEDICINE

Traditional healers use herbal medicines in myriad ways as part of an overall system or approach to wellness. Often, they rely on combinations of herbs called formulas, which they can tailor to the specific needs of a patient. Traditional healthcare systems that rely on whole plant medicines—herbal remedies in their most natural forms—include traditional Chinese medicine (TCM), Ayurvedic medicine, Tibetan medicine, and the traditional medicines of Africa, South and Central America, the Pacific Islands, and Australia. Some of these healing systems have existed for millennia. Whole plant medicines are also used in Western herbalism, a system of herbal therapeutics that evolved in Europe and North America.

HERBS IN MODERN HEALTH CARE

Herbal medicine is finding its way into modern Western health care through the fields of integrative medicine (IM) and complementary and alternative medicine (CAM). Both IM and CAM combine mainstream medical practices with "complementary" approaches—including herbal remedies, when appropriate—that have some evidence of effectiveness. In some nations, such as China, traditional herbal medicine exists side by side with Western medicine, and many physicians are trained to use both traditional Chinese and conventional (allopathic or "mainstream") medical treatments. In the United States and Canada, most conventional physicians receive little, if any, training in the use of herbal medicines, and some are skeptical about their use. But this is beginning to change, as more than 50 academic institutions and affiliated centers now offer formal IM training programs.

In many European nations, health agencies have approved hundreds of herbs as official medicines. Conventional physicians there often receive training about botanicals in medical school, and they prescribe certain herbal medicines as low-cost, nontoxic alternatives to standard pharmaceutical treatments for common ailments. Saw palmetto (*Serenoa repens*), for instance, is now a preferred treatment in Europe for benign prostatic hyperplasia (enlarged prostate), a common health problem for men over the age of 50. European physicians also commonly prescribe black cohosh (*Actaea racemosa*) for symptoms of menopause, such as hot flashes.

Through global commerce, practitioners and consumers of conventional (Western) health care now have access to herbs from around the world. In Europe, physicians prescribe the Polynesian herb kava (*Piper methysticum*) for anxiety. Germany has approved the use of the Indian herb turmeric (*Curcuma longa*) for the treatment of indigestion. And physicians in the United States

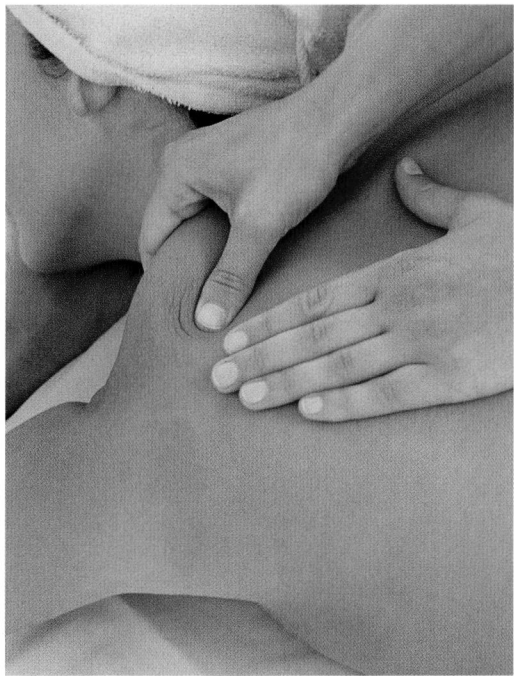

Holistic healers use methods, such as massage therapy with herbal oils, that promote the wellness of the whole person.

are recommending the Chinese medicinal herbs astragalus (*Astragalus membranaceus*) and shiitake mushroom (*Lentinus edodes*) for patients undergoing chemotherapy.

People all over the world also use herbs to treat themselves for minor illnesses and injuries—a practice often called folk medicine (the everyday medicine of the people). Herbal medicines are affordable; people who live in rural areas can even gather their own wild herbs locally and prepare the remedies at home. Pacific Islanders, for instance, use freshly squeezed juice from the root of a banana plant to help stop bleeding from a cut. Even city dwellers use herbs this way. If you've ever used aloe vera from a potted houseplant to soothe a burned finger or calmed an upset stomach by drinking ginger ale or chamomile tea, you've practiced herbal folk medicine.

Understanding Holistic Medicine

Holistic medicine is another term for an integrative approach to healing: The health-care professional treats the entire person—body, mind, and spirit—not just the symptoms of his or her disease. According to this definition, most (if not all) systems of traditional medicine are holistic, or "whole body" healing systems. Traditional Chinese medicine, Ayurveda, and Western herbalism all fall under the umbrella of holistic therapies.

All whole body systems of healing encompass diet, lifestyle, emotional well-being, spiritual considerations, and physical activity, in addition to the use of herbs or other medicines. Holistic healers believe that health and disease are products of a complex interplay among mind, body, and spirit. Each patient is considered a unique individual with specific issues and health-care needs. In holistic healing, the patient is a partner in the treatment process, not a passive bystander. A holistic herbalist expects patients to play an active role by making lifestyle choices that foster health.

Holistic healers seek to stimulate the body's own self-healing mechanism, or "vital force." When presented with an illness by a patient or client, holistic herbalists often recommend tonic herbs that nourish specific body systems and gently correct long-standing imbalances that they believe are the root cause of a disorder or disease. Holistic healers recommend plant remedies not because they provide rapid relief of symptoms, but because these nourishing tonics support your body's own efforts to heal itself. In contrast, conventional (Western) medicine adheres to what's known as the biomedical model, which asserts that all diseases have physical causes and should be treated accordingly with specific pharmaceuticals or surgical procedures.

Another hallmark of holistic herbal medicine is its focus on practices and behaviors intended to support health and prevent disease, rather than

Helping to Chart the Course of Modern Health Care

Tieraona Low Dog, MD, has been described as a "modern Eclectic physician." Eclectic medicine, which began in the United States in the early 1800s and was popular through the mid-1900s, focuses on the individual needs of the patient, using all therapies available—including, but not limited to, herbs.

Dr. Low Dog is trained as an herbalist, massage therapist, midwife, and medical doctor. An integrative physician with her own practice for many years, she now holds a faculty position at the Arizona Center for Integrative Medicine at the University of Arizona. Having lived and worked with many traditional cultures, she describes her practice as "a compilation of the wisdom and magic of many healers."

Dr. Low Dog's own journey as a healer began during her childhood. She was influenced by her family's belief that the body has "an amazing capacity for self-healing if we give it what it needs and don't get in the way too much." Early in life, Dr. Low Dog recognized the importance of a strong bond with nature, and she grew up spending long periods studying medicinal plants in the desert of the Southwest, as well as working with her grandmothers, who were very knowledgeable about healing and herbs.

Dr. Low Dog is a visionary who has labored tirelessly and effectively to improve health care in this country and internationally, and she has been recognized for her important contributions with dozens of awards and honors. She describes her role in life—a healer—as "the bridge

between the woman growing peppermint in her garden and the researcher isolating menthol and everything in between." See pages 346–349 for 25 of her favorite healing herbs.

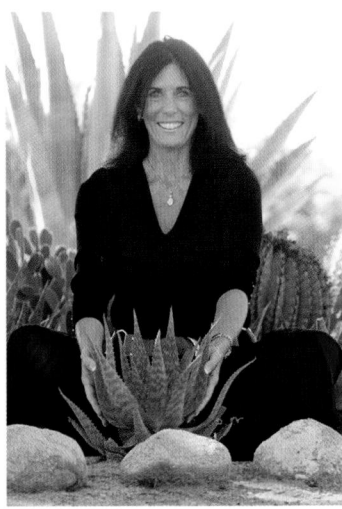

---

simply treating disease when it occurs. A holistic herbalist might advise a patient about the ways lifestyle can affect overall health—he or she would discuss not only herbs, but also dietary modifications, bodywork (such as massage or chiropractic), psychological counseling (to manage emotional issues and stress), and exercise (yoga, dance, tai chi, walking, or some other appropriate physical activity). Even conventional medicine can be part of holistic treatment, as long as the treatment considers the whole person: body, mind, and spirit.

Whole Plant Herbal Remedies and Phytomedicines

In the past, people used herbs only in their most naturally occurring form—as fresh or dried plants. They might have consumed the herb whole or made it into any of a variety of whole plant remedies—teas, tinctures (healing substances in an alcoholic solution), poultices, and many other traditional applications. Herbs are still used this way in traditional healing systems such as TCM and Ayurveda, as well as in folk medicine.

Holistic herbalists maintain that it's impossible

to understand the uses of plant parts separated from the whole and that plants are most beneficial when taken in their whole, natural form. In fact, this is part of the meaning of the word "holistic" in the context of herbalism. On the other hand, whole plants contain many hundreds of different chemical compounds, as explained in Chapter 3, and some of these can work in opposition to, in support of, or through synergy with each other. Plants grown in different places or under different conditions can contain varying concentrations of key chemical compounds. This means that it can be difficult, at times, to make absolute generalizations about how a mixture made from a whole herb will act in your body.

To solve this problem, some researchers use a concept known as "reductionism," which views a plant as a collection of individual compounds, one or some of which might be responsible for its overall effect. By isolating and concentrating the specific plant chemical they believe is responsible for the plant's medicinal effects (the so-called "active ingredient"), researchers can create a kind of phytomedicine. This highly processed herbal medicine, also called a standardized extract, contains a specified amount of one or two chemicals called "marker compounds." Having a product that contains verifiable quantities of the desired plant chemicals also makes it easier to ensure that future research on that species, for example studies with lab animals or humans, can be undertaken with herbal extracts that are consistent in their composition. The ability to replicate a scientific experiment and obtain identical results is an essential part of scientific methodology.

But isolating and increasing percentages of specific compounds can also have unintended consequences. The focus on one specific ingredient ignores many other chemical constituents that contribute to the whole plant's activity, and in some cases, these compounds temper or balance the very potent effects

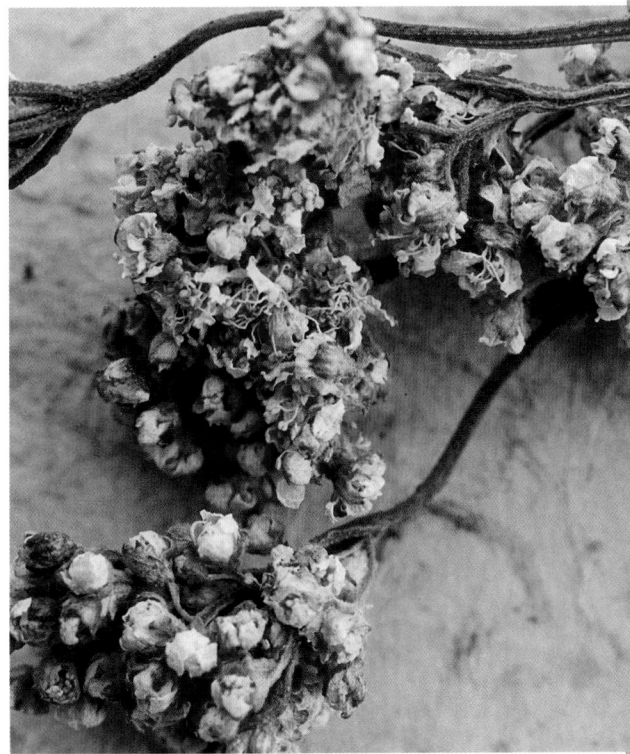

Meadowsweet (*Filipendula ulmaria*) was the original source for one of the world's most important and widely used drugs: aspirin.

of the remedy. In rare cases, when the standardized compound is increased to a very high percentage of the product's content—approaching the concentration of a pharmaceutical medicine—isolated constituents can be more likely to cause side effects that do not occur when the whole plant is used.

Modern Research on Herbs for Healing

Many people mistakenly believe that little or no scientific evidence exists to support the health benefits and safety of herbs. The truth is, thousands of scientific studies have been conducted on hundreds of herbs—from basic laboratory studies in test tubes (known as in vitro studies, these are experiments with a portion of an organism isolated from its natural biological surroundings, such as cancer cells studied in a cell culture dish) to long-term clinical studies with humans.

The gold standard of medical research is the double-blind test—meaning that neither the study participants nor the researchers know which group is getting which substance, a practice intended to eliminate bias. Double-blind, placebo-controlled clinical studies are considered the most reliable for testing the medicinal uses of herbs. These studies compare the effects of herbal medicine on two groups of human volunteers—one group takes the herb while the other takes a placebo (an inactive substance that resembles the test medicine). Studies in Europe (especially Germany) and Asia have begun to validate important traditional uses of some herbs and their clinical potential.

But more research is needed. Although many herbs have a long history of use, only a small fraction of them has been thoroughly evaluated for safety and effectiveness. Just as prescription pharmaceuticals can cause unexpected adverse effects among certain individuals, herbal remedies can also affect people in different ways. Whether your health-care professional is treating you with an herb or a pharmaceutical drug, be sure to work closely with him or her to understand the medicine's properties and possible side effects.

HEALING THERAPIES

Plant remedies play an important role in traditional healing systems. Here are several major traditional healing systems and some of their most important herbs.

WESTERN HERBALISM

Western herbalism (the use of herbs by North American and European herbal healers) has roots not only in the works of the classical Greek and Arab physicians, but also in the folk-healing systems of Europe and North America. European settlers brought their favorite medicinal plants with them to the New World on the North American continent. But they also eagerly learned the uses of North American plants from Native American healers. European physicians readily adopted native North American plants, including echinacea (*Echinacea* spp.), saw palmetto (*Serenoa repens*), and black cohosh (*Actaea racemosa*). (See Chapter 1 for more about Western herbalism in Europe and the Americas.)

TRADITIONAL CHINESE MEDICINE

Traditional Chinese medicine (TCM) is an ancient healing system that originated in China but is used today to treat millions of people all around the world. TCM applies treatments including acupuncture and herbs according to a highly developed, holistic philosophy of health and disease. Treatment is based on balancing and regulating the flow of qi (pronounced "chee")—the body's life energy or vital force. Japan, Korea, and Vietnam have all developed traditional medicine systems of their own, based on concepts and practices begun in China at least 3,000 years ago.

Principles of TCM

The principles of traditional Chinese medicine are deeply rooted in the Chinese philosophy and way of seeing the universe. Some Westerners have difficulty fully understanding the concepts of TCM, which do not conform to conventional (Western) ideas about science and medicine. Traditional

(continued on page 350)

THE IMPORTANCE *of* HERBAL MEDICINE

"Integrative medicine just makes sense—each patient is a whole human being, a person with a rich story, a history and set of beliefs and a culture that must be considered in the co-creation [by physician and patient] of a treatment plan."

As an herbalist and physician, I have long valued the role plants play in maintaining our health. Herbal medicine is ancient, and it gave birth to the modern sciences of botany, pharmacy, perfumery, and chemistry. Some of our most useful and beneficial medicines originate from plants, including aspirin (salicylic acid derivatives from willow bark and meadowsweet), quinine (from cinchona bark), digoxin (from foxglove), and morphine (from opium poppy). Just 100 years ago, the United States Pharmacopeia was filled with plant-based drugs, but today, few physicians are well versed in botany and few botanists deeply understand medicine.

This is unfortunate because there are times when an herbal remedy could offer a safer alternative. Take chamomile: The flowers have been used for centuries as a gentle calmative for young and old alike. It is non-habit-forming and well tolerated. A study sponsored by the University of Michigan found that chamomile extract had roughly the same efficacy as many prescription sleeping medications when given to adults with insomnia. Peppermint oil has been shown to be as effective as pharmaceutical drugs for relieving irritable bowel syndrome, but without the ofttimes dangerous side effects. Clinical studies have shown that ginger relieves morning sickness, sage can relieve a sore throat, and hibiscus tea gently lowers blood pressure. I believe it's better to use mild remedies for minor health problems and save the more potent, and risky, prescription medications for more serious conditions.

Sometimes an herb can fill a niche for which there is no pharmaceutical equivalent. Milk thistle is a classic example. Numerous scientific studies show that the extract can prevent liver damage caused by environmental toxins, alcohol, and medications like acetaminophen (Tylenol). A Columbia University study of children with acute lymphoblastic leukemia (ALL) found that milk thistle could reverse the liver toxicity that resulted from chemotherapy, allowing children to receive their treatments on time. Milk thistle protects the liver without interfering with the effectiveness of medications—and nothing currently in our modern pharmacy can match it. Some herbal remedies (such as the antidepressant St. John's wort), however, can interact with medications. So if you're taking a prescription medication, talk to your pharmacist and/or health-care provider before you take any herbal remedy or dietary supplement.

Consumers want to know about alternatives to conventional approaches; health-care practitioners and pharmacists should be able to answer their questions and provide appropriate guidance. Centuries of use and human clinical studies confirm that herbal remedies can be safe, effective, and economical options for many common conditions. For me, herbal medicines unquestionably play a unique and important role in modern health care.

—*Tieraona Low Dog, MD*

DR. TIERAONA LOW DOG'S FAVORITE HEALING HERBS *and* THEIR USES

Tieraona Low Dog, MD, frequently prescribes these 25 herbs for common health conditions. All are effective, have few safety concerns, and have a long history of traditional use. The dose recommendations are for adults. Read more about these herbs in Part II, beginning on page 80. (For more about making healing herbal teas, see "Herbal Infusions and Decoctions" on page 365.)

HERB	USES
Ashwagandha (*Withania somnifera*)	Rejuvenating tonic, anti-inflammatory, reduces anxiety, boosts immune health.
Black Cohosh (*Actaea racemosa*)	Relieves menstrual cramps and arthritic pain; commonly used to ease menopausal symptoms.
Calendula (*Calendula officinalis*)	Flowers have long been used to relieve inflammation in the mouth, throat, and stomach; popular as a topical cream or ointment to relieve rashes and irritation and to help heal wounds.
Catnip (*Nepeta cataria*)	Soothes an upset stomach; reduces anxiety and tension.
Chasteberry (*Vitex agnus-castus*)	Premiere herb for relieving PMS symptoms.
Cranberry (*Vaccinium macrocarpon*)	Well-established treatment for reducing the risk of bladder infection; could also be beneficial for chronic prostatitis.
Echinacea (*Echinacea* spp.)	Antiviral and immune-enhancing properties; popular for relieving colds and upper respiratory infections (approved in Europe for these uses).
Elderberry (*Sambucus nigra,* *S. canadensis*)	Flowers valued as a remedy for colds and fever for centuries; fruit extracts have been shown to have significant antiviral activity, especially against the flu.
Garlic (*Allium sativum*)	Potent antimicrobial; often used to combat colds, ease sinus congestion, and stave off traveler's diarrhea. Studies show that regular use can help gently lower blood pressure.
Ginger (*Zingiber officinale*)	Premiere remedy for easing nausea, vomiting, and upset stomach; fresh teas relieve cold and flu symptoms
Ginseng (*Panax quinquefolius;* *P. ginseng*)	Helps relieve and prevent mental and physical fatigue; shown to reduce the frequency and severity of colds; possibly beneficial for erectile dysfunction.
Hibiscus (*Hibiscus sabdariffa*)	Lowers blood pressure and has mild diuretic activity; traditionally used to ease sore throats and colds.

PREPARATIONS AND DOSES	CONCERNS
Tea: Simmer 1 tsp dried and sliced root in 1 cup water or milk for 10 minutes. Strain. Drink one or two times per day. **Standardized extract** (2-5% withanolides): Take 500 mg two or three times per day.	Can cause mild sedation; potential to stimulate thyroid hormones.
Tincture: Take 1–2 ml three times per day. **Standardized extract:** Take 20–80 mg two times per day.	Very rare case reports of liver damage (likely due to misidentified herb); purchase only from reputable supplier.
Tea: Pour 1 cup boiling water over 2 tsp petals. Steep for 10 minutes. Strain. Use as needed as a mouthwash, gargle, or tea. **Ointment:** Apply to skin two or three times per day as needed.	None known.
Tea: Pour 1 cup boiling water over 4 or 5 fresh or 1 tsp dried leaves. Steep for 5 minutes. Strain and sweeten, if desired. Drink one or two times per day.	None known.
Capsules: Take 250–500 mg dried fruit once per day. **Tincture:** Take 2–3 ml each morning.	None known.
Juice: Drink ½ to ¾ cup twice per day. **Capsules:** Take 300–500 mg concentrated juice extract two times per day.	None known.
Tea: Simmer 1 tsp dried and sliced root in 1 cup water for 10 minutes. Strain. Drink 1–3 cups per day. **Tincture:** Take 5 ml three to six times per day at onset of cold symptoms.	Rare allergic reactions.
Tea: Pour 1 cup boiling water over 1–2 tsp flowers. Steep for 10 minutes. Sweeten if desired and drink hot two or three times per day. **Berry extracts:** Use as directed.	None known.
Eat: Eat 1–2 cloves fresh daily. **Capsules:** Take 4–8 mg allicin per day; enteric-coated products may be superior if specifically treating diarrhea.	May interact with warfarin.
Tea: Steep ¼–½ tsp dried ginger or simmer 1 tsp fresh ginger root in 1 cup hot water for 10 minutes. Strain and sweeten, if desired. Drink 1–2 cups per day. **Capsules:** Take 250–500 mg two times per day.	Very safe in small amounts; heartburn and stomach upset can occur with high doses. Pregnant women should not take more than 1,500 mg per day of dried ginger.
Tea: Simmer 1 tsp dried and sliced root in 1 cup water for 10 minutes. Strain. Drink 1–2 cups per day. **Standardized extract** (4–7% ginsenosides): 100–400 mg per day.	Purchase from a reputable manufacturer, as ginseng has often been adulterated in the past.
Tea: Pour 1 cup boiling water over 1–2 tsp dried flowers. Steep for 10 minutes. Strain and sweeten, if desired. Drink 2 cups per day. **Capsules:** Take 1,000 mg two times per day.	Talk to your health-care provider if you have high blood pressure.

HERB	USES
Hops (*Humulus lupulus*)	Excellent sleeping aid; smaller, daytime doses used to ease tension, restlessness, and anxiety; might help reduce hot flashes during menopause.
Horse Chestnut (*Aesculus hippocastanum*)	Seed extracts shown to be highly effective for treatment of varicose veins and chronic venous insufficiency (blood pools in lower leg veins after standing or sitting); topical gels can reduce swelling and tenderness due to injury.
Kava (*Piper methysticum*)	Clinical trials have shown kava to be highly effective for relieving anxiety. Also has significant muscle relaxing effects.
Lemon Balm (*Melissa officinalis*)	Gentle calmative; eases tension, digestive upset, and colic; topical creams used for fever blisters.
Licorice (*Glycyrrhiza glabra*)	Excellent anti-inflammatory; soothes mucous membranes; useful for sore throats and coughs; protects and heals gastrointestinal tract.
Marshmallow (*Althaea officinalis*)	Root and leaf are rich in mucilage, a substance that coats the lining of the mouth and throat, as well as the tissue that lines the gastrointestinal tract. Used for sore throat, heartburn, and minor GI inflammation.
Milk Thistle (*Silybum marianum*)	Protects the liver from damage caused by environmental toxins, medications, and alcohol. Recent studies suggest it protects the kidneys similarly.
Mullein (*Verbascum thapsus*)	Leaves commonly used to relieve coughs, sore throats, and chest congestion; steeped in oil, the flowers relieve earache.
Nettle (*Urtica dioica*)	Fresh, freeze-dried leaves relieved seasonal allergy symptoms in one human trial. Impressive research supports use of the root for easing symptoms of enlarged prostate. Tea widely recommended for its nutritive value.
Sage (*Salvia officinalis*)	Excellent for sore throats, coughs, and colds; recognized in Germany as a treatment for excessive sweating; studies show it can help reduce menopausal hot flashes and night sweats.
Slippery Elm (*Ulmus rubra*)	FDA-approved as a safe, nonprescription remedy for minor throat irritation; also very useful for relieving coughs and occasional heartburn.
St. John's Wort (*Hypericum perforatum*)	More than 40 studies have confirmed its effectiveness for relieving mild to moderate depression; may also relieve PMS symptoms and menopausal hot flashes, especially when combined with black cohosh.
Thyme (*Thymus vulgaris*)	Highly regarded for relieving coughs, colds, and congestion; rich in volatile oils that have significant antimicrobial and antispasmodic activity.

PREPARATIONS AND DOSES	CONCERNS
Capsules: Take 200–300 mg one to three times per day. **Tincture:** Take 2–4 ml before bed.	Can cause sedation.
Seed extract (containing 100–150 mg aescin/escin): Take 600 mg per day in divided doses.	Unprocessed horse chestnut seeds can be toxic; use only appropriately prepared seed extracts.
Tea: Simmer 1 tsp dried and sliced root in 1 cup water for 10 minutes. Strain. Drink 1–2 cups per day. **Extract of root:** Take 100–200 mg two or three times per day. (Do not exceed 210 mg per day of kavalactones.)	Rare cases of liver toxicity; do not use if you have liver disease, frequently drink alcohol, or are taking acetaminophen or prescription medications.
Tea: Pour 1 cup boiling water over 5 or 6 fresh or 1 tsp dried leaves. Steep for 5 minutes. Strain and sweeten, if desired. Drink several times per day.	None; suitable for all ages.
Tea: Simmer 1 tsp dried and sliced root in 1 cup water for 10 minutes. Strain. Drink two or three times per day for up to 7 days. **Capsules:** Take up to 3,000 mg per day for 7 days. Do not exceed 500 mg per day if taking for longer than 7 days.	Do not use high doses for longer than 1 week as it elevates blood pressure and causes potassium loss. (DGL, a special preparation commonly used for heartburn, is safe for prolonged use.)
Tea: Pour 1 cup hot water over 1 tsp dried and sliced root or 2 tsp leaf. Steep for 2 hours. Strain and drink as desired.	Take other drugs 1 hour prior to or several hours after consuming marshmallow, as it could slow absorption of oral medications.
Extract (guaranteed minimum of 70% silymarin): Take 400–700 mg per day in divided doses.	None known.
Tea: Pour 1 cup boiling water over 1–2 tsp leaves. Steep for 10 minutes. Strain, sweeten, and drink as desired. **Ear oil:** Use as directed.	None known.
Tea: Pour 1 cup boiling water over 2 tsp leaves. Steep for 10 minutes. Strain. Sweeten if desired. Drink 1–3 cups per day. **Freeze-dried nettle capsules:** Take 300–500 mg two times per day. **Nettle root:** Take 250–400 mg two or three times per day.	Wear gloves when handling fresh nettles to avoid stinging and irritation (sting is lost with cooking or drying); very safe herb.
Tea: Pour 1 cup boiling water over 1 tsp leaves. Steep for 10 minutes. Strain. Drink, or use as a sore throat gargle. **Capsules:** Take 500 mg dried leaf two times per day.	Do not use therapeutic doses during pregnancy; do not use sage essential oil internally.
Lozenges: Take as directed. **Tea:** Pour 1 cup boiling water over 1–2 tsp powdered bark. Steep for 5 minutes. Drink two or three times per day.	Take other drugs 1 hour before or several hours after consuming, as it could slow absorption of oral medications.
Standardized extract (standardized to 0.3% hypericin and/or 3–5% hyperforin): Take 300–600 mg three times per day.	Talk to your physician or pharmacist before using if you are taking prescription medications; the chance for herb-drug interaction is high.
Tea: Pour 1 cup boiling water over 1 Tbsp fresh or 1 tsp dried leaves. Steep for 10 minutes. Strain and sweeten, if desired. Drink ⅓ cup three times per day.	None known.

Chinese healers believe that human beings are subject to the same laws that govern nature and that disease results from imbalances or lack of harmony in forces that influence the workings of the body.

The concept of "complementary opposites," known as yin and yang, is at the heart of Chinese philosophy and TCM. In extremely simplified terms, yin and yang are idealized polarities: yin represents dark and yang represents light; yin represents the female and yang the male; and so on. In the Chinese worldview, however, the concept is much more complex than this. Yin and yang are not at odds or in conflict with one another, but instead represent a constant flow and exchange of energy from one to the other. They exist only in relation to one another. But at the same time, they constantly blend with and become one another. In an idealized state, yin is the absence of yang—but in reality, there is always some yang in yin, and vice versa.

The original Chinese character for yang, which depicts the sun and a mountain, means "the light side of the mountain." The original character for yin depicts a cloud and a mountain and means "the dark side of the mountain." So while the characters are opposites, they have the mountain in common. Each is incomplete without the other, and together they represent the "whole"—known in Chinese as the tao.

In traditional Chinese medicine, the body is divided into yin parts and yang parts. Herbs, foods, and even activities are classified along a spectrum from those that are most yin to those that are most yang. The attraction and tension between yin and yang creates qi, the body's life force.

Yin elements are earth, moon, dark, female, expansive, passive, cold, night, slow, moist, and winter. The associated yang elements are the heavens, sun, light, male, contractive, aggressive, hot, day, fast, dry, and summer.

The Chinese Five Elements (*Wu Xing*), also known as Five Element Theory, is another governing concept in TCM. Each element—wood, fire, earth, metal, and water—is associated with specific body functions, organs, and senses, as well as emotions, activities, foods, flavors, and temperatures.

THE FIVE ELEMENTS *of* TRADITIONAL CHINESE MEDICINE *and* THEIR ASSOCIATIONS

The Five Elements represent fundamental relationships among the forces and cycles of nature and their effects upon the human body. Each element is associated with specific organs and emotions.

ELEMENT	SEASON	TASTE	EMOTION	BODY PARTS
Wood	Spring	Sour	Anger	Liver, gallbladder, eyes, tendons
Fire	Summer	Bitter	Joy	Heart, small intestine, tongue, blood vessels
Earth	Indian summer	Sweet	Worry	Spleen, stomach, mouth, muscles
Metal	Fall	Pungent	Grief	Lungs, large intestine, nose, skin
Water	Winter	Salty	Fear	Kidneys, bladder, ears, bones

The Practice of TCM

A TCM practitioner's first step is to pinpoint imbalances that have resulted in a person's physical problems. In TCM, all disease is viewed as the result of energetic imbalances (excess or deficiency) caused by a person's way of life and relationship with the universe. The six external causes of disease are wind, cold, heat, dampness, dryness, and summer heat. The seven internal causes, or emotions, that contribute to physical manifestations of disharmony are joy, anger, sadness, pensiveness, grief, fear, and fright. So, for example, a TCM practitioner might conclude that a patient's disease is caused by excessive "wind" in the body, too much "heat" in a specific organ, or by "qi deficiency" or "deficient spleen yang."

A traditional Chinese physician uses a unique array of diagnostic techniques. In addition to carefully questioning a patient about his health, lifestyle, and behavior, the doctor examines his tongue for signs of illness, observes all aspects of his appearance, palpates his abdomen, and analyzes his pulse. Chinese pulse diagnosis is a highly refined art that takes many years to master.

Acupuncture and herbs, often used in combination, are the two most important components of TCM practice. Other treatments include nutritional therapies, restorative physical exercises such

IMPORTANT HERBS *in* TRADITIONAL CHINESE MEDICINE

These are only a few examples of the many thousands of different herbs that are important in traditional Chinese medicine (TCM). As in many traditional medical systems, combinations of herbs are also an integral part of the pharmacopoeia.

ASTRAGALUS
(*Astragalus membranaceus*)

Astragalus root, called *huang qi* in Chinese, is an important qi tonic that is considered slightly warming and sweet. It is used to treat conditions characterized by deficient qi. These include frequent colds, general weakness and fatigue, weak digestion and lack of appetite, and chronic weakness of the lungs with shortness of breath. For use as a daily tonic, pieces of astragalus root can be cooked into soups or other foods. Healers often prescribe a combination of astragalus and ginseng roots (called *bu zhong yi qi tang*) for debility and fatigue.

DONG QUAI
(*Angelica sinensis*)

Practitioners of TCM consider dong quai root (also called *dang gui,* or Chinese angelica) warm, sweet, acrid, and bitter. It is the most important "blood tonic" in traditional Chinese medicine, and healers use it to invigorate blood and relieve blood stagnation. Dong quai is often called the female ginseng because in TCM, women's health relates closely to blood. Practitioners prescribe it widely in combination with other herbs to treat women's health conditions, such as irregular menstruation, menopausal symptoms, and postpartum debility (weakness after giving birth). Four Things Soup, a classical Chinese formula, is a women's tonic widely prescribed throughout China. This formula contains dong quai, Chinese peony (*Paeonia lactiflora*), rehmannia (*Rehmannia glutinosa*), and ligusticum (*Ligusticum sinense*) in equal parts, prepared by simmering the herbs.

GINSENG
(*Panax ginseng*)

TCM classifies ginseng root, known as *ren shen* in Chinese, as a "superior" herb, or one of the most useful and safest remedies available. An important qi tonic, it is considered warming, sweet, and slightly bitter. Traditional healers use ginseng to treat extreme fatigue, debility caused by illness or old age, and heart and blood pressure problems. They generally prescribe it only for people over the age of 45 or 50 and treat young people with it only if they have severe qi deficiency.

as qigong or tai chi, meditation, and massage.

Acupuncture, which originated in China at least 2,000 years ago, remains one of the most commonly used medical procedures in the world. Acupuncture involves the insertion of tiny needles in specific places along the body's meridians—pathways that serve as channels for the flow of qi. There are 12 major meridians and more than 1,000 acupuncture points along the meridians.

Through the precise placement of needles on these points, the skilled acupuncturist manipulates the flow of qi to reduce excess, counteract deficiency, or otherwise correct underlying energetic imbalances to treat disease. Modern clinical studies conducted in China and in the West indicate that acupuncture can be an effective treatment or supportive therapy for health problems including addictions, asthma, carpal tunnel syndrome, fibromyalgia, headache, low-back pain, menstrual cramps, osteoarthritis pain, postoperative dental pain, postoperative and chemotherapy-related nausea and vomiting, and stroke rehabilitation.

Chinese Herbal Formulary

TCM classifies herbs according to four energies (cold, cool, warm, and hot) and five flavors (spicy, sweet, sour, bitter, and salty). Healers might prescribe cooling herbs to relieve conditions caused by excess heat in the body, for example, or sweet herbs to tonify qi and nourish the blood. TCM practitioners rarely use herbs singly; instead, they compound herbs into formulas. A single herb can have many different effects, so practitioners carefully choose and combine them with other herbs in a prescription designed to address myriad health issues at the same time.

TCM practitioners can choose from nearly 6,000 herbs to create an herbal formula that could contain 20 or more herbs. The traditional Chinese pharmacopoeia lists hundreds of different formulas for specific patterns of disharmony. The practitioner adjusts these formulas, which usually contain at least 10 different herbs, to suit the unique characteristics and needs of the patient.

Chinese practitioners often prescribe a formula as a decoction (a tea made by simmering dried herbs) to be brewed and consumed several times a day. Patients can also take an herbal formula as a powder, pill, or alcohol-based tincture, or they can add the roots, leaves, or other parts of the plant to a soup, porridge, or other food. Some classic Chinese formulas are mass-produced as ready-to-use "patent remedies" made according to a specific formula. These are usually sold in pill form.

An external herbal treatment called moxibustion is often used in combination with acupuncture. To perform moxibustion, the practitioner applies heat to acupuncture points by burning moxa (a dried herb, usually *Artemesia vulgaris,* or mugwort) near or on the skin. The heat is believed to penetrate into the meridians to influence qi and blood flow. Moxa is available in a variety of forms—including loose powder, cones, and sticks—for different applications. Moxa cones can be burned directly on the skin, but moxa is often applied indirectly, such as by wrapping a ball of the herb around the end of an acupuncture needle before lighting it.

AYURVEDA

One of the ancient healing systems of India, Ayurveda combines diet, herbs, physical activity, and spiritual practice to preserve health and promote longevity. The practice of Ayurvedic medicine goes back at least 5,000 years. Today, this holistic system is becoming increasingly popular outside India among people attracted to its emphasis on balancing body, mind, and spirit for optimal health and well-being.

The word *Ayurveda* comes from the Sanskrit

words *ayur* (meaning "life" or "longevity") and *veda* (meaning "knowledge" or "wisdom"). The practice of Ayurveda is based upon several ancient works, including the *Atharva Veda,* the fourth in the series of Hindu books of knowledge called Vedas. *Atharva Veda* contains ancient wisdom about healing and sickness. Other major foundational works that have guided the practice of Ayurveda are *Sushruta Samhita* (with information on surgery, more than 700 medicinal plants, and more than 100 formulas from mineral and animal sources) and *Charaka Samhita* (which includes information on medicines, foods, and internal medicine, written in a poetic style to facilitate memorization). Modern Ayurvedic healers continue to follow the traditional philosophies and techniques of *Charaka Samhita.*

The "Science of Life"

Ayurveda, often called "the science of life," treats the whole person—body, mind, and spirit—to ensure optimal health. It addresses all aspects of everyday life to achieve and maintain good health (*swasthavritta*) through daily and seasonal lifestyle regimens. These regimens, which incorporate diet, herbs, exercise, hygiene, and spiritual and mental health, are designed to balance vital forces to maintain physical well-being as well as a harmonious relationship between the body and the mind.

Ayurveda believes the body has a vital energy, called *prana,* which activates the body and mind. This is similar to the concept of qi in traditional Chinese medicine; other healing systems have related concepts of vital energy. Breath is the

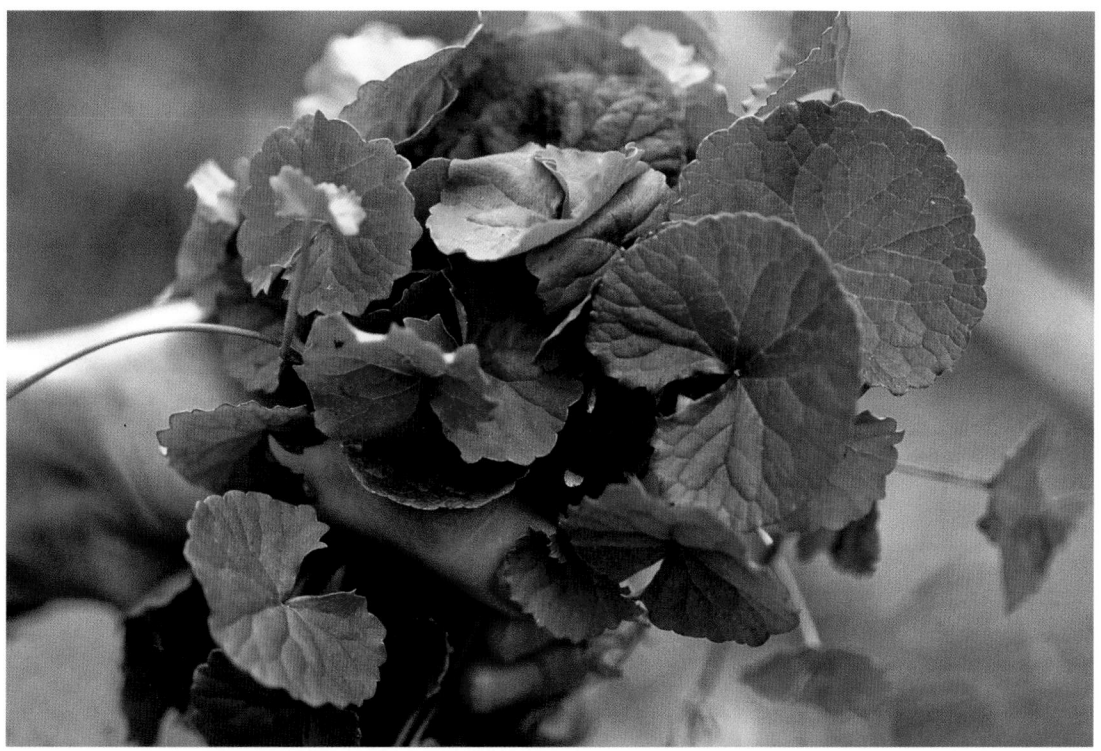

One of the many important herbs in Ayurveda, gotu kola (*Centella asiatica*) is used to revitalize the nervous and immune systems. It is believed to improve memory and concentration and to promote longevity.

bodily manifestation of prana. Seven energy centers called chakras keep prana flowing smoothly through the body. According to Ayurveda, the human body and the whole universe are composed of five basic substances that occur in various combinations and proportions. These five great elements (*panchamahabhutas*) are space (*akasha*), air (*vayu*), fire (*agni*), water (*jala*), and earth (*prithvi*). The five elements symbolize the physical substances that give the human body form. Each is associated with different physical properties, actions, and sensory functions.

The Three Doshas

Ayurveda recognizes three primary life forces or energies, called *doshas: vata, pitta,* and *kapha.* Each dosha is composed of a combination of two of the five great elements. These constantly fluctuating energies are essential components of the body and are responsible for a person's health. Each person displays a unique combination of doshas that determines their main physical strengths and weaknesses, personality, and intellectual function. One or two doshas tend to dominate for each individual; a person might be

THE THREE DOSHAS *of* AYURVEDA

According to Ayurveda, each person displays a unique combination of life energies, called doshas. To be healthy, a person must manage the daily fluctuation of his or her doshas by using the appropriate foods, herbs, and forms of exercise.

	VATA	PITTA	KAPHA
Element	Air/space	Fire/water	Water/earth
Body type	Thin build; narrow shoulders; may be very tall or short	Well-proportioned, muscular; fair or ruddy coloring; average height	Thickset, strong; graceful, slow-moving; may be prone to weight gain
Personality	Creative, enthusiastic, vivacious, imaginative, anxious; may make quick, nervous movements; tendency to waste	Sharp-witted, intense, driven, confident, quick to anger, impatient, ambitious; can be aggressive and competitive	Stable, patient, tranquil, affectionate, complacent; can be possessive
Basic body function	Movement	Metabolism	Structure
Seat	Colon	Small intestine	Lungs
Season	Fall/early winter	Summer	Middle of winter
Time of day	Dawn	Midday	Evening
Tastes/foods that aggravate	Pungent, bitter, astringent; raw foods	Sour, salty, pungent; red meat	Sweet, sour, salty; dairy products
Tastes/foods that pacify	Sweet, sour, salty; moist, warming foods; cooked root vegetables	Sweet, astringent, bitter; cooling foods, such as salads; mushrooms, fish, chicken, and tofu	Pungent, bitter, astringent; hot and spicy foods; leafy vegetables, legumes, apples, and pears

primarily vata, for example, or a combination of vata-pitta. This proportion of doshas determines a person's basic nature from birth (called *prakriti*) and affects the way prana flows through the body. To achieve optimal health, a person must harmonize the doshas with his or her basic nature.

Ayurvedic practitioners believe that the levels of the doshas in individuals fluctuate daily according to numerous influences, including foods eaten, time of day, season, stress level, and emotions. Each dosha has a "seat" in the body that helps keep imbalances in check. Chronic imbalances in the doshas, however, disrupt the flow of *prana* and can result in disease. For optimal health, a person must take responsibility for managing imbalances and fluctuations by "pacifying" excesses in the doshas with foods, herbs, exercise, and various stress-reducing techniques.

Diet, Herbs, and Lifestyle

Before prescribing treatment, the Ayurvedic practitioner determines a patient's *tridosha* (doshic constitution) and diagnoses any imbalances. Diagnosis begins with a detailed history that takes into account lifestyle factors as well as physical symptoms. As in traditional Chinese medicine, the

---

EXAMPLES *of* IMPORTANT HERBS *in* AYURVEDA

Depending on your doshic constitution, an Ayurvedic practitioner might prescribe one or more of these important herbs to help you maintain good health. They are just a few of the many herbs and herb combinations used in Ayurveda.

ASHWAGANDHA
(*Withania somnifera*)
Ayurveda uses ashwagandha to treat debility and weakness in the elderly, people with chronic illnesses, and those exhausted by overwork or lack of sleep, much the way traditional Chinese medicine uses ginseng. Considered the best rejuvenating herb for the vata constitution, ashwagandha often is prepared as a milk decoction with sweetener and rice. Ashwagandha is bitter and astringent, calming and clarifying to the mind, and it promotes restful sleep.

INDIAN FRANKINCENSE
(*Boswellia serrata*)
Indian frankincense is a tree resin that hardens into a gum. The gum was traditionally used to treat arthritis, digestive disorders, pulmonary conditions, and ringworm. Recent studies have shown that Indian frankincense limits the production of leukotrienes, which cause inflammation.

GINGER
(*Zingiber officinale*)
Pungent, sweet, warming ginger pacifies kapha and vata, increases pitta, and has been called "the universal medicine" (*vishwabhesaj*) by Ayurvedic practitioners. Dried ginger is considered hotter and better for relieving kapha, while fresh ginger is a more effective diaphoretic (fever reducer) and better for relieving vata. Ayurvedic practitioners use ginger extensively to treat digestive and respiratory conditions, including colds and flu. It is also valued for relieving menstrual and abdominal cramps, for treating arthritis, and as a heart tonic.

GOTU KOLA
(*Centella asiatica*)
Ayurvedic practitioners consider gotu kola to be one of the most important rejuvenating herbs. They use it to revitalize the brain, nervous system, and immune system and to strengthen the adrenal glands. In Ayurveda, gotu kola clarifies the mind, improves memory, and promotes longevity. Himalayan yogis consume the herb as food or brew it into a tea to enhance their meditation practice. Bitter and cooling, gotu kola is a rejuvenating tonic for pitta people, but it also reduces excessive kapha and calms vata.

Ayurvedic practitioner examines the patient's pulse and tongue, and also could look at the eyes, listen to the organs, and palpate the abdomen to pinpoint doshic imbalances.

The Ayurvedic practitioner then considers all physical and lifestyle factors to custom-design an individualized formula—called a *rasayana*—to balance the patient's doshas for optimal health and well-being. The practitioner might instruct the patient to change various lifestyle practices—for example, how much sleep to get or how and when to eat. A practitioner also might recommend yoga, meditation, massage, or breathing exercises to help reduce the effects of stress and further pacify the doshas.

Herbal rasayanas incorporate herb, food, and mineral mixtures. As in TCM, Ayurveda uses herbs and foods according to what is known as a system of "energetics"—properties of foods and healing substances. This system takes into account flavor and energy (heating and cooling properties). Ayurveda classifies foods according to six primary tastes: sweet, sour, salty, pungent, bitter, and astringent. Each of these tastes has specific effects on the doshas. Ayurvedic remedies can contain as many as 20 different herbs, foods, and minerals.

An Ayurvedic herbal preparation could be a fresh juice, crushed pulp or paste, decoction (made by boiling herbs in liquid), hot infusion (made by steeping herbs in hot liquid), or cold infusion (made by steeping herbs in cold liquid). People also take herbs in powders, milk decoctions, and medicated wines, jellies, jams, ghee (clarified butter), and confections. Medicated oils, usually made by heating herbs in sesame oil, are used in massage or as ointments, douches, or internal remedies.

Many Ayurvedic practitioners also advise patients to undergo purification practices such as *panchakarma* (five actions). This is a rigorous multistep detoxification process that aims to help your body eliminate impurities (*ama*) to further balance the doshas. It includes specialized treatments such as oil therapy, sweating, purging, enemas, bloodletting, and nasal drops.

AROMATHERAPY

The use of highly concentrated aromatic essential oils for healing is often called aromatherapy. While the term aromatherapy is relatively new, the use of fragrant plant oils as medicines, perfumes, and cosmetics is ancient. People in the Middle East devised distillation methods to extract essential oils from plants as early as 1000 BCE. By the Middle Ages, many people throughout Europe used essential oils as perfumes and medicines.

Plants produce essential oils, also called volatile oils, in specialized oil glands located within or on their leaves, flowers, roots, fruit, seeds, or other parts. Long important in commercial perfumery, these oils are still used to create exquisite and expensive perfumes, but they have many other uses, too. Commercial food and beverage makers use essential oils as flavorings. Other industries incorporate essential oils with antiseptic properties into products designed to kill germs. Essential oil of thyme, for example, is a main ingredient in some mouthwashes. Pure plant essential oils are popular in the manufacture of natural cosmetics because they have properties, including anti-inflammatory and antiseptic abilities, that help soothe and rejuvenate your skin.

Scientific research has shown that aromas can have a profound effect on human emotions, and plant essential oils (aromatherapy) are often used to improve mood or state of mind. Some plant oils, such as peppermint, have uplifting and invigorating effects, helping to refresh and clear the mind. Others, like lavender, are calming and can help induce relaxation or even sleep. A growing body of research supports the clinical use of aromatherapy to treat certain conditions, such as anxiety. One small clinical study, for example, showed that massage with lavender essential oil reduced patient anxiety in a hospital intensive care unit. Other clinical studies have confirmed the traditional use of lavender essential oil to treat insomnia. Hundreds of laboratory studies have documented the antiseptic and anti-inflammatory properties of other essential oils.

How Aromatherapy Works

Essential oils are composed of molecules of aromatic compounds. One essential oil might contain hundreds of these aromatic compounds, which contribute to the oil's unique aroma and physiological actions. Chemists call these "volatile compounds" because their molecules easily evaporate, or volatilize, into the air. This is contrasted with fixed oils, such as cooking oils, which do not evaporate as quickly.

Essential oils can enter your body via absorption through your skin. In addition, the aromatic molecules floating around in the air enter your nose and are picked up by olfactory receptors. These transport information to the olfactory bulb located at the top of the nasal passage at the base of your brain. From there, scent information is passed on to the limbic system, a primitive part of your brain responsible for very basic body functions. The limbic system communicates with the hypothalamus and pituitary, master glands that affect and regulate fundamental body processes including the secretion of hormones and the regulation of moods, digestion, appetite, sexual arousal, and heartbeat. Aromas also stimulate the parts of your brain that control memory.

Important Cautions

Essential oils are extremely concentrated and must be treated with respect. A good rule of thumb is that *more is not better!* Never use undiluted essential oils directly on your skin—always use them in a diluted form (in a carrier oil, cream, or water), or vaporize them and gently inhale them. Never take essential oils internally, and keep them away from your eyes. Be sure to use only high-grade, pure plant essential oils (not synthetic fragrance oils), and become educated on the use of essential oils by reading a reputable book devoted to the subject or consulting a trained aromatherapy professional. (See "Resources" on page 472.)

Essential oils are estimated to be about 50 times stronger than the whole herbs from which they are extracted, but the concentration depends on the species from which they are derived. Also, be aware that some herbs that are perfectly safe to eat or to drink as a tea contain very strong, potentially toxic essential oils that must be used with caution. Examples include cinnamon bark (*Cinnamomum verum*), clove (*Syzygium aromaticum*), oregano (*Origanum vulgare*), savory (*Satureja* spp.), and thyme (*Thymus vulgaris*). Other essential oils, such as tansy (*Tanacetum vulgare*), are so toxic that they should not be used at all in aromatherapy. Essential oils made from flowers (such as rose or orange blossom) generally are the mildest essential oils.

Using Essential Oils

Two of the most popular ways to use essential oils are by inhaling them (smelling them) and by applying them to the skin (in a massage oil or facial oil). To obtain the benefits of aromatherapy, essential oils can also be added to bathwater, skin creams, and lotions; used to scent bedding, clothing, and laundry; and incorporated into homemade air-fresheners. A diffuser (a device specially designed to disperse essential oils into the air) can be used to fill an entire room with fragrance.

Inhaling essential oils: Add a few drops of essential oil to a piece of cloth or a cotton ball. To make a steam inhalation, add three to five drops of essential oil to a pot of steaming water. Steam provides a vehicle not only for inhaling essential oils,

ESSENTIAL OILS *and* THEIR PROPERTIES

Essential oils are highly concentrated sources of plant compounds. Many of them have healing properties, but they should never be taken internally.

HERB	PROPERTY
Carrot seed (*Daucus carota*)	Stimulates and regenerates skin cells; good for dry and mature skin
Chamomile, German (*Matricaria recutita*)	Anti-inflammatory; soothes sensitive skin and sore muscles; relaxing, uplifting aroma; might help ease insomnia
Clary sage (*Salvia sclarea*)	Eases muscle tension and menstrual cramps; helpful for oily skin; relaxing, euphoric aroma
Eucalyptus (*Eucalyptus globulus*)	Antibacterial, decongestant; clears sinuses and bronchial tubes; stimulating aroma
Geranium (*Pelargonium graveolens*)	Anti-inflammatory, antibacterial, antifungal; stimulates and regenerates skin cells; helpful for mature skin; relaxing aroma
Lavender (*Lavandula angustifolia*)	Anti-inflammatory, antibacterial, antifungal; general first aid; stimulates and regenerates skin cells; helpful for sensitive and mature skin; calming and relaxing, might help ease insomnia
Lemon (*Citrus limon*)	Antibacterial, antifungal; helpful for oily skin; uplifting aroma; might help ease stress and insomnia
Peppermint (*Mentha × piperita*)	Antibacterial; uplifting, stimulating aroma
Rose (*Rosa × centifolia or R. × damascena*)	Antiseptic, anti-inflammatory; stimulates and regenerates skin cells; helpful for mature skin
Rosemary (*Rosmarinus officinalis*)	Soothes muscle aches; stimulates circulation; helpful for mature skin; stimulating aroma
Tea tree (*Melaleuca alternifolia*)	Antibacterial, antifungal, anti-inflammatory

but also for carrying the essential oils to your skin. Position your face about 12 inches over the steaming water, drape a towel over your head, and breathe the steam for a moment or two. Remove the towel and take a few breaths of fresh air. Repeat the process for a maximum of 5 to 10 minutes.

Applying essential oils to your skin: To protect your skin from irritation, always dilute essential oils in a carrier oil (a vegetable or nut oil) such as sweet almond, grapeseed, sunflower, olive, jojoba, apricot kernel, kukui nut, or hazelnut oil.

Aromatic waters are another easy and pleasant way to use essential oils on your skin. To make aromatic water, add 10 drops of essential oil to 1 ounce of water in a spray bottle. To use, thoroughly shake the mixture, then mist your body and face, being sure to close your eyes before you spray.

How Essential Oils Are Produced

All plant aromas can be attributed to the presence of essential oils, which perform vital functions in the life cycles of plants. Some aromas produced by essential oils serve to attract pollinators. Some aromas repel pests or discourage grazing animals from eating the plant. Others protect plants against infection by bacteria, viruses, and fungi.

For commercial use, huge amounts of plant material are needed to produce small quantities of essential oils, which explains why some essential oils are so costly to buy. For example, 3 to 6 pounds of eucalyptus leaves are used to make 1 ounce of its essential oil. Ten to 20 pounds of lavender flowers are used to make 1 ounce of its essential oil. Production of 1 ounce of jasmine oil requires 160 to 280 pounds of flowers. And 2,000 rose petals are needed to make a single drop of rose oil.

Several different techniques can be used to extract essential oil, depending on the plant.

Steam distillation: Approximately 80 percent of plant essential oils are obtained by steam distillation—a process that uses steam, heat, and condensation to separate a plant's essential oils from its solid and water components. This technology uses no solvents, so the product is very pure. Essential oils produced this way include lavender, rosemary, peppermint, and eucalyptus.

Solvent extraction: For very delicate plants easily damaged by heat, other extraction techniques are available. Solvent extraction uses liquid solvents to dissolve and extract essential oils from the plant; the solvent is then evaporated under pressure. The initial product, called a concrete, is a sticky substance that contains plant waxes and pigments in addition to essential oils. The concrete can be sold as is or further refined to create a product called an absolute. This process is expensive, so it's generally used only to extract desirable and costly fragrances (like jasmine) that can't be produced through distillation. Solvent-extracted concretes and absolutes can contain traces of the solvents used to make them, so they aren't appropriate for therapeutic use but are fine to use as perfumes.

Supercritical carbon dioxide (CO_2) extraction: This newer technology uses carbon dioxide gas under low heat conditions to extract essential oils. Because less heat is used, the aroma of the essential oil is very close to that of the original plant. The final product is also free of solvent residues and is considered very pure. But the equipment needed for CO_2 extraction is expensive, as are the oils produced.

DILUTIONS *for* COMMON USES *of* ESSENTIAL OILS

Essential oils are extremely concentrated. You can benefit from just a few drops diluted in water or a carrier oil, lotion, or cream. Good carrier oils include sweet almond, grapeseed, and olive oils.

USE	DILUTION
Aromatic water (body mist)	10 drops per 1 oz water
Bathwater	3–6 drops per tub
Body or facial oil	6–8 drops per 1 oz carrier oil
Footbath	5 drops per basin of water
Massage oil	6–8 drops per 1 oz carrier oil
Room spray	15–20 drops per 1 oz water
Skin cream or lotion	6–8 drops per 1 oz lotion or cream
Steam inhalation	3–5 drops per 1 quart steaming water

Two types of essential oils are produced through CO_2 extraction, using slightly different technologies. One, called a selective extract, is a liquid composed mainly of volatile compounds. Oils produced this way include frankincense and myrrh. The other type, called a total extract, contains volatile components as well as fats, waxes, and pigments with medicinal properties. This technology is used to produce essential oil extracts of carrot seed, calendula, chamomile, and vanilla. It's also used to manufacture high-quality herbal extracts.

Cold expression: The essential oils of citrus fruits such as lemons, grapefruits, oranges, and limes are found in special oil glands in the rinds of these fruits. These oils are often extracted through a process called cold expression, which involves crushing the rinds to press out the oil, much like the way olive oil is produced. Citrus oils can also be produced through distillation.

Enfleurage: The oldest method for producing essential oils, rarely used today, is called enfleurage. The procedure involves placing fragrant blossoms on solid sheets of animal or vegetable fat and allowing the scent of the flowers to permeate the oil. When the fragrances in the blossoms are exhausted—having been absorbed by the fat—they are removed and replaced with fresh flowers. This process is repeated until the fat is saturated with volatile oils. A solvent can be used to extract the oils from the fat, or the fat can be used as is, in the form of an enfleurage pomade. Before the advent of solvent extraction, enfleurage was the only method available for extracting essential oils from delicate flowers such as rose, jasmine, and tuberose. This is a very old system of extraction that traces its origins to ancient Egypt, where fragrant flowers were extracted in animal fat and used to perfume the body.

Hydrosols: Hydrosols—true "flower waters"—are by-products of the steam distillation of essential oils. A hydrosol is the water component left behind when a plant's essential oil is separated out in the distillation process. Hydrosols contain water-soluble compounds that make them fragrant and soothing to the skin.

Two of the best-known and most popular hydrosols are orange flower water and rose water. Both have traditionally been used in cosmetics and for culinary flavorings. Hydrosols also make refreshing, aromatic body mists and skin toners, and these are sold in spray bottles. Some commercially available hydrosols include lavender, geranium, chamomile, rose, neroli (or orange blossom), and rosemary. When purchasing a hydrosol, look carefully at the label to be sure it is a true hydrosol and not aromatic water, which is a blend of water and essential oils.

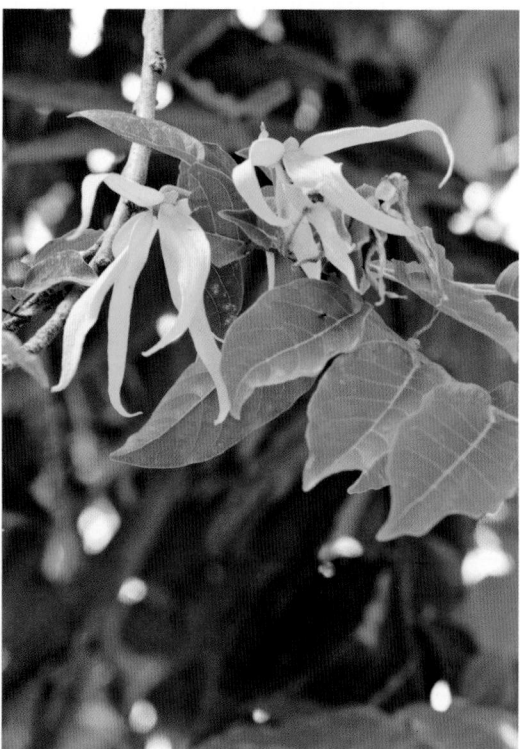

Intensely fragrant ylang-ylang blossoms are frequently used to scent perfumes, soaps, and candles. The aroma of this herb's oil can vary from floral to fruity.

How to Make Natural Perfumes

Using essential oils to create original fragrance blends for homemade cosmetics, air fresheners, or perfumes is fun and easy. And by making your own formulas you can avoid the harmful chemical compounds, such as phthalates, commonly used in commercial perfumes and beauty-care products. (Recent research has linked phthalates to serious health conditions.)

Start by choosing one essential oil to serve as the backbone of the fragrance, and then add small amounts of other oils, sniffing to judge the effect after each addition. You could use a fixative, such as glycerin, to help slow the evaporation rate of the essential oils. But before you add a fixative to any fragrance, test it on a small area of your skin, as it could cause an allergic reaction. Pay attention to the intensity of each oil, and use extremely strong-smelling oils sparingly so their presence does not overwhelm the others. A good rule of thumb is to use only one drop of very strong-smelling oil—such as jasmine, patchouli, rosemary, or ylang-ylang—for every 5 to 10 drops of milder-smelling oil, such as citrus or lavender.

Make small batches of fragrance until the process becomes comfortable. Take notes so that you can duplicate your favorites later. To make a perfume, add about 12 drops of a blend to 1 ounce of a carrier oil. (Jojoba oil makes a good perfume base.)

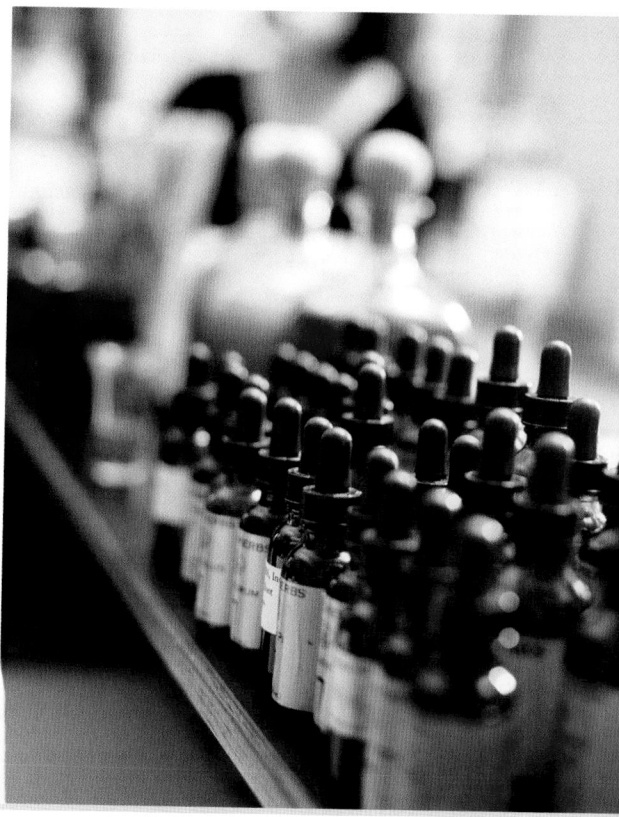

Medical providers are learning to incorporate herbal treatments, including homeopathic remedies, into their practices. Many are advising the use of herbal extracts that have been clinically proven to be safe, such as saw palmetto.

HOMEOPATHY

The medicinal practice of homeopathy is very different from herbal medicine. It is often included in discussions of herbs, however, because many homeopathic remedies contain tiny dilutions of plant substances.

Homeopathic remedies are preparations of highly diluted plants, or other natural substances, administered to stimulate your body's own healing responses. In contrast, herbal medicine uses relatively larger doses of plants to achieve therapeutic effects. The homeopathic system was developed in the early 19th century by the German physician and chemist Samuel Hahnemann (1755–1843). Discouraged by the practice of conventional medicine—which at the time relied in large part on the prescription of highly toxic drugs, purging, and bloodletting—Hahnemann embarked on a series of experiments with plant medicines that led to the development of the first homeopathic remedies.

In the first of these experiments, which came to be known as "provings," Hahnemann dosed himself with cinchona bark, a plant medicine used to treat malaria. Hahnemann was surprised to find that after taking cinchona bark, he developed symptoms similar to those of malaria. He eventually developed the Law of Similars, a guiding principle of homeopathy (see below). In his lifetime, Hahnemann proved the effectiveness of about 100 remedies; currently, more than 3,000 remedies are available.

Homeopathy is most widely practiced in Europe and North America, with approximately 5 million people in the United States reporting having used a homeopathic product in 2006. In Europe, the practice is supported by legislation passed in 1997 by the European parliament. Both conventional physicians and professional homeopaths (those trained primarily in homeopathy) are legally permitted to practice in most European countries. In the United States, homeopathy is often practiced along with a licensed medical discipline, such as conventional medicine, naturopathy, chiropractic, or veterinary medicine. Homeopathy is a regular part of training for naturopathic doctors; other health practitioners receive training through diploma and certificate programs. Since 1938, homeopathic remedies have been regulated as over-the-counter (nonprescription) drugs in the United States, unlike herbs, which are currently regulated as dietary supplements.

Numerous modern studies have investigated the clinical use of homeopathy, and positive results have been demonstrated in some studies on influenza, allergies, allergic asthma, acute childhood diarrhea, vertigo, and osteoarthritis pain. However, many clinical studies have had conflicting or negative results, and some research on homeopathy has been criticized as not being sufficiently rigorous. Although many theories have been proposed, researchers have not yet been able to find any conclusive scientific explanation for how homeopathic remedies work. This is a subject of ongoing controversy and debate in the scientific community. Skeptics claim the benefits of homeopathy can be attributed to the placebo effect—an improvement due only to the expectations of the patient. At a minimum, this shows the importance of the mind-body connection.

Other researchers believe homeopathy's effects

FLOWER REMEDIES

Flower remedies are a type of homeopathic remedy intended to work not on physical problems, but rather on psychological and emotional disturbances. (Flower remedies are called flower essences in the United States to comply with regulatory requirements.)

The Bach Flower Remedies constitute the original flower remedy system, introduced in the early 20th century by the English physician, pathologist, and immunologist Edward Bach (1886–1936). Bach's system of 38 flower remedies is still widely used. Practitioners of the Bach system can be found all over the world, especially in the United Kingdom, Germany, and the United States. Numerous other flower remedy systems have been developed in more recent years, using flowers that are indigenous to different regions of the world.

To make a flower remedy, an "essence" of a plant is first prepared, either by floating blossoms in pure water in a clear glass bowl set in the sun for several hours or by boiling the plant material. The essence is then preserved in brandy to create a stock from which individual medicines are made. An individual medicine consists of 2 drops of the stock medicine mixed with 1 ounce (30 ml) of pure water in a dropper bottle. According to Dr. Bach, a patient should take 4 drops of a remedy four times a day.

can be explained by quantum physics, an area of science that is still evolving. Whatever might be the most accurate explanation, millions of people around the world rely on homeopathy to treat a variety of conditions.

Principles of Homeopathy

Homeopaths believe that every person has a "vital force" or self-healing ability that can be called upon to treat or prevent disease. Homeopathic medicine aims to stimulate your body's own self-healing response through the use of carefully chosen homeopathic remedies.

Homeopaths base diagnosis and treatment upon an in-depth case history that provides a complete picture of an individual's current and past physical symptoms, as well as many other factors, including outlook on life, emotional temperament, food preferences, and reactions to stress. Treatment is based upon the Law of Similars, or "like cures like." (The word homeopathy comes from the Greek words *homeo*, meaning "similar," and *pathos*, which means "disease" or "suffering.")

A simple explanation of this principle is that a substance that causes a certain symptom when given in a large dose can be used in minute amounts to treat that same symptom. For example, the pungent compounds in onions cause watery eyes and nose, throat irritation, coughing, and sneezing. Therefore, in homeopathy, a diluted preparation of onion is used to treat colds or allergies that cause similar symptoms.

Practitioners of homeopathy believe that self-treatment with homeopathic remedies is appropri-ate for minor acute problems and injuries, but that a qualified homeopath should be consulted for more serious problems.

Homeopathic Remedies

Homeopathic remedies are preparations made from highly diluted natural substances. These natural substances can come from plants, minerals, or animals. Even bacteria and very poisonous substances, such as arsenic and cadmium, can be used. In most highly diluted remedies, however, not even a molecule of the original substance can be detected in the finished product. For this reason, homeopathic remedies are generally considered safe and nontoxic.

A homeopathic remedy is created through a multistep process. First, the plant, mineral, or animal material being used to make the remedy is extracted in alcohol to create what is called a "mother tincture." Next, 1 drop of this mother tincture is added to 99 drops of an alcohol-water solution and then "succussed" (shaken vigorously). This process of dilution and succussion is repeated until the desired dilution has been attained.

Homeopathic remedies are sold in liquid, tablet, pellet, powder, and ointment forms. The strength of the remedy, known in homeopathy as potency, is indicated on the label on a scale from highest potency (3c or 3x) to lowest potency (30c or 30x). The higher the number, the lower the potency. Potency is usually determined by the amount of times the solution is shaken and diluted during preparation. The lower the potency (in other words, the more dilute the remedy), the more effective the remedy is believed to be.

USING HERBS AS MEDICINE

The most basic way to obtain the health benefits of a beneficial herb internally is to put the appropriate plant part (leaf, flower, root, etc.) in your mouth and chew it. But this is rarely the most convenient or pleasant way to take an herbal remedy. In most cases, the desirable compounds first must be extracted or converted into a form that's easy to take. Some herbal preparations—those that contain alcohol, for example—also help preserve the herbs.

Extracting medicinal compounds from a plant generally requires a solvent—a substance capable of separating out the desired constituents and leaving the rest behind. Boiling water functions as the solvent for herbal infusions and decoctions (teas). But not all plant compounds are soluble in water—some require alcohol or even oil for effective extraction. Other solvents include vegetable glycerin and vinegar.

HERBAL PREPARATIONS

Medicinal herbal preparations run the gamut from do-it-yourself "kitchen medicines" made from fresh, whole plants to high-tech standardized extracts produced in modern, high-quality manufacturing facilities. Today, many people enjoy the convenience and uniformity of commercially prepared herbal remedies, although it's easy to prepare your own simple remedies, too.

Commercially available herbal preparations include tablets, capsules, cough syrups, ointments, creams, suppositories, and lotions. Tablets are made by eliminating the water from a plant or extract, powdering it, and pressing it into the form of a tablet, sometimes along with fillers or excipients (inert substances that help hold shape). Hard-shelled capsules are two-part shells (made of gelatin, starch, or cellulose) filled with powdered herb. Soft-shelled capsules are often made of a single piece designed to hold oil-based extracts or pure oils.

PLANT FOODS *as* MEDICINES

Noncommunicable diseases (NCDs), such as cancer, asthma, diabetes, and heart disease, are some of the world's leading causes of mortality and affect most regions around the globe. They are known as "lifestyle" diseases because poor diet, physical inactivity, and other lifestyle choices are major contributors to their development. The World Health Organization (WHO) estimates that by 2020, NCDs will contribute to 7 out of every 10 deaths in developing countries, killing 52 million people annually worldwide by 2030.

Researchers at the Institute of Economic Botany at The New York Botanical Garden have discovered that a potential solution to this epidemic might be found in the traditional uses of plant medicines.

Ina Vandebroek, PhD, and her colleagues are conducting studies about the ethnomedical traditions of Latino and Caribbean immigrant communities in New York City. Since 2005, her research has focused on understanding the cultural practices of immigrants from the Dominican Republic who self-medicate with plants they purchase from specialized stores called *botánicas*. The study, initially funded by the National Institutes of Health/ National Center for Complementary and Alternative Medicine (NIH/ NCCAM), found that plant foods, such as lime, bitter orange, garlic, onion, shallot, watercress, and radish, become more important as medicines for Dominicans after immigration to New York City. The popularity and use of these medicinal foods can contribute to addressing the NCDs epidemic, although much more laboratory and clinical research into these foods' potential preventive and therapeutic activities for specific conditions is needed. We have a lot to learn from the communities who come to this country, bringing many of their plant foods and medicines with them, along with their healing knowledge and practices.—M. J. B.

Standardized Extracts

Standardized extracts must contain a specified amount of one or more chemical constituents, often called marker compounds. (For more about this, see "Whole Plant Herbal Remedies and Phytomedicines" on page 342.) Chemists test for marker compounds using sophisticated laboratory technologies, such as high-pressure liquid chromatography (HPLC). With HPLC, a solvent-containing extract is pumped over a solid material that separates compounds by physical and/or chemical properties. This provides a chemical profile that shows exactly what compounds an extract contains and in what proportions.

Standardized extracts are usually sold as capsules or tablets, labeled with the percentage of marker compounds they contain. Milk thistle (*Silybum marianum*), for example, is usually standardized to contain 70 to 80 percent silymarin. Saw palmetto (*Serenoa repens*) is standardized to 85 to 95 percent fatty acids and sterols. Some standardized extracts are also concentrated to increase the levels of certain constituents. For example, standardized *Ginkgo biloba* extract is a 50:1 concentrated extract standardized to contain 24 percent ginkgo flavone glycosides and 6 percent terpene lactones.

Standardized extracts offer several advantages. They allow herbal product manufacturers to ensure that the extract contains the same quantity of marker compounds each and every time they make it. (In nature, the amount of chemicals produced by a given plant can vary according to weather, altitude, soil composition, and other factors.) And doctors and clinical researchers appreciate standardized extracts because they can administer the same dosage to a patient time and time again, ensuring consistent results.

But standardized extracts have drawbacks, too. As mentioned earlier, the beneficial effects of many herbs appear to be due to many constituents working together. Because of this, identifying the active ingredients, or marker compounds, for a standardized extract can be challenging. Another disadvantage is that they're usually more expensive than simpler, traditional herbal preparations, and they can't be made at home. Some herbalists and consumers are uncomfortable using standardized extracts because they seem more like high-tech pharmaceuticals than natural plant remedies.

Herbal Infusions and Decoctions

Herbal infusions and decoctions, commonly called "herb teas," are two of the simplest and most effective ways to take herbs that have water-soluble constituents, and you can easily prepare them yourself. Herbal infusions can also be added to baths or used in compresses, douches, enemas, gargles, and mouthwashes.

Infusion is a gentler extraction method than decoction. It's best for delicate leaves and flowers that could be destroyed by too much heat, such as mints (*Mentha* spp.), lemon balm (*Melissa officinalis*), bee balm (*Monarda* spp.), and chamomile (*Chamaemelum nobile*). Decoction is used to extract water-soluble compounds from harder plant materials such as roots, like astragalus and ginger, seeds, and bark. Roots with a particularly high content of volatile oils, such as valerian, should not be decocted, however, but instead ground into a fine powder and steeped as an infusion to prevent the loss of volatile oils.

To make an infusion: Pour boiling water over dried or fresh leaves or flowers, and cover the container tightly to prevent the escape of volatile oils. Steep for 10 to 15 minutes, strain, and drink. The exact proportion of plant material to water will vary with the herb used, but a general rule of thumb is to use 1 cup of water to 1 teaspoon of dried herb. Fresh herbs have a high water content, so you'll need to use about three times as much fresh herb for a similar concentration.

To make a decoction: Place herbs (roots, bark,

or seeds) and water in a pot. Cover, bring to a boil, lower the heat, and simmer for about 20 minutes. Strain and drink. General proportions for decoctions are 1 cup of water to 1 ounce of dried herb.

Tinctures

Tincturing is a method for extracting and preserving the medicinal constituents of herbs in a solution of alcohol and water. Black cohosh (*Actaea racemosa*), echinacea (*Echinacea* spp.), passionflower (*Passiflora incarnata*), cat's claw (*Uncaria tomentosa*), nettle (*Urtica dioica*), and valerian (*Valeriana officinalis*) are frequently prepared this way. Properly made and stored, tinctures can last for 5 years or more. While many high-quality commercially prepared tinctures are available, you can make them at home, too. For the home medicine-maker, vodka is an excellent solvent for most herbs because it has a mild flavor and contains enough alcohol to serve as a good preservative. To reduce the chance of spoilage, use 100 proof (50 percent) vodka.

To make a tincture: Finely chop the fresh or dried herb. Fill a 1-quart glass jar about two-thirds full with the herb. (If you're using roots, fill the jar only one-third full.) Add the vodka to within ½ inch of the jar rim, completely covering the herb. Stir gently to release any air bubbles. Cap the jar tightly. About twice a week, shake the jar to help extract the medicinal compounds; also check the liquid level and top off with more vodka if necessary. Allow the mixture to extract for 6 weeks. Drain the resulting mixture through a coffee filter or a strainer lined with muslin or cheesecloth, pressing as much liquid as possible out of the herb. Label and store the tincture in a dark-colored glass bottle, out of the reach of children and pets.

Herb-Infused Oils

Infused oils—vegetable oils in which dried herbs have been steeped (or macerated)—have therapeutic benefits when applied directly to your skin. Infused oils can also be used as bases for healing salves, ointments, and other preparations.

Organic olive oil is an excellent base for therapeutic infused oils; grapeseed, sweet almond, and other oils can also be used. Olive oil infused with the flowers of St. John's wort makes an effective massage oil for treating sciatic nerve pain. Mullein flower oil is useful for treating skin conditions, earaches, and joint pain. Arnica, calendula, chamomile, chickweed, comfrey, and many other herbs can also be infused in oil for external use.

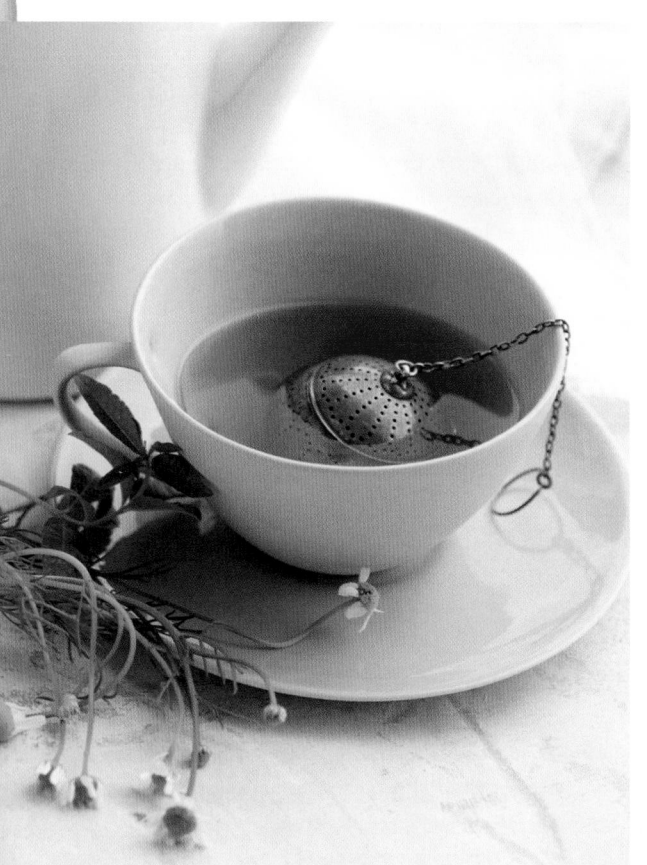

An infusion of chamomile flowers tames tension and aids digestion.

To make a therapeutic herb-infused oil: Fill a jar about three-quarters full with dried herbs (fresh herbs are more likely to cause spoilage), and then pour the olive oil over the herbs to fill the jar. Be sure the herbs are completely submerged in the oil, because any plant material exposed to air can generate spoilage. Cap the jar. Allow the herb to soak (macerate) in the oil in a warm, sunny location for 4 to 6 weeks, and then strain carefully through cheesecloth or muslin, pressing out as much oil as possible from the herb. Pour the oil into clean, dry, amber bottles. Label and store them in a cool, dark location for up to 1 year.

Salves

Oils infused with herbs can be used—alone or in combination—to make healing salves. Try any of those listed in "Healing Herbs Used Externally" on page 369.

To make a healing salve: Gently heat ½ cup of herb-infused oil in a double boiler. Add ½ ounce of grated beeswax to the oil. Stir, and remove from the heat when the mixture is blended and the wax has melted. Add the contents of two vitamin E capsules (as a preservative). Cool for 2 to 3 minutes, then pour into a small, wide-mouth jar. The salve will become semifirm as it cools. When it has cooled completely, cap the jar, label, and then store it in a cool, dry location. Apply the salve externally, directly to your skin, to treat skin irritation and muscle or joint pain.

Liniments

Liniments are similar to herb-infused oils but use rubbing alcohol as a base rather than oil. Eucalyptus and peppermint are often included for their cooling effect. The liquid or spray is rubbed into your skin to soothe muscle aches, sprains, joint pain, and bruises.

To make a liniment: Fill a jar about two-thirds

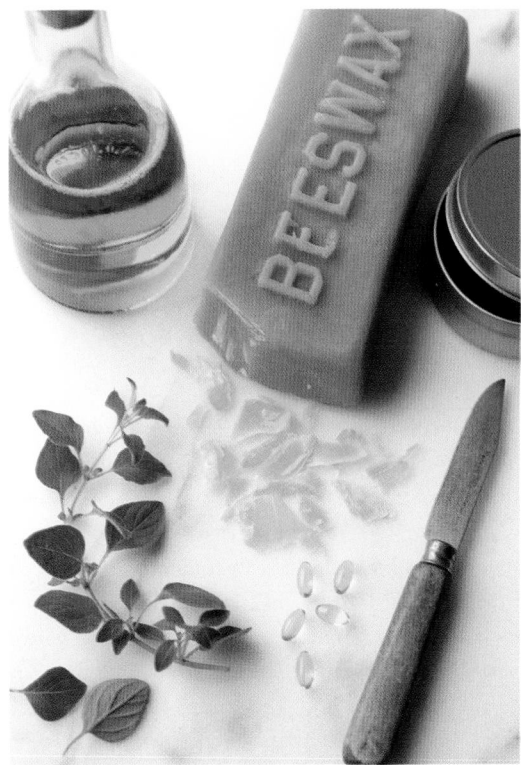

The ingredients for a healing salve include herb-infused oil, beeswax, and vitamin E.

full with dried herbs, such as peppermint, rosemary, and lavender. Cover the herbs with rubbing alcohol, then seal the jar tightly. Macerate (soak) the herbs in the alcohol for 4 to 6 weeks, shaking the jar every few days. Strain the liquid into glass bottles with mister tops. Label and store in a cool, dry place.

Compresses

A compress can be applied externally to treat pain and inflammation, strains, sprains, chest congestion, or sunburn. In Thailand, hot herbal compresses have been used for thousands of years. Ginger, turmeric, and lemongrass are commonly used. The herbs are wrapped in muslin and then steamed to moisten and heat them. The hot compresses are then pressed onto the skin or applied in circular motions to treat muscle pain and cramping, arthritis, tendonitis, stress, and anxiety, and to increase the flow of energy.

To prepare a compress: First make a strong infusion or decoction. Dip a cloth into the liquid, then apply it to the affected area for up to 1 hour. Reapply several times a day, as needed.

Poultices

A poultice is a paste prepared from moistened herbs. It can be applied, cold or hot, directly to the skin to treat inflammation, bruises, or chest congestion, or to draw out toxins. (The technical name for a hot poultice is a fomentation.) Herbs traditionally used in poultices include St. John's wort (for inflammation and muscle or nerve pain), yarrow (for skin irritations and bruising), plantain (for cuts, burns, eczema, poison ivy, and insect bites and stings), and mullein (for sore throat, chest congestion, hemorrhoids, and skin irritations including sunburn). Mullein poultices are usually prepared with a hot liquid, such as cider vinegar, sometimes diluted with water.

To prepare a poultice: Use a mortar and pestle or a blender to crush the herbs. Slowly add enough distilled water to make a thick, spreadable—but not watery—paste. Clean the affected area with hydrogen peroxide, than apply the paste. Loosely cover it with a bandage or gauze and tape. Reapply the poultice as needed when it has dried.

USING HERBS SAFELY

Herbs are best used in moderation to gently support and maintain health while protecting the body against disease. Used sensibly, most, but not all, herbs have an excellent safety record based on centuries of human use as medicines and foods. However, always use these powerful plants under the supervision of a qualified health-care practitioner—self-medication carries risks.

To put the issue of safety in relative terms, consider that every ingested substance carries some degree of risk. As with any substance, including foods, it's possible for one person to have an allergic or otherwise unusual reaction to an herb that most people can use without problems. This is a common phenomenon in medicine as well as in the culinary arts. Documented herb allergies are uncommon, but not unknown. For example, people who are allergic to ragweed and other plants in the family Asteraceae are cautioned to avoid chamomile, but only a relatively few cases of chamomile allergy have actually been reported.

The vast majority of herbs are safe and nontoxic when used as directed by a knowledgeable health-care professional—but note that this does not include a helpful clerk in a health food store or content on a Web site. Most professionals who work with herbs have undertaken many years of formal training to learn all there is to know about the plants they use and their effects—both beneficial and potentially harmful—on people, as well as the interactions of herbal remedies with other medications a person could be taking. That professional will advise you when to begin taking an herb and when to suspend use, if need be.

Certain individuals, including pregnant women, children, people with serious health conditions (such as high blood pressure, chronic illnesses, liver problems, or kidney disease), and those taking pharmaceutical drugs *should always consult a physician before using herbs.*

Many of the problems reported with herbs in recent years can be attributed to what amounts to "herb abuse"—such as taking large doses of ephedra (*Ephedra sinica*) for weight loss or energy enhancement. Using herbs in high doses to enhance weight loss or sports performance is not a wise use of plant remedies, nor is it in keeping with traditional herb applications.

HEALING HERBS USED EXTERNALLY

These are just a few of the many healing herbs that can be applied topically in oils, salves, liniments, and creams. (*Note:* Oils, salves, and other external herbal preparations should not be applied to broken skin or open wounds unless your practitioner has advised otherwise.)

Arnica flowers: muscle and joint pain

Calendula flowers: rashes, insect bites, minor burns

Chamomile flowers: itching, eczema, inflammation

Chickweed leaves: eczema, psoriasis, dryness, itching

Comfrey leaves: minor cuts, scrapes, insect stings, muscle and joint pain

Eucalyptus leaves: insect bites, stings, wounds, and blisters; analgesic and anti-inflammatory for muscles and joints

Jewelweed leaves and stems: rash, minor cuts, poison ivy, nettle stings

Lavender flowers: itching, insect bites, minor burns, muscle aches

Mullein flowers and leaves: skin irritation, joint pain, hemorrhoids, earache, sore throat, chest congestion

Oregano leaves: insect bites, athlete's foot

Plantain leaves: insect bites and stings, pain, poison ivy, itching, rashes, sores

Rosemary leaves and flowers: muscle and nerve pain, such as sciatica

St. John's wort flowers: burns, insect bites, nerve pain

Thyme leaves: minor cuts and scrapes, muscle pain

Yarrow flowers: bruises, cuts, eczema, rashes, sprains, wounds, and areas with swelling and bleeding

---

With some herbal remedies, such as stimulant laxatives, the same chemical compounds that offer medicinal effects in small doses can cause harmful side effects in larger doses or with chronic use. Use stimulant laxatives in moderation. Occasional short-term use is fine, but long-term use can cause your bowels to lose their ability to function without help. Chronic use can also lead to dangerous fluid depletion, electrolyte imbalances, and other problems. Herbal stimulant laxatives include cascara sagrada (*Rhamnus purshiana*), senna (*Senna alexandrina*), purging buckthorn (*R. cathartica*), alder buckthorn (*R. frangula*), Chinese rhubarb (*Rheum officinale, R. palmatum*), and the dried latex from the leaves (not the gel) of the aloe plant (*Aloe vera*).

Some herbs are toxic if used in large doses, and certain herbs are so potent that they simply shouldn't be used as remedies under any circumstances. So become as educated as possible about an herb before you take it. If in doubt about the safety of any herb or herbal remedy, be sure to consult a qualified herbalist, reputable herbal guidebook, or your local poison control center, which can provide information about the toxicity of plants ingested by people.

From the earliest days of human civilization, settlement, and agriculture—and certainly for many millennia before the advent of recorded history—plants have been essential to humans. From what undoubtedly were our first food sources—wild grasses, leaves, fleshy roots, and fruits—to the herbs that healed us and soothed our souls, plants have influenced our development as a species.

Modernization has taken many of us far from the gardens, fields, forests, and wilderness areas where so many healing plants can be found. Today, through movements such as integrative medicine and a rebirth of interest in traditional practices, many people are taking more responsibility for their health and wellness. Herbs and botanical remedies are an essential part of the path to a higher quality of life.

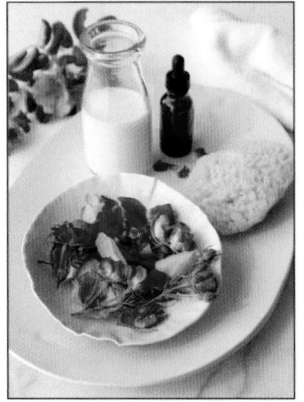

CHAPTER 6

HERBS FOR BEAUTY *and* BATH

Since the earliest days of recorded history, people have used herbs and other plant ingredients to beautify and scent their skin, hair, and nails. Ancient records reveal recipes for fragrant hair treatments, healing herb-infused oils, and tonics for longevity and youthful appearance. Botanical cosmetics have been discovered in the tombs of ancient Egyptians, and legendary beauties Cleopatra and Nefertiti are reputed to have claimed aloe as one of their antiaging secrets. For centuries, Indian women have decorated their hair and skin with henna and anointed their bodies with fragrant botanical oils and herbs such as turmeric. Hippocrates (460–377 BCE), an ancient Greek physician, studied the link between health and beauty and is credited with developing the science of dermatology.

Today, herbs are no less popular as cosmetic ingredients. Herbs and other botanical ingredients—from gentle, emollient vegetable oils to fruits rich in skin-softening plant compounds—offer an alternative to the harsh chemicals found in many synthetically based commercial beauty and hair- and skin-care products. Equally important, they provide exquisite natural fragrances that uplift the spirit, rejuvenate the body, and add to personal allure.

SKIN HEALTH

Beautiful skin is healthy skin. Used on the outside of your body, herbs and other botanical ingredients can help keep skin looking fresh and youthful by exfoliating dead skin cells, improving skin tone and blood circulation, and keeping skin supple and hydrated. They can soothe irritated skin, combat inflammation, fight skin infections, and help to heal wounds, sores, and burns. The botanical world is also rich in alpha hydroxy acids (AHAs). These acidic plant compounds help exfoliate and soften skin and are used in many of today's antiaging skin products.

Having radiant, healthy skin does not depend solely on what we put on our skin—what we put *into* our bodies matters, too. Taken internally, many herbs—including burdock, nettle, and red clover—have a long history of traditional use for treating skin problems. Drinking plenty of water is also essential to keeping skin hydrated and looking its best. Skin, hair, and nail health all require and benefit from a balanced diet that includes plenty of plant-based foods—nutrient-rich fruits, vegetables, legumes, whole grains, and healthful oils, and especially those foods that are rich in antioxidants and essential fatty acids. Regular exercise promotes blood flow, resulting in a healthy glow that keeps skin looking fresh and youthful. And never underestimate the cosmetic value of adequate sleep—it's called "beauty rest" for a reason.

Other lifestyle choices are just as important to healthy skin as proper diet and exercise. Exposure to the sun's rays and cigarette smoke are recognized as two of the leading causes of skin wrinkling and other signs of premature aging. Experts advise using adequate sun protection, such as sunscreen and a wide-brimmed hat, whenever you're exposed to the damaging rays of the sun. Avoid secondhand smoke, and if you yourself smoke, give it up—your entire body will thank you for it.

BEAUTY THROUGH THE AGES

The desire to look and feel our best is universal. All over the world, people have spent time and energy—and money—to develop herbal products for cosmetic and medicinal use.

When other civilizations were still in their infancy, Chinese herbalists were experimenting with the possible uses of plants, seeking the combination of herbs that would do the most to nourish and cure. The ancient Egyptians used eye pencils, depilatories, deodorants, hair tonics, and cleansing creams made from limes, lilies, frankincense, and myrrh. In India, both men and women used makeup and perfumes to adorn themselves for religious ceremonies, as early as the second century BCE.

Ancient Romans used lavender to scent bathwater and linens and to soothe wounds—in fact, this herb's name comes from the Latin *lavare*, meaning "to wash." In biblical times in the Middle East, perfumes and bath oils were made from saffron, cassia, cinnamon, and camphire (henna). By the 9th century, Arab scientists had perfected the process for extracting an herb's essential oil via

(continued on page 374)

HERBS *for* HEALTHY, BEAUTIFUL SKIN *and* HAIR

The following herbs have properties that can protect, heal, and beautify your skin and hair. Depending on their effects, you can use them to make gentle cleansers, stimulating rinses, soothing salves, and much more. (For how to make healing salves for skin, see Chapter 5 on page 367.)

HERB	EFFECT
Aloe (*Aloe vera*)	Antifungal, anti-inflammatory, emollient; helps heal wounds and burns
Bay (*Laurus nobilis*)	Antibacterial, antifungal; used in shampoos, hair rinses, and hair tonics to treat dandruff and possibly stimulate hair growth
Burdock (*Arctium lappa*)	Antifungal, anti-inflammatory, emollient; used externally and internally for acne, eczema, and psoriasis; good for oily skin
Calendula (*Calendula officinalis*)	Antifungal, antiseptic, anti-inflammatory, astringent, styptic; helps heal wounds and burns, relieves sunburn; good for normal, dry, and sensitive skin types; good all-purpose hair rinse
Chickweed (*Stellaria media*)	Helps relieve itching
Citrus (*Citrus* spp.)	Antibacterial, antifungal, anti-inflammatory, astringent; helps heal insect bites and wounds; good for oily skin
Comfrey (*Symphytum officinale*)	Emollient; stimulates cell growth, helps in wound healing; good for dry skin
Echinacea (*Echinacea* spp.)	Fights infection, helps in wound healing
Elder flower (*Sambucus* spp.)	Anti-inflammatory, astringent, emollient; good for both dry and oily skin types
Fennel (*Foeniculum vulgare*)	Anti-inflammatory, aromatic; good for dry skin
German chamomile (*Matricaria recutita*)	Anti-inflammatory and antiseptic; used for minor burns, cuts, eczema, and other skin irritations; good for normal, dry, and sensitive skin types
Ginger (*Zingiber officinale*)	Analgesic, antibacterial, anti-inflammatory, astringent, stimulating; used to relieve bruises, muscular aches and pains, and poor circulation
Gotu kola (*Centella asiatica*)	Helps promote wound and scar healing, encourages production of collagen
Grand Fir (*Abies grandis*)	Antiseptic, astringent, deodorant, stimulant, tonic; good for burns, cuts, muscle aches and pains, and wounds
Henna (*Lawsonia inermis*)	Enhances hair color
Jasmine (*Jasminum grandiflorum*)	Analgesic, anti-inflammatory, tonic; soothes irritated skin
Kelp (*Laminaria* spp.)	Emollient, nutritive; good for dry skin
Lavender (*Lavandula* spp.)	Antiseptic, anti-inflammatory, aromatic; good for normal and sensitive skin types

HERB	EFFECT
Lemon balm (*Melissa officinalis*)	Antiseptic, aromatic
Marshmallow (*Althaea officinalis*)	Anti-inflammatory, emollient; good for sensitive skin
Neem (*Azadirachta indica*)	Antifungal, anti-inflammatory; helpful against dandruff
Nettle (*Urtica dioica*)	Astringent, nutritive; helpful against dandruff; used in hair rinses
Oats, oatstraw (*Avena sativa*)	Emollient, nutritive; good for dry and sensitive skin types
Passionflower (*Passiflora incarnata*)	Sedative; relieves irritated skin; can be used to make a relaxing bath
Peppermint (*Mentha × piperita*)	Antiseptic, astringent, cooling, stimulating; good for oily skin
Plantain (*Plantago major*)	Antiseptic, anti-inflammatory, astringent, emollient; helps with wound healing
Red clover (*Trifolium pratense*)	Anti-inflammatory; used externally and internally for acne, eczema, and psoriasis
Roman chamomile (*Chamaemelum nobile*)	Analgesic, anti-inflammatory, antiseptic; used to treat burns, cuts, insect bites, and other skin irritations; adds shine to hair
Rose (*Rosa* spp.)	Antiseptic, aromatic, astringent, emollient; good for normal, dry, and sensitive skin types
Rosemary (*Rosmarinus officinalis*)	Antiseptic, aromatic, astringent, stimulating; good for oily skin and hair
Sage (*Salvia officinalis*)	Antiseptic, aromatic; used to treat acne; good for oily skin and hair
Spearmint (*Mentha spicata*)	Analgesic, antiseptic, astringent, stimulant; good for oily skin and hair
St. John's wort (*Hypericum perforatum*)	Anti-inflammatory; helps heal wounds and burns (avoid sun exposure after applying to skin)
Tea tree (*Melaleuca alternifolia*)	Antibacterial, antifungal, antiseptic; used to treat fungal infections, acne, dandruff, and eczema
Witch hazel (*Hamamelis virginiana*)	Anti-inflammatory, antiseptic, astringent, styptic; helps relieve itching; good for oily skin
Yarrow (*Achillea millefolium*)	Anti-inflammatory, antiseptic, astringent, styptic; good for oily skin
Ylang-ylang (*Cananga odorata*)	Antifungal, anti-inflammatory, antiseptic; used to heal insect bites, scars, and wounds

Your skin is your body's largest organ. Its surface area can be as much as 3,100 square inches. Although we tend to think of our skin as a barrier to the outside world, it's really more like a living sponge. Skin can absorb thousands of chemicals, feed them into your bloodstream through the network of tiny blood vessels just below its surface, and immediately circulate them through your body. When these compounds are toxic, they can do damage over both the short and long term.

To experience how easily and quickly compounds can be absorbed into your skin, try this simple test: Place a drop of spearmint or pepper-mint oil on your forefinger and rub it with your thumb. Be careful not to smell the oil—hold your hand as far from your nose as possible. Look at a clock with a second hand. If you are like most people, you will feel a small sensation—I call it a "puff"—of peppermint taste at the back of your throat or inside your mouth in less than a minute. Your skin has absorbed a fragrant compound, and the compound has circulated through your body, where you sense it in your throat.

No peppermint or spearmint oil lying around the house? No worries—just rub a crushed clove of garlic on the bottom of your foot. A few min-utes later, you will have a mild taste of garlic in your mouth.

The toxic and irritating compounds in the personal-care products and household cleansers you use enter your body in the same manner. But the truth is, so many known or suspected toxins are allowed to be used in personal-care products and household cleaners (to name just two categories) that we all need to exam-ine labels carefully and choose prod-ucts wisely. Opt for those with simple, natural ingredients—or make your own. You can reduce your toxin load a bit by making some of the herbal products discussed in this chapter. —M. J. B.

---

distillation. Over the centuries that followed, much of the Arab world was using aromatic baths, powders, and salves to cure a variety of ills.

Some plants have had special significance for hundreds of years. One introduced to Europe from the Middle East during the Crusades was the dam-ask rose. Roses and the fragrant oils they produce have been supremely important in the Muslim world since the time of Mohammed (570–632). As early as the 7th century, Arab alchemists used roses and their fragrant extracts to purify mosques, infuse prayer beads with fragrance, sprinkle guests as they entered houses, and flavor foods ranging from sherbet to candy. In fact, one of the books by the Arabic herbalist Abu 'Ali al-Husayn ibn 'Abd Allah ibn Sina, known in the Western world as Avicenna (980–1037), was devoted entirely to roses. Today, rose oil continues to be an impor-tant ingredient in beauty products, as well as aromatherapy.

HERBAL BEAUTY PRODUCTS

A walk through the cosmetics aisle of your grocery or health food store can reveal a bewildering array of products—shampoos and conditioners, soaps, cleansers, and antiaging face creams—promoting the benefits of the botanical ingredients they con-tain. But be aware that many commercial skin- and hair-care products touted as "natural" contain synthetic ingredients, including preservatives and surfactants. Preservatives give a product a longer shelf life but don't have an impact on its effective-ness. Some surfactants are thought to be harmful to the environment and are banned in Europe.

If you are purchasing herbal beauty products from a store, it's a good idea to become educated about the ingredients they contain—or do not contain in sufficient quantities to have an effect. Read the labels carefully: Be sure the products can deliver the benefits they promise, and seek out clinical studies that can back up their claims. How many of the plant ingredients do you recognize? You will find many common garden flowers and herbs—such as aloe, chamomile, lavender, rose, and rosemary—listed, as well as more unusual and exotic plants such as ginger, passionflower, ylang-ylang, and yucca.

An easy, economical, and in some cases more healthful approach is to make herbal skin- and hair-care products in your own kitchen. Herbs can be incorporated into beauty products in many ways. Whole, dried herbs can be added to facial steams; ground herbs can be used to make facial scrubs. Herbal infusions or decoctions (teas) can be used as rinses to add shine to hair or to bring therapeutic benefits to a bath or foot soak. Infused in oil (such as sweet almond or grapeseed oil), herbs can be applied directly to your skin or incorporated into creams, lotions, and salves with soothing, emollient properties. All kinds of botanicals and kitchen ingredients, including fruits and milk products, can be used to make rejuvenating facial masks. By choosing herbs and ingredients recommended for specific skin types or problems (see pages 372–373), you can easily customize herbal beauty products to not only enhance your appearance, but also to improve the health of your skin.

You can further personalize homemade beauty products by scenting them with aromatic herbs or essential oils, which are much more concentrated than herbs. (See pages 357–360 for more information and cautions about using essential oils.) Floral scents, such as jasmine, lavender, orange blossom, and rose, are generally more popular with women than with men. To give homemade herbal beauty products a masculine flair, focus on plants with woodsy, spicy, or "green" scents, such as bay, fir, peppermint, and rosemary. By choosing herbs with clean, light, or neutral aromas, such as calendula, lavender, or citrus, you can make natural skin-care products that will appeal to both men and women.

Because homemade herbal beauty products do not contain chemical preservatives, they will have a shorter shelf life than their commercial counterparts. To reduce the risk of spoilage, make sure that all the equipment you use to make herbal cosmetics is absolutely clean. Avoid dipping your fingers directly into these mixtures; instead, use a small spatula or other clean utensil. Make herbal beauty products in small batches, and store them in your refrigerator to keep them fresh for as long as possible.

AN HERBAL FACIAL

A homemade herbal facial is a gentle and wonderful way to cleanse, exfoliate, and enhance blood circulation to your facial skin. Performed once a week, it can keep skin looking vibrant and feeling supple. Customize the treatment to meet the needs of your particular skin type.

1. **Cleanse your skin.** Use a mild cleanser.
2. **Steam your pores open.** Use an herbal steam. (Or, for very sensitive skin, use a warm washcloth.)
3. **Exfoliate with an herbal scrub.** Be careful not to rub too hard; avoid the delicate skin around your eyes.
4. **Rinse and apply a mask.** Choose a mask appropriate for your skin type (a clay-based mask for oily skin or a cream and avocado mask for dry skin).
5. **Tone and moisturize.** Carefully remove the mask with cleanser and warm water. Finish by splashing with toner. Blot your face dry and apply a moisturizer.

To avoid an allergic reaction, test any new herbal product on the inside of your arm before applying it to your face, and avoid getting any cosmetic product in your eyes.

CLEANSERS AND SCRUBS

Routinely removing accumulated oil, pollutants, and bacteria from your face is essential for obtaining clear skin that glows with good health. Gently cleanse your face once or twice daily.

Use a scrub less often—about once a week—to slough off dead skin cells and stimulate circulation. The mild exfoliating action of an herbal scrub will leave your face looking radiant and feeling baby soft. Be careful, though: Scrubbing too vigorously can leave unsightly blotches, although these will fade with time. If you have sensitive skin, be extra gentle.

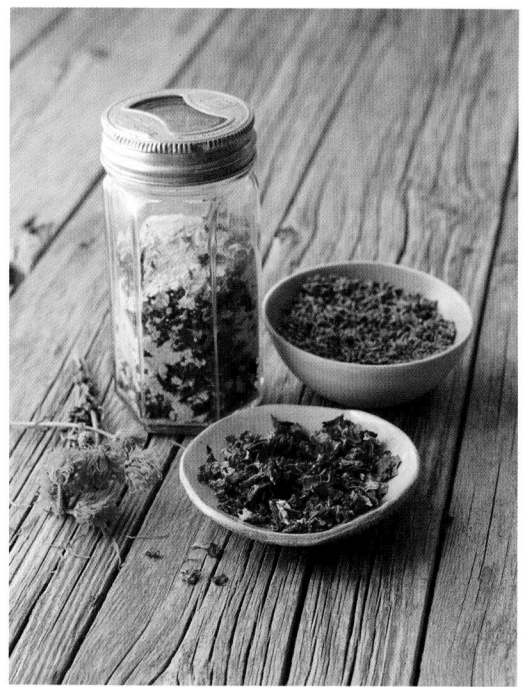

Oatmeal, lavender, rose petals, calendula, and cornmeal make an invigorating homemade facial scrub.

Mild Herbal Skin Cleanser

1 teaspoon dried herb or a handful of fresh herbs (see the chart on pages 372–373 for suggested herbs)

1 tablespoon powdered milk

Make an infusion with the herb and 1 cup of water (see page 365). Allow it to cool to a comfortable temperature. Mix in the powdered milk. Apply the liquid to your face with a cotton ball or cloth, then rinse with cool water. Immediately refrigerate any unused portion; discard after 48 hours.

Herbal Facial Scrub

1 cup rolled oats

⅓ cup cornmeal

⅓ cup dried herbs (such as calendula, lavender, peppermint, rose petals, or a mixture of herbs)

Almonds, clay, or sugar (optional; use alone or in combination to total 1 tablespoon)

In a clean coffee grinder, combine the oatmeal, cornmeal, herbs, and almonds, clay, or sugar (if using). Grind the mixture to a fine powder. (You could also use a mortar and pestle.) Store the scrub in a tightly sealed container in a cool, dry location for up to 3 months. To use, place some of the mixture in the palm of your hand. Add enough water to make a paste. Apply the mixture evenly over your face, avoiding your eyes. Massage the scrub gently into your skin, using circular motions. Rinse thoroughly.

HAND-MILLED HERBAL SOAP

Fragrant, soothing, all-natural soap can make a facial or a shower feel like a trip to the spa. Why do without it? Hand-milled herbal soap is easy and fun to make, and the creative possibilities are almost endless. Dozens of herbs are fragrant, gentle on your skin, and have antimicrobial powers—use your imagination to combine essential oils, herbal flowers, and other ingredients for fragrance and beauty. Lavender, rosemary, peppermint, and citrus-scented herbal soaps are just the beginning.

Hand-milled soap (also called "rebatched soap") is especially easy to make because you start with premade, unscented soap—no lye required. As you become more comfortable with the process of making hand-milled soap, you might want to try making soap from scratch using freshly harvested and dried herbs. Many good books are available; see "Resources" on page 472.

Basic Soap-Making Technique

You can use this basic method for making many other kinds of herbal soaps. Calendula, used in this recipe, has cleansing and anti-inflammatory properties and is a favorite for treating skin problems. For gift giving, wrap several soaps in a washcloth and tie with a ribbon.

½ cup dried calendula petals, divided

16 ounces unscented castile bar soap, grated

¼ cup finely ground rolled oats

1 teaspoon calendula essential oil

1. To give this soap a pale yellow color, bring 1½ cups of water to a boil in a small pot over high heat, then infuse ¼ cup of the calendula petals in the hot water. Remove from the heat and allow the liquid to cool to room temperature. Strain, discard the petals, and reserve the liquid.

2. In a heavy pot over low heat, combine the grated soap and the calendula water. Slowly heat the mixture, stirring often with a wooden spoon. Be sure the soap does not boil or stick to the bottom of the pot. It will take about 30 minutes for the soap to melt completely.

3. When the soap has completely melted and blended with the liquid, stir in the remaining

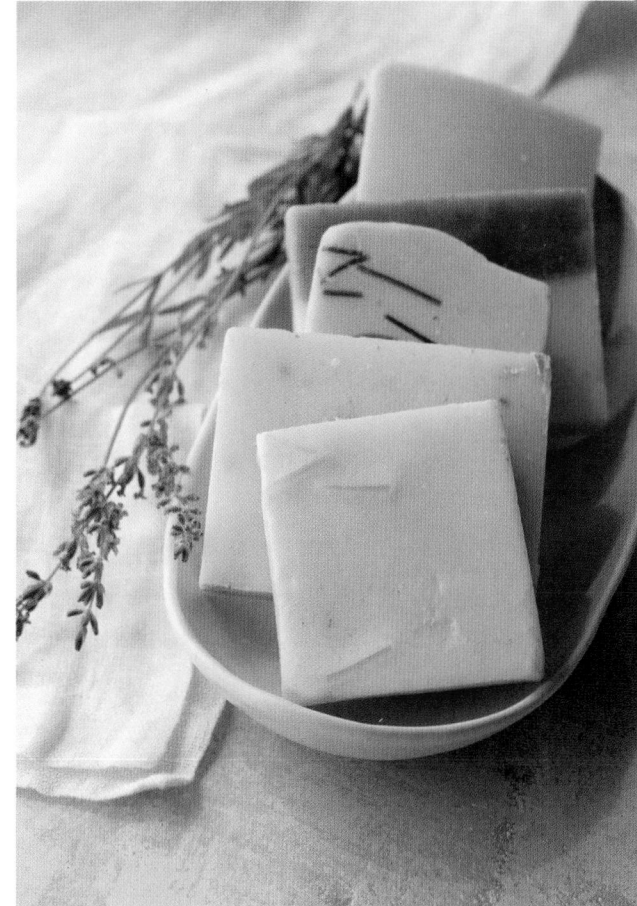

Pamper yourself and your family with hand-milled soaps made with skin-soothing herbs.

¼ cup of calendula petals and the oatmeal. The mix should have the consistency of a thick dough. Turn off the heat and stir in the essential oil. Mix thoroughly, scraping down the sides.

4. Make a test ball. Scoop out a small amount of the soap and put it on a plate to cool. When you are able to hold it, use your hand to squeeze the soap into a ball. If it is too sticky to roll into a ball, you'll need to add a bit more oatmeal to the pot; if it won't hold together, you'll need more water. Return the soap to the pot, place the pot over low

heat, and adjust as needed, until the squeeze test shows it's reached the right consistency.

5. Shape the soap. Remove the pot from the heat and allow it to cool. When it's cool enough to handle, shape the soap into 2½-inch-diameter balls by rolling it firmly between the palms of your hands.

6. Line a tray with waxed paper, place the soap balls on the tray, and cure the soap for 3 to 6 weeks. Turn the balls every few days so that they dry evenly. The longer the curing period, the longer the soap will last when you use it. When the soaps have finished curing, they're ready to use—or to give as gifts.

Nature's Body Wash

Some plants contain compounds known as saponins—these are a type of glycoside that can be irritating or even toxic if ingested, but which form a soapy froth when shaken in water. Long ago, people recognized the value of this froth for cleaning their bodies as well as objects they used, such as clothing or cooking implements.

Some Native American people used the fresh or dried flowers and fruits of species in the genus Ceonanthus, a group of small trees and shrubs in the buckthorn family, for washing and as a detergent. Another important cleaning plant in North America was the genus Yucca, the root of which was collected and pounded for use in bathing, shampooing, and washing clothes. In Europe, soapwort (Saponaria officinalis), so named for its use for washing, was a common cleanser. A diluted extract of soapwort root, produced by boiling it in water, was used for cleaning delicate textiles.

My favorite saponin-rich plant is the shampoo ginger (Zingiber zerumbet), found in many areas of the tropics. I first saw it on Pohnpei, in the Federated States of Micronesia, where it is called oanginpele. People squeeze the slimy sap from the shiny red inflorescences and rub it into their hair as a shampoo and conditioner, which is then washed out with water. It's easy to use and produces immediate results!—M. J. B.

Zesty Peppermint Rosemary Soap

Wake up to the stimulating scents of peppermint and rosemary! Both are also excellent cleansers with antiseptic properties. And because both are astringent, this recipe is especially good for oily skin.

16 ounces unscented castile bar soap, grated
¼ cup dried rosemary leaves
¼ cup dried peppermint leaves
1 teaspoon peppermint essential oil

In a heavy pot over low heat, combine the grated soap with 1½ cups of water. Melt the soap, stirring often with a wooden spoon to prevent sticking. After about 30 minutes, when the soap has completely melted to a uniform consistency, stir in the rosemary and peppermint. Turn off the heat and stir in the oil. Finish by following steps 4 through 6 of "Basic Soap-Making Technique" on pages 377–378.

HERBAL STEAMS

An herbal steam opens pores and stimulates blood circulation. But for people who have extremely sensitive, damaged, or dry skin, or those who are prone to developing tiny broken veins or capillaries, herbal steams can be irritating and should be avoided unless suggested by a doctor or other health-care provider.

Simple Herbal Facial Steam

½ cup dried herbs (such as calendula, German or Roman chamomile, lavender flowers, orange or other citrus peel, peppermint, rosemary, or rose petals)*

Bring a 3-quart pot of water to a boil, then remove it from the heat. Add the herbs to the pot of steaming water. Wait a few minutes to allow the water to cool slightly. Place your face about 12 inches above the pot and drape a towel over your head. Allow

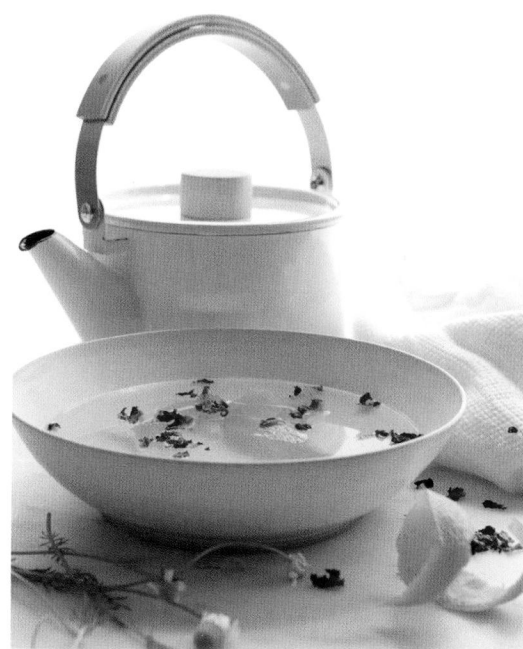

Dried herbs and flowers, such as chamomile, orange peel, and rose petals, can be added to homemade facial steams.

the steam to bathe the skin of your face for a moment or two. Remove the towel, raise your head, and take a few breaths of fresh air. Repeat the process for a maximum of 5 to 10 minutes. As the herbs steep, the rising steam will open your pores and carry the aromatic volatile oil components of the herbs to your facial skin. To finish, use a cleanser, scrub, or mask (if desired), and then splash your face with cool (not cold) water or toner to close your pores.

* See the chart on pages 372–373 for suggested herbs.

FACIAL MASKS

Depending on your skin type, a botanical mask can be designed to be either a hydrating, emollient, deep-moisturizing treatment or an astringent, skin-tightening treatment.

You'll find most of the ingredients you'll need

in your refrigerator or kitchen pantry. Many fruits and milk products are rich in skin-softening alpha hydroxy acids (AHAs), which make them an excellent addition to facial masks. Other good ingredients for facial masks are aloe vera gel, eggs, pumpkin pulp, and unsweetened cocoa powder. If your skin is dry, choose ingredients with moisturizing benefits, such as avocado, coconut oil, cream, egg yolks, honey, oats, olive oil, powdered milk, or plain yogurt. If your skin is oily, choose ingredients with astringent or toning effects, such as apple cider vinegar, banana, citrus or cranberry juice, egg whites, green clay (also called bentonite, available in natural food stores), strawberries, or witch hazel. Once mixed, the mask ingredients won't keep well, so discard any leftovers.

Simple Mask for Dry Skin

2 tablespoons plain thick yogurt

1 egg yolk or 1 tablespoon liquid honey

Few drops coconut or olive oil

In a small bowl, whisk together the yogurt, egg yolk or honey, and oil. Use a cotton ball to apply the mask to your face, avoiding the eye area. Leave the mask on for 10 to 15 minutes. Cleanse thoroughly with warm water, then splash your face with cool water.

Simple Mask for Oily Skin

1 ripe banana

1 egg white

1 teaspoon apple cider vinegar or citrus juice

In a blender, combine the banana, egg white, and vinegar or juice. Blend to form a smooth paste. Use a cotton ball to apply the mask to your face, avoiding the eye area. Leave the mask on for 10 to 15 minutes. Cleanse thoroughly with warm water, then splash your face with cool water.

TONERS

Applying a toner after cleansing your skin helps restore its acid pH and tighten pores. Hydrosols (flower waters created during the manufacture of essential oils) also make soothing, aromatic toners. Witch hazel is an excellent toner for oily skin.

Basic Herbal Skin Toner

1 tablespoon apple cider vinegar or lemon juice

1 cup water

In a small jar, combine the vinegar or lemon juice and water. Splash or spray your face with the toner, avoiding your eyes. There's no need to rinse; the toner will evaporate quickly. Vinegar toners will keep indefinitely at room temperature. Keep lemon juice toner in the refrigerator for up to 10 days.

HERB-INFUSED OILS

Applied directly to your face or body, infused oils—vegetable oils in which herbs have been steeped—have moisturizing and other therapeutic benefits. Infused oils are also important ingredients in other herbal cosmetics and skin-care prod-

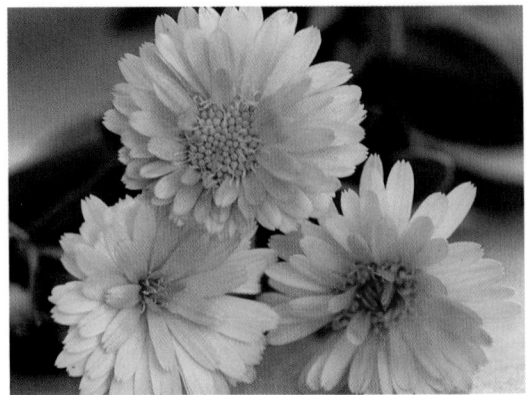

Calendula is a common ingredient in creams, salves, and soaps that soothe skin irritations.

ucts, such as moisturizing face creams, body lotions, and healing salves.

Good choices of oils for cosmetic use include grapeseed, kukui nut, and sweet almond oils. These oils tend to be lighter and feel less greasy than many other vegetable oils. Olive oil is often used to make infused oils for therapeutic application. For example, olive oil infused with the flowers of St. John's wort makes an effective massage oil for treating sciatic nerve pain.

QUEEN *of* HUNGARY'S WATER

Handed down through the generations, Queen of Hungary's water is a classic vinegar-based skin toner that tightens pores, balances pH, and improves skin tone. Herb-infused vinegars, such as this one, provide myriad cosmetic benefits and are remarkably easy to make. Although some modern women may shy away from using vinegar as a skin-care ingredient, herb-infused vinegars have been treasured cosmetics for

centuries. In fact, few ingredients are as effective at balancing your skin's pH. The aroma of the vinegar dissipates quickly and does not linger on your skin.

The ingredients and proportions used in Queen of Hungary's water can vary according to what you have on hand, but the basic ingredients are dried calendula, chamomile, comfrey, elder flower, lemon balm, lemon peel, rose petals, rosemary,

and sage. Place the herbs in a jar, cover them completely with apple cider vinegar, and let them soak (macerate) in the vinegar for at least 2 weeks. Strain. To each cup of herb-infused vinegar, add ½ cup of rose water (available from health food stores, natural grocers, and online herb suppliers). Store Queen of Hungary's Water in the refrigerator for up to 10 days.

To make an herb-infused oil for external or cosmetic use, fill a glass jar about three-quarters full with dried herbs (calendula flowers, for example; see the chart on pages 372–373 for other suggestions). Pour the oil of your choice over the herbs to fill the jar. Be sure the herbs are completely submerged in the oil; any plant material exposed to the air can cause spoilage. Cap the jar. Allow the herbs to soak in the oil in a warm, sunny location for 4 to 6 weeks, and then strain it carefully. Pour the oil into clean, dry, amber bottles. Label and store them in a cool, dry location for up to 1 year.

You can use your herb-infused oils—alone or in combination—as the base of a soothing salve or skin cream. Beeswax solidifies the mix; vitamin E acts as a preservative. You'll also need small tins to contain your salve. The beeswax and tins are available from herbal products suppliers and health food stores.

Lavender Hand Salve

8 ounces lavender-infused sweet almond oil

1 ounce beeswax, grated

4 vitamin E capsules

10 drops lavender essential oil

10 drops rosemary essential oil

In a double boiler over low heat, gently heat the infused oil. Add the beeswax and stir until melted. Remove the pan from the heat, and stir in the contents of the vitamin E capsules and the essential oils. Pour the salve into clean, dry tins. When the salve has cooled completely, put the caps on the tins. Label and store them in a cool, dry location for up to 1 year.

HERBAL BATHS

Soaking in bathwater infused with aromatic herbs is an excellent way to experience the cleansing and healing benefits of plants. It's also an unbeatable way to relax and ease away the tensions of a stressful day at work!

Because your body is able to absorb some medicinal compounds through your skin, herbal baths have as many therapeutic uses as they do cosmetic benefits. "Hydrotherapy" and "balneotherapy" are terms regularly used to describe the use of baths to treat physical ailments, including damaged skin. Among many other applications, therapeutic herbal baths can help soothe itchy or irritated skin, ease sore muscles, treat stress and insomnia, reduce fevers, and heal problems in anal and genital areas.

Frequent hot baths can be drying to your skin, however. When treating dry skin, include colloidal oatmeal or other emollient herbs (such as seaweed), or add herb-infused vegetable oils directly to your bathwater. If you're adding oil, be careful not to slip on the oily surface when getting in and out of the tub.

Because herbs are so easily absorbed through the soles of your feet, foot soaks can also confer therapeutic benefits. Simply add an herbal infusion of your choice to a large basin of warm water and soak your feet for 10 minutes.

How to Make an Herbal Bath

There are two main methods for making an herbal bath. One is to start by making a strong herbal infusion (or tea) by steeping dried herbs in boiling water: Use 1 to 2 tablespoons of dried herbs, or several handfuls of fresh herbs, per 2 cups of water. Then add the prepared infusion to your bathwater.

Another easy way to make an herbal bath is to place a mixture of herbs in a cloth bag (muslin and cheesecloth both work well), and suspend this from the bath tap so that the hot water flows through it and soaks the herbs as the bath fills. After your bath, discard the herbs and save the bag for future herbal baths.

To take advantage of one of the best-kept beauty secrets of the ancients, add about 1 cup of powdered milk to your bathwater. Milk products exfoliate and tone your skin, leaving it feeling exceptionally soft and supple.

HERBAL HAIR CARE

Herbs have long been held in high esteem for natural hair care. Throughout history, herbs and other botanicals have been used in all kinds of hair-care products, from hair rinses and deep-conditioning treatments to remedies for dandruff, hair loss, and other scalp problems.

Herbs recommended for oily hair include sage and burdock. Herbs traditionally used for treating dry hair include calendula, comfrey leaf and root, and marshmallow root. Herbs appropriate for all hair types include chamomile, lavender, nettle, rose, and rosemary. Scalp irritations can be soothed with calendula, comfrey, or German chamomile, while dandruff can be helped with burdock, sage, nettle, or rosemary.

Rinses and Conditioners

Rinses and conditioners are the best ways to bring the benefits of herbs to your hair. Many commercial shampoos tout the benefits of the herbs they contain. Although these herbal shampoos smell wonderful (and can lift your mood), they do little to truly improve hair health because they remain on your hair for just a short time.

For more lasting benefits, select herbal rinses and deep conditioners, which are left on your hair for a longer period of time and are therefore better able to coat and penetrate the hair shaft. Dry hair benefits from oil- and protein-rich deep-conditioning treatments.

You can use an herbal tea, or infusion, as a simple homemade hair rinse. Nettle, considered appropriate for all hair types, is one good choice. Or experiment with calendula, rosemary, sage, or other herbs. Adding vinegar or lemon juice to the infusion will help restore your hair's natural pH. The vinegar scent dissipates quickly and will not remain in your hair.

Simple Herbal Hair Rinse

1 teaspoon dried herb or handful of fresh herbs (see the chart on pages 372–373 for suggested herbs)

1 tablespoon apple cider vinegar or lemon juice

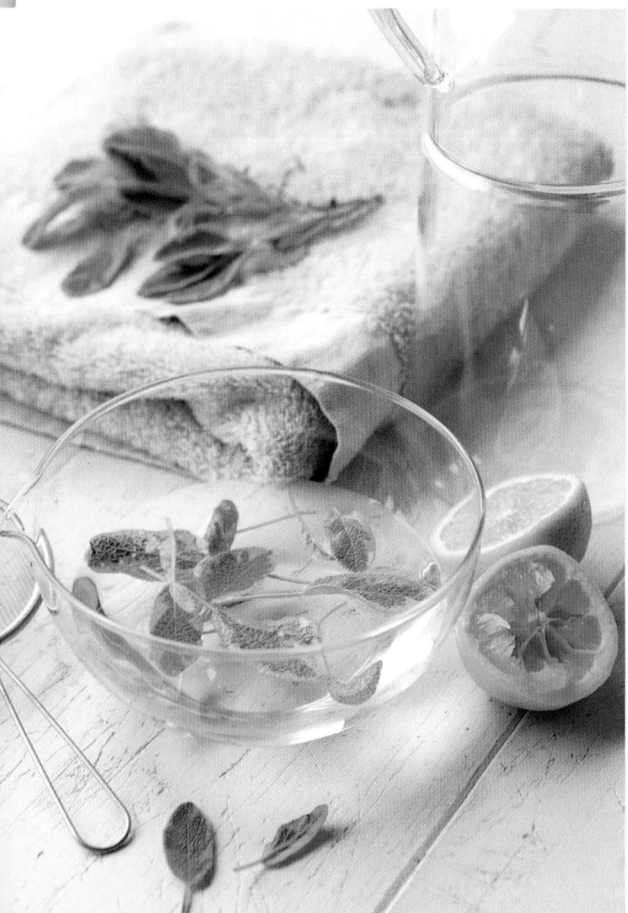

Teas made from fresh herbs and herb flowers along with lemon juice can be used as hair rinses.

Place the herb or herbs in a bowl and pour 1 cup of boiling water over the top. Add the vinegar or lemon juice and steep, covered, for 10 to 15 minutes. Strain, let the infusion cool to a comfortable temperature, and pour it through freshly shampooed hair. (Makes enough for one use.)

Moisturizing Deep-Conditioning Treatment

½ avocado (mashed), 1 tablespoon plain yogurt, or 1 tablespoon powdered milk

Egg yolk

1 to 2 tablespoons olive oil, coconut oil, or shea butter

In a medium bowl, combine the avocado, yogurt, or powdered milk and the egg yolk. Stir to thoroughly combine. Moisten the mixture with the olive oil, coconut oil, or shea butter. Work the conditioner thoroughly through your hair, paying special attention to the ends. Cover your head with a shower cap or plastic bag, and relax for 10 to 20 minutes. Rinse, then wash your hair thoroughly with a pH-balanced shampoo.

Herbal Hair Coloring

Herbs can be used to enhance hair color. The most important herbal hair dye comes from henna (*Lawsonia inermis*), used in Egypt, India, and the Middle East for at least 8,000 years to provide hair with shine and striking red highlights. Other herbs, such as turmeric and saffron (for yellow) and nettle (for green), were also used. Commercial henna hair dyes come in a variety of colors, but only true, unadulterated henna creates the red color. Black henna, for example, contains a synthetic black hair dye.

Henna is also used to create temporary tattoos that are an important part of traditional Indian wedding ceremonies. The longer the henna remains on your skin, the darker and longer lasting the tattoo will be. The henna dye soaks into the outermost layer of skin and coats the hair shaft, but it does not permanently stain skin or hair.

Various other herbs can be used to enhance natural hair color, even though they are not true dyes. For example, hair rinses that contain German and Roman chamomile are used to add shine and bring out highlights in blond hair. Rosemary and sage rinses are believed to help enhance the natural beauty of brunette hair. (See "Simple Herbal Hair Rinse" on page 382.)

Folk Remedies for Hair Loss

Hair loss (alopecia) can be a distressing problem for both men and women, although the condition is much more common in men. Herbal folk remedies reputed to help with hair loss abound, but there's little scientific evidence that any one of them works. When a hair follicle stops producing hair, it's difficult—if not impossible—to reverse the process.

Herbs that have garnered a traditional reputation for stimulating hair growth (or at least slowing hair loss) include aloe, burdock, chamomile, nettle, peppermint, rosemary, and sage. One small clinical study suggested that saw palmetto can help reverse genetic hair loss, including male-pattern baldness.

A traditional remedy for treating hair loss recommends massaging your scalp daily with an oil (such as olive oil) infused with rosemary. The biggest benefit of the treatment, however, could be the massage itself, which stimulates circulation to your scalp and hair follicles.

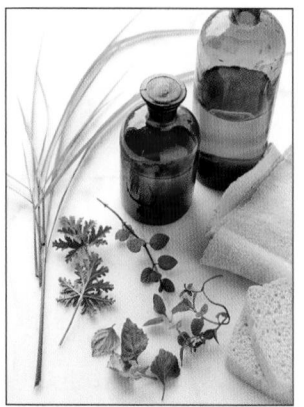

CHAPTER 7

USING HERBS
in YOUR HOME

Ancient people noticed that using herbs throughout their living

areas offered many benefits—the scent of some plants was able to

cover noxious smells, clean the air or water, or repel pests such as fleas and

mice (a big plus in sleeping areas, which often were directly on the floor).

Ancient Romans cleansed and scented their bathwater with aromatic lavender,

an herb that science now knows has powerful antimicrobial properties. Later,

Medieval and Renaissance Europeans scattered herbs across the floors of their

dwellings—a practice known as using "strewing herbs"—to repel pests and

improve their harsh living conditions.

In North America, native people cleaned cooking items with horsetail (*Equisetum* spp.)—one of the oldest groups of plants on earth—by rubbing the plants' silica-rich stems on dirty pots. When North American settlers learned to use the plants this way, they referred to them as "scouring rushes."

In ancient China, people burned the bark of fragrant herbs such as sandalwood and cinnamon to produce a purifying smoke that was often used during ceremonies and rituals. And as long as 5,000 years ago, Egyptians burned aromatic plants to cover bad odors in their dwellings, repel harmful spirits, and enhance sacred rituals.

People have always used herbs—especially those with strong and pleasant fragrances—in their homes to create a more pleasant living environment. Learning about these ancient uses of herbs is not only fascinating, but it can also offer healthy alternatives for modern living.

CLEAN AND GREEN HOUSEHOLD HELPERS

Ever wonder if those commercial cleaning products and indoor pesticides you use might do more harm than good? You're not alone. Natural home-care products (many of which contain herbs) are growing in popularity as more homemakers become aware of indoor toxins. The use of certain cleaning products has been linked to higher rates of asthma—inducing the condition in some people, as well as aggravating the condition in those who already have this chronic inflammatory disease. And although you can buy many excellent non-toxic products for your home, it's easy and fun to make your own. Just remember that even plant products can be toxic under some circumstances, and the same cautions given for other herbal uses also apply here. For specific cautions, see the individual plant entries in Part II of this book.

SIMPLY CLEAN SOLUTIONS

With just a few basic ingredients, you can make safer "green" cleaning products for a fraction of the cost of the commercial products and without the scary ingredients. Distilled white vinegar (which contains acetic acid) has antifungal and antimicrobial properties and can eliminate mineral deposits from sink and bathtub fixtures, as well as cookware. Acidic lemon juice kills germs on countertops, cutting boards, and more. Baking soda deodorizes and dissolves grease and dirt. Mixed with other ingredients, it makes a gentle but effective scrub. All-natural castile soap, made for centuries with olive oil, not only washes dirt and grease from your body, but also from household surfaces and laundry.

Many herbs have potent disinfectant properties, too. Basil, bay, cardamom, clove, coriander, eucalyptus, ginger, hyssop, lavender, lemongrass, oregano, peppermint, rose geranium, rosemary, sage, spearmint, and thyme are cleaning powerhouses. All contain a multitude of plant chemicals that possess antibacterial, antifungal, antiseptic, and antiviral actions. By adding a few drops of these essential oils to your homemade cleaning products, you can boost their cleaning power and impart a delightful fragrance that makes cleaning more pleasurable.

Because essential oils break down plastic over time, it's best to store your homemade cleaning products in labeled, dark glass containers (see "Resources" on page 472). Plastic spray bottles are fine for short-term storage of smaller quantities. Also, remember to store all cleaning products—even those made with natural ingredients—in a cool, dark location where children and pets cannot reach them.

Kitchen Countertop Spray

Use this fragrant solution to disinfect counter-tops, refrigerator shelves, and painted surfaces, including walls and wood trim. Feel free to experiment with other antibacterial essential oils, such as basil, thyme, or lemon.

½ cup distilled white vinegar

½ cup water

10–12 drops rose geranium essential oil

In a small, dark glass jar, combine the vinegar, water, and oil. Stir. Pour small amounts into a spray bottle as necessary.

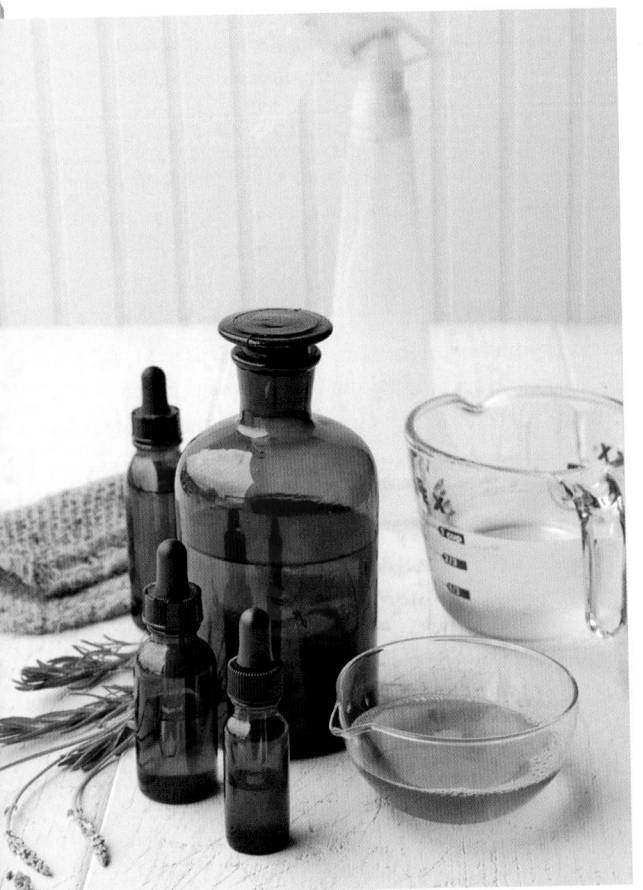

Make a fragrant countertop cleaner with vinegar, water, and essential oils, such as lavender.

Gentle Spearmint Scrubber

This nonscratching, chlorine-free paste is perfect for cleaning cookware, countertops, and porcelain sinks and tubs. Lemon and lemon verbena essential oils also work well in place of the spearmint.

1 cup baking soda

1 tablespoon liquid castile soap

10–12 drops spearmint essential oil

Warm water (90° to 110°F)

In a small, dark glass jar, combine the baking soda, soap, and enough warm water to form a thick but pourable paste. Stir in the essential oil. Apply to surfaces, wait for 5 minutes or more, then scrub with a sponge. Rinse off the residue with water.

Antibacterial Bathroom Cleaner

Use this fragrant spray to disinfect bathroom surfaces. Tea tree (*Melaleuca alternifolia*) oil—which has antibacterial, antiviral, and antifungal powers—helps clean and control mildew. Lavender and hyssop, which were once used as disinfectant strewing herbs, have antibacterial and antiviral properties.

½ cup distilled white vinegar

1½ cups water

2 tablespoons liquid castile soap

8–10 drops tea tree essential oil

8–10 drops lavender essential oil

8–10 drops hyssop essential oil

Combine the vinegar, water, soap, tea tree oil, lavender oil, and hyssop oil in a dark glass jar. Stir. Pour a small amount into a spray bottle to use as needed. Rinse off any residue with water.

Chlorine-Free Grout Cleaner

This all-natural paste removes mildew but has no harsh fumes.

- 1 cup baking soda
- 10 drops tea tree oil
- Water

In a dark glass jar, combine the baking soda and oil with enough water to make a thick paste. Apply the paste to grout, then wait 1 to 2 hours. Scrub with a stiff nylon brush, then rinse with water.

Fragrant Floor Cleaner

Mop floors with this fresh-smelling liquid; the eucalyptus and rosemary oils have antiviral properties. Make a fresh mixture each time you need it.

- 1 cup distilled white vinegar
- 1 gallon hot water (at least 130°F)
- 1–2 tablespoons liquid castile soap (optional)
- 1 teaspoon lavender or eucalyptus essential oil
- 1 teaspoon rosemary essential oil

In a bucket, combine the vinegar, hot water, soap (if using), and lavender or eucalyptus oil and rosemary oil. If you include the soap, rinse with clear water after using.

Lemon-Scented Furniture Polish

Remove dirt as you add shine to furniture with this naturally lemon-scented formula. Shake well before using; buff dry with a clean cloth.

- 1 cup olive oil
- 2 tablespoons distilled white vinegar
- ½ cup water
- 1 teaspoon lemon or lemongrass essential oil

In a dark glass jar, combine the olive oil, vinegar, water, and lemon or lemongrass oil. Pour a small amount into a spray bottle to use as needed.

Magic Carpet Deodorizer

The spicy fragrance of this deodorizer will remind you of an island breeze.

- 1 cup baking soda
- 10 drops grapefruit essential oil
- 10 drops ginger essential oil

In a dark glass jar, combine the baking soda, grapefruit oil, and ginger oil. Sprinkle the mix over your carpet, wait an hour, and then vacuum.

Fresh Air Laundry Detergent

This powdered mix will clean and brighten your laundry naturally and give it a fresh outdoor scent. The recipe makes enough to last several months.

- 8 cups baking soda
- 6 cups borax
- 4 cups grated castile soap
- 1 tablespoon lavender essential oil
- 1 teaspoon clary sage essential oil

In a large bucket, combine the baking soda, borax, and soap. Whisk in the lavender and clary sage oils. Store in a dark, covered container in a cool, dark location. Use ⅛ cup per medium-size load.

Aromatic Fabric Spray

Refresh upholstered furniture, drapes, linens, and mattresses with this herbal spray.

- 15 drops lavender, lemongrass, patchouli, or other fragrant essential oil
- 1½ cups distilled water

In a dark glass jar, combine the essential oil and water. Pour a small amount into a spray bottle to use as needed.

INDOOR PEST CONTROL

When flies, ants, or moths make your house *their* house, put the pest-fighting properties of plants to work for you, instead. Basil, black pepper, calamint, clove, eucalyptus, fennel, garlic, hyssop, mugwort, rosemary, sage, southernwood, thyme, and tansy are among the many herbs that contain chemical compounds with insect-repelling properties. Here are a few tried-and-true remedies.

Ants: Defend your home against invading ants by spraying ant trails with equal parts white vinegar and water, mixed with a few drops of eucalyptus oil. You can use the same solution to wash countertops, floors, and other areas where you see ants. Sprinkle freshly ground black pepper in doorways, on windowsills, and around other areas where ants are entering. Sliced, fresh garlic cloves; mint leaves; tansy leaves; and whole cloves are also reported to drive away indoor ants. Try guarding entryways by placing a pot of tansy by the doorway, or grow the herb in a window box. Be cautious: Tansy is invasive in the garden, and when ingested, it can be toxic to people and pets.

Flies and mosquitoes: The chemical compound d-limonene, found in citrus fruits, is used in many commercial fly and mosquito repellents. Grapefruit, lemon, and orange are particularly high in this compound, but basil, hyssop, calamint, fennel, and black pepper also have high concentrations of d-limonene. Citronella oil (steam-distilled from *Cymbopogon nardus* and *C. winterianus*), popular in candles, contains several other compounds known to repel insects. Diffusing any of these fragrant, insect-repellent oils can make summer evenings on the deck or patio more pleasant.

Clothing moths: Protect clothing from moth damage with pest-repellent *Artemisia* species (such as mugwort or southernwood), eucalyptus, hyssop, sage, rosemary, tansy, and thyme. Fill small muslin or cheesecloth bags with the dried herbs, and tuck them into drawers or hang them inside closets. Or

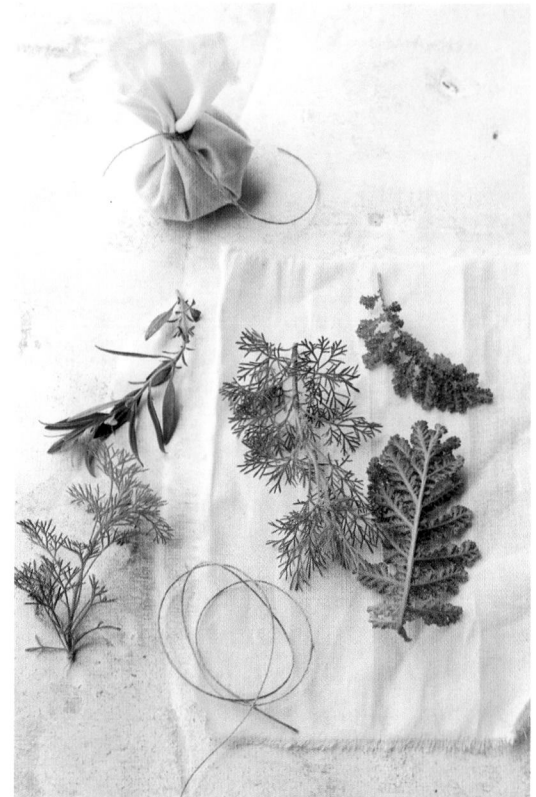

Protect clothing from moths with bags of pest-repellent herbs, such as mugwort, southernwood, hyssop, and tansy.

make natural mothballs: Soak cotton balls in a few drops of the essential oil of one or more of these herbs. Hang bags of the cotton balls, or set them on a shelf in your closet, being careful to keep them from touching your clothes.

Pantry moths: The larvae of several different moths (commonly grouped together as "pantry moths" or "flour weevils") can ruin stored rice, cereal, flour, birdseed, and more. Keeping cupboards clean and free of crumbs and loose grains, as well as storing grains and seeds in sealed containers, will go a long way toward preventing infestations of these pests. For added insurance, tuck bay leaves inside canisters and other places you store grain products. Bay contains several chemical compounds known to repel insects.

SCENTING YOUR HOME WITH HERBS

Scents affect us profoundly. Brushing by lemon verbena or roses in your garden can instantly lift your mood or evoke long-forgotten memories. With potpourris, sachets, and incense, you can enjoy delightful herbal aromas—some pungent, some spicy, some sweet—indoors, year-round.

POTPOURRIS

A potpourri is a mixture of dried aromatic herbs stored in a closed container. When the container is opened, the herbal mix perfumes the air.

What to include: When making potpourri, choose plant materials with fragrance, shape, and color in mind. Also, consider herb and garden flowers that aren't especially fragrant but that are colorful and easy to dry, such as baby's breath, calendula, delphinium, elecampane, goldenrod, hydrangea, larkspur, marigold, pansy, statice, sunflower, tansy, yarrow, and zinnia. Small conifer cones, conifer needles, dried fruit peels, flower buds, and whole spices add visual appeal and texture.

Essential oils can intensify or accent the main fragrance of your potpourri. To complement a woodsy blend, for instance, you might add a few drops of bayberry or rosemary oil. Essential oils can also be used to refresh the fragrance of a potpourri when it begins to fade.

Including a fixative, such as orris root, is important to slow the evaporation of essential oils and retain fragrance. Made from the ground roots of *Iris × germanica* var. *florentina*, orris root is a commonly used fixative, but it can cause an allergic reaction. Other plant-based fixatives include angelica root, clary sage, oak moss (*Evernia prunastri*, a lichen), Australian sandalwood (*Santalum spicatum*), and vanilla beans.

Washing Pots in the Rainforest

When you wash dishes today, notice that little scrubber in your hand. Whether it be a nylon pad, piece of steel wool, or brush, the rough edges are essential for removing dirt and grime. While Victorians used metal-tipped brushes, and scrubbing pads were developed and patented in the 20th century, the real inventors of these types of products were preindustrial traditional peoples.

The Maya people of Belize taught me about a plant family (Dilleniaceae) with exceptionally rough leaves, which they have always used to scrub dishes, pots, and other household objects. Spanish-speaking people in this area refer to these forest plants as lava platos—meaning, "wash dishes"—referring to one of their traditional uses. The bushmasters (forest guides) I worked with showed me just how tough these leaves are by rubbing them on my skin and scraping a layer right off—hence one of the English names, "sandpaper tree."

Nature's scouring pads grow throughout the forest. Parts of certain bromeliads are also used this way: The roots of Aechmea tillandsioides make a handy scrub brush, as do the dried flower stalks of Androlepis skinneri. Many other household items also derive from nature's diversity of designs and materials. In the Belizean tropical forest, nature has even provided a horsetail-shaped brush for swatting away flies—fibers from the leaf bases of a large tree, the Attalea cohune palm. The plant world is rich with inspiration and delight for so many of the basic needs of life.—M. J. B.

Harvesting and drying herbal ingredients: Cut herbs on a sunny day, working early in the morning, just after the dew has dried. Gather flowers just after they have opened, when their essential oils will be at their peak.

Be sure your herbs are thoroughly dry before you mix them. Gently remove flower petals and strip the leaves from their stems, then spread the leaves on a screen in a warm, dark, airy location. Stir the herbs often. If you are gathering and drying herbs over several seasons, store the dry ingredients in airtight containers until you are ready to mix them.

Mixing: In a glass or ceramic bowl (not metal, which can alter the fragrance), use your hands or a wooden spoon to toss together the ingredients. Stir in the fixative and a few drops of the essential oils, if you are using them. Pour the mix into a large, wide-mouthed ceramic or glass container, then cover it tightly. Store the container in a cool, dark location for about 6 weeks, to allow the scents to blend. About once a week, shake or stir the contents. At the end of the 6 weeks, you'll have a delightful potpourri for your home or to give as a gift.

Floral Bouquet Potpourri

This blend captures the heady fragrances of a flower garden in full bloom.

1 cup dried rose petals

1 cup dried lavender buds

1 cup dried clary sage (leaves and flowers)

1 cup dried rose-scented geranium (leaves and flowers)

1 tablespoon powdered orris root

Few drops of clary sage, jasmine, rose, and/or sandalwood essential oils

Herb Basket Potpourri

Bring the fresh, clean scent of your herb garden into your kitchen or bath.

1 cup dried rosemary leaves

1 cup dried peppermint leaves

1 cup dried lavender buds

1 cup dried lemon verbena leaves

Handful dried rosemary or peppermint flowers

Handful dried calendula petals

Several sprigs dried sweet Annie (*Artemisia annua*) foliage

1½ tablespoons powdered orris root

Few drops essential oil of the above herbs and/or basil, geranium, or thyme

Walk in the Woods Potpourri

The perfect winter scent; set the container near a fireplace and enjoy the earthy aroma as it wafts through the room. Whole dried cloves, allspice berries, and cinnamon sticks are sold as kitchen spices. (*Note:* As a precaution, wear gloves when handling the oak moss. Some people experience an allergic skin reaction upon contact with this botanical.)

2 cups dried bayberry leaves

1 cup dried rose hips

½ cup dried miniature pinecones

½ cup dried pine or fir needles

½ cup dried cut oak moss

1 tablespoon whole dried cloves

1 tablespoon whole allspice berries

Few cinnamon sticks, broken

Few drops bayberry, cedar wood, juniper, and/or winterberry essential oils

SWEET DREAMS PILLOW

Dream pillows are similar to sachets and potpourris, but the herbs are chosen to help you fall into a pleasant, fragrant slumber. Some claim they can even induce more vivid or lucid dreams (sweet ones, of course!). Make the pillow from a natural fabric, such as cotton or silk. Slip it inside your pillowcase, right above your regular pillow. Dream pillows make great gifts, too.

Materials: 2 pieces of prewashed fabric, each 9 x 9 inches; sewing machine or hand-sewing supplies; ¼ cup dried hops flowers; ¼ cup dried lavender flowers; ¼ cup dried mugwort leaves; ¼ cup lemon balm or catnip leaves; 1 teaspoon powdered orris root; few drops essential oil of lavender and/or rose; cotton batting; optional Velcro strips

1. Make the pillow: If your fabric has a "right" side, layer the two pieces with their right sides together. Using ½-inch seams, sew along three sides of your pillow. Leave one side open. Turn the pillow right side out.

2. Fill the pillow: In a glass or ceramic bowl, mix together the hops, lavender, mugwort, lemon balm or catnip, and orris root, then stir in the essential oils. Fill the pillow with the herb mix, then add a handful or two of cotton batting for comfort.

3. Close the pillow: Sew the remaining side of the pillow, or fold the raw edges to the inside and follow the package directions to attach Velcro strips (if using) so that you can replenish the herbal filling when the fragrance fades. Pleasant dreams!

HERBS and SCENTS for POTPOURRIS

Depending on the type of scent you want (earthy, spicy, floral, or a combination), you can make potpourri with seeds, bark, leaves, roots, flower petals, or fruit peels, along with essential oils to enhance and complement the main fragrance.

WOODSY/EARTHY SCENTS	SPICY SCENTS	FLORAL SCENTS	FRUIT SCENTS
Bayberry	Allspice	Clary sage	Bergamot
Frankincense	Angelica root	Hops flower	German chamomile
Marjoram	Anise	Jasmine	Grapefruit
Myrrh	Basil	Lavender	Lemon balm
Patchouli	Bay	Neroli	Lemongrass
Rosemary	Cardamom	Palmarosa	Lemon thyme
Southernwood	Cinnamon	Rose	Lemon verbena
Sweet woodruff	Clove	Scented geranium (rose)	Mandarin
Thyme	Ginger	Violet	Scented geranium (lemon)
Wormwood	Hyssop	Ylang-ylang	
	Mint		
	Vanilla		

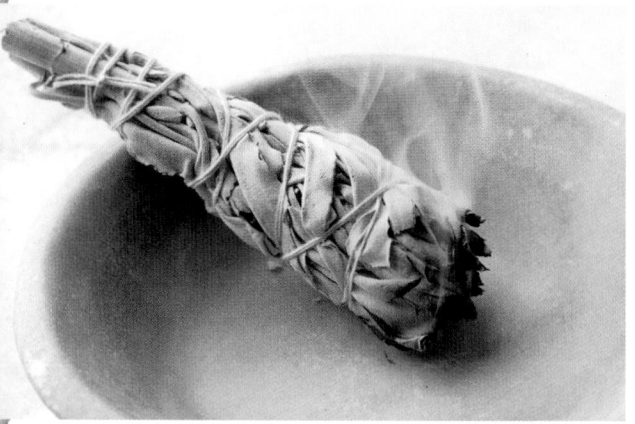

A smudge stick or smudge bundle contains various dried herbs tied with string, made into a small bundle, and lighted with a flame until it smolders, giving off an aromatic smoke used to cleanse the home or other living areas.

INCENSE

Long before incense became popular in the 1960s, people of many cultures burned plants to scent their homes, keep away disease, and perfume their clothing. Early physicians advised their patients to inhale incense for medicinal purposes. The word "perfume" means "through smoke," suggesting that burning incense was probably one of the first ways people used fragrances.

Incense is quite easy to make with powdered herbs, a binding agent, and water. Kits also are available.

HOLIDAY GIFTS INCENSE

Makko (incense powder) is made from the bark of the tabunoki tree (*Machilus thunbergii*), an Asian evergreen. It works as a binding agent to hold the other ingredients together. You can buy makko from natural foods stores and specialty herb suppliers. This recipe makes about 12 cones.

MATERIALS: 1 teaspoon frankincense powder; 1 teaspoon myrrh powder; 1 teaspoon cardamom; 2 teaspoons makko powder; 5 to 10 drops cypress or mandarin essential oil

1. Mix the ingredients. In a mortar and pestle, grind together the frankincense, myrrh, cardamom, and makko. Stir in the essential oil. Slowly add warm water, a few drops at a time, mixing thoroughly after each addition until the mixture is soft and pliable—but not runny or crumbly.

2. Form cones. Make small, ½-inch-diameter balls, then shape one side of each ball into a point and flatten the opposite side. (Each cone should be about 1 inch tall and ½ inch across at the base.)

3. Dry the cones. Set the cones upright on waxed paper, and allow them to dry. When the sides of the cones feel dry, turn them over to dry the bases. Total drying time will be about 1 week. To use, set a cone upright on a ceramic plate. Light the top of the cone, and allow it to burn naturally. Store cones in a cool, dry location.

THE TRADITION *of* INCENSE

The word incense is derived from the Latin *incendere*, meaning, "set on fire." The practice of burning plants to release their fragrant smoke can be traced back to the earliest history of religion. For some species, the leaves and stems were burned; for others, the resin or hardened sap was burned. The smoke that wafted into the air aided meditation, freed the mind, pacified the spirits, and warded off evil.

Scientists have recorded nearly 400 species of plants used as incense around the world. To mourn the loss of his wife, Emperor Nero of Rome (37–68 CE) ordered thousands of tons of frankincense and myrrh to be burned.

The very sacred Native American practice of smudging involves burning plants such as sage, sweetgrass, and other species during prayer and for purification. The dried plants are not burned to produce a flame, but only to release smoke, filling the air with the plant's aromatic essential oils. It is thought that from our earliest days, as people watched smoke ascending to the heavens, they considered this a link between earth, its people, and the world above.

BRINGING NATURE'S BEAUTY INTO YOUR HOME

Herbs are more than just practical plants: Their rich colors, textures, and fragrances can add natural beauty to your home. You can use herbs to create living works of art, such as a topiary or living wreath, fresh or dried arrangements, botanical prints, and much more. And the pleasure is not all in the final result; you'll find the process of making art with herbs is itself relaxing and fun. Each piece becomes a personal, local, and distinctive expression of nature's beauty. Here are a few fun and easy projects.

HERBAL STANDARD

If you enjoy the simple pleasure of caring for plants, you'll enjoy making and maintaining an herbal standard—a simple decorative form that consists of a single straight stem and a head of smaller stems and leaves. Using a perennial herb with pliable stems, you can create a kind of living sculpture by training and pruning the growing sprigs. Good choices for this technique include bay laurel, French lavender, lemon verbena, scented geraniums (especially 'Little Gem' and 'Toronto'), rosemary (especially 'Arp', 'Ken's Prostrate', and 'Tuscan Blue'), and thyme (especially 'Argenteus', also known as silver). In general, the smaller the herb's leaves, the smaller the standard should be. A silver thyme standard might be 6 inches tall, for instance, while a large-leaved bay standard could be several feet tall. As with bonsai, the routine care is a pleasant way to relax. A potted herbal standard makes a beautiful and fragrant centerpiece or patio accent.

Rosemary is an easy plant for beginners to work with. Start with a 3- to 4-inch-tall plant that has a single, straight stem. Mail-order herb suppliers will send a suitable plant if you tell them you'll be training it as a standard.

MATERIALS: 3- to 4-inch-tall rooted rosemary plant; 3- to 4-inch-diameter pot; 5- to 6-inch-diameter pot; light potting medium; wire or bamboo stakes; green floral tape; garden twine or old pantyhose; pruning shears

1. Pot, prune, and stake. If the rosemary isn't already potted, plant it in the center of the 3- to 4-inch pot. Prune away any side branches so that you have a single, straight stem. For this first potting, the stake should be 8 to 10 inches long. If you're using a wire stake, wrap it with the green floral tape. Insert it into the soil, pushing it to the bottom of the potting medium, about ½ inch away from the stem.

2. Secure the stem. Secure the stem loosely to the stake at one or two places—be careful not to damage the tender young stem. As the plant grows, add additional ties to keep it growing straight. Loosen the ties if they appear to be constricting the growing stem.

3. Repot, restake. When the stem reaches the top of the stake, repot the plant into a 5- to 6-inch-diameter pot. Remove the ties and existing stake and replace the stake with a sturdier one that's 12 to 15 inches long. Insert it into the soil about 1 inch away from the stem and push the stake to the bottom of the potting medium. Loosely secure the stem, at about 1-inch intervals, with the ties.

4. Clip to form the "trunk." When the rosemary reaches the height you want the standard to be, pinch off the tip (called the leader). Also prune away the stems and leaves from the bottom two-thirds of the main stem. (For example, if the plant is 6 inches tall, remove the bottom 4 inches of leaves.) This pruning will encourage strong, bushy growth at the top of the stem.

5. Shape the head. Over the coming months, more top growth will appear. Gradually form the round, globe shape by clipping new growth—twice a month during the growing season, less often during fall and winter. Continue to remove growth from the lower stem. Try to maintain a 2:1 ratio of stem length to head, for pleasing proportions.

LIVING WREATH

Living wreaths are like having an herb garden on your wall, door, or tabletop. Start them in spring, when small plants are readily available at the garden center or from your renovated outdoor plantings. Good plant choices for living wreaths include lavender, marjoram, oregano, prostrate rosemary, sage, scented geranium, and thyme (especially creeping wooly thyme). The wreath will be fully covered with herbs about 6 weeks after planting.

MATERIALS: Sphagnum moss (coarse textured, not milled); 12 x 30-inch rectangular piece of chicken wire (1/2-inch mesh); small, rooted herbs—some with creeping stems about 6 inches long

1. Prepare the moss. Soak several handfuls of sphagnum moss in water until thoroughly wet, about 15 minutes.

2. Make the planter. Bend the long sides of the chicken wire so they curl up to form a 30-inch-long trough. Squeeze enough water out of the sphagnum so that it remains wet but isn't dripping, and pack it tightly into the trough. (A good dense mass of sphagnum will give the plants a firm base and will hold water well.)

3. Form the wreath. Form a cylinder by bending the top edges of the trough together until they overlap slightly. Fasten the edges together by bending the loose prongs (they'll be sticking out where the mesh was cut) to form little hooks that catch in the mesh holes on the opposite side of the seam. Do the same with the ends of the cylinder, connecting them to form a wreath.

4. Plant the herbs. Poke through the wire to make seven little wells in the sphagnum, spacing them evenly about the wreath. Plant a young herb in each, anchoring wayward runners with hairpins, if necessary.

5. Hang the wreath in strong but indirect sunlight. When the moss starts to dry out, soak the whole wreath for 15 minutes in a basin of water that has a few drops of fish emulsion in it. Prune back or wire wayward stems as the plants grow.

DRIED FLOWERS AND FOLIAGE

By drying the cut stems of many herbs, you can create beautiful arrangements with echoes of summer: clumps of golden or burgundy blooms, tiny blue petals, silvery foliage, dark brown seedpods, and much more.

The easiest way to dry herbs and flowers is just like Mother Nature does: Provide warm air, a light breeze, and a couple of days for it to happen.

How to Air-Dry Herbs for Arranging

Air drying is the simplest way to preserve herbs and flowers for arranging, but you must choose plants that will dry easily with this method, and you have to pick them at the proper stage.

- Goldenrod, pokeweed, and safflower: Cut stems before the flowers fully open.

- Chives, echinacea, lavender, mint, rosemary, sage, and witch hazel: Cut just after the flowers have opened.

- Tansy and yarrow: Pick only after the flowers have become very dry on their stems.

- Rue seed heads: Gather them either green or dry.

- Hops: Gather the female cones when they are still green.

- *Artemisia* species: Harvest and air-dry the silvery green foliage, which makes great filler, almost anytime.

- Bayberry, bay laurel, boxwood, juniper, and sage: Harvest the foliage sprigs anytime and use them as neutral accents or background.

If you plan to use only the flowers in your arrangement, strip the leaves from the stems before you dry them: The less plant material on each stem, the faster it will dry. Tie 8 to 10 stems in a bundle and hang them upside down in a dark, well-ventilated area. Air movement is key. During summer, flowers dry in about 10 days. As soon as the flowers are dry, pack them in labeled boxes (one type per box) until you are ready to use them.

How to Dry with Desiccants

Use a desiccant for drying finicky flowers such as carnation, delphinium, forget-me-not, hollyhock, larkspur, marigold, rose, and zinnia. Desiccants are moisture-absorbing materials such as sand, borax, and cornmeal. You can use pure, clean sand; borax mixed with sand (use a 2:1 ratio); or cornmeal mixed with borax (equal parts). The process usually takes 1 to 4 weeks, depending on the type of flowers you're drying and the humidity level in your home.

Silica gel, another desiccant, is a chemical compound that resembles sea salt. Compared to other desiccants, silica gel works faster (in about 3 to 5 days) and preserves colors better. The fine granules are also less likely to damage delicate leaves and petals. Silica gel is reusable and widely available at craft stores. Wear a dust mask and gloves when working with it, and never use it to dry culinary herbs.

Here's the basic drying process when using a desiccant.

1. Pick flowers when they're not quite fully open. Cut off the stem right below the blossom.

2. Poke a piece of florist's wire into the center of the flower. Then pull it through to form a wire stem. Bend one end of the wire into a little hook so it won't pull out. (It's important to do this now; the flowers will be too fragile to wire after they're dried.)

3. Cover the bottom of a wide, low container. Use a 1-inch layer of the desiccant, then nestle the flowers into it. Don't let the blossoms touch. Gently pour in additional desiccant to completely cover the flowers with another 1-inch layer. Cover the container tightly, and store it in a warm, dry location.

4. Gently remove the flowers. The time to remove them is when they're still colorful but not so dry that they fall apart. If you're using silica gel, check the flowers in 3 days; wait 1 week to check flowers dried in other desiccants. Flowers with thin petals will dry faster than those with fleshier petals. If a petal breaks off, reattach it with a spot of white glue.

Arranging Dried Herbs and Flowers

Here's how expert florists make beautiful, long-lasting arrangements with dried flowers, foliage, and herbs.

1. Work with dried plants on a dry day. On rainy days, the plants can absorb moisture and become difficult to handle. If you find the arrangement "wilting" as you put it together, just turn up the heat in the workroom, or set the herbs in silica gel for several hours, overnight, or until they recover.

2. Consider plant shapes and colors. Vary the shapes. To achieve arrangements of rich texture, use some dried flowers that are spike-shape (like mints or lavender); some that are round and fairly large (like yarrow); and some small, dainty flowers (like safflower).

Choose two or three shades of the same color. For example, use a red and a pink, or three flowers of various shades of yellow. That range will make the colors seem richer.

3. Fill the containers with sand. This will hold the flowers and give them some stability. For little finger vases, use plugs of florist's foam.

4. Arrange from the bottom up. Begin working with the low core of the arrangement. Dried flowers are fragile, so you don't want to reach among the tall stems any more than necessary. Since dried flowers don't have the substance of fresh flowers, make a fairly dense mass at the base for a more dramatic effect, perhaps with a lot of goldenrod or artemisia. After constructing a dense core for the arrangement, insert airier plant material higher up.

DRIED HERB WREATH

Your imagination and flower supply are your only limitations in making this wreath. To vary the look a bit over the season, wire in several florist's tubes so you can replace faded herbs and flowers with fresh ones.

MATERIALS: Straw or Spanish moss wreath base (available at garden centers or craft stores); florist's wire and tubes; selection of dried herbs and flowers

1. Choose a "base" plant. This should be something you have in quantity and that will go well with the other flowers you intend to use. 'Silver King' artemisia, for example, makes an excellent background. Insert it in the wreath base, stem by stem, until the whole wreath is covered.

2. Add the accents. These could be little bunches (about 3 inches across) of colorful dried flowers; use florist's wire to make bunches of the smallest blooms. Space them around the wreath, alternating with larger spaces of a more neutral color. For best results, keep the composition simple, using no more than three main colors, such as gray (artemisia), purple (lavender), and pink (rose).

PRINTING WITH HERBS

Using plants to create printed impressions—sometimes called nature printing—combines scientific practicality with decorative art. Leonardo da Vinci (1452–1519) recorded the process in his manuscript *Codex Atlanticus* (ca. 1500), which includes a print of a sage leaf. In the 18th century, Ben Franklin, a printer by trade, printed leaves on the back of currency to deter counterfeiting. The unique pattern of their veins made them almost impossible to duplicate by hand.

Today, herbs can be used to make beautiful botanical prints for display on walls, fabrics, or note cards—or to record your own botanical observations in a study journal. You can experiment with all kinds of herbs and herb parts—flowers, foliage, and roots. Before inking thick sprigs (like thyme) or feathery leaves (like yarrow), press them in a book for about an hour to get a more even printing surface. With practice, you'll learn to adjust the amount of ink and pressure you use depending on the plant. Don't be surprised if the ink picks up delicate features that you missed with your eyes!

MATERIALS: Water-soluble pigment or block-printing inks; palette; soft wedge sponge (or dabber); fresh herbs; tweezers; print-making paper, art paper, or note cards

1. Apply ink. Put a small amount of ink on the palette. Dip the bottom of the sponge into the ink several times, until the base is evenly covered. Use the sponge to gently ink the part of the plant you wish to print.

2. Make the print. Using the tweezers, gently position the herb, inked side down, on your paper or card. Cover the herb with a piece of newspaper or waxed paper. Hold the paper in place with one hand, and use your other hand to gently press over the entire area of the herb.

3. Dry. Remove the paper and use the tweezers to carefully remove the herb. Allow the print to dry undisturbed overnight.

MAKING AND USING HERBAL DYES

Nature provides beautiful living color in thousands of hues, ranging from vibrant reds to soft golden yellows to tranquil azure blues. With herbal dyes, you can surround yourself with the colors of nature. Processing the leaves, flowers, roots, bark, or fruit of many plants unlocks hidden pigments that you can use to dye yarns or fabric.

People began making and using dye for textiles thousands of years ago. Written records show that plant dyes were used in China as early as 2600 BCE, and tests revealed the use of a pigment from madder in the Egyptian King Tutankhamen's (ca. 1341–1323 BCE) tomb. Indigo was also used in ancient Egypt—possibly as early as 4,000 years ago. By the late 16th century, three inexpensive dyes were commonly used in Europe: yellow from the foliage of weld (*Reseda luteola*), red from the roots of madder (*Rubia tinctorum*), and blue from the foliage of woad (*Isatis tintoria*). In North America, Native Americans used plants such as bloodroot (*Sanguinaria canadensis*), mountain alder (*Alnus tenuifolia; A. incana; A. viridis* ssp. *crispa*), and sumac (*Rhus* species) for red or orange dyes; honey locust (*Gleditsia triacanthos*) and yarrow (*Achillea millefolium*) for yellow dyes; and pokeweed (*Phytolacca* species) and mulberry (*Morus* species) for blue or purple dyes. Most plants yielded multiple hues depending on the part used and the processing method. In 1856, the English chemist William H. Perkins accidentally discovered how to make a synthetic dye, and interest in natural dyeing waned over the next 100 years. In recent years, though, interest in natural dyes has returned as artisans have rediscovered the rich range of color possible from herbs.

USING MORDANTS IN DYEING

When using dyes for fibers and textiles, you'll want to consider using mordants—fixatives—to help set color so that it won't fade or bleed. Mordants also help the color adhere to the yarn or fabric, and they may affect the hue. A few plant dyes (such as black tea and turmeric) don't require a mordant to hold their color. These are called substantive dyes. But even with these dyes, using a mordant can be helpful because it often allows a greater range of potential shades. Mordants are usually applied before dyeing by simmering the yarn in water combined with the mordant. Our ancestors used salt, vinegar, baking soda, wood ashes, tannic acid (from sumac or oak leaves), cream of tartar, and alum—as well as blood and even urine—as mordants.

Today, dyers still use some of these agents, but they also use the highly toxic metals chrome, copper, and tin. You can achieve good results using just alum, cream of tartar, or, in some cases, iron.

Alum (potassium aluminum sulfate), which is also used in baking powder, is considered the most stable and one of the least-toxic chemical mordants. You can buy it at a pharmacy. Pickling alum, available at the supermarket, isn't considered as effective but can be substituted.

Cream of tartar not only fixes color, but also brightens it. It's also sold at the supermarket.

Iron (ferrous sulfate) grays or darkens the color of yarn (called "saddening") after it's been dyed. You can buy it online.

You might also try adding some copper pennies to the dye bath as a less-toxic alternative to copper mordant. Or experiment with old rusty nails in place of ferrous sulfate to sadden colors. Some dyers dye in an iron pot to achieve the same effect.

Safety note: Although alum, cream of tartar, and iron are much less toxic than other mordants, it's best to be cautious when using them. Wear gloves, a respirator, and goggles throughout the entire mordanting and dyeing processes, and store unused powdered mordants and used mordant baths in a safe location. Reserve your dyeing equipment for this use only; don't use the same pots to prepare food.

HOW TO DYE WOOL: STOVE TOP METHOD

You can dye wool, cotton, linen, or silk fibers, but wool is easiest. Most, but not all, dyes require a mordant to help set the color (see "Using Mordants in Dyeing"). Some herbs—such as safflower, turmeric, and tea—do not need a mordant, but using one can increase the range of shades possible. Changing the pH of the water by adding vinegar, lemon juice, or baking soda to the dye pot can greatly affect color, too.

Making herbal dyes is both an art and a science, and many excellent books are available on the topic (see "Resources" on page 472). Here's a basic step-by-step process for dyeing wool yarn in an herbal dye bath heated on the stove. Allow 4 to 6 hours, start to finish, if you're working with flowers, foliage, or berries. For bark and roots, the process takes longer because you must presoak these tough-textured herbs the night before you dye the wool.

Note that the herb quantities are approximate; the amount may vary depending on the plant you use. In general, fresh herbs produce the best results. For the dye bath, many dyers prefer to use soft rainwater or distilled water because the mineral content and pH of some tap water can affect the dye color.

MATERIALS: 1 pound (four 4-ounce skeins) undyed wool yarn; 20-quart or larger stainless steel or enamel stockpot; cotton thread; mild soap; large towel; 1-quart stainless steel or enamel pan; plastic or wooden stirring rod; 4 ounces alum;

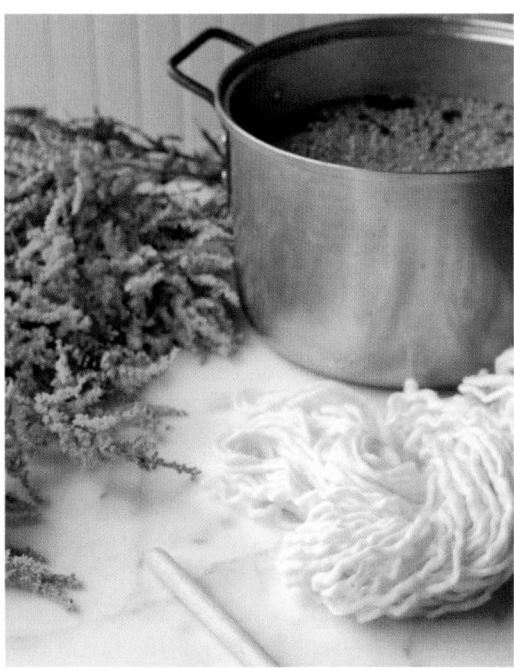

Goldenrod flowers are a natural source of golden yellow for dyeing.

1 ounce cream of tartar; insulated rubber gloves; respirator mask; safety goggles; plastic bag; herbs for dyeing (per pound of yarn, use about 8 quarts fresh flowers or foliage, or 1 pound bark or berries, or ½ pound roots); large sieve; ½ ounce iron; 1 additional ounce cream of tartar (optional for saddening); and nonreactive container

1. Wash the yarn. To keep the yarn from becoming tangled while it's washed and dyed, first wrap the skeins with cotton thread in a figure eight pattern. Keep the thread loose enough to allow the dye to flow around the individual yarn strands. Wash the skeins for several minutes in warm water (95°F) with mild soap to remove all traces of dirt or oil that would repel the dye. Rinse with warm water, gently squeeze out the water (don't wring or twist), and then roll the skein of yarn in a towel to absorb more moisture.

2. Mordant the wool. To help set the dye color, simmer the wool in a mordant bath. Heat 4 gallons of water in the large pot. Meanwhile, heat 1½ cups of water in the 1-quart pan over medium heat. While wearing safety goggles, a respirator, and gloves, dissolve the mordant—in this case, alum and cream of tartar—in the smaller pan of hot water. Stir the solution into the larger pot. When the water in the larger pot is lukewarm, add the yarn. *Slowly* increase the heat level to bring the water to a boil, then lower the heat and let it simmer for 1 hour. Let the mordant bath cool, then remove the wool. Place the wet yarn in a plastic bag until you're ready to add it to the dye bath. Discard the mordant bath, or save it for reuse. If you save it, store it in a labeled, covered, glass container.

3. Prepare the herbs and dye bath. Depending on the plant you are using, either chop the leaves, stems, and roots; mash the berries; separate the petals from the flowers; or break up the bark. (If you're using tough-textured roots or bark, presoak them overnight.) After you prepare the plant material, add it to the large pot, along with 4 gallons of fresh water (some dyers prefer soft

HERBS *for* DYEING

These are just a few of the many plants that will yield colorful dyes. Using different parts of the same plant, along with different mordants, can result in very different colors.

HERB	COLOR	PART USED	MORDANT
Agrimony (*Agrimonia eupatoria*)	Brassy yellow	Leaves, stems	Alum
Betony (*Stachys officinalis*)	Chartreuse	All	Alum
Bloodroot (*Sanguinaria canadensis*)	Red-orange	Roots	None
Calendula (*Calendula officinalis*)	Yellow	Flowers	Alum
Chamomile, Roman (*Chamaemelum nobile*)	Bright yellow	Flowers	Alum
Dandelion (*Taraxacum officinale*)	Soft yellow	Flowers	Alum
	Magenta	All	None
Dock (*Rumex* spp.)	Deep yellow	Roots	Alum
	Yellow	Leaves	Alum
	Dark green	Leaves	Iron
Elder (*Sambucus* spp.)	Violet	Berries	Alum
	Soft yellow	Leaves	Alum
	Gray	Bark	Iron
Foxglove (*Digitalis purpurea*)	Chartreuse	Flowers	Alum
Goldenrod (*Solidago* spp.)	Yellow	Flowers	Alum
Goldenseal (*Hydrastis canadensis*)	Mustard yellow	Roots	None
Indigo (*Indigofera tinctoria*)	Blue	Fermented leaves	None
Madder (*Rubia tinctorum*)	Red	Roots	Alum
Nettle (*Urtica dioica*)	Greenish yellow	Leaves	Alum
Plantain (*Plantago major*)	Dull gold	Leaves	Alum
Pokeweed (*Phytolacca americana*)	Pink to red	Berries	Alum
Pomegranate (*Punica granatum*)	Yellow to brown	Rind	Alum
Rosemary (*Rosmarinus officinalis*)	Yellow-green	Leaves, flowers	Alum
Safflower (*Carthamus tinctorius*)	Pink-red or yellow	Flowers	None
Sweet woodruff (*Galium odoratum*)	Tan	Leaves	Alum
	Red	Roots	Alum
Turmeric (*Curcuma longa*)	Golden yellow	Roots	None
Uva-ursi (*Arctostaphylos uva-ursi*)	Camel	Leaves	None
	Green	All	Alum and iron
Woad (*Isatis tinctoria*)	Blue	Leaves	None

rainwater). Over high heat, bring the water to a boil, and then reduce the heat and let it simmer for 30 to 60 minutes, until the herbs have released their color. Use the sieve to strain out the herbs. Allow the dye to cool to a lukewarm temperature (90° to 110°F).

4. Dye the wool. Place the dye over low heat and then add the skeins of wet yarn. (The yarn must be wet to absorb the dye.) *Slowly* raise the heat level until the dye reaches a simmer. Slowly lift and turn the yarn with the stirring rod; don't stir or agitate it, which could mat the fibers. The yarn should be covered by the bath but move around freely on its own. Simmer for about 1 hour, until the yarn is the color you want—or slightly darker. (The color lightens as the yarn dries.) Dyes made from flowers might take only half an hour; those made from roots or bark could take 2 hours.

Optional (to sadden the yarn color): Remove the yarn from the dye bath. Dissolve the iron and cream of tartar in 1 cup of boiling water in a non-reactive container, then stir the liquid into the dye bath. Put the yarn back into the bath and let it simmer for 20 to 40 minutes.

5. Rinse and dry the yarn. Fill a large clean bucket, utility tub, or laundry sink with warm water (90° to 110°F). Transfer the yarn from the dye bath into the rinse water. Gently lift and turn the skeins to release excess dye. Drain the water, then repeat the process two or three more times, using successively cooler water until the rinse water looks clear. Roll the skeins in a towel, then gently press out the water. Finish drying the yarn in the shade.

HOW TO DYE WOOL: SOLAR METHOD

With solar dyeing, there's no need to stand over a hot stove for several hours and no need to pretreat the wool with a mordant bath. The sun's heat does the work, gradually releasing the plant pigments over several days. This method works best with delicate flowers, leaves, and berries, sometimes producing brighter colors than the stove top method does. You can dye 8 ounces of yarn in a 2-gallon glass jar with a lid (available from restaurant supply stores or online).

MATERIALS: 8 ounces clean wool yarn (to clean, see Step 1 in the stove top method, page 398); 2-gallon wide-mouth glass jar with lid; 4 to 5 quarts fresh flowers, leaves, or berries; 1-quart pan; 4 teaspoons alum; 2 teaspoons cream of tartar; stirring rod

Presoak the wool in warm water for at least 1 hour. Meanwhile, add the prepared herbs to the jar, then add lukewarm water to cover the herbs. In a 1-quart pan, heat 1½ cups of water over medium heat, then dissolve the alum and cream of tartar in the hot water. Add the water to the jar, and use the stirring rod to stir. Add the wet wool to the jar, then add more warm water to within 1 inch of the top of the jar. Stir gently. Cap and set the jar in the sun for several days or as long as a week, shaking the jar daily, until the wool has reached a shade you like. Remove the wool carefully, squeeze out the water, then rinse several times in lukewarm water. Squeeze and blot dry. Finish drying the wool in the shade.

HERBAL PET CARE

Just as we use herbs to enhance our own lives, we can do the same for our four-legged family members—our pets. A growing number of veterinarians take a holistic approach to health care for animals, and that includes the use of herbs to promote wellness and increase the quality and length of our pets' lives. At home, you can use herbs to supplement your pet's diet and make healing preparations for them. But remember: *Always work with a veterinarian who is trained in the use of herbs for pets.*

FOOD FIRST

The holistic approach to pet health begins with a healthy and balanced diet that provides essential nutrients, vitamins, and minerals. In the wild, our pets' ancestors got protein and fat from meat, calcium from crunching on bones, and vegetables from the digestive tracts of their prey.

The commercial pet foods we feed our pets today often lack nutrients that cats or dogs need to be healthy at different times in their lives. Or they contain meat by-products or vegetable sources of protein, which aren't always easy for pets to digest. Commercial foods may also contain things your pet doesn't need, like preservatives and coloring agents. After consuming a steady diet of packaged food for several years, dogs and cats frequently begin to show signs of poor health, such as bad breath, itchy skin, intestinal gas, and dull or dry coats.

Often, simply giving your pet a more balanced natural diet is enough to reverse skin problems, digestive disorders, kidney problems, depression, and other conditions. While commercial natural foods are preferable to their mainstream counterparts, many holistic veterinarians recommend bypassing commercial foods altogether and making your pet's food at home, using the freshest, most wholesome natural ingredients. Whole foods, such as uncooked meats and plants, come much closer to the diet our pets' ancestors consumed, and herbs can play an important part in your pet's natural diet.

The most important step in planning a natural diet is to make sure you'll provide the right mix of nutrients. For adult dogs, that usually means one-third protein, one-third vegetables, and one-third grains. Cats need more meat protein: Their diets should include 50 to 80 percent meat, with the balance made up of vegetables and grains. Of course, every pet has different needs (puppies and kittens need more protein, for example), so it's a good idea to discuss these proportions with your vet. Here are the basic ingredients of a natural diet for dogs and cats.

- **Meat:** Holistic veterinarians recommend beef, poultry, lamb, pork, venison, and occasionally seafood to provide the protein and fats that all dogs and cats require. Some holistic vets favor fresh, raw meat because cooking can destroy healthful proteins, bacteria, and enzymes, and it can make meats harder to digest. If you're concerned about salmonella or other pathogens, lightly steam or boil the meat. Always cook pork or fish, which could contain harmful parasites. To ensure that your cat receives enough of the critical amino acid taurine, include small amounts of raw poultry heart, mackerel, or clams in her diet. But limit her intake of tuna—an all-tuna diet can lead to a deficiency of vitamin E.

- **Vegetables and fruits:** Cats and dogs get vitamins, minerals, fiber, and immune-supporting antioxidants from plant foods. Good choices include carrots, celery, broccoli, zucchini, cucumber, leafy greens, and bean and alfalfa sprouts. Go easy on the spinach; it contains oxalic acid, which can bind with calcium and cause bladder and kidney stones. Unsalted pumpkin seeds and peanut butter, as well as apples, oranges, bananas, and watermelon are also good dietary additions. You don't need to cook the vegetables or fruits—grate, puree, blend, or juice them. *Never feed them* avocado, chocolate, garlic, onions, grapes, macadamia nuts, green potatoes, and green tomatoes. These foods can cause serious problems or even death.

- **Grains:** Unless your pet has a known grain allergy, whole grains are good to include because they are a natural source of the carbohydrates needed to fuel your pet's brain and muscles. Dogs and cats don't digest grains as easily as they do meats, so be sure to cook grains to unlock their nutrients.

- **Calcium:** A homemade natural pet food *must* provide calcium, either in the form of steamed bonemeal (human food quality) or baked eggshell powder. To make eggshell powder, bake eggshells in a 400°F oven for about 5 minutes, then use a rolling pin or mortar and pestle to crush the shells into a fine powder. Dark leafy greens, such as kale and chard, are also good sources of calcium.

- **Herbs:** Many herbs are rich in vitamins, minerals, antioxidants, and essential fatty acids. Adding these nutritive herbs (see "Nutritive Herbs for Pets" on page 404) to your pet's daily diet will help ensure that he receives all of the nutrients necessary for a long, healthy, active life. Herbs supply nutrients in an easy-to-assimilate, natural form without stressing your pet's liver or kidneys and without creating imbalances the way megadoses of vitamins and minerals can.

As a dietary supplement, herbs especially benefit older dogs and cats. Astragalus (*Astragalus membranaceus*), which supports the immune system and increases vitality, is a good general tonic for older animals. Nettle (*Urtica dioica*), dandelion (*Taraxacum officinale*), and parsley (*Petroselinum crispum*) benefit senior pets' kidneys, livers, and digestive systems. For older animals who show symptoms of nervous system impairment, your holistic vet might suggest ginkgo (*Ginkgo biloba*), gotu kola (*Centella asiatica*), peppermint (*Mentha × piperita*), or oat straw (*Avena sativa*). To support your older pet's heart, hawthorn (*Crataegus laevigata*), yarrow (*Achillea millefolium*), and ginkgo can be used. Dandelion leaves (either minced or made into a tea and added to food) are very effective for removing excess fluid from the body, associated with congestive heart failure.

HEALTHY HERBAL TREATS

Instead of buying dog and cat treats with questionable ingredients, you can make your own natural biscuits and cookies for your pet. Experiment by adding or substituting some of the nutritive herbs found on page 404. Use a cookie cutter to make fun shapes.

Cheese and Herb Dog Biscuits

1¾ cups all-purpose flour

1 cup rolled oats

1 cup finely grated cheese

3 tablespoons ground flaxseed

1 tablespoon finely chopped fresh parsley

1¼ cups water

1. Preheat the oven to 300°F. Coat a baking sheet with cooking spray.

2. In a medium bowl, combine the flour, oatmeal, cheese, flaxseed, and parsley. Pour in the water and mix thoroughly to form a dough. Flour a clean surface and roll out the dough on it. Cut the dough into shapes using a floured cookie cutter. Use a spatula to transfer the biscuits to the baking sheet. Bake for 30 to 45 minutes, until the biscuits are lightly browned. Cool the biscuits on the tray, and store them in an airtight container.

Nippy Kitty Cookies

1 tablespoon ground flaxseed

3 tablespoons water

1¼ cups all-purpose flour

¼ cup milk

2 tablespoons finely chopped fresh parsley

2 tablespoons molasses

2 tablespoons vegetable oil

1 tablespoon fresh (or 1 teaspoon dry) chopped catnip (*Nepeta cataria*)

1. Preheat the oven to 350°F. Coat a baking sheet with cooking spray.

2. In a small bowl, combine the flaxseed with the water, and let the mixture sit for 2 minutes. In a medium bowl, combine the flour, milk, parsley, molasses, oil, and catnip, then stir in the flaxseed

mixture. Flour a clean surface and roll out the dough on it. Cut the dough into shapes with a floured cookie cutter or knife. Transfer the cookies to the baking sheet. Bake for 20 minutes. Cool the cookies on the tray, and store them in an airtight container.

HERBAL HEALING FOR PETS

Even with a healthy diet and regular exercise, your cat or dog could be plagued by parasites, be stung by a bee, or could develop an acute or chronic disease. A holistic veterinarian might treat the problem in a variety of ways, but the treatment will likely include the use of herbs. Here are a few of the most common problems dogs and cats experience and the herbs used to treat them. Work with your vet to determine the best preparation and dosage for your pet. To find a holistic veterinarian in your area, contact the American Holistic Veterinary Medical Association (www.ahvma.org). Many of these practitioners use herbs as part of an integrated approach to pet health.

Allergies: Allergies result when the body's immune system becomes overactive in response to an allergen. Besides identifying and avoiding the triggering substance, treatment could include the use of herbs that help the body filter toxins, such as burdock (*Arctium lappa*) and dandelion (*Taraxacum officinale*) root. Diuretic nettle (*Urtica dioica*) and dandelion leaf help rid the body of waste. (Nettle also has antihistamine properties, making it useful against seasonal allergies.) Immune system modulators, such as astragalus (*Astragalus membranaceus*), can also be helpful. Also, be sure your pet is receiving adequate amounts of essential fatty acids, found in flaxseed and borage seed oil.

Anxiety and nervous disorders: For acute anxiety, such as may be caused by travel, for instance, your pet's practitioner might recommend Roman chamomile (*Chamaemelum nobile*), passionflower (*Passiflora incarnata*), or valerian (*Valeriana officinalis*) to help the pet relax. If anxiety and nervousness are chronic, work with your vet to determine the underlying causes. Adaptogenic herbs such as astragalus can help a chronically anxious pet manage stress. Use sedative herbs, such as valerian, only occasionally—not routinely.

Arthritis: The pain of joint degeneration and the inflammation that accompanies it can be eased with anti-inflammatory herbs such as boswellia (*Boswellia serrata*), licorice (*Glycyrrhiza glabra*), and alfalfa (*Medicago sativa*). Nettle, dandelion, and burdock help rid the body of toxic wastes. Dogs may also benefit from a warm compress of comfrey (*Symphytum officinale*) leaves or yarrow, applied externally to sore joints.

Digestive troubles: Recurrent diarrhea and vomiting can be symptoms of other, more serious conditions, such as pancreatitis, liver disease, or cancer. To relieve occasional colon pain and spasms (colic) and eliminate excess gas, try fennel seed (*Foeniculum vulgare*), chamomile, dill (*Anethum graveolens*), peppermint (*Mentha ×

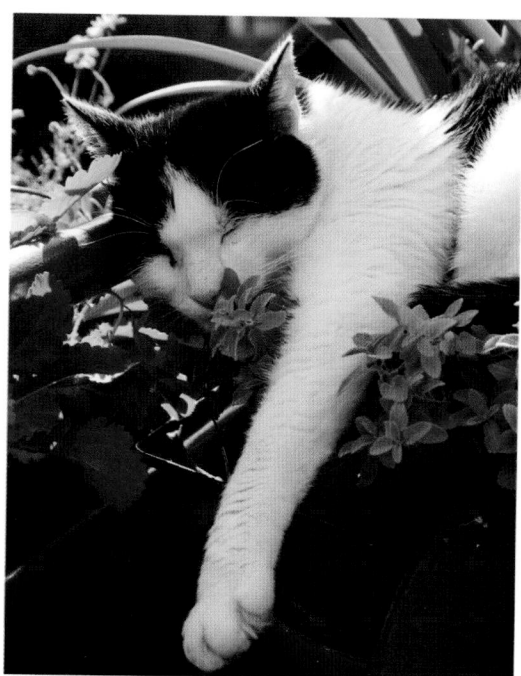

Don't be surprised to find your cat napping after an active play session in the catnip.

piperita), or marshmallow root (*Althaea officina-lis*). For a bout of diarrhea, gentle astringent herbs, such as chamomile, slippery elm (*Ulmus rubra*), or plantain (*Plantago major*), or mucilaginous marsh-mallow root, are helpful. For constipation, dande-lion root or marshmallow root are effective.

Ear mites: Ear mites and bacterial or fungal infections of the ear can be treated with oil that's infused with garlic (*Allium sativum*) or calendula (*Calendula officinalis*) or mullein (*Verbascum thapsus*) flowers. Apply three to seven drops of the oil into the ear canal daily for up to 4 weeks.

Fleas and ticks: If your pet suffers from flea-bites despite having a healthy diet, supplementing his diet with a small amount of dry or blanched nettle leaves could help reduce the severity of his allergic response. Besides being nutritious, nettle has antihistamine properties. To remove fleas indoors, vacuum frequently and wash pet bedding. Use a flea comb on your pet. Be sure to use the kind sold in pet supply stores.

As a preventative, treat your pet with an herbal spray that contains natural insect-repelling com-pounds. (See "Fleas-Be-Gone Spray or Shampoo" on page 405.) If your pet already has a flea prob-lem, you can use the same formula to make a flea shampoo. *Do not use products that contain pennyroyal or pyrethrins, which can be toxic to pets—especially cats.*

Urinary problems: Antimicrobial and soothing to irritated mucous membranes, marshmallow root tea (given in very small quantities) is a good treatment for urinary tract infections, kidney stones, and inflammation. Immune-stimulating and antimicrobial echinacea (*Echinacea* spp.) can help reduce or prevent infections. Nettles,

NUTRITIVE HERBS *for* PETS

The following herbs are excellent daily additions to your pet's diet. Finely mince the fresh, organic herbs and sprinkle them over food just before serving. Grind the seeds into a powder and add just a pinch to food before serving. Decoct (simmer in water for 10 to 15 minutes) the burdock root, and pour some of the liquid over your pet's food.

PARSLEY

(*Petroselinum crispum*) leaves—
Supplies protein; also rich in vitamins A and C, calcium, riboflavin, potassium, iron, magnesium, niacin, and phosphorus.

DANDELION

(*Taraxacum officinale*) leaves—
Rich in protein, potassium, vita-min A, iron, manganese, and other trace minerals; supports the liver.

NETTLE

(*Urtica dioica*) leaves—
Rich in protein, phosphorus, iron, magnesium, and potassium, as well as vitamins A, C, D, and B complex. (Note: Nettle leaves must be dried or cooked to destroy the plant's stinging qualities.)

PURSLANE

(*Portulaca oleracea*) leaves—
An excellent source of omega-3 fatty acids and antioxidants, as well as vitamins A and C and the minerals iron, magnesium, and calcium.

BORAGE

(*Borago officinalis*) seeds, eve-ning primrose (*Oenothera biennis*) seeds, or flax (*Linum usitatissimum*) seeds—
Provide essential fatty acids, nec-essary for the development and maintenance of the brain, liver, heart, and immune system.

BURDOCK

(*Arctium lappa*) root—
Abundant source of calcium, phosphorus, and thiamine; excel-lent liver tonic, cleanses the body of toxins.

dandelion, and goldenrod (*Solidago* spp.) will stimulate urine flow, and gingko improves blood circulation in the kidneys. If your pet's kidneys have been damaged by a poor diet, liver disease, or other problems, your vet will probably recommend a reduced-protein diet, as well.

Skin problems: Calendula (*Calendula officinalis*) flowers prepared as a spritz (an infusion applied as a spray), oil, or salve is one of the safest, most effective treatments for minor skin inflammations, scrapes, itches, and burns. Lavender (*Lavandula angustifolia*), St. John's wort (*Hypericum perforatum*), yarrow (*Achillea millefolium*), and chamomile (*Chamaemelum nobile*) also have skin-healing properties and can be used in sprays, oils, or salves. They also make good additions to calendula preparations. Try aloe juice for burns and fresh yarrow leaves for wounds with minor bleeding. For abscesses or infected wounds that require draining, first apply a poultice of macerated plantain (*Plantago major*) mixed with a bit of olive oil or witch hazel; after the wound has drained, apply calendula oil or salve.

Fleas-Be-Gone Spray or Shampoo

Any combination of the following herbs totaling 2 tablespoons fresh or 1 tablespoon dried:

Rosemary leaves (*Rosmarinus officinalis*)

Oregano leaves (*Origanum vulgare*)

Lemon verbena leaves (*Aloysia citriodora*)

Lavender buds (*Lavandula angustifolia*)

Spearmint leaves (*Mentha spicata*)

Calendula petals (*Calendula officinalis*)

2 cups boiling water

1 tablespoon baby shampoo or liquid castile soap (if making shampoo)

Place the herbs in a medium pot or heatproof bowl. Cover the herbs with the boiling water, and let them steep until the tea has cooled. Strain out the herbs.

For a repellent spray: Fill a spray bottle with the herbal liquid. Spray your pet, rubbing the liquid into her fur. Begin using this spray at the beginning of flea and tick season, and repeat several times each week.

For a shampoo: Combine the shampoo or liquid castile soap with the herbal liquid. In a bathtub filled with warm water, massage the shampoo into your pet's damp fur and lather well. Wait 10 minutes, then rinse with water. The shampoo will cause fleas to jump off and drown in the water. Reapply once or twice each week until the fleas are gone.

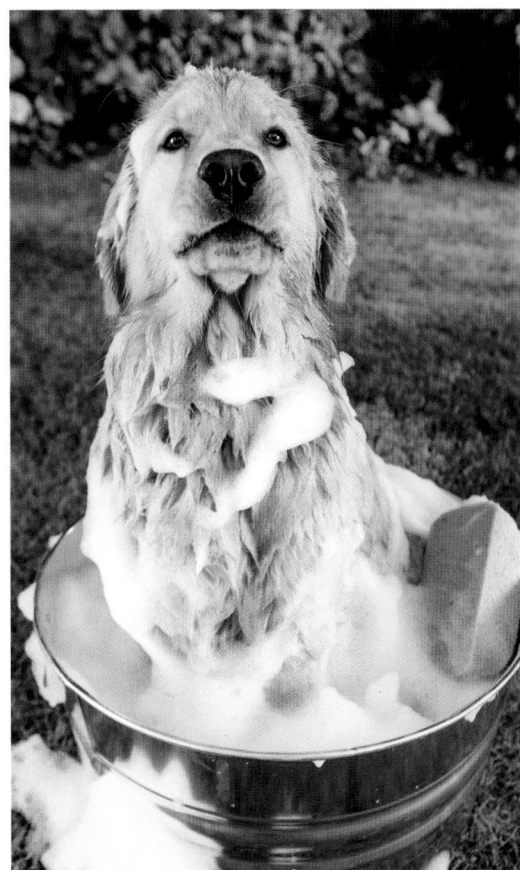

Some insect-repelling herbs make effective and fragrant flea treatments for pets.

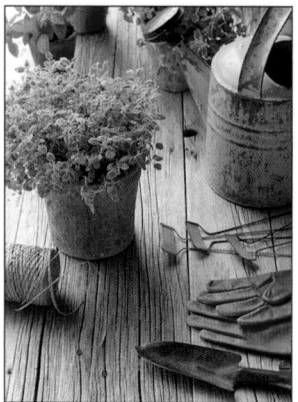

CHAPTER 8

GROWING HERBS

People grow herbs for so many different reasons: to enjoy their beauty and fragrances in the garden . . . to harvest medicinal plants as needed . . . to have easy access to fresh culinary ingredients . . . to admire the birds and insects attracted to these plants. Whatever your intention or level of gardening knowledge, growing herbs at home can be both an enjoyable hobby and an excellent way to ensure a ready supply of fresh, sometimes hard-to-obtain plants.

Herbs blend well with other garden plants in formal and informal gardens and in containers. They are relatively care free—the chemicals they contain naturally help protect them against insect pests and plant diseases. And no matter what your growing conditions—wet or dry, sunny or shaded, dense clay or sandy loam—you'll find dozens of species that will thrive, giving back so much for the minimal effort they require.

CHOOSING HERBS TO GROW

Besides choosing herbs for their practical purposes—for use in medicine, cooking, crafts, etc.—consider what they can add to your garden and landscape. Many herbs have colorful flowers, interesting foliage, or unusual forms.

Also consider the life cycles of the potential selections for your garden: annuals, perennials, or biennials. Annual plants die away at the end of the growing season, but new plants can be grown from the seeds borne during the preceding season. Some self-sow, producing "volunteers" that return year after year. Popular annual herbs include basil (*Ocimum basilicum*), chamomile (*Chamaemelum nobile*), coriander (*Coriandrum sativum*), dill (*Anethum graveolens*), and borage (*Borago officinalis*).

Perennials are plants whose upper portions die during the dormant season while their underground portions remain alive. These plants make new stems and foliage at the beginning of each growing season, and their root systems usually grow larger year after year. Common perennial herbs include bee balm (*Monarda* spp.), catnip (*Nepeta cataria*), chives (*Allium schoenoprasum*), lemon balm (*Melissa officinalis*), and echinacea (*Echinacea* spp.). Some herbs, such as lavender (*Lavandula* spp.) and rosemary (*Rosmarinus officinalis*), retain a woody, aboveground portion throughout the dormant months of the year. At the beginning of the growing season, new foliage forms on these older woody stems. Perennials don't require replanting year after year, but they perform best if you give them some light annual maintenance.

Biennials have a 2-year life cycle. They grow from seed their first season; in their second season, they die after sending up flowers and making seeds. Angelica (*Angelica archangelica*), caraway (*Carum carvi*), evening primrose (*Oenothera biennis*), and parsley (*Petroselinum crispum*) are biennial herbs.

Herb gardens often contain a mix of annuals, perennials, and biennials. When planning your home herb garden, consider how you will combine these different types of herbs in a single space. Even within a mixed bed, it's often best to segregate annuals and perennials, since their maintenance requirements can differ. (For more about garden planning and design, see Chapter 9.)

WHERE TO GROW HERBS OUTDOORS

Many gardeners choose to grow herbs in a dedicated garden space. But versatile herbs can be grown most anywhere: mixed into vegetable beds and ornamental borders, as edgings and groundcovers, in rock gardens and atop stone walls, and in indoor and outdoor containers. The ideal site for herbs depends somewhat on their purpose. You might want basil, thyme, oregano, and other culinary herbs close to your kitchen. If you want your garden to serve primarily as a contemplative retreat, the best site would be a tranquil distance away from daily human activity.

Before planting, assess the growing conditions of your potential garden space. How much sunlight does it receive? Does the sunlight vary from season to season? Is the soil naturally moist or dry? Is it heavy clay or sandy loam? Is the location protected from driving winds and rain?

Most outdoor spaces consist of several microclimates—small areas with unique environmental characteristics such as levels of sunlight and soil moisture. Some areas of a garden might receive direct, intense sunlight all day, while others are in dappled or full shade or receive indirect, reflected light. The amount of sunlight can also vary from

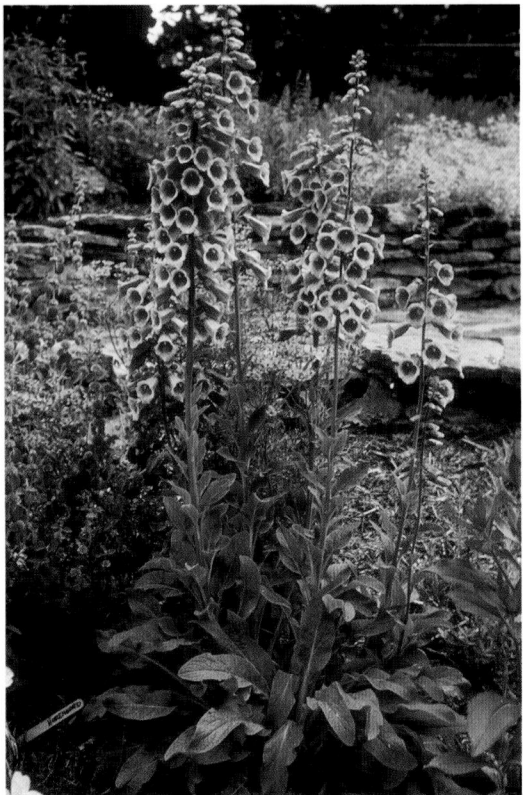

Even a garden area that receives only partial sun can be beautiful; many plants and herbs, such as this foxglove, thrive in part or full shade.

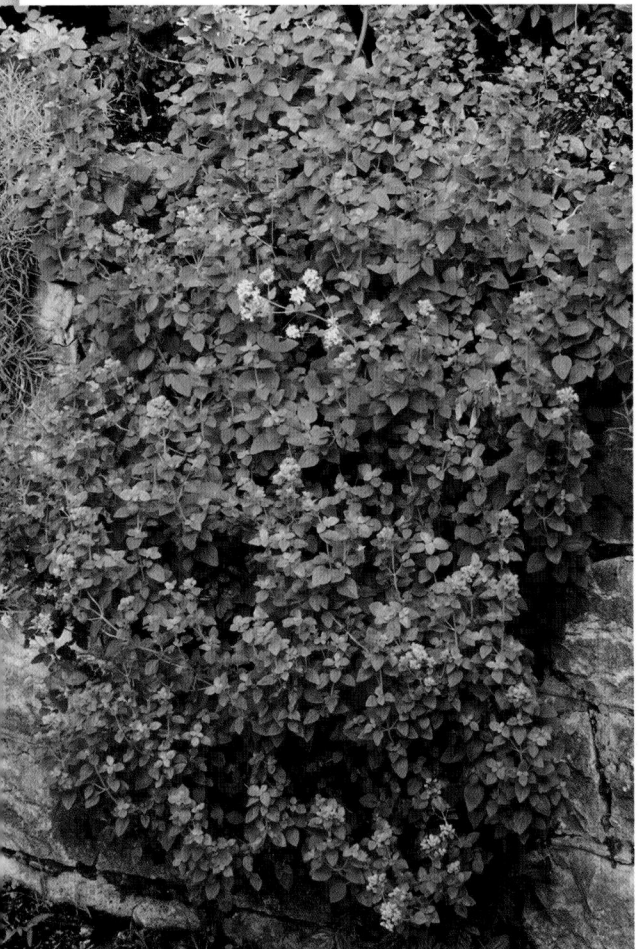

Matching herbs to a garden's microclimate will help ensure healthy plants. Oregano plants thrive in dry, rocky conditions.

season to season. The area beneath a densely leaved deciduous tree, for instance, would be sunny from fall through spring but shady during summer.

Some microclimates have drier soil than others. Elevated spots have less soil moisture than low-lying areas, and plantings beneath a leafy canopy or the eaves of a house receive significantly less precipitation than those in open areas. Soil exposed to wind and sun also rapidly loses moisture. Soil composition and pH can vary widely among microclimates, too. Sandy soil drains and warms quickly, but it's usually low in nutrients because water rapidly leaches them out. Heavy

BEST HERBS *for* SPECIAL SITES

If you are limited to a garden site with very specific growing conditions, choose herbs that will thrive there. (Find out more about these herbs in the species entries in Part II, beginning on page 82.)

PARTIAL SHADE/SHADE

Alpine strawberry (*Fragaria vesca*)

Angelica (*Angelica archangelica*)

Black cohosh (*Actaea racemosa*)

Black hellebore (*Helleborus niger*)

Bloodroot (*Sanguinaria canadensis*)

Blue cohosh (*Caulophyllum thalictroides*)

Chervil (*Anthriscus cerefolium*)

Epimedium (*Epimedium* spp.)

Foxglove (*Digitalis purpurea*)

Mint (*Mentha* spp.)

Passionflower (*Passiflora incarnata*)

Partridge berry (*Mitchella repens*)

Sweet cicely (*Myrrhis odorata*)

Sweet woodruff (*Galium odoratum*)

Tarragon (*Artemisia dracunculus*)

Wintergreen (*Gaultheria procumbens*)

DAMP/WET

Angelica (*Angelica archangelica*)

Bee balm (*Monarda didyma* only)

Elderberry (*Sambucus nigra*)

Elecampane (*Inula helenium*)

Goldenseal (*Hydrastis canadensis*)

Gotu kola (*Centella asiatica*)

Lovage (*Levisticum officinale*)

Mayapple (*Podophyllum peltatum*)

Meadowsweet (*Filipendula ulmaria*)

Mint (*Mentha* spp.)

Sweet flag (*Acorus calamus*)

Valerian (*Valeriana officinalis*)

DRY

Anise hyssop (*Agastache foeniculum*)

Catnip (*Nepeta cataria*)

Chaparral (*Larrea tridentata*)

Ephedra (*Ephedra sinica*)

Evening primrose (*Oenothera biennis*)

Horehound (*Marrubium vulgare*)

Hyssop (*Hyssopus officinalis*)

Marjoram (*Origanum majorana*)

Milk thistle (*Silybum marianum*)

New Jersey tea (*Ceanothus americanus*)

Oregano (*Origanum vulgare*)

Rosemary (*Rosmarinus officinalis*)

St. John's wort (*Hypericum perforatum*)

Wood betony (*Stachys officinalis*)

Wormwood (*Artemisia absinthium*)

ALKALINE SOIL

Ashwagandha (*Withania somnifera*)

Bee balm (*Monarda* spp.)

Boswellia (*Boswellia serrata*)

Cowslip (*Primula veris*)

Goji berry (*Lycium barbarum*)

Lavender (*Lavandula angustifolia*)

Maca (*Lepidium meyenii*)

Rue (*Ruta graveolens*)

Scented geraniums (*Pelargonium* spp.)

Summer savory (*Satureja hortensis*)

ACID SOIL

Alpine strawberry (*Fragaria vesca*)

Bilberry (*Vaccinium myrtillus*)

Birch (*Betula* spp.)

Blueberry (*Vaccinium angustifolium* and others)

Blue cohosh (*Caulophyllum thalictroides*)

Cranberry (*Vaccinium macrocarpon*)

Epimedium (*Epimedium* spp.)

Grape (*Vitis vinifera*)

Horsetail (*Equisetum arvense*)

Mountain arnica (*Arnica montana*)

Partridge berry (*Mitchella repens*)

Sweet woodruff (*Galium odoratum*)

Wintergreen (*Gaultheria procumbens*)

Witch hazel (*Hamamelis virginiana*)

clay soil tends to contain more nutrients, but it drains poorly. As a result, plant roots grow shallowly and might not get enough oxygen, leaving plants susceptible to disease. As much as possible, match the growing conditions to the growing requirements of the herbs you want for your garden. Nearly all herbs benefit from soil that contains a good level of organic matter.

START WITH THE SOIL

The most important thing you can do to ensure the success of your herb garden is to care for the soil. Soil provides nutrition, water, and structural support for plants.

Most herbs prefer loose, well-drained soil that contains some organic matter, is moderately fertile, and has a pH of 6.5 to 7.0—although some herbs have other requirements. (See "Best Herbs for Special Sites" on page 409.)

If your soil hasn't been tested recently, contact the Cooperative Extension Service to obtain a soil testing kit. A soil test conducted by a lab will give you a detailed analysis of your soil's pH, organic matter, and nutrient content.

Soil pH can range from 4.0 or less (acidic) to 9.0 and above (alkaline); neutral soil pH is 7.0. Soil pH affects the availability of nutrients within your soil. The nutrient nitrogen, for example, is readily available in soil with a pH above 5.5. Below a pH of 6.0, the availability of phosphorous, potassium, calcium, and magnesium decreases, and the availability of the metallic micronutrients zinc, manganese, copper, and iron increases—a condition that can be harmful to plants. A very high pH, on the

ORGANIC FERTILIZERS MADE EASY

Plant nutrients such as nitrogen, phosphorus, and potassium are essential to plant growth, root development, and disease resistance. If a soil test indicates a deficiency of a key nutrient, such as phosphorus or potassium, add an organic fertilizer for peak performance. One of the main advantages of organic fertilizers is that they release their nutrients slowly, providing more nutrients over time. Chemical fertilizers are highly soluble and wash through your soil quickly. If your plants don't use them, they can end up as pollutants in groundwater, and they can be harmful to earthworms and other beneficial soil organisms.

Here's a quick overview of essential plant nutrients and the organic fertilizers that provide them.

- **Nitrogen.** Promotes leafy growth, but too much of it can inhibit flowering. Plants respond quickly to this nutrient, so use it sparingly. Manure, fish meal, and bloodmeal are organic sources of nitrogen.

- **Phosphorus.** Helps plants develop strong root systems and promotes flowering. It does not move easily in the soil, so dig it into the soil where plant roots can reach it. Organic sources include bonemeal and rock phosphate.

- **Potassium.** Helps plants withstand disease, drought, and temperature extremes. It also helps with fruiting and seed formation. Greensand and sulfate of potash-magnesia (a mined mineral) supply potassium.

How much fertilizer should you use? Soil test reports usually advise adding a specific number of pounds of a nutrient for every 1,000 square feet of garden soil. The label on the fertilizer will tell you the percentage of nutrients it contains. Many high-quality organic fertilizer blends are available. Apply fertilizer in small amounts when the soil is moist, and follow up with a light watering.

THE BEAUTY *of* COMPOST

Compost is made from plant matter that decomposes into a porous, spongy substance called humus. Indispensable to your garden, compost benefits soil and plants in so many ways.

- Helps soil retain air and moisture around plant roots, offering protection during periods of drought
- Allows water to circulate freely around plant roots, decreasing the chance of root rot
- Buffers pH and nutrient imbalances
- Protects plants from disease
- Releases a slow, steady supply of nutrients
- Darkens soil so that it warms earlier, extending your growing season
- Supports beneficial bacteria, which break down organic matter and make nutrients more available to plants
- Supports beneficial insects that help control plant pests and worms that burrow through soil to keep it well aerated.

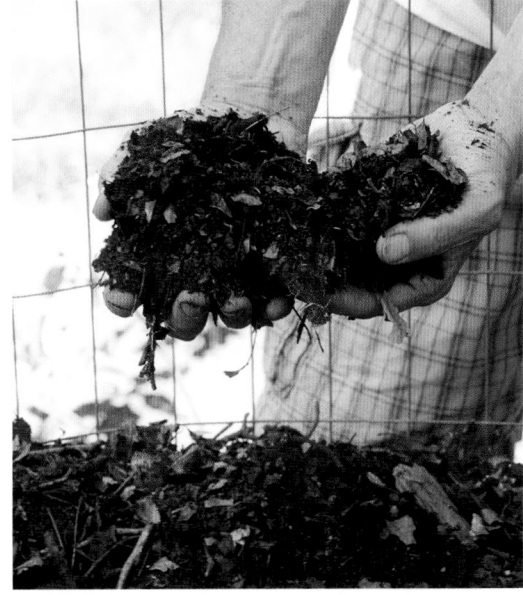

Recycling yard and kitchen waste as compost creates fertile growing material for herbs and other plants.

other hand, can result in deficiencies of these micronutrients, as well as of phosphorus. Soil microorganisms are also affected by pH; a pH of 6.6 to 7.3 is favorable for microbial activities that contribute to the availability of nitrogen, sulfur, and phosphorus in soils.

Soil pH can be raised by adding ground agricultural limestone, sold as either calcitic or dolomitic limestone—natural materials available from most garden supply stores. Calcitic limestone supplies mostly calcium; dolomitic limestone also provides magnesium. Apply limestone at the rate suggested by your soil test. Because limestone does not dissolve easily in water, it's important to mix it thoroughly into the top 8 to 10 inches of soil.

If a soil test shows your soil to be very alkaline (a pH of 8.0 or above), add elemental sulfur to a depth of 6 inches to lower the pH. Because soil

bacteria are needed to help lower pH, the soil should be moist, well aerated, and warm. Elemental sulfur works fast, but be careful not to add too much. It will work over a period of several weeks to months.

Compost is also an excellent buffer for soil pH, bringing both acid and alkaline soils closer to neutral over time, while also adding organic matter, beneficial microbes, and trace minerals.

THE COMPOST ADVANTAGE

There are several ways to change and improve soil quality. The very best thing you can do to improve soil structure is to add compost. Like the spongy, dark humus that covers the forest floor, compost is black gold: It is nature's perfect recycling method for transforming organic waste, such as leaves and

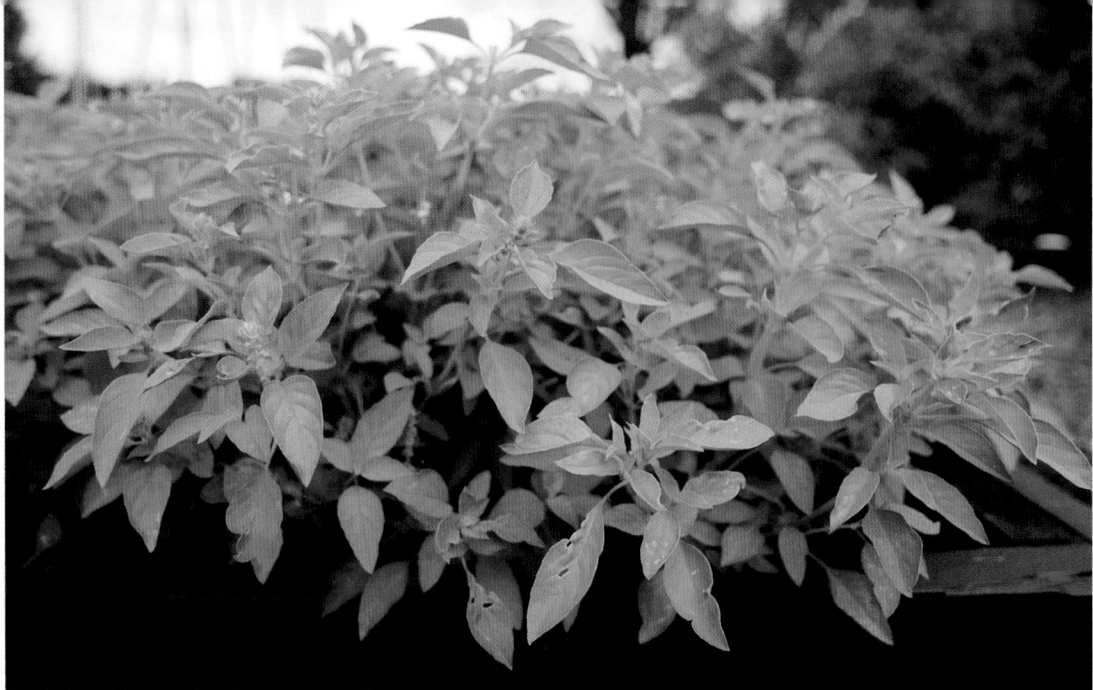

Basil and many other herbs thrive in the loose, well-drained soil of a raised bed.

decaying bark, into an almost magical substance for soil and plants. Compost benefits all kinds of soils—wet, dry, sandy, heavy clay, low pH, high pH, depleted, and imbalanced.

Compost can be made from yard waste, such as grass clippings, pine needles, wood chips, and leaves, as well as from straw, manure, and kitchen waste. Coffee grounds, fruit and vegetable peels, and eggshells are all excellent for composting, but avoid using meat and dairy products, which can attract insects and animals.

To make a simple compost pile, combine high-nitrogen materials (sometimes called "greens"), such as grass clippings, kitchen scraps, and manure, with carbon materials (sometimes called "browns"), such as dry leaves, wood chips, and sawdust. For best decomposition, the pile should be a minimum of 27 cubic feet (3 feet tall by 3 feet wide by 3 feet deep). Keep the materials damp but not saturated, and turn the mixture periodically with a shovel or pitchfork to admit air into the center of the pile. The more often you turn your compost, the faster it will break down. Mature compost is dark brown and sweet smelling—like humus.

Add finished compost to garden beds and containers before planting, or spread it on top of your soil as mulch.

BOOSTING RESULTS WITH RAISED BEDS

Raised beds provide ideal growing conditions for many herbs. In raised beds, soil not only drains more freely, but it also thaws and warms faster—allowing you to plant earlier in the season. The soil in raised beds also tends to remain looser and more friable because it is never walked upon.

A raised bed can be as simple as a mound of soil in any shape. But many gardeners prefer enclosed, rectangular raised beds—basically a bottomless box filled with soil. Garden suppliers sell a variety of premade enclosures for raised beds, or you can easily construct your own from wooden boards, stones, concrete blocks, or bricks.

Don't use pressure-treated lumber, which could

GREENING *the* BRONX

In the borough of the Bronx, New York City, between a brick apartment building and a lot overgrown with waist-high weeds, Victoria Cabrera cuts *papalo* (*Porophyllum ruderale*) from her urban garden plot. Papalo is a Central American culinary herb with a distinctive flavor, sometimes described as "cilantro on steroids." It's also used as a traditional medicine to lower blood pressure. Victoria will either use the herb in homemade *tortas* for her family or sell bunches of it at La Familia Verde farmers market.

Called the "Garden of Happiness," Victoria's garden is part of Bronx Green-Up, a community garden outreach program launched by The New York Botanical Garden (NYBG). The program began in 1988, when the NYBG donated plants to help with the cleanup of an abandoned urban lot. Through educational programs and on-site guidance, Bronx Green-Up now supports an ever-growing number of community horticulture projects, currently totaling more than 150 Bronx school and community gardens. According to a 2010 survey I conducted with Katherine Herrera of The New York Botanical Garden's Institute of Economic Botany, 66 percent of Bronx urban gardeners grew plants for culinary purposes, 14 percent grew them for medicinal purposes, 18 percent grew them for ornamental purposes, and 1 percent grew them for ritualistic purposes.

Today, a green renaissance is sweeping New York City. Take an elevator to the top of an office building or walk over a bridge to Brooklyn, Queens, or the Bronx, and you will see green roofs; planted schoolyards, parks, and ball fields; community gardens; and even commercial farms. The contributions of urban gardeners and their rural counterparts are showing up on the menus of some of the city's finest restaurants, which boast of the flavor and freshness of locally grown, sustainably raised food. You can even drop off food scraps at a Greenmarket—they will be composted and then used as the growing medium for a variety of crops, as well as medicinal and ornamental plants, thanks to the hard work of many urban herbal pioneers. Together, these greening efforts contribute to the sustainable management of land, economic empowerment, and improved nutrition.

If you wish to try growing papalo yourself, check the Internet for sources of seed.

—Sara Katz,
Community Horticulturist,
Bronx Green-Up at
The New York Botanical Garden

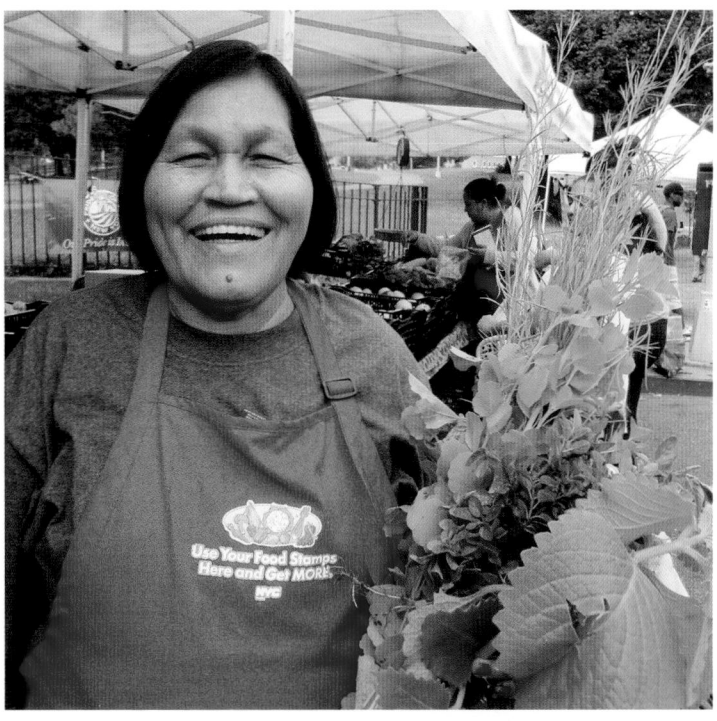

Community gardener Victoria Cabrera sells culinary and medicinal herbs, some of which are native to her home country, Honduras, at the La Familia Verde farmers' market in the Bronx.

contain heavy metals that can leach from the wood. Chromated copper arsenate, creosote, and pentachlorophenol—chemicals used as timber preservatives—are not only toxic to insects and fungi that attack wood, but also to people, pets, and garden plants. And as attractive and "green" as recycled wood might sound, stay away from it because you won't be able to tell whether it's pressure treated or not. Cedar is a good choice for constructing raised beds because it is naturally resistant to rot and insect damage.

Over time, the soil can push apart the sides of wood-framed beds if the corners are not securely fastened. Building your beds with prefabricated metal corners, available from many garden supply companies, can solve this problem.

HOW TO START HERBS

Herb plants and seeds can be purchased from mail-order suppliers (see "Resources" on page 472) or at local plant nurseries or greenhouses. When buying plants, make sure they are robust and healthy. Always choose the bushiest plants with the most intensely colored foliage. Avoid those with pot-bound roots or pest-infested leaves.

Many plant nurseries will ship seeds, young plants, shrubs, and even trees to distant locales. Trees and shrubs purchased this way usually arrive in dormant, bareroot form. Their roots should be full and slightly moist. Plants with dry brown or soggy black roots and those with any indication that they carry insects or disease are unlikely to grow well. Don't hesitate to return unhealthy plants for a refund.

Besides purchasing herb plants from a nursery or other retailer, you can start herbs from seeds, either directly in your garden or indoors. Herbs can also be propagated from cuttings and by division and layering.

GROWING HERBS FROM SEEDS

Many herbs are easy to grow from seeds sown directly in your garden, and once established, they will resow themselves freely year after year. Others have very specific germination and growing requirements.

Sowing Seeds Outdoors

Some annual herbs, such as basil, borage, and German chamomile, grow easily from seeds sown directly in the ground outdoors. Others, like caraway, chervil, cilantro, and dill, have sensitive roots, which prompt the plants to bolt—meaning go to seed—if disturbed. To grow these herbs from seeds, start them where they will grow outdoors, or sow the seeds indoors in peat pots, which later

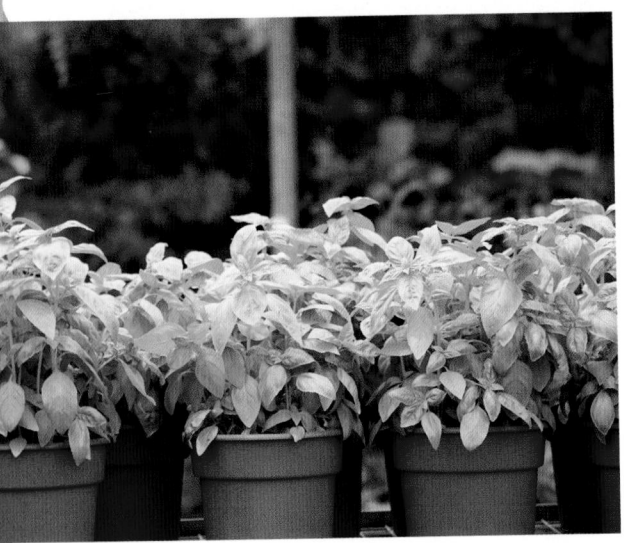

When buying herbs at a garden center, choose bushy, multistemmed plants that are brightly colored and strongly fragrant—these are signs of good health.

can be transplanted to the garden without disturbing the plant roots.

Perennials are generally more difficult to start from seeds, but there are some exceptions: angelica, anise hyssop, chives, fennel, lemon balm, lovage, sage, and summer savory are relatively easy to sow outdoors.

To prepare a garden bed for seeds, remove stones and clumps of soil. Dig in some compost, turn over the soil, and break it up using a hoe, rake, or similar garden tool. For optimal germination, the soil should be finely textured and lightweight. Follow the seed packet instructions for planting depth. If small seeds are planted too deep, they can run out of energy before the sprouts reach the soil surface. Some seeds require light for germination and must be pressed into the soil surface but not covered. Other seeds germinate only in the absence of light and so must be planted deeper: as deep as three or four times their width. Lightly water the seeded bed and keep the soil moist (but not saturated) until the seeds sprout.

Starting Seeds Indoors

To give plants a jump on the growing season, you can germinate seeds indoors before the weather warms and then transplant the seedlings outdoors when conditions are favorable. Seeds can be started in a variety of container types, as long as the container allows excess water to drain out of it. Commercially available "seedling trays" allow seedling roots to draw water from a bottom tray. Some, called plug trays, have thimble-sized soil "plugs" that pop out for easy transplanting.

For best results, germinate seeds in a medium specially formulated for seed starting. Seed-starting mixes are lightweight so that delicate seedling roots can grow easily, and they're sterile, or free of pathogens, pests, and weeds. You can buy a commercial blend at a garden supply store, or prepare your own seed-starting mix at home by combining

SEED STARTING

Starting herbs from seed is fun, easy, and thrifty. Here's how to do it.

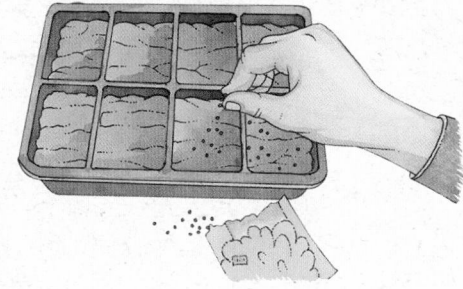

STEP 1: To start seeds in trays, sprinkle the seeds evenly over the surface of your moistened medium.

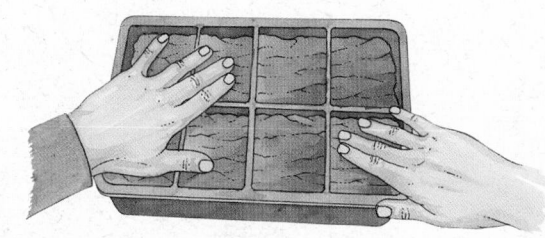

STEP 2: Cover the seeds with more planting medium, according to the specifics on the seed packets.

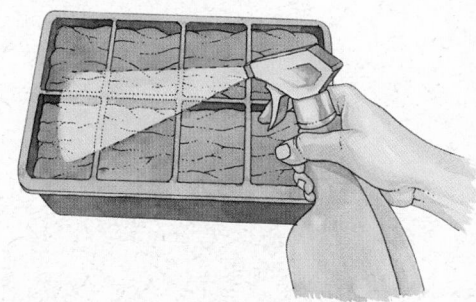

STEP 3: Gently water to moisten the surface. Cover your trays with plastic to retain moisture until the seeds sprout.

2 parts sand, 2 parts perlite, and 1 part well-aged compost.

Moisten the medium with warm water before filling your seed-starting containers. When sowing seeds, follow the instructions on the seed packets. A general rule is that seeds should be planted no more than three to four times as deep as each seed is wide. Until the seeds germinate, keep the growing mix consistently moist—not too wet or dry—by covering the seedling trays with clear plastic wrap or a plastic dome.

Check the seed packet for the herb seeds' ideal germination temperature; many (but not all—see "Stratification" on page 418) germinate most readily in consistently warm soil. To provide gentle warmth, set your seedling trays atop a heat-generating appliance, such as a refrigerator, or on a seedling germination mat.

When your seeds sprout, move the trays to a spot where they will receive 14 to 16 hours of light each day. Windowsills are not usually bright enough for good seedling growth; instead, use a grow light fixture. Although many types of lights are sold and used for starting seeds and growing plants indoors (including metal halide, high pressure sodium, and LED), a standard fluorescent "shop" light fixture will work just fine for starting seeds. Keep the lights very close to the seedlings—1 to 3 inches above the leaves is optimal.

When the first true leaves appear above the seed leaves (cotyledons), it's time to transplant the seedlings into larger containers—pressed peat pots, peat pellets, or cell packs—filled with moistened growing mix. To transplant, first make planting indentations in the growing mix of the larger containers. Use a small fork or craft stick to gently lift out the seedlings with their roots and the surrounding soil. Place the roots in the new planting holes, carefully press down the soil around them, and gently water. Feed the seedlings weekly with an organic fertilizer, such as fish emulsion that's diluted to half-strength.

After 6 to 8 weeks, when outdoor conditions have stabilized, begin acclimating your indoor seedlings to wind, sun, and varying temperatures. This process, called "hardening off," encourages the plants' tender new growth to become more firm and less susceptible to damage. To do this, place seedlings in a shady outdoor location with a temperature between 45° and 50°F. Over the next few days, move the seedling containers into sunlight for increasing periods of time. After 10 days, the seedlings should be hardy enough to plant in your garden.

Special Seed-Starting Techniques

A few herbs require special but very simple seed-starting methods.

Scarification: **Scarification** simply means "scarring" or nicking the seed coat. It is used to promote the germination of hard seeds, such as

SEEDLINGS

After seeds sprout, it's time to move them to a larger container.

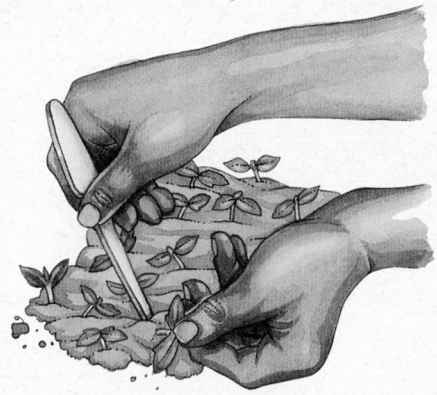

Transplanting seedlings requires a delicate touch. Use a small fork or craft stick to gently lift them out, along with their roots.

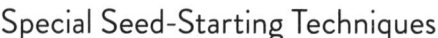

THE BEST METHODS *for* STARTING PLANTS

Your very first garden herbs no doubt will be young plants started by a local or mail-order nursery. But within a year or two, you'll find that starting your own herbs is a fun and inexpensive way to fill your garden with old favorites and new varieties. Use the following methods for starting specific herbs.

HERBS TO START FROM SEED

Angelica (*Angelica archangelica*)

Anise (*Pimpinella anisum*)

Anise hyssop (*Agastache foeniculum*)

Basil (*Ocimum basilicum*)

Borage (*Borago officinalis*)

Calendula (*Calendula officinalis*)

Caraway (*Carum carvi*)

Chervil (*Anthriscus cerefolium*)

Chile peppers (*Capsicum annuum*)

Chives (*Allium schoenoprasum*)

Cilantro (*Coriandrum sativum*)

Dill (*Anethum graveolens*)

Fennel (*Foeniculum vulgare*)

Hyssop (*Hyssopus officinalis*)

Lemon balm (*Melissa officinalis*)

Lovage (*Levisticum officinale*)

Marjoram (*Origanum majorana*)

Oregano (*Origanum vulgare*)

Rosemary (*Rosmarinus officinalis*)

Sage (*Salvia officinalis*)

Salad burnet (*Sanguisorba minor*)

Summer savory (*Satureja hortensis*)

Thyme (*Thymus vulgaris*)

Valerian (*Valeriana officinalis*)

HERBS TO START FROM CUTTINGS

Basil (*Ocimum basilicum*)

Catnip (*Nepeta cataria*)

Lavender (*Lavandula angustifolia*)

Mint (*Mentha* spp.)

Oregano (*Origanum vulgare*)

Pineapple sage (*Salvia elegans*)

Rosemary (*Rosmarinus officinalis*)

Sage (*Salvia officinalis*)

Thyme (*Thymus vulgaris*)

HERBS TO GROW FROM LAYERING

Creeping thyme (*Thymus serpyllum* cv. 'Coccineus')

Lavender (*Lavandula angustifolia*)

Lemon balm (*Melissa officinalis*)

Marjoram (*Origanum majorana*)

Mint (*Mentha* spp.)

Oregano (*Origanum vulgare*)

Roman chamomile (*Chamaemelum nobile*)

Rosemary, prostrate (*Rosmarinus officinalis* var. *prostratus*)

Sage (*Salvia officinalis*)

Tarragon (*Artemisia dracunculus*)

Thyme (*Thymus vulgaris*)

Winter savory (*Satureja montana*)

HERBS TO START FROM DIVISION

Bee balm (*Monarda* spp.)

Catnip (*Nepeta cataria*)

Chives (*Allium schoenoprasum*)

Germander (*Teucrium chamaedrys*)

Hyssop (*Hyssopus officinalis*)

Lemon balm (*Melissa officinalis*)

Lemongrass (*Cymbopogon citratus*)

Mint (*Mentha* spp.)

Oregano (*Origanum vulgare*)

Rue (*Ruta graveolens*)

Saffron (*Crocus sativus*)

Sweet woodruff (*Galium odoratum*)

Tarragon (*Artemisia dracunculus*)

those of astragalus. To scarify seeds, use a sharp knife to gently nick the outside of the seed, or rub seeds over a piece of fine sandpaper. Small seeds can be rubbed between two pieces of fine sandpaper.

Stratification: This is a method of chilling seeds to encourage germination, just as the seeds of many plants in nature require a period of chilling before they can germinate—breaking their dormancy by going through cold winter temperatures. Echinacea (*Echinacea* spp.), gentian (*Gentiana lutea*), jewelweed (*Impatiens capensis*), lavender (*Lavandula angustifolia*), myrrh (*Myrrhis odorata*), osha (*Ligusticum porteri*), and sage (*Salvia officinalis*) seeds respond well to stratification. Put seed packets in a zipper-lock bag (to keep them from drying out), mark the date on the bag, then refrigerate the sealed bag for 4 to 6 weeks, or the recommended period for your specific seeds. Start seeds according to the packet directions.

GROWING HERBS FROM CUTTINGS

If you or a friend already has mature herb plants, you might be able to start new plants quickly and easily by taking cuttings and then rooting them in water or a growing medium. See the chart on page 417 for suggested herbs to start from cuttings.

Rooting Cuttings in Water

Cuttings of basil, mint, and pineapple sage root quickly in water. The best time to take the cuttings is early in the growing season, when your plants have just begun to produce new growth. Use scissors or pruning shears to clip pieces of stem that are about 6 inches long and have several leaf nodes. Clip just below a node. Place the cuttings in a clean, water-filled glass container, and set it in a sunny window. Remember to change the water

ROOTING CUTTINGS IN A MEDIUM

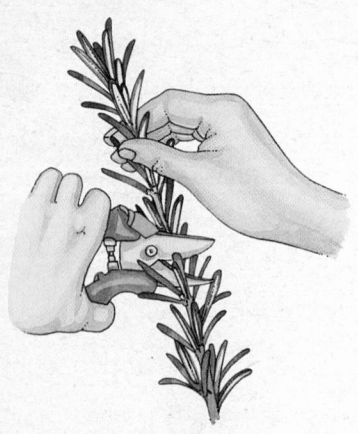 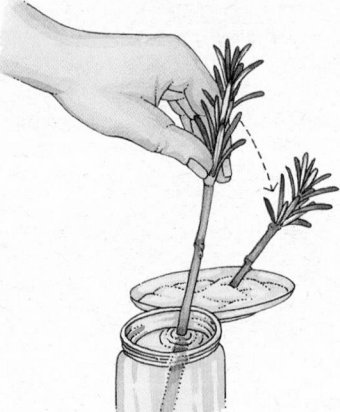 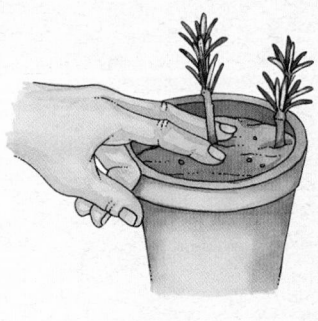

STEP 1: Take 6-inch cuttings that have several leaf nodes.

STEP 2: Strip the bottom 4 inches of leaves, then dip the cutting in a rooting solution.

STEP 3: Sink the bottom 3 inches into a premoistened medium; maintain a humid environment until cuttings form roots.

daily. Roots should soon form along the lower portion of the cutting. When the roots are about ¼ inch long, plant the new herbs in potting soil or directly in your garden. (Follow the instructions for "hardening off" seedlings before transplanting the rooted cuttings to your garden.)

Rooting Cuttings in a Growing Medium

Stem cuttings of basil, catnip, lavender, oregano, rosemary, sage, and thyme can be rooted directly in a growing medium, such as a combination of peat moss and sand, or a store-bought mixture. Use sharp scissors or pruners to take 6-inch stem cuttings that have several leaf nodes. Strip the bottom two-thirds of the leaves from the cuttings, then dip them into a rooting hormone solution. Stick the cut ends about 3 inches deep in a pot filled with premoistened growing medium; space the cuttings about 4 inches apart. Provide indirect light and keep the medium consistently moist.

To encourage rooting, maintain a humid environment by loosely covering the cuttings with clear plastic until they form roots—about 4 to 6 weeks. Occasionally lift an edge of the plastic to mist the plants with water. When the cuttings begin to grow new leaves, transplant them to individual containers filled with regular potting soil, or to your garden. (Follow the instructions for "hardening off" seedlings before transplanting the rooted cuttings to the garden.)

GROWING HERBS FROM DIVISIONS

Another easy way to multiply herbs is to divide large, established plants. Three types of herbs can be propagated by division: (1) herbs that form bulbs, cloves, or corms (such as chives and saffron); (2) herbs that creep (such as mint, oregano, and sweet woodruff); and (3) herbs that form clumps (such as germander, catnip, and lemon

DIVIDING

Herbs that creep, clump, or form bulbs are easy to multiply by division.

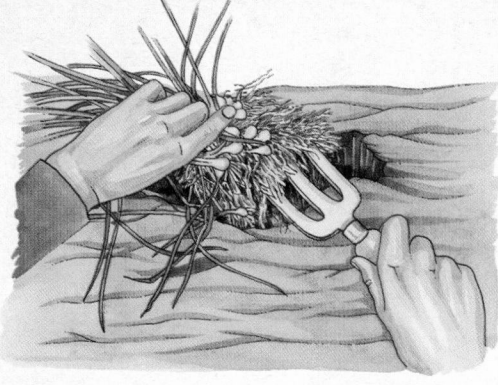

STEP 1: To start new chive plants, use a garden fork to lift the roots of a 3- to 4-year-old plant.

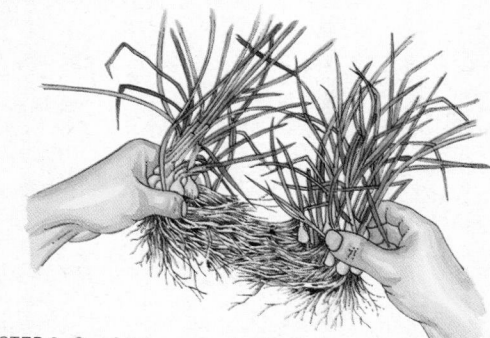

STEP 2: Carefully separate the plant into smaller sections, each with healthy roots and shoots.

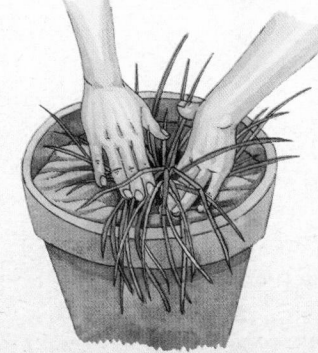

STEP 3: Replant the divisions immediately, then water well.

LAYERING

Plants that sprawl or creep, such as mint or oregano, are easy to propagate by layering.

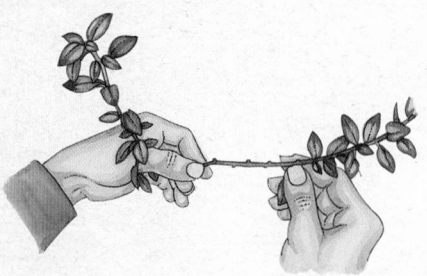

STEP 1: To layer a low, creeping herb such as mint, choose a long, flexible stem low to the ground. Starting 3 to 4 inches from the tip, remove the leaves from a section that is a few inches long.

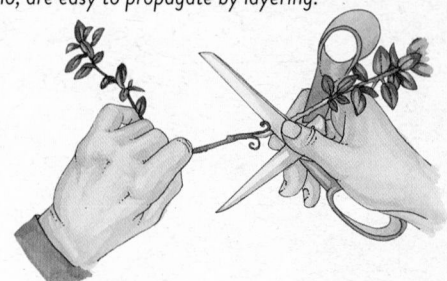

STEP 2: Use a pair of sharp scissors to gently scrape the outside layer from that section of stem. This will encourage the stem to make roots at that point.

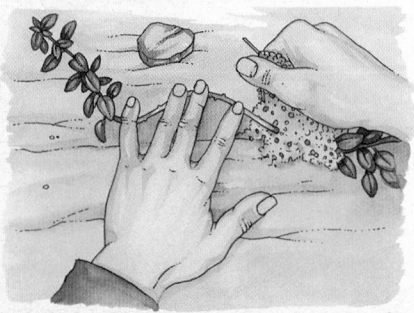

STEP 3: Carefully bend the stem to the ground and cover the scraped section with soil. Anchor it in place with a small rock, then water thoroughly.

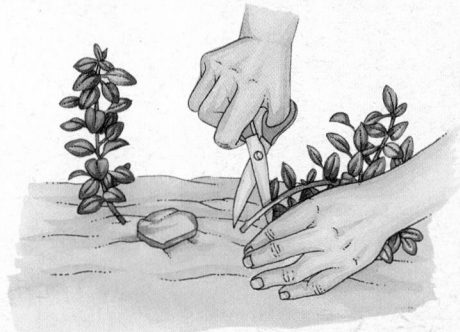

STEP 4: Keep the area moist until roots grow—usually within 4 to 6 weeks. The following spring, clip the "mother stem" and dig up a new plant. Transplant it to its new garden location.

balm). At the beginning of the growing season (for peak- or end-of-season bloomers) or at the end of the growing season (for early season bloomers), use a garden fork to carefully dig up an entire plant. Gently separate the roots into smaller sections. Each new, small plant should contain a good set of roots and some strong, healthy shoots. Replant these immediately, or store bulbs, corms, or tubers in a cool, dry spot for planting later.

GROWING HERBS BY LAYERING

When the stems of some herbs (especially mint, thyme, and oregano) touch the soil, the plant might sprout roots at the point of contact. When this occurs naturally in your garden, the new plantlets can be separated from the main plant, dug up, and relocated. You can use this same process, called layering, to propagate lavender, lemon balm, prostrate rosemary, Roman chamomile, sage, tarragon, and winter savory.

TRANSPLANTING

Ease young herbs' transition to the garden to avoid any setback in their growth.

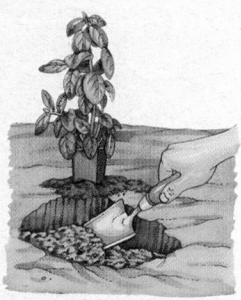 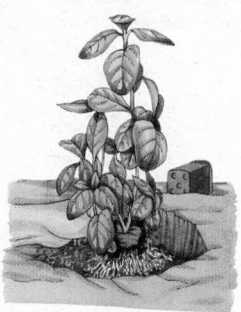 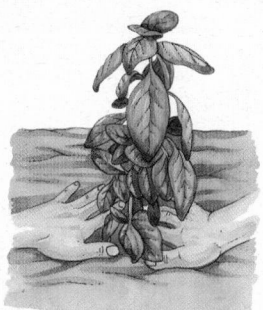 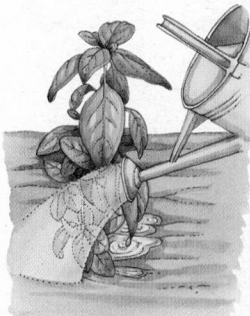

STEP 1: To transplant herbs such as basil, dig a hole deeper and wider than the size of the seedling's container.

STEP 2: After removing the plant from its container, place it in the hole so that the tops of the roots are level with the soil surface.

STEP 3: Fill in the hole, cover the roots with soil, pressing down firmly to eliminate any air pockets.

STEP 4: Water well, so that the soil is soaked, ensuring that the roots receive enough water to encourage new growth.

PLANTING HERBS

Whether you are starting herbs from seeds, cuttings, or division, or purchasing plants from a garden center or mail-order supplier, your plants will grow best if they're properly planted. This is especially important for shrubs and trees, which are usually a larger financial investment than annuals and perennials.

PLANTING SEEDLINGS

Plant annuals, such as basil, in your garden after the last expected spring frost date; perennials can be planted 1 or 2 weeks earlier. If possible, plant on an overcast day or during the late afternoon or evening, when sunlight is less intense, to reduce stress on your plants. Water annuals and perennials several hours before you transplant them. Also soak the roots of bareroot plants for an hour or two prior to transplanting.

Prepare the site before planting by mixing compost, limestone, and other necessary amendments uniformly throughout the soil. To plant seedlings of annuals and perennials, dig a hole slightly deeper and wider than the container. Next, remove the plants by inverting their containers and gently pushing from the bottom. If the roots have become compacted within the pot, use the tip of a trowel to make shallow vertical cuts into the outside of the rootball. This will encourage new root growth into the surrounding soil after planting. Avoid holding seedlings by their tender stems or leaves, which can put unnecessary stress on these fragile plant parts. Instead, grasp the root ball.

Set the plants into the holes so the tops of the roots are level with the ground. Cover the roots with soil, pressing down firmly to eliminate any air pockets around the roots. Water the plants immediately. When working with plants grown in peat pots or peat pellets, place the entire container directly into the ground—the plant's roots will grow right through the walls of the pot, which will disintegrate. Be sure to cover the tops of peat pots completely, or tear off their top lips. An edge sticking out of the soil can act as a wick, drawing water away from the plant's roots.

To help plants recover from the shock of being transplanted, soak them well and then shelter them from wind and sun for a few days by covering them with a flowerpot, basket, or small tree branch with leaves. If rainfall is insufficient the first week after transplanting, water the plants daily. During the second week after transplanting, water the plants every other day, and then every third day the third week. Steady watering is especially important for seedlings because their roots haven't developed enough to reach deep soil moisture.

PLANTING SHRUBS AND TREES

Shrubs and trees are sold in one of three forms: balled-and-burlapped (also called B&B), containerized, or bareroot. Most mail-order nurseries ship deciduous trees, bushes, and roses in bareroot form, wrapped in sphagnum moss, to reduce shipping charges. When bareroot plants arrive by mail, unpack them as soon as possible and soak the roots in water for several hours.

Plant shrubs and trees as soon as possible after you receive them in the mail or buy them at a nursery. If immediate planting isn't possible, hold the plants temporarily in a shady spot; cover bare roots with moist soil, sand, or peat moss. Moisten the soil of B&B or containerized plants that you are unable to plant immediately.

The best time to plant shrubs and trees is at the end or the very beginning of the growing season, when they are most likely to generate new roots and least likely to lose moisture through their leaves. The bareroot stock shipped by mail-order nurseries is usually dormant (without leaves), and could be small in size. Smaller shrubs and trees are usually more economical than larger plants. They also adapt more quickly to their surroundings, are less likely to suffer transplant shock, and quickly catch up to larger plants.

Before planting, be sure to site shrubs and trees far enough from foundations and paths so that, when fully grown, these plants will not block windows, crowd or damage buildings, or interfere with foot traffic. Once you've chosen your spot,

CONTAINING INVASIVE HERBS

Certain herbs grow so enthusiastically that they can take over a garden if not monitored. Mint, which sends out rhizomes below the surface of the soil, can sneak through a garden and choke out other plants. Horseradish, sweet woodruff, and tarragon can spread similarly. Prolific seeders such as borage, catnip, lemon balm, and mugwort generously spread their offspring all around a garden.

To keep creeping herbs such as mint under control, plant them in containers sunk into the soil, but leave a bit of the containers' rims above the ground. Pull up a pot periodically and check to make sure the roots of the plant have not escaped through a drainage hole. If they have, pull the roots gently out of the soil, getting as much of them as possible, and remove them from the bottom of the pot. Aboveground, you may have to remove plants as they spread out of the pot and begin to colonize the surrounding area. In addition, to help reduce the spread of borage, catnip, lemon balm, and other prolific seeders, remove their flower heads before they go to seed.

dig a hole twice as wide but only as deep as the plant's roots (or its pot).

For potted and bareroot plants: If the plant is in a container, ease it out and then use clean, sharp pruning shears to remove any damaged or diseased roots. Place the roots or rootball in the hole. When planted, the top of the roots or rootball should be level or slightly above the surface of the surrounding ground.

For B&B plants: Pull the burlap off of the rootball, leaving it in the hole. If the rootball is enclosed in a wire basket, cut the wires so they are below the surface of the soil and will not interfere with raking or cultivation.

Fill the hole three-quarters full with soil. Make sure the plant is standing up straight, and then gently press down the soil around it. Add water to eliminate any air pockets, and then fill the hole to ground level. Use additional soil to build a ring, or berm, about 6 inches from the outside edge of the hole. Water heavily again.

Finally, add a 2- or 3-inch layer of organic mulch, such as bark chips or shredded leaves, around the base of the plant to reduce moisture loss and discourage weed growth. Do not let the mulch come in direct contact with the trunk, however; this can damage the bark and encourage insect and disease troubles. In addition, a big pyramid of mulch around a tree can limit gas exchange in the soil, cutting off its supply of air and harming its growth. (For more, see "The Magic of Mulch" on page 425.)

During the first growing season, water shrubs and trees once a week if there is no rain, slowly soaking the soil. The water should reach the top of the berm so it will penetrate deeply and encourage root development. Watering is particularly crucial for B&B and container-grown shrubs and trees. In the nursery, the roots of these plants become concentrated in a small cluster. Until the roots are able to spread into the surrounding soil, these plants draw water mostly from their rootballs, which will dry out more quickly than the soil around them.

HERB GARDEN MAINTENANCE

Maintaining a healthy, vibrant garden of any kind means paying attention to the water and nutrient needs of your plants; managing competing weeds; and preventing or stopping disease and insect problems before they get out of hand. Fortunately, herbs are among the easiest plants to grow—typically, they need much less maintenance than other garden plants. By following these basic tips and techniques, your herb garden will practically care for itself.

WATER WISELY

In most areas, rainfall provides adequate moisture for herbs. Covering the surface of your garden beds with a 1- to 3-inch layer of organic mulch (such as shredded bark, leaves, or compost) will

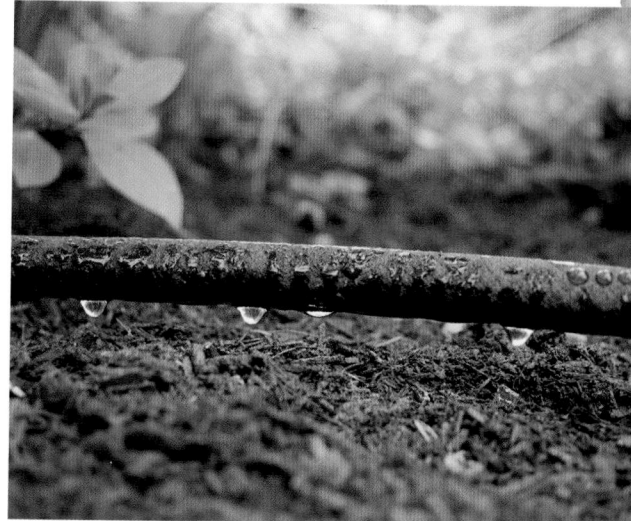

Soaker hoses deliver water efficiently to plant roots; less moisture is lost to evaporation.

help retain soil moisture, suppress weeds, and prevent soil erosion. Water is essential to plant growth. When rainfall isn't enough, deep watering once or twice a week can help.

If an extended drought causes some plants to wilt, deep watering (permeating 1 to 3 inches below the surface) can help them recover. Deep watering ensures healthier root development than shallow daily watering, which simply encourages the growth of roots upward toward the bit of moisture that is being provided. Before watering, loosen the soil that surrounds the plants to encourage easier absorption and discourage runoff. Water in the morning, if possible, so that any droplets that splash onto foliage can evaporate during the day. Using a soaker hose or drip irrigation will also keep foliage dry, protecting your plants from diseases (such as fungal infection) promoted by dampness. By releasing water close to the root zones of plants, drip systems also foster deep root growth and minimize runoff and evaporation.

A HEALTHY DIET

For most herbs, a yearly application of compost is enough to keep their soil in good condition. But some herbs—especially fast-growing annuals such as basil, cilantro, and dill—benefit from an occasional boost of organic fertilizer, such as fish emulsion or liquid seaweed. Avoid feeding plants too much nitrogen (such as in manure) because it can encourage weak growth that's more susceptible to disease and the ravages of cold weather.

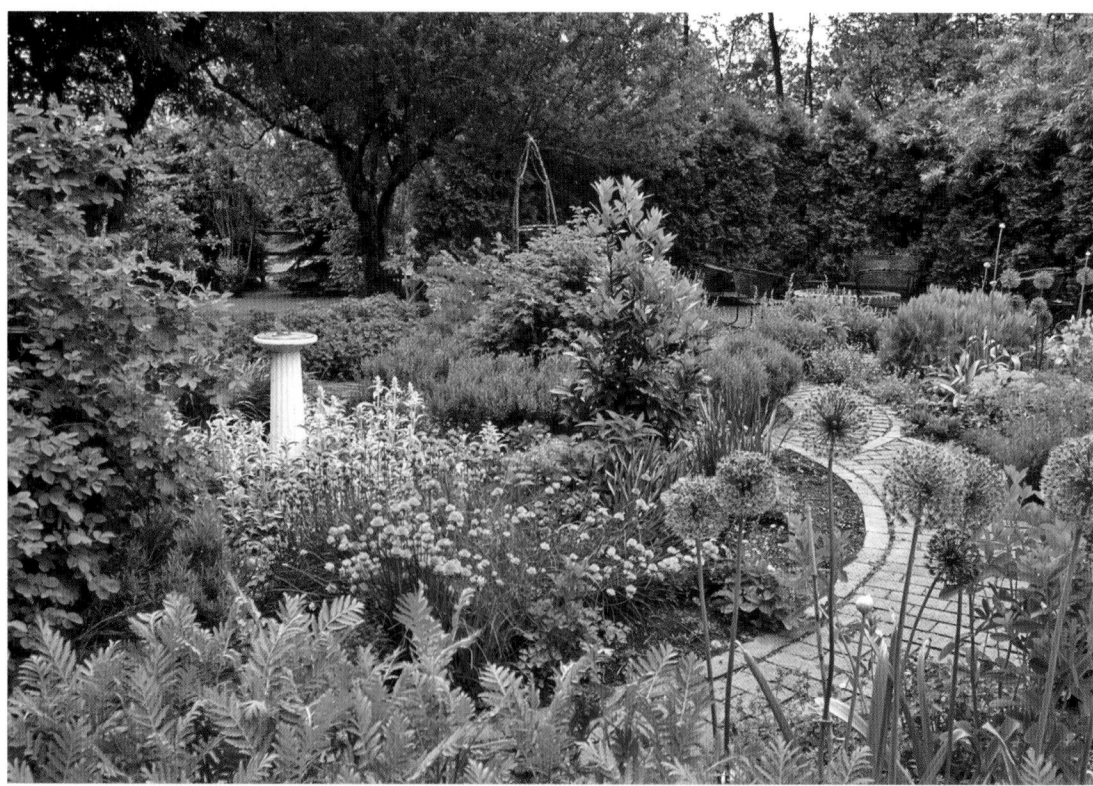

Routine garden maintenance—weeding, pruning, and watering—keeps an herb garden healthy and beautiful.

Once or twice a month, from spring to midsummer, treat your herbs to some compost "tea"—an effective liquid fertilizer and preventive for some mildew diseases. To make compost tea, place 1 quart of finished compost in a 5-gallon bucket, and then fill the bucket halfway with water. Steep the mixture for 5 to 15 days, then strain out the compost. Reserve the liquid and dilute it until it is the color of a cup of black tea. Spray the liquid on plant leaves early in the morning, or apply it to the soil around fast-growing herbs.

THE MAGIC OF MULCH

Mulch—a thin layer of organic or inorganic matter laid on the soil's surface—helps keep soil cool during the growing season and provides insulation during the dormant months. Mulch also slowly releases nutrients into the soil, retains moisture, and suppresses the growth of weeds around plantings.

The best organic mulches for garden plantings are shredded leaves, pine needles, and compost. Compost provides the added benefit of protecting plants against diseases. Studies at Ohio State University showed that a 2-inch layer of compost mulch blocked weeds while greatly enhancing plant growth. High-carbon materials, such as wood chips and sawdust, can inhibit plant growth in the garden, but they're perfect for mulching pathways. A double-layered mulch of damp newspapers topped with chipped bark or gravel works even better for stopping pathway weeds.

Apply a 2- to 4-inch layer of mulch over garden beds, but keep it several inches away from plant stems and trunks so that it doesn't damage the bark and encourage insects and disease. Replenish organic mulches every few years.

If mulch isn't enough to stop the growth of aggressive, unwanted plants, use a trowel or shovel to carefully remove these plant by their roots. Continue to inspect the area because new plants can sprout from root fragments or seeds.

PROPER PRUNING

Proper pruning encourages plants to produce healthier, bushier growth. Follow these guidelines to keep your herbs growing strong for years to come:

- *In midspring to late spring, prune woody, aromatic herbs* such as lavender, sage, southernwood, and rosemary. Use clean, sharp gardening shears to remove older, leggy growth. This will prompt the plant to generate young, healthy stems.

- *In early summer, prune flowering stems to promote extended foliage production* of such herbs as basil, Roman chamomile, chervil, costmary, lemon verbena, oregano, and tarragon. The flowering stems of these herbs will divert the plants' energy from the formation of fragrant or flavorful foliage. To prevent or delay flowering, use gardening shears to cut the

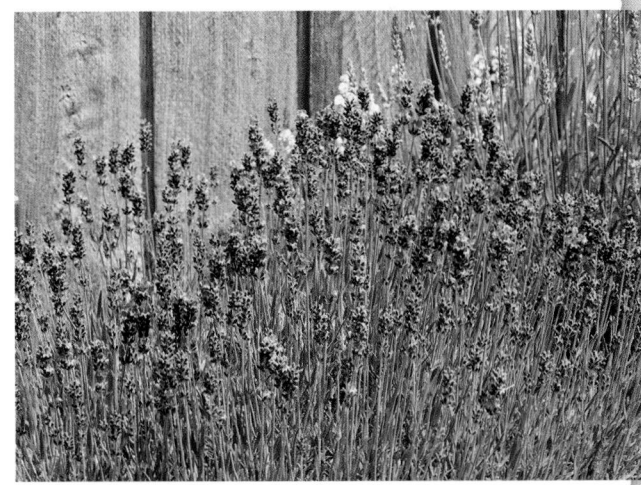

Planting in a protected area, such as next to a fence or building, can help herbs at the limit of their cold-tolerance survive winter. Mulch, row covers, and cold frames also offer protection against cold.

flower stems at their bases. For tender herbs such as basil, pinch off flowers as they form to prolong the production of aromatic foliage.

- *In the middle of the growing season, after they have flowered,* cut back catnip, comfrey, lemon balm, marjoram, mint, sweet cicely, and salad burnet. These herbs produce less-flavorful and tougher foliage later in the season. Cut the plants back by one-third to one-half to encourage a burst of tender new foliage.

EXTENDING THE GROWING SEASON

For annuals and tender-leaved perennials in temperate regions, the first and last frosts of the year generally signal the beginning and the end of the growing season. Neither annuals nor tender perennials tolerate temperatures below freezing: A night of frost can turn a healthy plant into a cluster of blackened, shriveled sticks. On the other end of the spectrum, plants accustomed to cool weather can fail to germinate under a blistering sun.

Sheltering structures can help moderate soil and air temperatures below and around plants, protecting individual plants or whole beds. In hot areas, a shade net of woven polypropylene fabric stretched over wire hoops or a movable wooden frame can keep soil cool and moist. Shade netting can be placed over newly sown seedbeds and transplanted seedlings to shield them from drying winds and to buffer the intense heat and light of the sun.

In cool weather regions, a cold frame can be used to trap the sun's heat and begin the growing season a few weeks earlier in spring and extend it a few weeks later in fall. A cold frame is a low, bottomless, boxlike structure that acts like a greenhouse. It usually has a higher south-facing back wall, a white interior to reflect light throughout the box, a glass or clear plastic cover that allows the sun's rays to penetrate, and a thermometer to monitor the interior temperature. You open the cover to reduce the temperature when it climbs too high for the plants inside. Cold frames are good for starting seedlings in spring, for hardening off seedlings that have been started indoors, and for extending the harvest season of cold-sensitive plants. A cloche or a bell-shaped cover (made from such materials as a plastic milk jug) can also be used to protect individual plants from cold temperatures in spring and fall.

In all climates, strong winds can prevent herbs from developing sturdy root systems, thereby preventing healthy growth. A wooden fence or row of planted shrubs can act as an effective windbreak, providing enough shelter to allow some marginal plants to survive otherwise.

GROWING HERBS IN CONTAINERS

Pots, planters, and half barrels overflowing with colorful and flavorful herbs add appeal to any garden or home. Growing herbs in containers can serve a variety of practical purposes, as well. If you live in the city and have limited growing space, containers of herbs can turn your balcony into a productive garden. If your yard is shaded, you can locate containers in sunny areas more conducive to plant growth. If you want to grow herbs right outside your kitchen door but your garden is many steps away, containers can solve that problem, too.

Container-grown plants also add versatility to gardens large and small. A pair of matching containers on either side of the front walk can serve as a welcoming decoration, while groups of pots on a deck can provide privacy as well as color, fragrance, and texture. You can position containers on the ground or on a pedestal, mount them on a windowsill, or hang them from your porch. Plant them with a single species, such as rosemary, bay, or thyme, for a stunning garden accent, or experiment by combining herbs of different forms and colors. The possibilities are almost endless.

CHOOSING CONTAINERS

Pots and planters are available in a wide range of sizes, shapes, materials, and styles. You can also modify containers such as bowls, barrels, buckets, wheelbarrows, and wagons to be planters. It's worth investing in attractive, well-made planters, even if they cost a little more. They will add beauty to your garden's decor, while inferior planters could detract from it, no matter how appealing the plants they contain.

For the growth and even survival of most plants, bigger pots are better. Those 10-inch hanging baskets—the ones so popular at garden centers in spring—require constant watering in summer. If you go away for the weekend, you're likely to find a shriveled plant upon your return. But with a larger container and more soil, your herbs can grow a larger root mass that will support lush, healthy, aboveground growth. Larger pots also retain soil moisture longer and are better insulated against temperature fluctuations.

To determine how large and deep a container should be, consider the size and shape of the herbs you wish to grow, as well as the plant types—annuals, perennials, or shrubs—and how rapidly they will grow. Rootbound plants dry out rapidly and won't grow well. For a mixed planting, choose a planter with enough root space for all of the plants you want to grow.

The maximum size (and weight) of a container will be limited by how much room you have, whether or not you plan to move the container, and the strength of the supporting structure. If your container garden is located on a balcony or deck, be sure to check how much weight the struc-

ture will safely hold. If you aren't sure, contact a structural engineer for an opinion. Remember that a fully watered large clay pot with plants can easily weigh 50 pounds or more.

Whatever container you choose, drainage holes are essential. Without drainage, the soil will become waterlogged, and your plants could die.

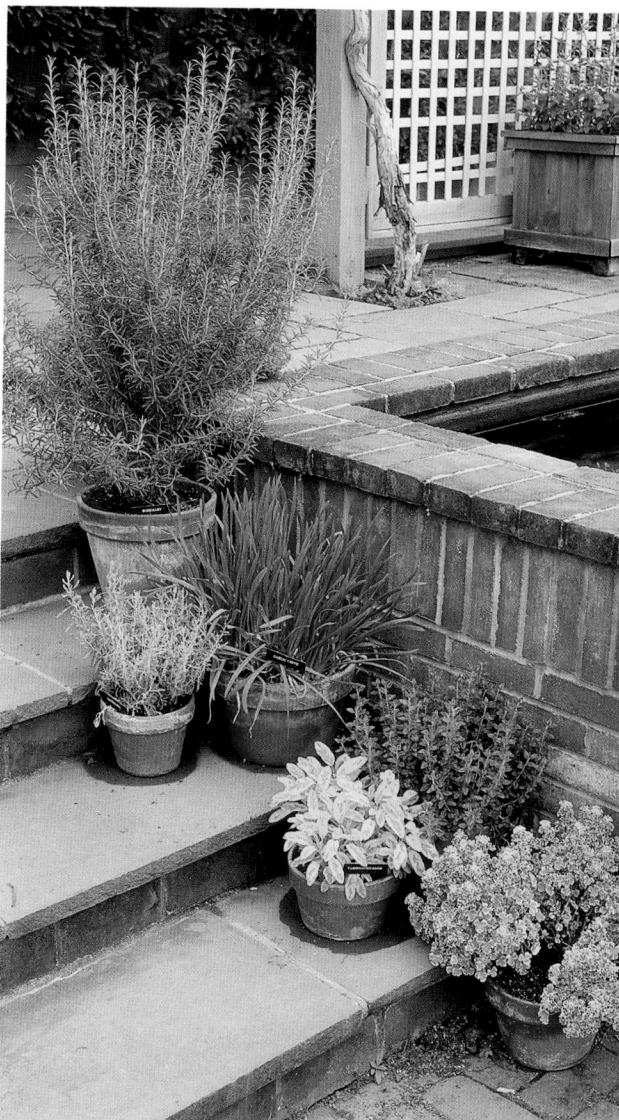

Potted herbs can lend instant color, provide a focal point, or help link the architecture of your house to your garden.

The holes need not be large, but there should be enough of them to allow excess water to drain out. If a container has no holes, try drilling some yourself (if the container can be drilled). A container without holes is best used as a cachepot, or cover, to hide a plain pot.

Cachepots (with holes or without them) are useful for managing large plants and heavy pots:

Porous terra-cotta pots allow air and moisture to penetrate. This means plants are less likely to drown if overwatered, but they could suffer if you forget to water.

Grow your plant in an ordinary nursery pot that fits inside a decorative cachepot so you can move them separately. Self-watering double-walled containers, hanging baskets, and window boxes are also available. These are useful for dealing with smaller plants that need frequent watering.

Containers are made from a variety of materials, and each type has advantages and disadvantages concerning their durability, appearance, weight, and initial cost.

- *Clay or terra-cotta* containers are attractive but breakable and are easily damaged by freezing and thawing. In northern areas, store these pots in a frost-free location to prevent cracking. They are not suitable for hardy perennials or hardy shrubs kept outdoors year-round.

- *Cast concrete* is long lasting and comes in a range of sizes and styles. These can be left outside in all weather and temperatures. You can even make attractive ones yourself. Plain concrete containers are very heavy, so they're difficult to move and not suitable for use on decks or balconies.

- *Stone* planters provide both durability and beauty, and they come in many different colors and textures. These containers require little maintenance but are very heavy and best used on firm ground.

- *Plastic, resin,* and *fiberglass* planters are lightweight, relatively inexpensive, and available in many sizes and shapes. Choose sturdy and somewhat flexible containers and avoid thin, stiff ones—they become brittle with cold or age.

- *Wood* is natural looking and protects roots from rapid temperature swings. You can build wooden planters yourself. Choose a naturally rot-resistant wood such as cedar, and never use wood treated with a preservative, which could leach into your soil, enter the roots of your herbs, and ultimately end up in your body. If you're purchasing a premade container, be sure it was made with untreated wood.

- *Metal* containers are strong, but they conduct heat, exposing roots to rapid temperature fluctuations. Also, metal must be lined with plastic if you're growing edibles.

- *Hayrack planters* with coir liners are attractive and easy to maintain, and they provide good drainage. They're great for annuals but not usable for perennials.

PREPARING CONTAINERS FOR PLANTING

Before you fill and plant your containers, decide where they will be located and move them there. If you plan to move heavy or large pots indoors in fall or to follow the sun during the day, platforms with wheels are available. If you'll have difficulty watering daily, look for sites that receive morning sun and are shaded during the hottest part of the day, even if you are growing plants that like full sun. Afternoon shade will reduce the amount of moisture your plants need.

Your containers must have drainage holes. If a pot is too deep for a very shallow-rooted plant, you can put a layer of gravel or lightweight packing peanuts in the bottom to reduce the amount of potting soil required.

Plain garden soil is usually too heavy for container plantings. For growing herbs in containers, use a commercial soil mix for houseplants, or make your own lightweight mix. (See the following potting mix recipes.)

Many of the components of potting soil are lightweight, dust-producing materials that can irritate your eyes, skin, and lungs. In some cases, vermiculite—which is in certain soil mixes—has been found to contain low levels of asbestos, and compost and peat moss can contain mold spores. Therefore, when you work with potting soil, observe the following precautions:

- Work outdoors or in a well-ventilated garage or garden shed.

- Wear a dust mask and gloves.

- Dampen individual ingredients before mixing them together to minimize the amount of dust released.

- After combining the ingredients, add more water to the mix, then stir to ensure that the medium is evenly moist before you fill the containers. After potting, store any leftover mix in a plastic bucket with a lid.

- If you've been working with vermiculite, be aware that the dust can cling to your clothing. Remove and wash dusty clothing as soon as possible to avoid dispersing asbestos inside your house.

Organic Potting Mix

This simple potting mix provides good drainage, air, and nutrients for growing plant roots.

1 part garden soil

1 part well-aged compost

1 part coarse sand or shredded pine or fir bark

1 part perlite (optional)

Enriched Potting Mix

Slow-growing plants, which will remain in the same container for several years, benefit from a mix that contains slow-release organic fertilizers.

1 cubic foot (approximately 32 quarts) Organic Potting Mix (above)

3 ounces bloodmeal

3 ounces soft rock phosphate or colloidal phosphate

3 ounces greensand

2 ounces dolomitic limestone (optional for alkaline-loving plants)

SELECTING PLANTS

Almost any herb—including shrubs and small trees—can grow successfully in a container. Dwarf and compact cultivars are best, especially for smaller pots. Select plants to suit the amount of sun or shade the container will receive.

Use your artistic imagination, and combine upright and trailing plants, colorful foliage, and flowers for pleasure and delight. Grow your favorite combinations of culinary herbs. A "pizza garden" might contain individual plants of thyme, oregano, and basil. A "chili garden" might have several colorful cultivars of hot chile peppers. Container gardens can be enjoyed for one season and

GROWING HERBS INDOORS

Containers are a must if you wish to grow perennial and woody herbs native to tropical or subtropical regions in a temperate climate, such as throughout most of North America. Such herbs as galangal, pineapple, and vanilla must be grown either indoors in a sunroom or warm greenhouse year-round or in a container that can be moved indoors when temperatures fall below 40° to 60°F, depending on the plant.

Before moving potted herbs indoors, inspect them carefully for insects (or treat them with insecticidal soap as a precaution). Check the plant entries in Part II of this book (beginning on page 82) for more details on individual light, temperature, and moisture requirements. In spring, before moving your plants outdoors, check your pot sizes and root prune or repot if necessary. Acclimate plants gradually to outdoor conditions the same way you would harden off seedlings (see page 416).

Here are just a few tropical and subtropical herbs that can be grown in containers year-round in a warm greenhouse or grown outdoors and moved indoors when temperatures cool.

Allspice (*Pimenta dioica*)

Aloe (*Aloe vera*)

Annatto (*Bixa orellana*)

Black pepper (*Piper nigrum*)

Cinnamon (*Cinnamomum cassia* and *C. verum*)

Coffee (*Coffea arabica*)

Galangal (*Alpinia galanga*)

Ginger (*Zingiber officinale*)

Gotu kola (*Centella asiatica*)

Guarana (*Paullinia cupana*)

Kava (*Piper methysticum*)

Lemongrass (*Cymbopogon citratus*)

Maté (*Ilex paraguariensis*)

Patchouli (*Pogostemon cablin*)

Pineapple (*Ananas comosus*)

Stevia (*Stevia rebaudiana*)

Tea (*Camellia sinensis*)

Turmeric (*Curcuma longa*)

Ylang-ylang (*Cananga odorata*)

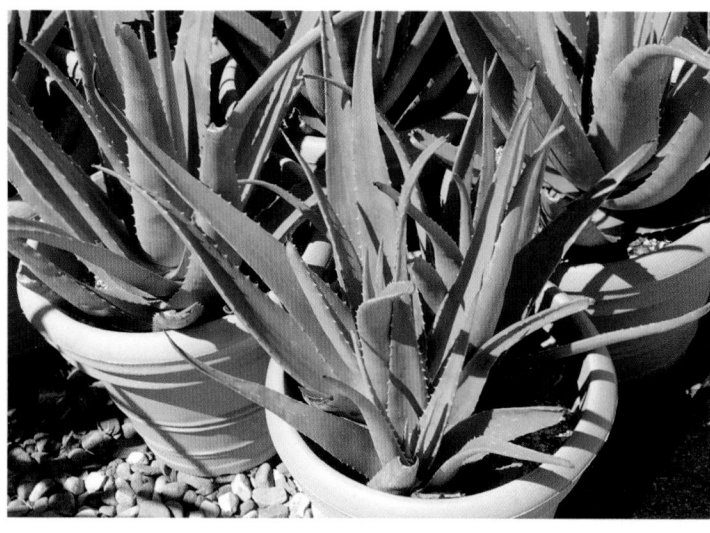

composed, to be replanted at the beginning of the next growing season, or they can be designed to last for years.

When designing permanent containers, remember that container plants will be less hardy than usual because their roots are more exposed to fluctuating air temperatures. Nonhardy plants will need outdoor protection or indoor shelter in winter, so consider how heavy the container will be and how you will move it before you plant.

Plant in containers as you would in your garden. If you are planting a mixed container, ignore spacing requirements and plant densely; you'll need to prune plants once they fill in. Depending on the size of the herb and its type—leafy or with very small leaves; tall or short; spreading or upright; annual, perennial, or shrub—you might need as many as four plants for an 18- or 24-inch container. For trees and shrubs, trim off any circling roots and cover the rootball to the same level

as it was set at the nursery. Firm the planting medium gently, and settle it by watering thoroughly. Don't fill pots all the way to the top with your soil mixture—leave space for watering. And, if you are gardening a few stories up in the air, remember that water follows the rules of gravity.

CARING FOR CONTAINER PLANTS

Water container plants thoroughly. How often you water depends on many factors, such as weather, plant size, and pot size. Don't let soil in containers dry out completely, as it is hard to rewet. To keep large containers attractive, spread a layer of mulch as you would in your garden. This will also help retain moisture. Be sure to keep mulch an inch or so away from plant stems and a few inches below the rim of the container.

Container plants need regular feeding, as the limited soil that nurtures the plant also has a

ROOT PRUNING

Root pruning rejuvenates pot-bound plants. Do this every 2 to 3 years for most potted plants; more aggressive growers (such as mints) may require annual root pruning.

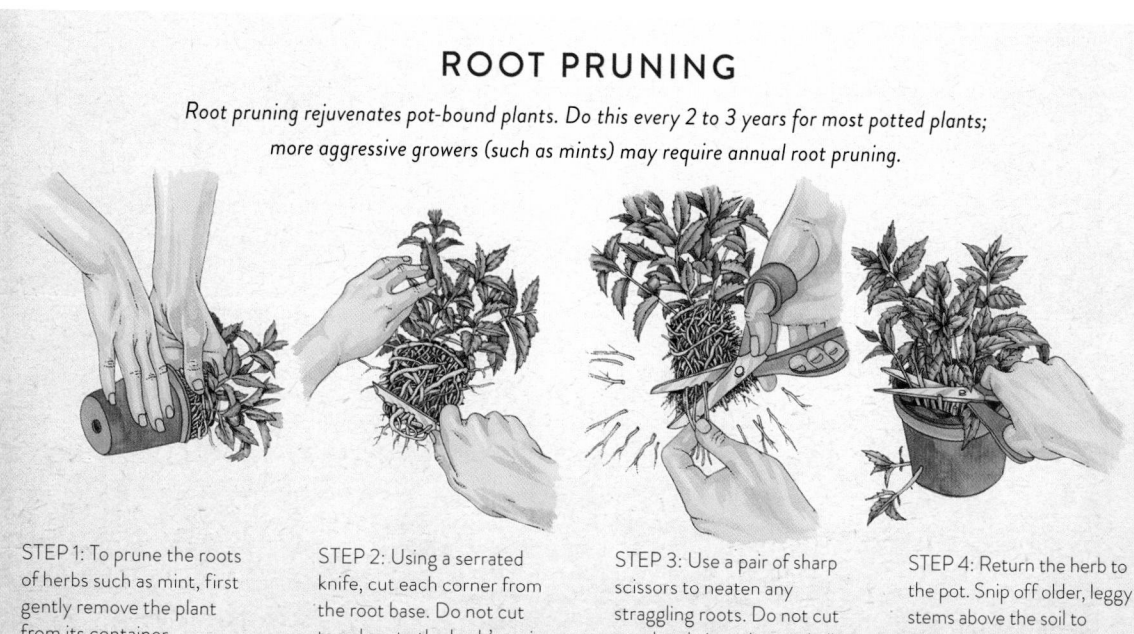

STEP 1: To prune the roots of herbs such as mint, first gently remove the plant from its container.

STEP 2: Using a serrated knife, cut each corner from the root base. Do not cut too close to the herb's main stem.

STEP 3: Use a pair of sharp scissors to neaten any straggling roots. Do not cut too deeply into the rootball.

STEP 4: Return the herb to the pot. Snip off older, leggy stems above the soil to encourage new, healthy growth.

limited supply of nutrients. Fertilize plants by watering them with diluted fish emulsion, seaweed extract, or compost tea. Start by feeding once every 2 weeks; adjust the frequency depending on plant response. Be careful not to pour fertilizer directly over the edible leaves of plants you harvest frequently, such as basil. (There's no need to dress your salad with fertilizer!)

Since containers are focal points outdoors and indoors, give them special attention to keep them looking their best. Remove tattered leaves and deadhead spent flowers. Prune back leggy plants and those that stop blooming. To keep mixed plantings attractive, dig out or cut back any plants that don't grow well or that go to war with other species, crowding them out aboveground or below-ground. Also keep an eye out for pests such as aphids and mites, and deal with them as soon as possible.

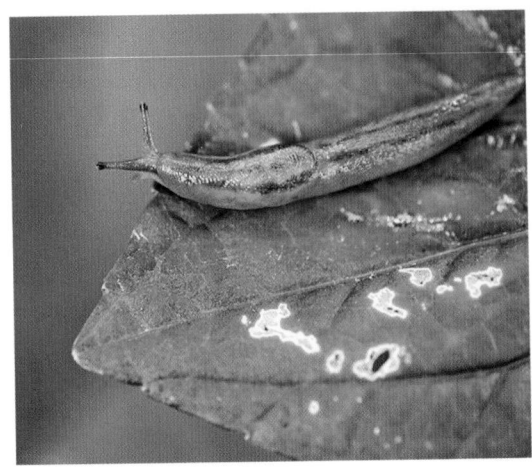

The damage caused by snails and slugs is obvious—holes that cause significant harm to leaves and impede overall plant growth. One way to control snails and slugs is to trap them with a shallow saucer of beer.

HARVESTING HERBS

Herbs can be harvested throughout the growing season—and even throughout the dormant season, if grown indoors. The following tools are useful to have on hand at harvesttime: pruning shears (remember that sharp shears are less likely to injure plants or you), rubber bands or twine (for tying bunches of stems together), and, on very hot days, a bucket of cool water in which to immerse herb stems.

If you're harvesting seed heads, bring along small paper bags to contain them. To harvest roots, you'll need a garden trowel or hand fork.

WHEN TO HARVEST

Small amounts of herbs can be harvested for immediate use throughout the growing season. Major harvests, however, should occur a few days before each plant flowers, when the concentration of essential oils in the leaves is highest. Flowering time varies among herbs, so observe your plants carefully. Perennials should not be pruned or harvested heavily during the last 30 to 45 days of your growing season, before your first seasonal frost is expected; this will ensure that your plants are strong enough to survive the dormant season. You can harvest annuals, such as basil, right up until they are killed by frost; after that, pull entire plants and compost them.

When harvesting a large amount of herbs for drying, making vinegars and potpourris, or other purposes, try to work during the cooler times of the day, when the herbs' essential oils are unlikely to evaporate and their foliage is less likely to wilt. The best time to harvest herbs is just after the morning dew has completely dried, because this moisture can cause the herbs to mold—making them useless for any kind of preparation.

HARVESTING LEAVES

It's important to remove herb leaves and stems in a way that will help promote new growth, rather than harming the plant. The method for doing that varies from herb to herb. Fortunately for the home gardener, most common herbs fall into just two of the more than 300 identified plant families, so it is relatively simple to learn the preferences of these two families.

- **Herbs in the mint (Lamiaceae) family,** including basil, bee balm, hyssop, lavender, lemon balm, marjoram, mint, oregano, and rosemary: Cut in the middle of their stems, just above a set of leaves, or pinch off the growing tips from the ends of the stems. Two new stems will form at these junctures, promoting abundant, bushy growth. Members of the mint family will produce vigorous new growth when cut back by one-third between the time they flower and set seeds, increasing their yield substantially. Tarragon and lemon verbena have growth habits similar to mint; harvest them the same way.

- **Plants in the parsley (Apiaceae) family,** including angelica, caraway, dill, fennel, parsley, and sweet cicely: Harvest by cutting stems at their bases from around the outside of the plant. This will encourage new shoots to grow from the center. Annuals in the parsley group (such as cilantro) produce leaves for a brief time before they flower. Harvest these leaves three to six times during the period before flowering.

Other types of herbs can be harvested and pruned using methods suggested by their growth habits. Chives, for example, sprout a dense cluster of blades from their bulbs. Cut individual chive blades close to the ground, or cut the entire plant to 1 inch above the soil level. New blades will generate from the bulbs. Bay (*Laurus nobilis*) and scented geranium both sprout leaves along their stems. Harvest these leaves individually. For herbs that produce both usable leaves and flowers, such as yarrow, feverfew, and tansy, wait to harvest the entire stem until just before the blooms open.

HARVESTING SEEDS

Gather seeds when they are ripe. On most plants (including caraway, coriander, dill, and fennel), the seed color changes from green to tan to light brown as ripening occurs. To harvest seeds,

HARVESTING

Proper harvesting techniques will help keep your herbs growing strong.

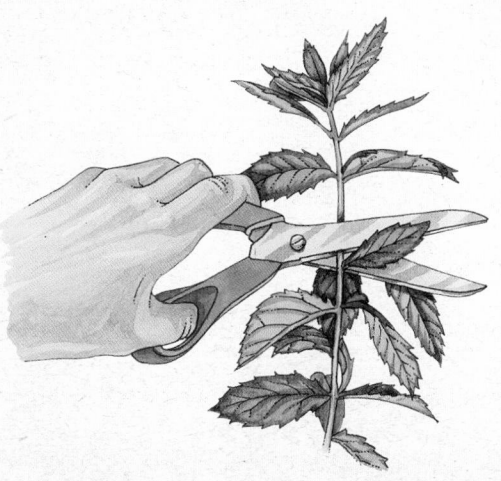

To harvest the leaves of herbs, including mint, cut the plant in the middle of its stem, just above a set of leaves.

pull up the whole plant from the soil when the seeds are barely ripe. Hang the plant upside down with a paper bag tied over the seed heads; as the seeds ripen and dry, they will drop into the bag.

Another way to collect mature seeds is to tie muslin bags over the seed heads of plants as they grow; the bags will catch seeds as they drop naturally. If the seeds haven't dried naturally on the plant, spread them out on paper towels and allow them to finish drying, Store dry, harvested seeds in a cool, dry place in cardboard boxes or in twists of aluminum foil.

HARVESTING FLOWERS

Herb flowers, such as those of calendula, lavender, and yarrow, should be picked just before they fully open. The flowers are more likely to lose their petals if you harvest them after they are completely open. But if you cut them before they are fully open, they will continue to open in the vase. Harvest flowers early in the day and transfer the stems to a vase or glass of water until you're ready to use them.

HARVESTING ROOTS

Most roots—including those of astragalus (*Astragalus membranaceus*), burdock (*Arctium lappa*), dong quai (*Angelica sinensis*), and echinacea (*Echinacea* spp.)—should be dug and harvested from mature plants at the end of the growing season, after a plant's leaves have yellowed and begun to die back. The roots of horseradish (*Armoracia rusticana*) are best dug when they are younger, before their flavor becomes too strong and their texture too coarse. Harvest roots using a garden fork: Carefully lift the root, then cut it away from the rest of the plant. Rinse roots with water, blot them dry, and then store them in a dry, well-ventilated area.

CLEANING HERBS

Plants that grow on long stems—basil, cilantro, and chives, for instance—are usually fairly free of soil or sand and so are relatively easy to clean before using. However, those that creep along the ground, such as thyme and oregano, can easily collect sand or mud on their leaves and stems, making them trickier to clean. In addition, herbs with crinkled leaves and those suffering from pest problems should be cleaned thoroughly under running water.

To remove grit, dust, or other residue, rinse the leaves under cold running water for a minute or two. Or fill your sink with cold water and immerse the herbs in the water. Swish them around, which will cause the debris to drop to the bottom of the sink. Repeat if necessary, then gently pat them dry.

PROBLEMS AND SOLUTIONS

Herbs are among the hardiest of plants. The very qualities that appeal to us—their intense fragrances and the flavors of their essential oils—also keep away most bothersome creatures. When all goes well, homegrown herbs—whether in your garden or in containers—provide a bountiful harvest for cooking, healing, crafting, and many other uses. But when stressed by too little water or light, insufficient nutrients, or poor air circulation, herbs become susceptible to disease and insect infestations that will reduce their productivity and usefulness.

Trouble can be signaled by symptoms that show up on leaves, stems, or fruit: yellowing, browning, or wilting; black or whitish powdery coatings; holes, bumps, or depressions. The symptoms of some conditions overlap those of others, so it's important to observe a plant carefully to correctly identify and address any underlying causes. The chart on pages 436–437 details the most common environmental conditions, pests, and diseases that can afflict herbs, along with treatments for each. Solutions for most problems include simple, nontoxic physical barriers and traps; insecticidal soap; horticultural oil; diatomaceous earth; and botanical pesticides. Always use the least-toxic approach before trying others.

PREVENTING GARDEN PROBLEMS

Of course, prevention is the best way to maintain a healthy, problem-free garden. Regular additions of compost will help make essential nutrients available. Plant only healthy herbs—those with consistent, deep foliage color and that show no signs of disease or infestation. Plant herbs only in well-drained soil in sites that receive appropriate light: shade-loving plants in shade, water lovers in moist areas, sun lovers in sun.

Diseases and insect infestations spread rapidly through related plants. As a deterrent, mix different herb species together in beds and other plantings. Lure natural predators of garden pests by planting herbs known to attract those beneficial organisms.

BRING *in the* GOOD BUGS!

The pollen- and nectar-rich herbs listed below will lure "beneficial" insects—parasitic wasps, ladybugs, lacewings, hoverflies, tachinid flies, and soldier beetles—that attack many common garden pests, including scale, aphids, and whiteflies. Planting them among vegetables and flowers, or in borders surrounding vegetable or flower gardens, will help keep pests in check.

Angelica (*Angelica archangelica*)

Anise (*Pimpinella anisum*)

Bee balm (*Monarda* spp.)

Borage (*Borago officinalis*)

Caraway (*Carum carvi*)

Catnip (*Nepeta cataria*)

Coneflower (*Echinacea* spp.)

Dill (*Anethum graveolens*)

Fennel (*Foeniculum vulgare*)

Lavender (*Lavandula* spp.)

Lemon balm (*Melissa officinalis*)

Marigold (*Tagetes* spp.)

Marjoram (*Origanum majorana*)

Onions, garlic, chives (*Allium* spp.)

Parsley (*Petroselinum* spp.)

Peppermint (*Mentha x piperita*)

Rosemary (*Rosmarinus* spp.)

Sage (*Salvia* spp.)

Spearmint (*Mentha spicata*)

Tansy (*Tanacetum vulgare*)

Thyme (*Thymus* spp.)

Yarrow (*Achillea millefolium*)

Beneficial insects are a boon to any garden, and herbs are among the best plants for attracting them.

HERB PROBLEMS *and* SOLUTIONS

ENVIRONMENTAL PROBLEMS

Symptoms	Possible Culprits	Susceptible Herbs	Solutions
Brown leaf tips	Excessive fertilizer, watering, high level of fluoride, boron, or copper in the water	All plants	Change watering and fertilizing habits. If symptoms persist, test water quality.
Poor growth, yellowing leaves, new growth shrivels and dies	pH imbalance, lack of nutrients, poor drainage	All plants	Check drainage; test soil. Amend with appropriate additives or repot plant to provide better drainage.

PEST PROBLEMS

Symptoms	Possible Culprits	Susceptible Herbs	Solutions
Stunted and deformed leaves and stems; plant parts covered with sticky, dark substance	Aphids: suck sap from plants, producing a sugary "honeydew"	Calendula, mint, oregano, and rosemary	Spray plants with water or insecticidal soap. Or wipe affected areas with a cotton swab soaked in rubbing alcohol.
Wilted leaves, possibly coated with sooty mold; plant loses vitality and eventually dies	Whiteflies: feed on undersides of leaves and can cause extensive damage	Calendula, lemon verbena, and rosemary	Spray plants with water. If indoors, lower growing temperature to decrease whitefly activity. *Encarsia formosa*, a species of tiny predatory wasp, can be an effective control outdoors.
Yellowish or silvery leaves; severe yellowing and rusty spots; fine webbing on leaves and stems	Spider mites: tiny pests puncture plant leaves and stems and feed on sap	Mint, oregano, parsley, rosemary, sage, and thyme	Apply horticultural oil or insecticidal soap. Wash plants with a mild solution of dish detergent and water. Prune heavily infested branches and isolate infested plants.
Holes at edges of leaves; plants are eventually defoliated	Japanese beetles: metallic green insect with copper-colored wings that feed on leaves	More than 200 plant species including basil, borage, and foxglove	Remove from leaves by hand. Control larvae with parasitic nematodes and the bacteria milky spore.
Yellow foliage; plants lose leaves, weaken, and die	Scale: minute, sap-feeding insects	Wide range of plants, including bay and rosemary	Remove with a soft-bristled toothbrush dipped in rubbing alcohol or insecticidal soap spray. Plant herbs to attract beneficials. Horticultural oils may help.

PEST PROBLEMS

Symptoms	Possible Culprits	Susceptible Herbs	Solutions
Irregular holes in the middle or at the edges of leaves; plants may be defoliated; shiny slime trails on and around plants	Snails and slugs: pests eat seedlings and soft-tissued parts at night and on cloudy, damp days	Bee balm, calendula, sage, and sorrel	Remove by hand daily, then weekly, when numbers drop. Edge beds with copper strips or diatomaceous earth. Trap with boards and rocks, or sink beer-filled saucers set into the ground with the rims at soil level.

DISEASE PROBLEMS

Yellow, drooping foliage; plants turn brown and die	Verticillium wilt: a fungal disease	Mint and many other plants	Plant disease-resistant varieties.
Weakened stems with flowers develop a fluffy gray or white growth, which spreads to fruits	Botrytis blight: a fungal disease	Rosemary, scented geranium, and many other plants	Destroy infected plant parts. Promote air circulation around plants by cutting back or removing plants that crowd each other.
Yellow or white spots on surface of leaves; crusty orange or yellow bumps on undersides; plants become stunted	Rust: a disease caused by 4,000 or so related fungi	Germander, mint, and yarrow	Destroy infected plant parts. Promote air circulation around plants by cutting back or removing plants that crowd each other.
Gray or white powdery growth on leaves; new leaves are distorted in shape; poor growth and low yield	Powdery mildew: a fungal disease that thrives in hot weather	Bee balm, catmint, germander, and lemon	Promote air circulation around plants by cutting back or removing plants that crowd each other. Spray affected plants with sulfur, lime-sulfur, horticultural oil, or a weak solution of baking soda and water.
Yellow foliage; brown coloration along leaf edges; plants wilt and become stunted; roots soft and waterlogged	Root rot: a fungal disease	Oregano, rosemary, sage, tarragon, and thyme	Use sterile potting soil when propagating plants. Avoid overwatering, but do not let plants dry out between waterings. Remove and destroy affected plants.
Yellow stunted leaves; wilting	Nematodes: microscopic wormlike creatures feed on roots, leaves, and stems and spread readily in water and on tools	Calendula and parsley	Remove and destroy infested plants. Amend soil with compost, organic fertilizers, and products containing seaweed.

HERB GARDENING TO-DO LIST BY SEASON

Late Winter through Early Spring

- **Start plants.** Start herb seeds indoors 6 to 8 weeks before your last expected frost. Also take cuttings from indoor herb plants to propagate new outdoor garden plants. Start herbs outdoors when nighttime temperatures exceed 55°F.

- **Prune.** Prune woody herbs such as lavender by removing leggy old growth to promote new stem growth and better form.

- **Weed.** At the beginning of the growing season, pull out weeds while their roots are still shallow.

- **Build soil.** Add compost or other organic material to your garden beds.

- **Rejuvenate beds.** Divide and transplant herbs that have outgrown their original sites. Add, remove, or move plants to refresh the design and appearance of your plantings.

Fall

- **Plant bulbs and seeds.** Plant bulbs of herbs such as garlic and saffron and seeds of caraway, dill, parsley, and sweet cicely, which will overwinter and begin growing in spring. In warm areas, plant seeds of cool-season herbs such as chervil, cilantro, and parsley in a cold frame for winter production.

- **Divide.** Divide and replant hardy perennials, or note which ones should be divided and moved in spring.

- **Clean up.** Rake leaves and pull weeds. Remove spent annuals; save their seeds for the next growing season. Leave some stalks and seeds of herbs such as chervil, echinacea, fennel, lavender, marjoram, rose, and sweet cicely to feed hungry birds during the dormant season.

- **Prepare for the dormant season.** Pot (if necessary) and move any nonhardy herbs indoors for the winter.

Spring through Late Summer

- **Plant.** After the weather stabilizes in spring, plant purchased herbs and transplant seedlings to the garden. Create container plantings. Continue to sow herbs that quickly go to seed (such as borage, cilantro, dill, and fennel) every few weeks to ensure a continuous supply throughout the growing season.

- **Mulch.** Cover beds with a layer of fresh organic mulch, such as compost, bark, or shredded leaves.

- **Water.** In arid climates and during dry periods, water herbs occasionally and deeply.

- **Weed.** Continue to dig up weeds as they appear. Also, monitor invasive herbs, such as mints, to prevent them from spreading beyond their containers.

- **Deadhead.** Remove spent flowers and seed heads of perennial herbs such as anise hyssop and catnip to encourage new flower production.

- **Harvest.** Pinch back rapidly growing herbs. Harvest according to herb type.

- **Preserve.** Dry herb foliage and flowers for later use. Prepare herbal vinegars, oils, infusions, and tinctures.

Winter

- **Care for indoor herbs.** To keep herbs alive indoors, be sure your plants receive adequate light, water, and nutrients. Monitor for pest and disease problems.

- **Propagate cuttings.** Take cuttings from indoor herbs and start them for the next growing season.

- **Plan for the new growing season.** Choose small or large projects for the next year: planting or moving a tree; rerouting paths; or adding new garden beds.

- **Make herb products.** Use previously harvested herbs to make herbal products and crafts such as potpourris, wreaths, and sachets.

- **Read and learn.** Now is the perfect time to read about new varieties and growing techniques. If some plantings failed to perform well last season, look for solutions. Also consider joining a garden club or taking a class.

- **DIY projects.** Build a potting bench, compost bin, coldframe, or enclosures for raised beds.

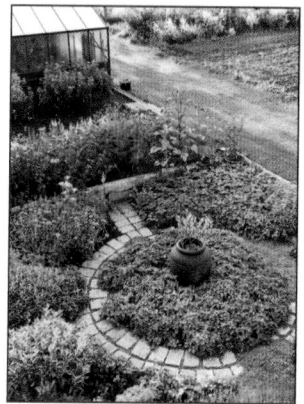

CHAPTER 9

DESIGNING YOUR HERB GARDEN

*F*or gardeners and plant lovers, the enormous selection of interesting herbs available at local nurseries and on the Web can seem both exhilarating and a bit overwhelming. Herbs are easy to work into an existing landscape—especially if you want to grow only a few of them. Culinary staples like parsley and basil can tuck neatly into a shrub border or large container outside your kitchen door. And flowering herbs like purple coneflower and bee balm are naturals for the perennial border.

But why stop there? With a dedicated herb garden, you can enjoy a full range of herbal colors, fragrances, and flavors—both outside and inside your home. Nature's most useful plants can provide the ingredients for delicious meals, healing teas and salves, refreshing facial scrubs and soaps, green cleaning preparations for your home, and so much more.

The style of your herb garden is up to you. An herb garden can be as formal as a 16th-century knot garden or as informal as a wild cottage garden, where these wonderful plants casually intermingle with flowering shrubs and vines. To help you begin, we've provided plans for 12 different herb gardens (starting on page 442). You can choose one of these to follow or draw inspiration from several of them to create an herb garden uniquely your own.

GARDEN DESIGN 101

Designing a garden can be great fun, as you consider potential plants and plant combinations, plant placement, and hardscape features (such as walls, pathways, and steps). The design and planning phase of a garden is also *critical* to its success—so take time to do it thoughtfully. It's a lot easier, and less expensive, to make changes on paper than in the garden.

Measure your garden site, then transfer the outline to graph paper, making the layout to scale. (Perhaps 1 foot can equal 1 inch on your graph paper.) Mark trees, buildings, and other obstructions, and note which direction is north. Be sure to leave enough space for comfortable paths, and keep your beds narrow enough to work in—4 to 5 feet across maximum—but wide enough to look both seductive and effective.

After you've established a design, choose the herbs that will bring it to life. Consider not only plant color, form, and texture, but also bloom time and mature height, as well as the conditions of the site. When planning where to place your plants, remember that herbaceous plants usually look best (and most natural) when planted in groups of a given type. Individual plants get lost, creating a blurred, jumbled effect, but masses of plants stand out and create a more unified design. The noted Brazilian landscape architect and artist Roberto Burle Marx once described plants in a garden not only as individual species, but also as "a color, a shape, a volume, or an arabesque in itself."

In your design, arrange plants so that taller and larger ones won't hide smaller ones. If your design features a border backed by a wall or fence, plant the tallest herbs in back and the lowest herbs in front. If you're planning an island bed, put the tall plants in the center and the low plants around the edges. Include a focal point, such as a large shrub or birdbath, to help anchor the planting.

Good design also considers perspective. For instance, if you're planning a knot garden—one of the styles in this chapter—make sure the garden "floor" contrasts with the knotted edging, or the pattern will be lost. If your design is meant to be viewed from a distance, use plants that will grab the viewer's eye—large ones with bright flowers or silver foliage.

Finally, a few words on maintenance. All gardens require some work, but keep in mind that the more formal your design and the larger its scale, the more weeding, clipping, mulching, and watering you'll need to do, and the more precise the planting will have to be. Herb gardens, like any others, look best when the plants are full and lush. This is vital when an herbal hedge or solid block of plants is integral to a design. It's a good idea to grow extra plants in a nursery area or greenhouse so you'll always have spares to fill in gaps.

PERIOD GARDENS

If you own a house with a distinct architectural style—such as Early American, Victorian, or Craftsman—you might want to echo the style of that period in your landscape and herb garden. Period gardens generally follow the designs, materials, techniques, and plants of a given era. Before you embark on a historical design, read up on the aesthetics and garden designs of that period. For a more formal look, you can draw inspiration from Renaissance gardens, which featured geometric patterns, topiaries, fountains, and even statues.

An enclosed medieval-style garden can make a tranquil refuge. You can enclose it with hedging, a tall wood fence, latticework covered with climbing plants, plaited wicker (wattling), or walls of brick or stone. Ideally, it should include a fountain. Surround the fountain with an herbal lawn studded with flowers—columbines, irises, lilies, pinks, primroses, and violets. If you have a tree in your garden, you can create a turf seat beneath an arbor. The turf seat—a medieval inspiration—is an earth-filled rectangular box surfaced with a creeping herb such as one of the prostrate thymes or creeping chamomile.

The symmetry of a colonial-style garden is also appealing. To make a colonial herb garden, lay out raised, board-sided beds along a central walk. The walk should lead to a sundial or bench. If possible, enclose the garden with a picket fence or a low hedge. Within the beds, you can mix vegetables and herbs or plant only herbs—such as angelica, borage, burnet, calendula, caraway, catmint, chamomile, chervil, comfrey, coriander, dill, fennel, lemon balm, licorice, lovage, madder, mint, nasturtiums, parsley, rue, sage, sweet cicely, tansy, tarragon, and woad. If you're attempting a true historical recreation, use only the materials available during that period. Wood, wattling, stone, gravel, brick, and clay were the usual building materials during the colonial period.

THEME GARDENS

Another approach to garden design is to focus on a common feature, or theme—such as herbs that are medicinal, herbs used for cooking, or herbs that attract butterflies. Theme gardens can also feature a common color—such as an all-white garden. You might even base your design on plants that have special significance. A Shakespearean garden, for instance, includes the Renaissance herbs mentioned in the plays of Shakespeare. Biblical gardens feature herbs from the Bible, such as anise, coriander, cumin, dill, mint, mustard, rose, rue, saffron, and wormwood. If you are a tea drinker, you might create a garden composed of chamomile, lemon balm, mints, basils, rosemary, and the natural sweetener stevia to make your own infusions. A collection of lemony herbs might include herbs that provide a citrus scent and flavor, such as lemon balm, lemon thyme, and lemon verbena.

On the following pages, you'll find garden designs that you can use as blueprints or as inspiration for your own herb garden. Many of the plants in the garden designs that follow are featured in Part II (see page 80), while other plants are wonderful companions that you may want to consider researching and adding to your collection. Most of the suggested plants are widely adapted, but feel free to experiment. (If you live in Zone 5 or colder, you might need to substitute more cold-hardy cultivars for some perennials.) Play in your horticultural sandbox by choosing plants better suited to your conditions and the environment you wish to create. By definition, all gardens, and gardeners, evolve over time—and experimenting with new plants and plant combinations is fun. For more design ideas, visit local public gardens. Many include outstanding period or theme herb gardens that are beautifully maintained. For more details about the individual plants in the following designs, see their entries in Part II, "Herbs to Know."

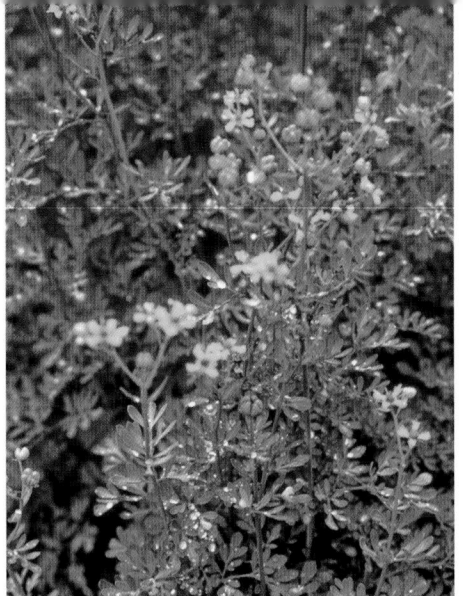
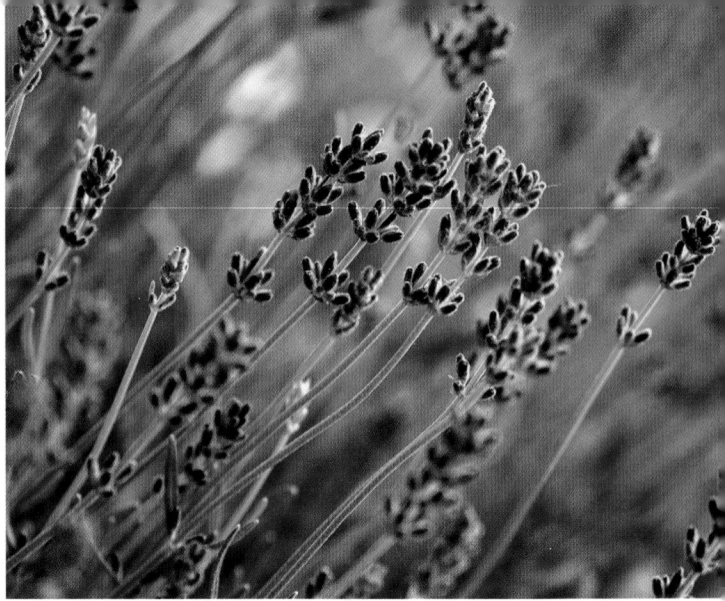

A Formal Knot Garden

During the 16th through 18th centuries, the grounds of many European and American estates featured formal knot gardens. The intricate, geometric pattern of the knot was meant to be viewed from above, so you could reflect on the pattern by looking down from a terrace or window.

Typically, knot plants are herbs that can be easily pruned to a uniform height, such as boxwood, germander, lavender, rosemary, sage, santolina, southernwood, winter savory, and wormwood. Accent plants within the knot add contrasting color or texture. You can play around with the background by using a contrasting mulch material—such as white marble chips or red crushed stone—to make the plants stand out. The entire garden can be framed in brick or stone.

1 **Green santolina** (*Santolina virens*): 2-foot-tall perennial with rich green, aromatic leaves and yellow flowers in early summer. Keep plants clipped to about 1 foot tall.

2 **Lavender 'Munstead'** (*Lavandula angustifolia*): Compact, 1-foot-tall perennial with aromatic gray foliage and bright lavender flower spikes in summer.

3 **Germander** (*Teucrium chamaedrys*): 18-inch-tall bushy perennial with dark green foliage and pink to purple flowers in midsummer to late summer. Keep plants clipped to about 1 foot tall.

4 **Lavender cotton** (*Santolina chamaecyparissus*): 2½-foot-tall mounding perennial with wide, finely cut, silver-gray foliage and yellow cotton ball–blooms in summer.

5 **Hyssop** (*Hyssopus officinalis*): 2- to 3-foot-tall perennial with aromatic green foliage and white, blue, or pink flowers in summer. Shear to desired shape.

6 **Rue 'Blue Beauty'** (*Ruta graveolens*): 2-foot-tall perennial with blue-green aromatic foliage and yellow flowers in summer. Shear to desired shape.

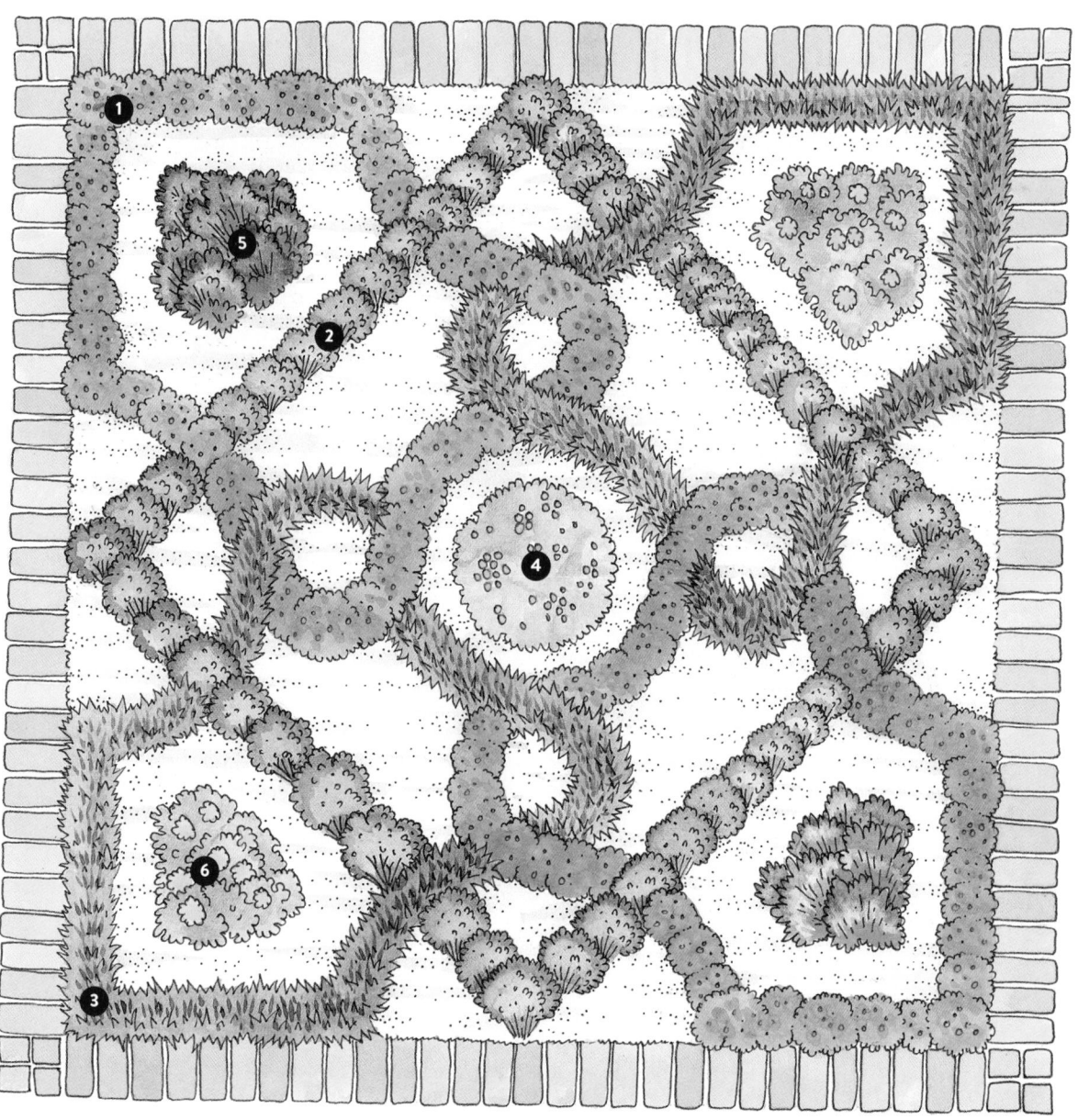

Cottage Herb Garden

Even a white picket fence can't contain the enthusiasm of a cottage garden. The climbing, creeping, and sprawling herbs seem to mingle randomly throughout the growing space. Self-seeding annuals reappear each year—often in surprising places—adding to the casual look.

Although this romantic style might look carefree, you'll need to do occasional maintenance to keep it from looking unruly. Space the plants tightly to inhibit weeds, use mulch, and remove volunteer seedlings that threaten to take over less-aggressive plants. Be sure to include a focal point—such as a sundial, bench, or birdhouse—to help unify the design. Also, remember to plant in groups to form masses of color, rather than jumbling together many different individual plants.

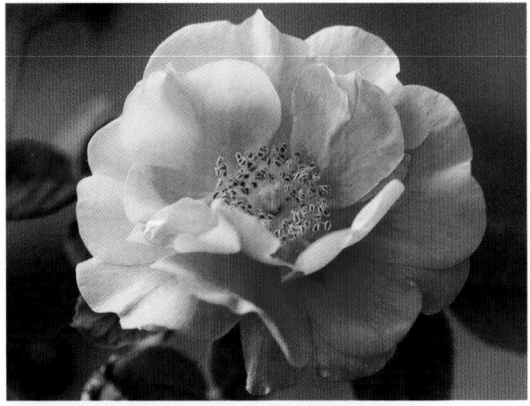

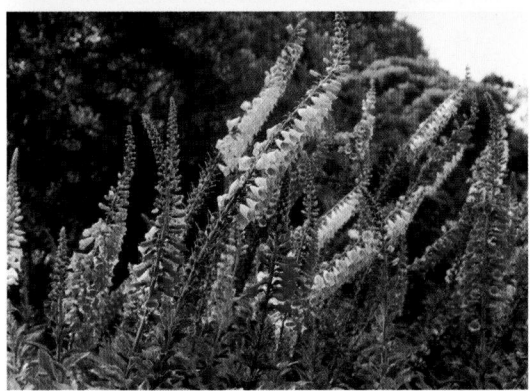

1 **Climbing nasturtium 'Moonlight'** (*Tropaeolum majus*): 6- to 8-foot climbing stems with pale yellow flowers in midsummer to fall; annual.

2 **English lavender 'Hidcote'** (*Lavandula angustifolia*): Deep purple, highly fragrant blooms cover 18-inch-tall perennial plants all summer; gray-green foliage.

3 **Foxglove** (*Digitalis purpurea*): Biennial plants bear 4- to 6-foot-tall spikes of purple, pink, or white blooms in late spring to midsummer; self-seeds.

4 **Calendula** (*Calendula officinalis*): 1- to 2-foot branching plants with orange or yellow flowers in summer; self-seeding annual.

5 **Bee balm 'Blue Stocking'** (*Monarda didyma*): 3- to 4-foot-tall perennial with violet-blue flowers in early to midsummer; aromatic leaves.

6 **Cowslip** (*Primula veris*): 10-inch-tall perennial bears fragrant, bright yellow, bell-shaped blooms in spring.

7 **Valerian** (*Valeriana officinalis*): 4- to 6-foot-tall sprawling perennial with fernlike leaves; clusters of white or pink, sweetly scented blooms in midsummer.

8 **Catmint 'Walker's Low'** (*Nepeta cataria*): 2-foot-tall perennial covered with small, lavender-blue flowers in spring to late summer; fragrant foliage.

9 **Violet** (*Viola odorata*): Creeping perennial to 6 inches tall with heart-shaped leaves and sweet-scented dark purple or white flowers in spring.

10 **Thyme 'Bressingham Pink'** (*Thymus praecox*): Evergreen perennial groundcover studded with tiny pink flowers in early summer; withstands light traffic.

11 **Apothecary rose** (*Rosa gallica* var. *officinalis*): Sprawling shrub, 3 to 4 feet tall and up to 6 feet across; fragrant, deep pink blooms in late spring to midsummer; orange hips in fall.

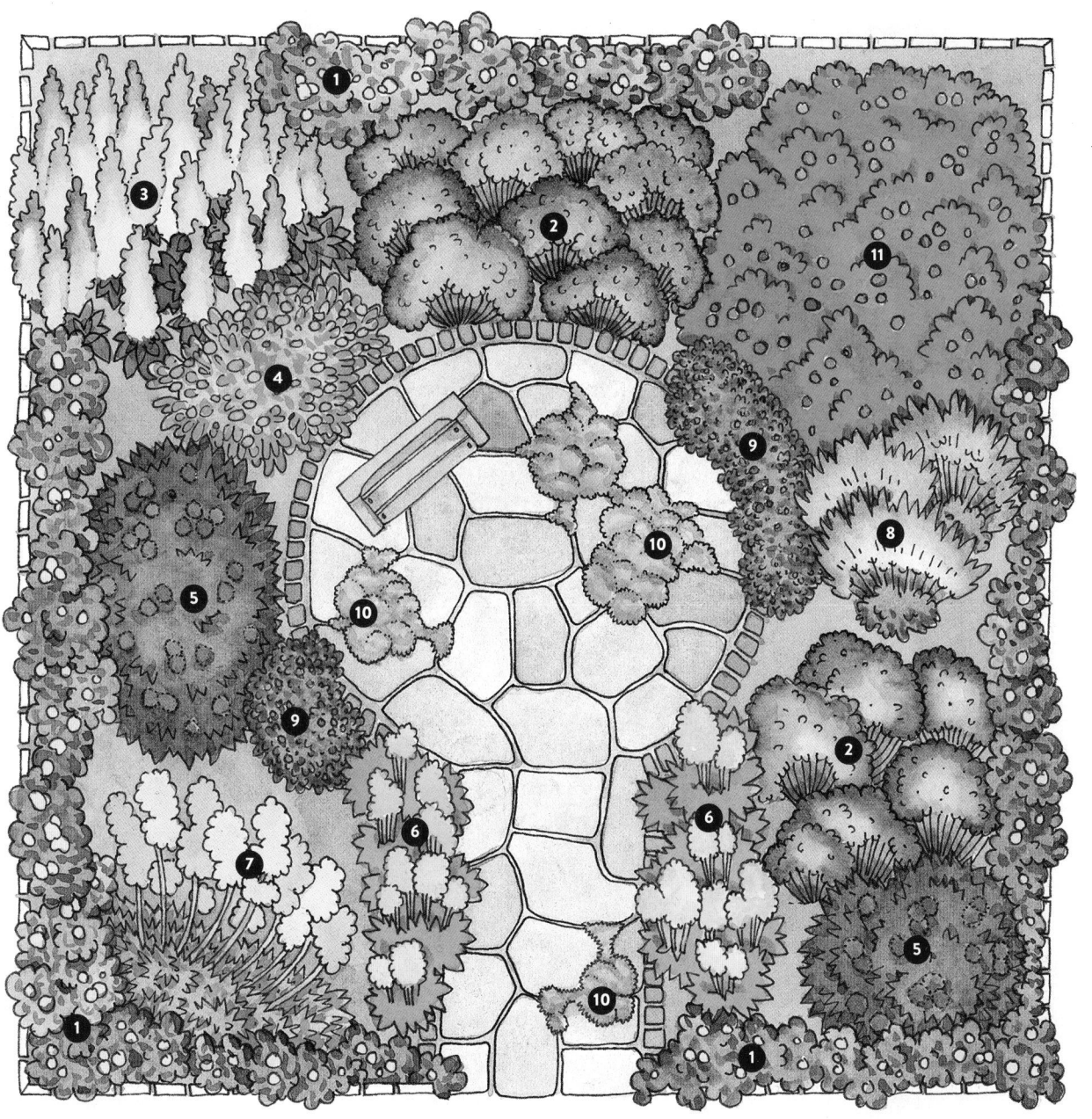

Kitchen Herb Garden

This kitchen garden includes the most common culinary herbs, arranged in an ornamental design. The borders of the central path are lined with the purple foliage and pink flowers of 'Dark Opal' basil and the green to purple foliage of purple sage. Large clumps of 'Genovese' basil fill the centers of both beds, but you could substitute a cut-and-come-again lettuce mix, arugula, or a salad tomato variety, or edible flowers, such as calendula.

A bark chip mulch accents the herbs' forms and foliage as it suppresses weeds and preserves moisture. To keep the aggressive mints from overtaking the entire bed, plant them in sunken, bottomless buckets, leaving an inch or so of the rims aboveground. Remove runners as soon as you spot them. Border your garden with bricks or flat stones for a clean finish and easy mowing.

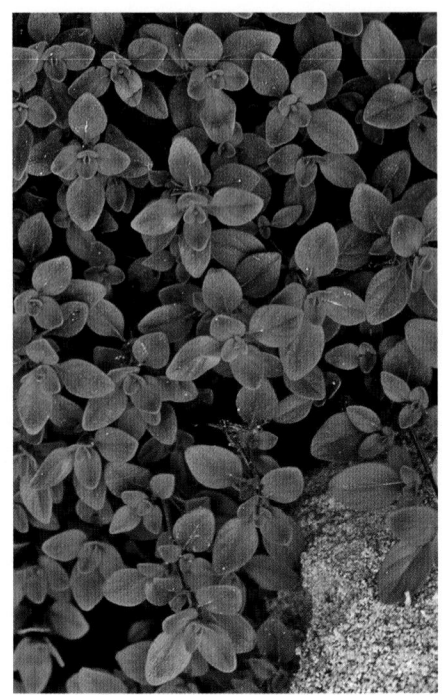

1 **Basil 'Dark Opal'** (*Ocimum basilicum*): Annual plants up to 15 inches tall with dark purple leaves and pink flowers in midsummer to late summer. For heaviest leaf production, pinch off flowers as they appear.

2 **Purple sage** (*Salvia officinalis* 'Purpurascens'): Perennial up to 10 inches tall; aromatic gray-green to purple leaves; purple flowers appear in June.

3 **Curly parsley** (*Petroselinum crispum*): Bushy, 12-inch-tall biennial plants with dark green, curled leaves. Replant annually.

4 **Chives** (*Allium schoenoprasum*): Perennial that forms spreading clumps up to 18 inches tall; tubular, deep green leaves with bright pink to lilac flowers in June.

5 **Garden thyme** (*Thymus vulgaris*): Sprawling, woody perennial, 6 inches tall with tiny, aromatic evergreen leaves and mauve to pink flowers in early summer.

6 **Lemon thyme** (*Thymus citriodorus*): Mounding evergreen perennial, 8 inches tall with pale pink flowers in midsummer; tiny leaves have a lemon scent and flavor.

7 **Rosemary** (*Rosmarinus officinalis*): Evergreen shrub up to 7 feet tall with needlelike gray-green leaves and blue flowers in early spring. Hardy to Zone 7; sink in pots to bring indoors for winter in colder climates.

8 **Oregano** (*Origanum vulgare*): Bushy, 2-foot-tall perennial with spikes of purple, pink, or white flowers in midsummer to late summer.

9 **Spearmint** (*Mentha spicata*): Spear-shaped, bright green leaves on 2-foot stems; pink, white, or purple flowers in midsummer; perennial. Confine the roots.

10 **Peppermint** (*Mentha × piperita*): 2-foot-tall perennial plants bear smooth, purple-tinged leaves and midsummer spikes of lilac-pink flowers. Confine the roots.

11 **Basil 'Genovese'** (*Ocimum basilicum*): The classic pesto variety. Annual, 2-foot-tall plants with bright green, aromatic leaves; white flowers in midsummer to late summer. Pinch off blooms to increase leaf production.

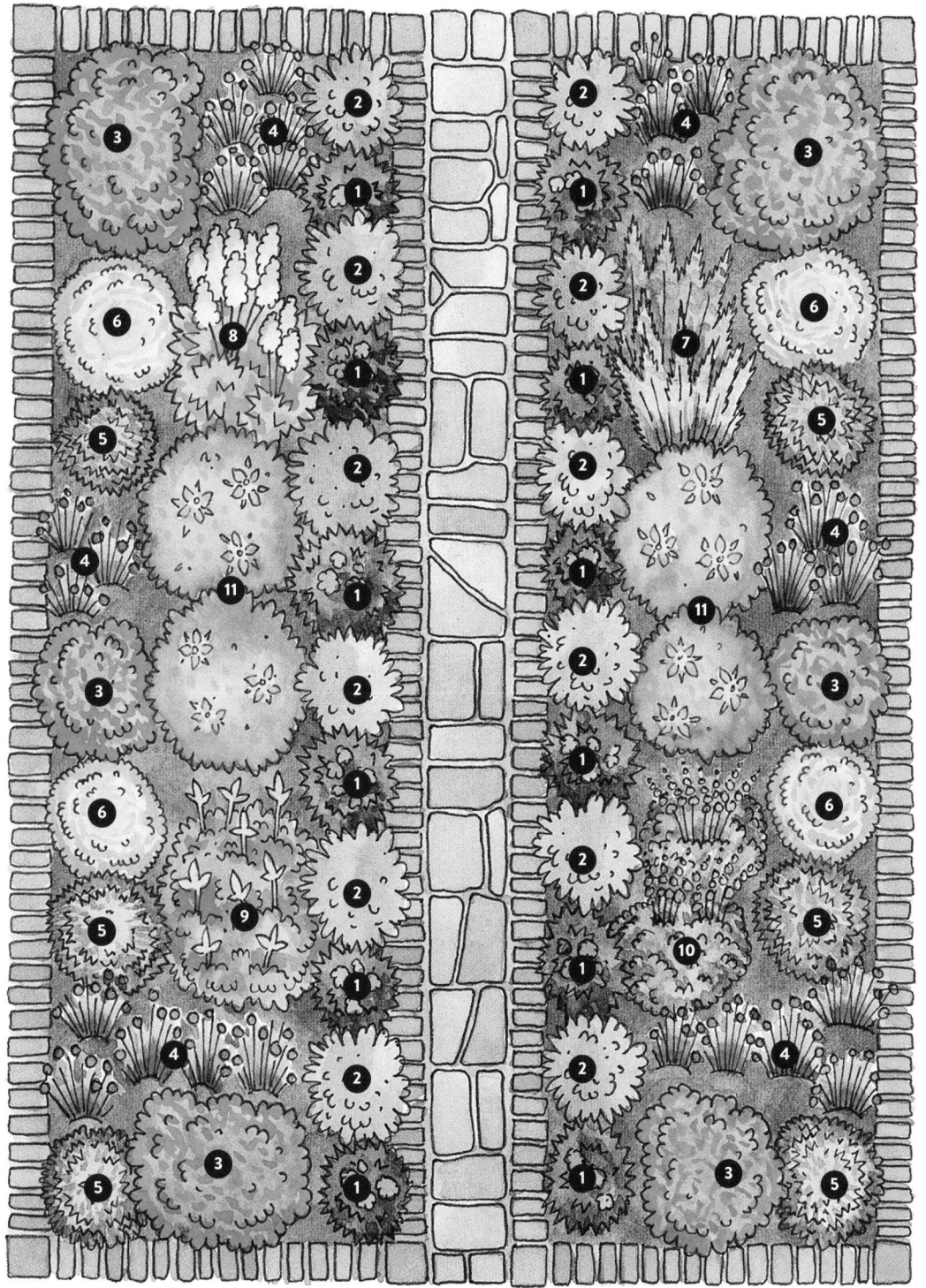

Healing Herb Garden

The leaves, flowers, or roots of the herbs in this garden can be used to make healing teas or salves. In this design, the herbs are loosely grouped by their healing properties: Tension tamers, such as valerian, marshmallow, and catnip, are grouped together; cold and flu fighters, like elderberry, horehound, garlic, and echinacea, are near each other; and muscle, joint, and skin savers, such as arnica and calendula, grow together. Most of these plants also add beauty to the landscape, so you'll enjoy their soothing qualities even when you aren't using them medicinally. Locating this border next to a fence or wall provides support for tall, rangy herbs like valerian.

For more details on using these herbs to make healing preparations, see Dr. Tieraona Low Dog's chart on pages 346–349 and the individual entries in Part II of this book.

1 **Elderberry** (*Sambucus nigra*): 10- to 12-foot-tall shrub; creamy white flowers in early summer, followed by deep purple-black berries. A tea from the flowers relieves colds and flu. The fruit, made into jam or juice, has antiviral properties.

2 **Horehound** (*Marrubium vulgare*): 24-inch-tall perennial with soft, hairy leaves; white flowers in early summer. A tea or syrup made from the leaves relieves coughs and sore throat.

3 **Marshmallow** (*Althaea officinalis*): A 4-foot tall perennial with soft, velvety, leaves; five-petaled pinkish white blooms in midsummer. A tea from the root or leaf soothes coughs and gastrointestinal troubles.

4 **Catnip** (*Nepeta cataria*): 2-foot-tall perennial covered with small, lavender-blue flowers in spring to late summer; fragrant foliage. The leaf tea soothes anxiety and indigestion.

5 **Valerian** (*Valeriana officinalis*): 4- to 6-foot-tall sprawling perennial with fernlike leaves; clusters of white or pink, fragrant blooms in midsummer. Root tea reduces nervous tension and promotes sleep.

6 **Sage** (*Salvia officinalis*): Up to 24 inches tall; aromatic leaves are gray-green; purple flowers appear in June. The leaf tea is excellent for sore throats, coughs, and colds. Also used to treat excessive sweating, menopausal hot flashes, and night sweats.

7 **Thyme** (*Thymus vulgaris*): Sprawling, woody perennial, 6 inches tall with tiny, aromatic evergreen leaves and mauve to pink flowers in early summer. The leaf tea is excellent for relieving coughs, colds, and congestion.

8 **Lemon balm** (*Melissa officinalis*): Bushy, 18-inch-tall perennial with lemon-scented leaves; white flower spikes in early to midsummer. The leaf tea eases tension, digestive upset, and colic. A topical cream can help fever blisters.

9 **Roman chamomile** (*Chamaemelum nobile*): Perennial evergreen groundcover with feathery leaves and white, daisylike flowers in late spring to late summer. A tea made from its leaves aids digestion and promotes relaxation and sleep.

10 **Garlic** (*Allium sativum*): Linear leaves arise from a bulb of 4 to 15 cloves; small white flowers in umbels on stems to 2 feet tall. Garlic has antiviral, anti-inflammatory, and antifungal properties.

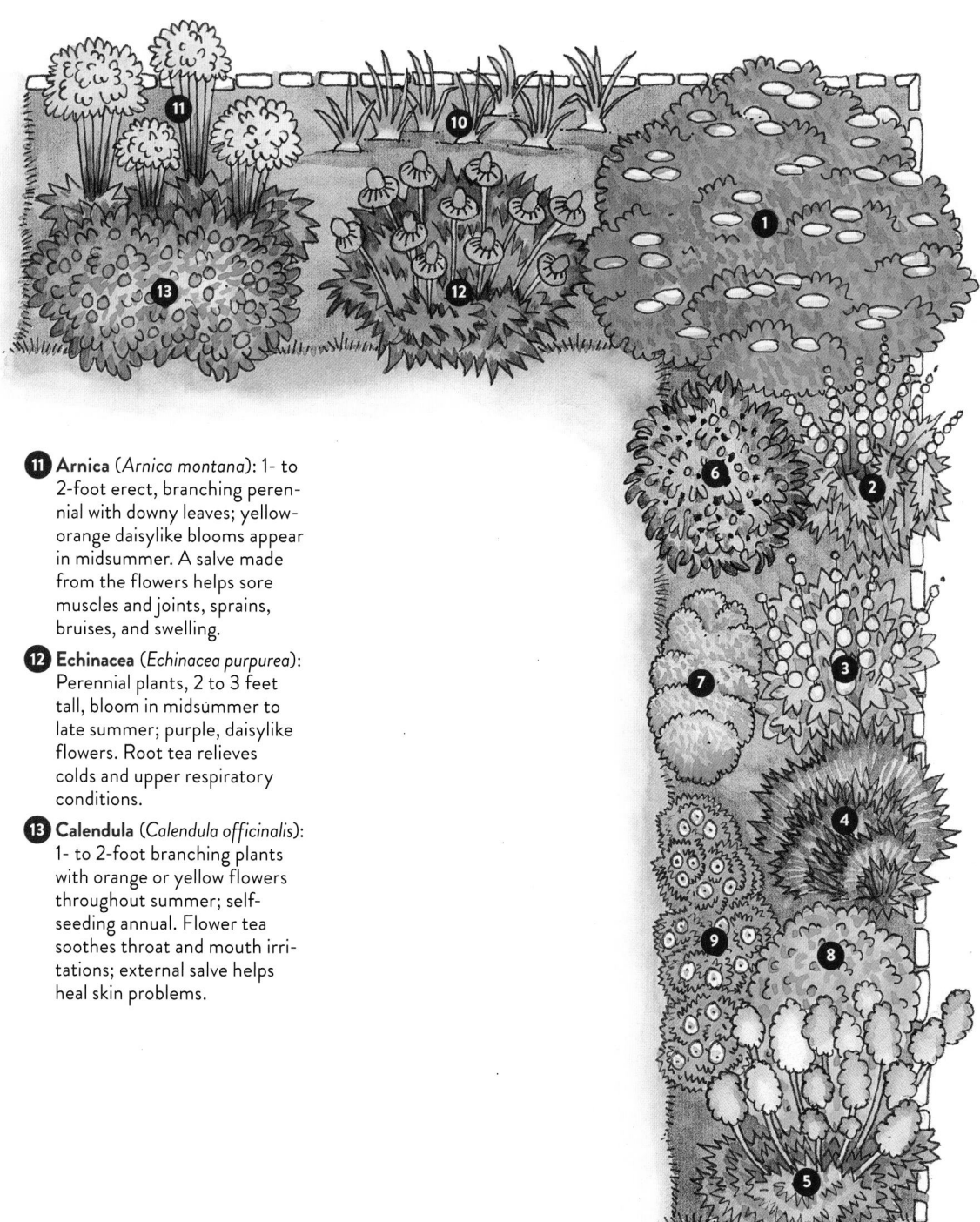

11 Arnica (*Arnica montana*): 1- to 2-foot erect, branching perennial with downy leaves; yellow-orange daisylike blooms appear in midsummer. A salve made from the flowers helps sore muscles and joints, sprains, bruises, and swelling.

12 Echinacea (*Echinacea purpurea*): Perennial plants, 2 to 3 feet tall, bloom in midsummer to late summer; purple, daisylike flowers. Root tea relieves colds and upper respiratory conditions.

13 Calendula (*Calendula officinalis*): 1- to 2-foot branching plants with orange or yellow flowers throughout summer; self-seeding annual. Flower tea soothes throat and mouth irritations; external salve helps heal skin problems.

Garden for Fragrance and Beauty

The bloom season of this fragrance garden extends from the first sweet violets in April until the last blooms of witch hazel in winter. A bench or swing below a rose-covered arbor provides a private spot to take in the scents. But fragrant flowers are only half the story. The aromatic foliage of scented geraniums, pineapple mint, and artemisia can be enjoyed spring through fall. Potted tropicals like ylang-ylang and patchouli come inside in autumn to scent the air until temperatures warm up again in spring. Besides stimulating your senses in the garden, many of these herbs can be used to make fragrant potpourris, sachets, soaps, and beauty-care preparations.

This design is located in a corner, backed by a fence or wall. If you don't have a fence or wall, you can expand the border a few feet in the back and fill that side with more low-growing herbs, such as calamint.

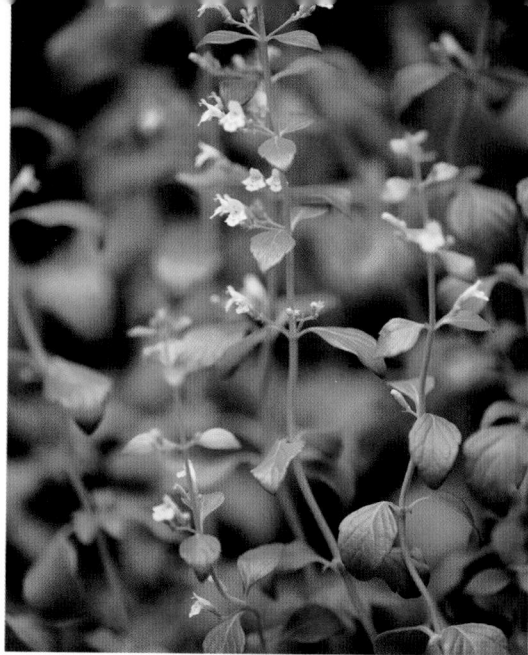
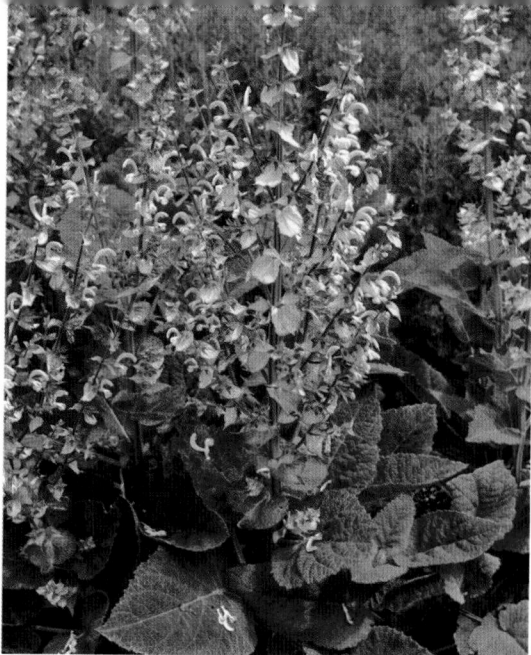

In the Garden

1 **Witch hazel 'Jelena'** (*Hamamelis × intermedia*): Woody shrub up to 15 feet tall; fragrant, copper-colored, threadlike flowers in early winter; coarsely toothed leaves turn orange-red in fall.

2 **Damask rose 'La Ville de Brux-elles'** (*Rosa × damascena*): Hardy, 5-foot-tall, rounded shrub with clusters of intensely fragrant, large pink double flowers; blooms late spring to early summer.

3 **Cabbage rose 'Dutch Provence'** (*Rosa × centifolia*): 8- to 10-foot climber with a profusion of pale pink, double, highly fragrant blooms in late spring to early summer.

4 **French lavender 'Grosso'** (*Lavandula × intermedia*): Woody, 2- to 3-foot-tall perennial, hardy to Zone 5; purple bloom spikes in late spring to midsummer.

5 **Clary sage** (*Salvia sclarea*): Erect biennial up to 4 feet tall; broad, opposite, heart-shaped leaves 6 to 9 inches long; spikes of purple or pale pink flowers in early summer.

6 **Calamint** (*Calamintha nepeta*): 15- to 18-inch perennial shrub forms a tidy mound of small, bright green leaves; lavender-pink bloom spikes last 6 weeks or more in midsummer to late summer.

7 **Southernwood 'Tangerine'** (*Artemisia abrotanum*): 3- to 4-foot perennial with finely divided, downy, olive green leaves; neat, upright form; citrusy scent.

8 **Artemisia 'Silver Brocade'** (*Artemisia stelleriana*): 6- to 12-inch perennial with velvety, divided, silvery leaves; drought-tolerant edging.

9 **Violet** (*Viola odorata*): Creeping perennial up to 6 inches tall; oval to heart-shaped leaves and dark purple or white springtime flowers. Let them wander below shrubs and around the bases of containers.

In Containers

10 **Dwarf ylang-ylang** (*Cananga odorata* var. *fruticosa*): 6-foot-tall tropical shrub with long, oblong leaves; scented yellow flowers throughout summer. Bring indoors to overwinter.

11 **Patchouli** (*Pogostemon cablin*): 2-foot-tall tropical perennial with handsome serrated leaves; white or pale pink flowers in autumn. Bring indoors to overwinter.

12 **Variegated pineapple mint** (*Mentha suaveolens* 'Variegata'): Perennial up to 2 feet tall; terminal spikes of tiny, purple-pink flowers; attractive light green leaves edged in white.

13 **Rose-scented geranium** (*Pelargonium graveolens*): Tender perennial up to 2 feet tall with frilly leaves and pink flowers. Bring indoors to overwinter.

14 **Lemon-scented geranium** (*Pelargonium crispum*): Tender perennial, 10 inches tall, with frilly leaves and pink flowers. Bring indoors to overwinter.

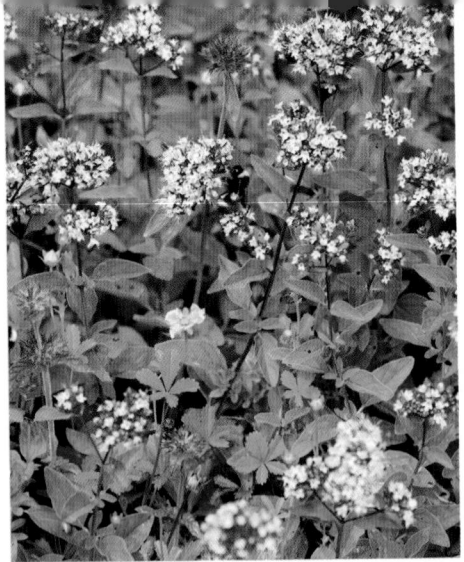
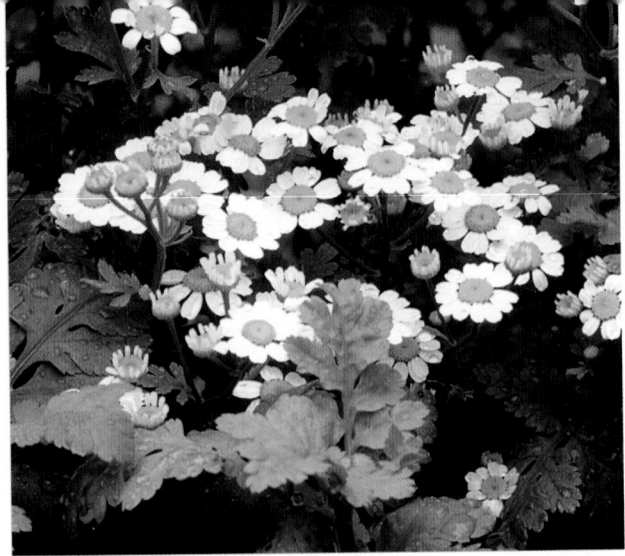

Garden of Everlastings

Featuring four different yarrow varieties, the perennial herbs in this circular garden will beautify your landscape and home year-round. Their flowers and foliage make gorgeous and long-lasting fresh or dried arrangements and wreaths. To dry the flowers or foliage, cut the stems on a dry day after the dew has evaporated. Because flowers continue to open as they dry, cut them before they are fully mature. (For information on drying herbs for crafts, see Chapter 7.)

1 **Artemisia 'Powis Castle'** (*Artemisia* hybrid): 26-inch-tall perennial grown for its feathery gray-green foliage; small yellow flowers in late summer to fall.

2 **English lavender 'Hidcote'** (*Lavandula angustifolia*): Deep purple, highly fragrant blooms cover the 18-inch-tall perennial plants all summer; gray-green foliage.

3 **Goldenrod 'Fireworks'** (*Solidago rugosa*): Brilliant yellow flowers on 3-foot stems in late summer.

4 **Yarrow 'Paprika'** (*Achillea millefolium*): 2-foot-tall perennial with erect stems and feathery foliage, topped with red-and-gold flower heads in midsummer to late summer.

5 **Purple marjoram** (*Origanum laevigata*): 2-foot-tall perennial with deep purple-red flowers in late summer to fall.

6 **Tansy** (*Tanacetum vulgare*): 3- to 4-foot-tall perennial with yellow button flowers in midsummer to late summer.

7 **Yarrow 'Moonshine'** (*Achillea* hybrid): 2-foot-tall perennial with erect stems and feathery foliage, topped with light golden flower heads all summer.

8 **English lavender 'Munstead'** (*Lavandula angustifolia*): 1-foot-tall perennial with gray-green foliage; bright lavender flower spikes throughout summer.

9 **Feverfew** (*Tanacetum parthenium*): Vigorous, hardy biennial or perennial 2 to 3 feet tall; small, white, daisylike flowers in tight, flat-topped clusters in midsummer to late summer.

10 **Yarrow 'Pomegranate'** (*Achillea millefolium*): 2-foot-tall perennial with erect stems and feathery foliage; topped with magenta-red flower heads all summer.

11 **Mountain mint** (*Pycnanthemum pilosum*): 30-inch perennial with fragrant leaves; white bloom spikes in late summer to fall.

12 **Yarrow 'Coronation Gold'** (*Achillea filipendulina*): 3-foot-tall perennial with erect stems and feathery foliage; topped with golden flower heads midsummer to late summer.

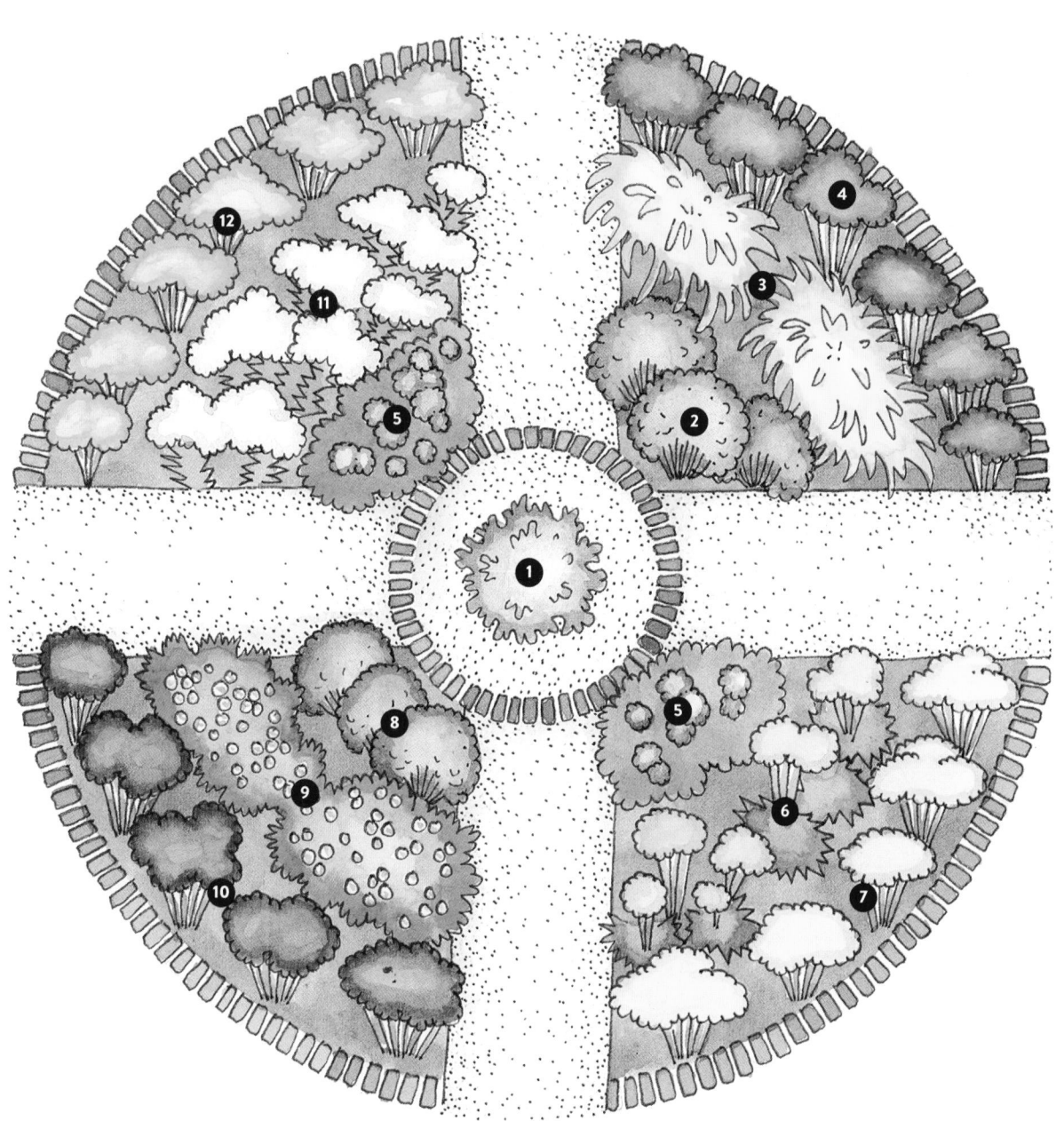

Garden for Birds and Butterflies

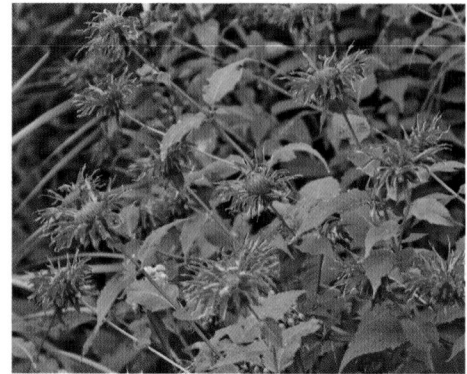

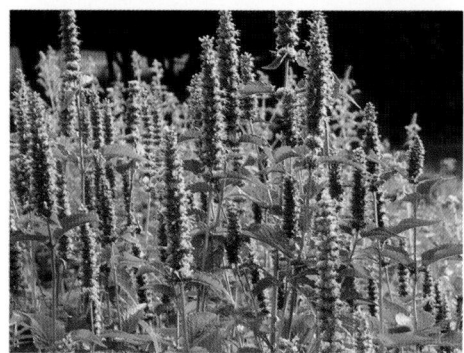

Create a haven for beautiful winged visitors with this garden of colorful herbs. Hummingbirds and butterflies can't resist sipping nectar from bright tubular blooms, like those of anise hyssop, calamint, and bee balm. Host plants meet the dietary needs of the caterpillars: Swallowtail larvae, for instance, feed on dill, parsley, and rue, while monarch caterpillars prefer milkweed—a showy native plant. The hawthorn tree anchors the planting, providing butterfly-attracting blooms in spring and bright red berries that feed birds in fall and winter. Look for a species native to your area.

A birdbath helps entice feathered friends to stop, splash, and play on hot summer days. For butterflies, provide shallow saucers of water at ground level.

1. **Calamint** (*Calamintha nepeta*): 15- to 18-inch perennial shrub forms a tidy mound of small, bright green leaves; lavender-pink bloom spikes in midsummer to late summer; fragrant.

2. **Anise hyssop** (*Agastache foeniculum*): Upright, 3- to 6-foot plant with maroon-tinted leaves; spikes of bright blue flowers in midsummer to late summer; aromatic.

3. **Bee balm** (*Monarda fistulosa*): Light purple flower heads atop 3-foot stems in midsummer to late summer; dark green leaves with toothed margins; aromatic.

4. **Purple coneflower** (*Echinacea purpurea*): Sturdy stems 2 to 3 feet tall; purple daisylike flowers in midsummer to late summer.

5. **Soapwort 'Rosea Plena'** (*Saponaria officinalis*): Erect leafy stem up to 2 feet tall; clusters of double pink blooms in midsummer to late summer.

6. **Curly parsley** (*Petroselinum crispum*): Bushy, 12-inch-tall biennial plants with dark green, curled leaves. Replant annually.

7. **Dill** (*Anethum graveolens*): 2- to 3-foot upright stems topped by yellow-green flower umbels up to 6 inches across; feathery leaves; aromatic.

8. **Milkweed** (*Asclepias syriaca*): Shrubby, 3-foot-tall perennial with showy pink blooms in early to midsummer; large, dark green leaves. A monarch favorite!

9. **Rue 'Blue Mound'** (*Ruta graveolens*): Compact evergreen shrub, 12 inches tall; grayish blue, spade-shaped leaves; bright yellow flowers in midsummer to late summer.

10. **New Jersey tea** (*Ceanothus americanus*): Deciduous shrub up to 3 feet tall; finely toothed, dark green leaves; airy white flowers on racemes in early to midsummer, followed by seedpods.

11. **Hawthorn** (*Crataegus* spp.): A member of the rose family, this deciduous, thorny, small tree bears clusters of aromatic white flowers in spring; bright red berries persist into winter.

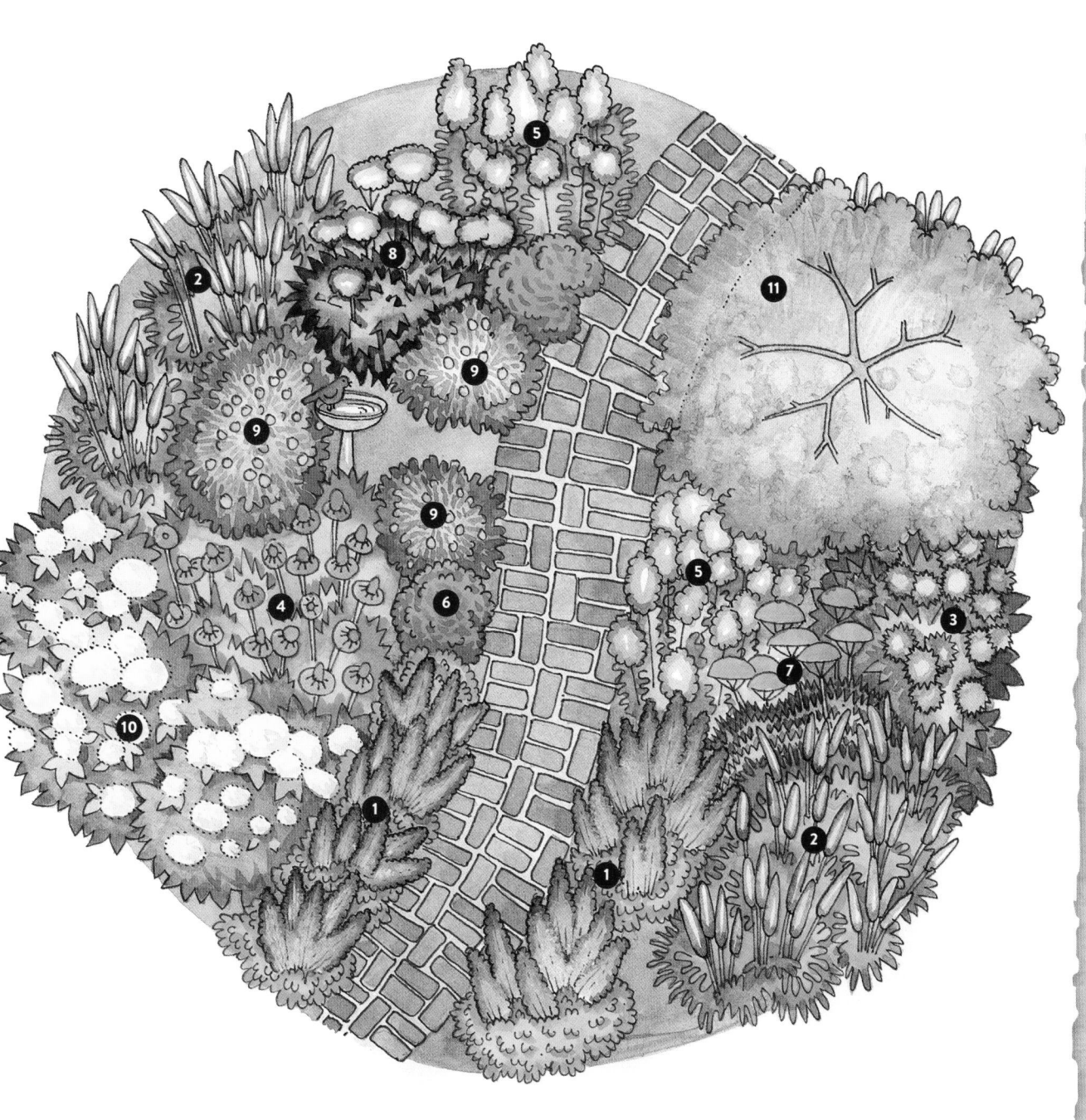

"Grand Opening" Entryway Garden

Say "good-bye" to boring foundation shrubs and "welcome" to visitors with this bright herbal entryway garden. Colorful blooms and refreshing scents make a positive first impression. And unlike many front-door landscapes, this one practically takes care of itself, requiring little upkeep once established. Many of these plants are drought tolerant, so they'll adapt well to the often-dry conditions around a home. Most of them also attract butterflies and hummingbirds!

When designing an entryway garden, plan for at least three layers, with the tallest plants closest to the house, medium-height plants in the middle, and the shortest plants farthest away from the house. Choose two or three dominant colors with a neutral background color, such as gray foliage, to unify the design.

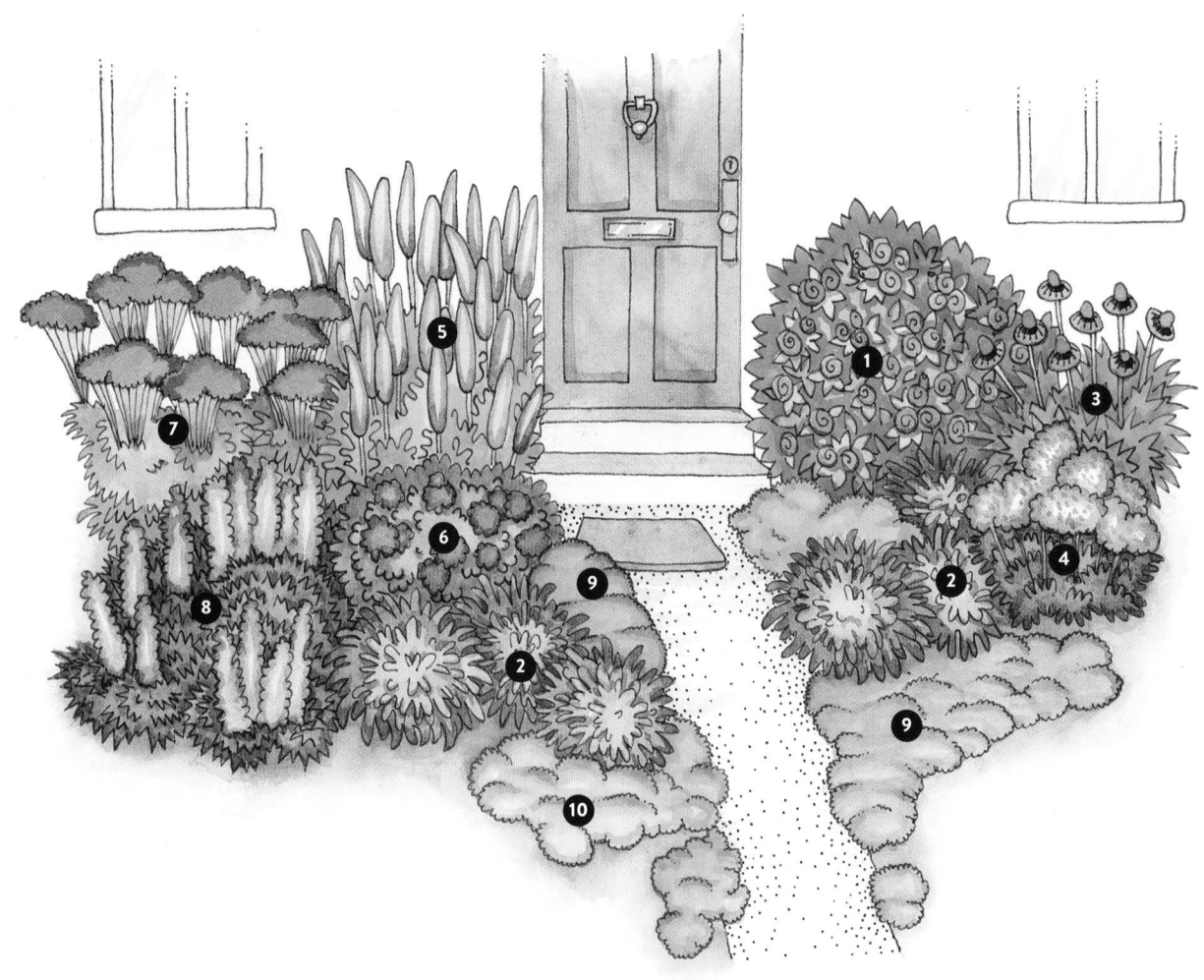

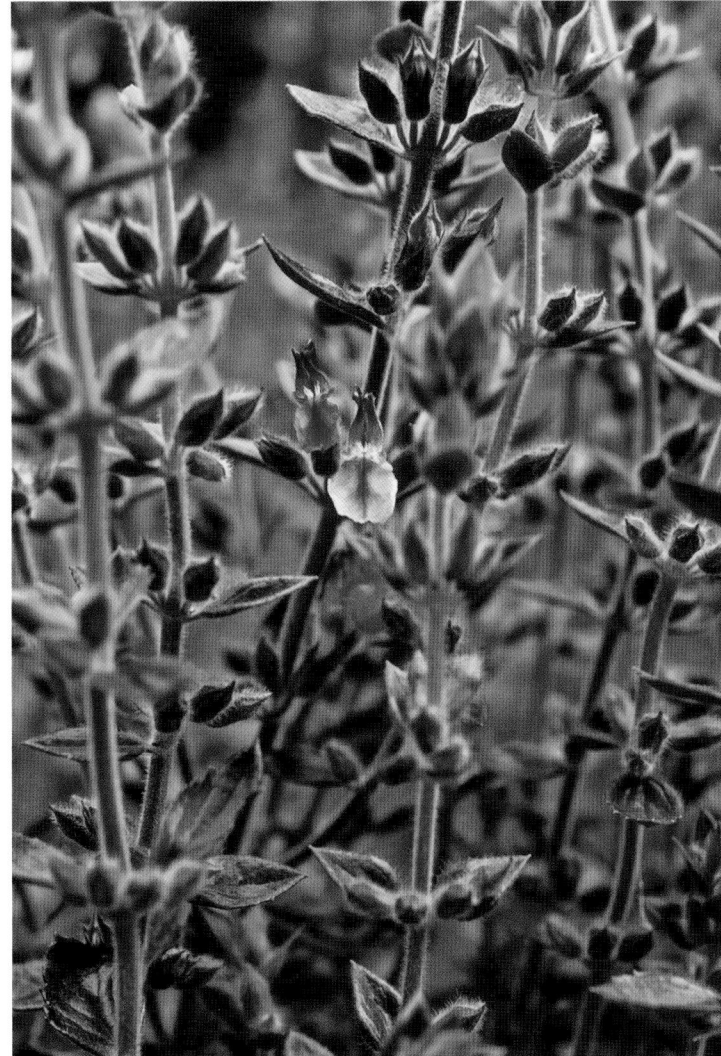

1. **Cabbage rose 'Pompon de Bourgogne'** (*Rosa centifolia*): Compact, 2 x 3-foot plant densely covered with foliage; bears a profusion of fragrant pale pink to purple double blooms in late spring to early summer.

2. **Purple sage** (*Salvia officinalis* 'Purpurascens'): Perennial up to 10 inches tall; aromatic, gray-green to purple leaves; purple flowers appear in June.

3. **Purple coneflower** (*Echinacea purpurea*): Sturdy stems 2 to 3 feet tall; daisylike flowers with cone center surrounded by purple rays in midsummer to late summer.

4. **Oregano 'Hopley's'** (*Origanum laevigatum*): Shrubby perennial up to 2 feet tall; spikes of deep purple blooms in midsummer to late summer.

5. **Anise hyssop 'Blue Blazes'** (*Agastache foeniculum* hybrid): 3- to 5-foot-tall perennial with upright form; lavender-purple flower spikes in midsummer to late summer; butterfly and hummingbird favorite.

6. **Purple marjoram** (*Origanum laevigata*): Shrubby perennial up to 2 feet tall; spikes of red-purple blooms midsummer to late summer.

7. **Yarrow 'Cerise Queen'** (*Achillea millefolium*): 1½- to 2½-foot-tall perennial with erect stems and feathery green foliage; flat-topped deep rose-pink flowers in early to late summer.

8. **Germander** (*Teucrium chamaedrys*): Shrubby perennial up to 18 inches tall; bright green leaves; rose to purple blooms on small spikes in midsummer to late summer.

9. **Thyme 'Pink Chintz'** (*Thymus serpyllum*): Creeping groundcover with tiny green leaves; forms a carpet of pink blooms in late spring to midsummer.

10. **Thyme 'Lime'** (*Thymus vulgaris*): Mounding groundcover with bright lime green, citrus-scented leaves; light pink flowers in midsummer.

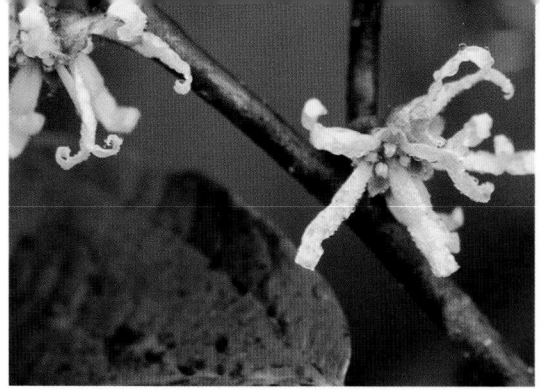
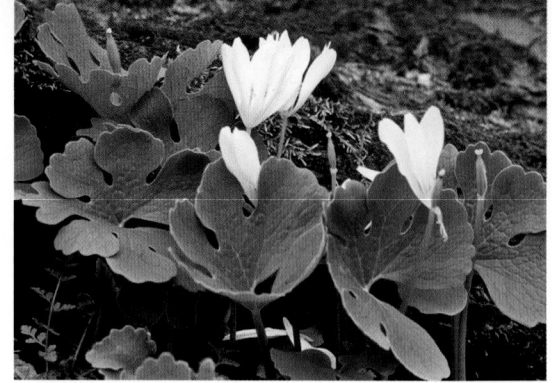

Four-Season Woodland Border

Most of the plants in this large border are native to the eastern woodlands of America. They provide four seasons of natural beauty—from the flowering of black hellebore in earliest spring to the brilliant fall foliage of sassafras and fragrant early winter blooms of witch hazel. Even through melting snow, the wintergreen groundcover provides bright red berries and glossy green leaves. In spring and summer, a variety of interesting and ornamental perennials and shrubs light up the shade. Watch for wildlife: You're sure to have visitors!

Over time, as the trees and shrubs mature and produce a larger canopy, the shorter perennials and groundcovers will naturalize to form an understory that thrives in the moist, acidic conditions created by decomposing leaves, twigs, and bark—much like a natural forest floor.

1. **Sassafras** (*Sassafras albidum*): Tree or large shrub 30 to 60 feet tall and 25 feet wide; leaves have two or three distinct lobes and brilliant fall color.

2. **Witch hazel** (*Hamamelis virginiana*): Woody, spreading shrub up to 15 feet tall and wide; fragrant, yellow, threadlike flowers in late fall; coarsely toothed leaves turn gold.

3. **Elder 'Black Lace'** (*Sambucus nigra*): 6- to 8-foot-tall shrub; deep purple-black stems and contrasting creamy pink blooms that appear in airy clusters in early summer; deep purple berries.

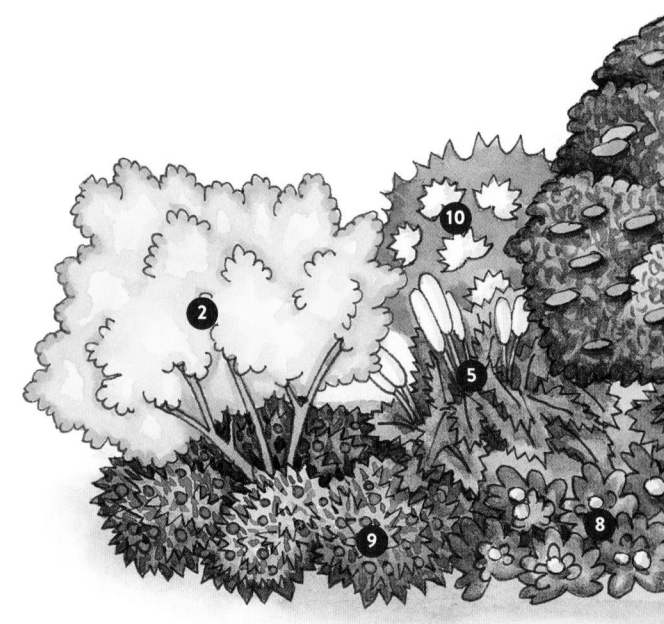

4 New Jersey tea (*Ceanothus americanus*): Deciduous shrub up to 3 feet tall; finely toothed, dark green leaves; airy white flowers on racemes early to midsummer, followed by seedpods.

5 Black cohosh (*Actaea racemosa*): Perennial with small, creamy flowers on 4- to 7-foot-tall bloom spikes in early to midsummer; broad, lacy leaves up to 2 feet long.

6 Foxglove (*Digitalis purpurea*): Biennial plants with 4- to 6-foot-tall spikes of purple, pink, or white blooms from late spring to midsummer. Self-seeds.

7 Blue cohosh (*Caulophyllum thalictroides*): Perennial with bluish green leaves and 1- to 3-foot-tall stems; dark blue berrylike fruit in autumn.

8 Black hellebore (*Helleborus niger*): Perennial up to 1 foot tall; deep green, divided evergreen leaves; pinkish white roselike blooms in late winter.

9 Wintergreen (*Gaultheria procumbens*): Creeping perennial up to 6 inches tall; glossy, evergreen leaves and tiny, bell-shaped white flowers in midsummer; round, red berries appear in late summer, persist through winter.

10 Bloodroot 'Multiplex' (*Sanguinaria canadensis*): 4- to 6-inch-tall perennial; naked stems topped with 1- to 2-inch white flowers in midspring; deeply lobed palmate leaves up to 8 inches across.

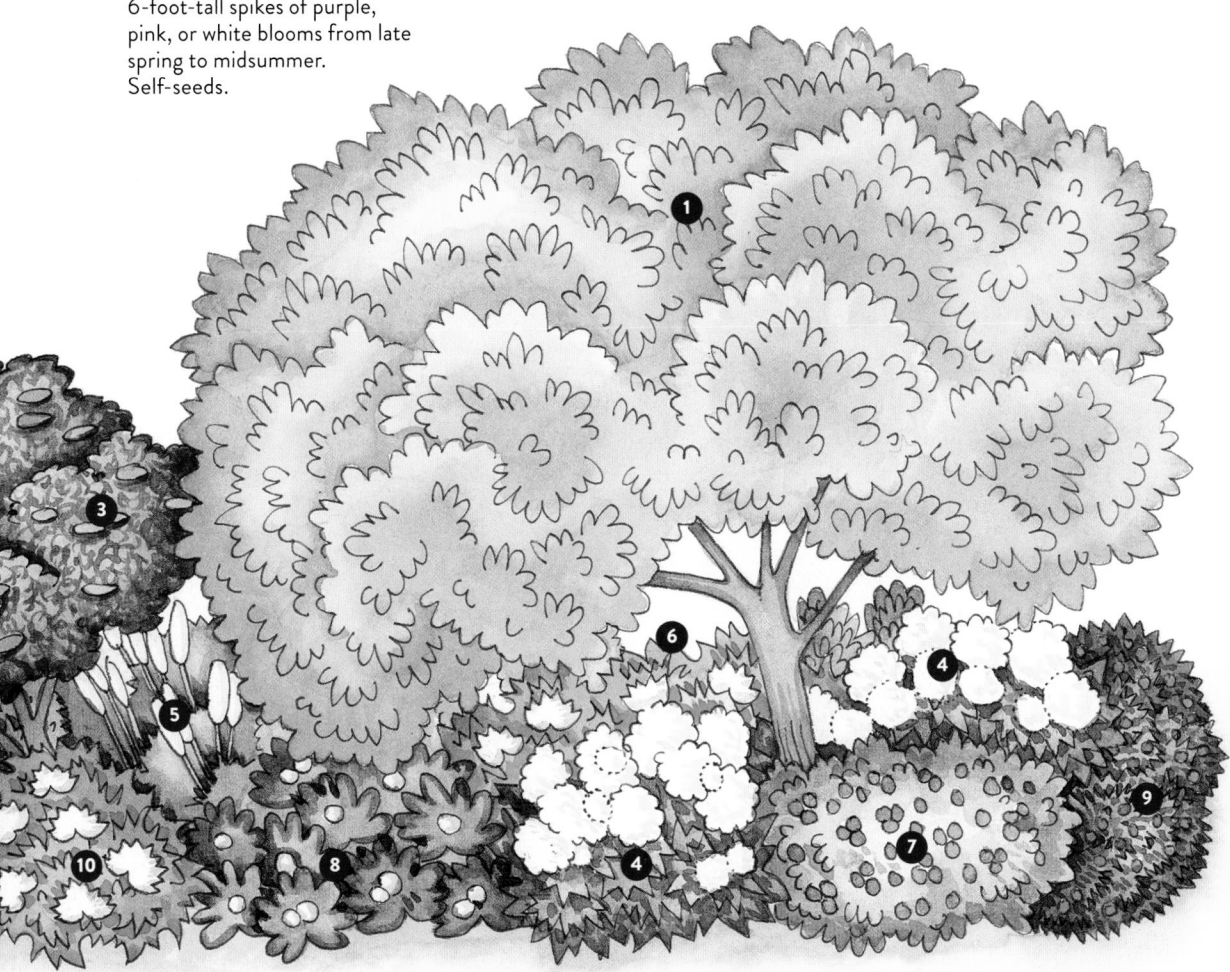

Rock Wall Herb Garden

Drought-tolerant, compact Mediterranean herbs—such as creeping thymes, prostrate rosemary, Roman chamomile, and many oreganos—can turn an ordinary stone wall into a wall of living color and fragrance. If you don't have a stone wall, you can plant this combination in a hillside rock garden or other sunny, dry location. In addition to the suggested plants, also consider aloes, portulaca, sedums, and other succulents. Some specialty suppliers offer "alpine plants" uniquely suited to these conditions.

To plant in the crevices of a stone wall, you'll need to make a growing medium of gravel, sand, and compost, then moisten it well with water. Use a trowel or small spatula to work the growing medium between the rocks; make indentations in the medium for planting. Tuck in your plants, and then tamp the medium firmly around them. Gently water the wall from the top down, and continue watering occasionally until the plants become established.

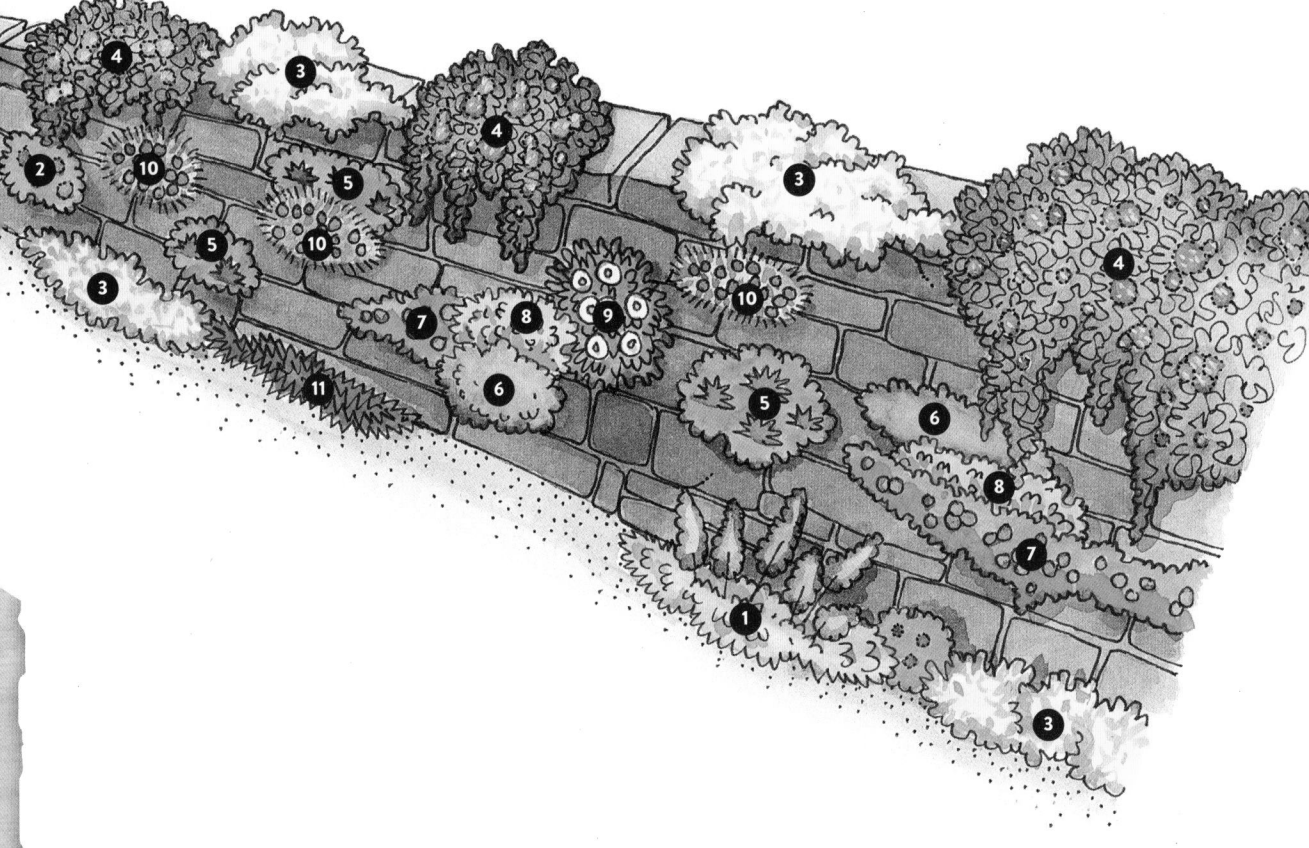

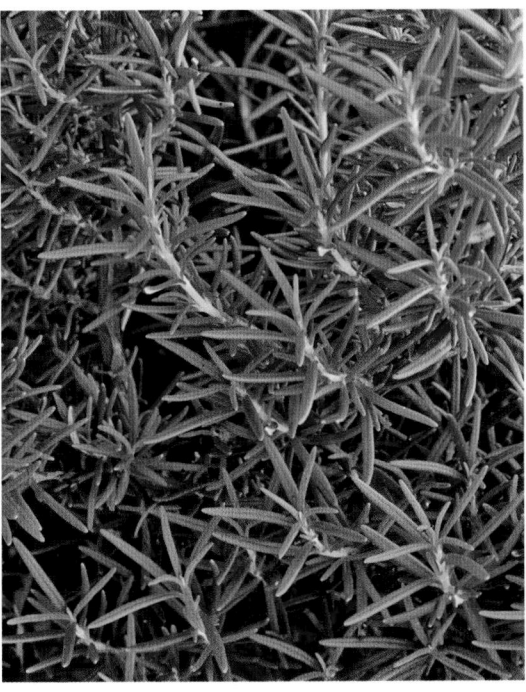
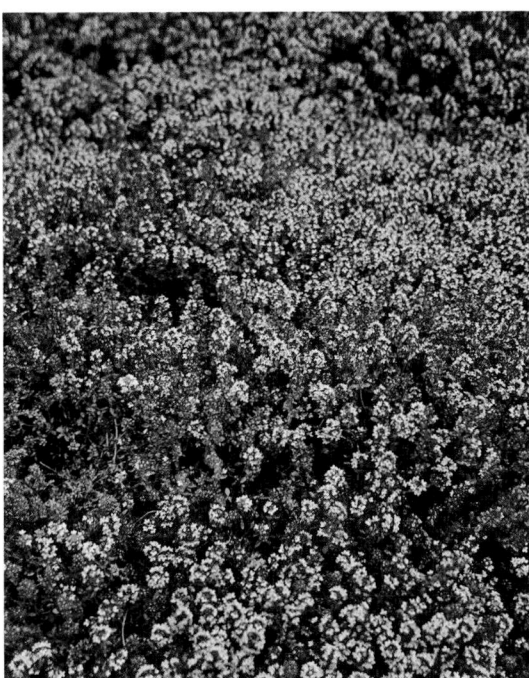

1 Golden oregano, also called 'Aureum' (*Origanum vulgare*): 4-inch-tall creeping perennial with golden leaves; white flowers in midsummer to late summer.

2 Compact oregano, also called 'Humile' (*Origanum vulgare*): 3-inch-tall creeping perennial with green leaves and purple flowers in midsummer to late summer.

3 Variegated oregano, also called 'Variegata' (*Origanum vulgare*): 8-inch-tall perennial with golden variegated leaves; pink-white flowers in midsummer to late summer.

4 Prostrate rosemary (*Rosmarinus officinalis*): Perennial with cascading form and short, deep green, needlelike leaves; deep blue, long-lasting blooms.

5 Sedum 'Dragon's Blood' (*Sedum spurium*): Creeping, 4-inch perennial plants with succulent green leaves; dark red flowers in midsummer to late summer.

6 Woolly thyme (*Thymus pseudolanuginosus*): Forms a thick, fuzzy carpet of gray-green leaves with pink-purple flowers in midsummer.

7 Nutmeg thyme (*Thymus praecox*): Forms a thick carpet of spicy-scented green leaves with lavender-pink flowers in early to midsummer.

8 Thyme 'Goldstream' (*Thymus praecox*): Low-growing groundcover with variegated green-gold leaves; pale pink flowers in early to midsummer.

9 Double Roman chamomile, also called 'Flore Pleno' (*Chamaemelum nobile*): Compact, 3-inch-tall form with double, white, daisylike blooms in early summer.

10 Dianthus 'Tiny Rubies' (*Dianthus gratianopolitanus*): 2-inch-tall clump-forming perennial with silvery blue foliage; bright pink, double fragrant (edible) blooms in late spring to early summer.

11 Creeping winter savory (*Satureja montana* ssp. *illyrica*): 4-inch-tall creeping perennial with bright green leaves; white to pale purple flowers in early to midsummer.

Silver Terrace Garden

This terrace or patio garden features herbs with light-reflecting silver-gray foliage, such as artemisia and sage. Their leaves seem to shimmer, creating a serene setting for an outdoor garden room. The blooms in the surrounding border and pots light up the area with contrasting hues of hot pink, vibrant purple, and creamy white. Simply brushing the herbal foliage releases a cloud of scents—providing the perfect ambience for relaxing summer evenings alone or with friends. Fragrant old-fashioned roses (small enough to grow in large containers) flank the steps.

Cover the sitting area with crushed white stone to reflect even more light, or set flagstone pavers in gravel. Between the flagstones, plant a creeping groundcover that can tolerate foot traffic, such as 'Annie Hall' thyme. Bring tender perennials, such as Mexican bush sage and scented geranium, indoors in fall to enjoy their beauty and fragrance throughout the winter.

In the Garden

1. **Artemisia 'Lambrook Silver'** (*Artemisia absinthium*): Finely cut silver-gray foliage on mounding, 30-inch-tall perennial plants; fragrant.

2. **Silver sage** (*Salvia argentea*): Big, bold biennial produces a 3-foot-wide mound of large (up to 12 inches long), downy silver leaves in its first year; 2-foot-tall white bloom spikes appear in early summer of the second year.

3. **Dianthus 'Firewitch'** (*Dianthus gratianopolitanus*): Forms neat, 8-inch mounds of silver-gray foliage; fragrant magenta-pink blooms in early summer.

4. **Foxglove 'Camelot Lavender'** (*Digitalis purpurea* ssp. *heywoodii*): 3- to 4-foot-tall biennial plants bear spikes of lavender-mauve flowers in early to midsummer.

5. **Silver corkscrew chives** (*Allium senescens* ssp. *glaucum*): Compact, 6-inch-tall variety with uniquely curled silver-gray leaves; lavender-pink blooms midsummer to fall.

6. **Thyme 'Annie Hall'** (*Thymus praecox*): Mat-forming groundcover variety fills crevices between stepping stones, withstanding foot traffic; covered with rose-red blooms from late spring to early summer.

In Containers

7. **Cabbage rose 'De Meaux'** (*Rosa × centifolia*): Compact 3-foot-tall plants with tiny buds that open in late spring to 1-inch pale to deep pink blooms. Intensely fragrant; excellent for potpourris.

8. **Scented geranium 'Grey Lady Plymouth'** (*Pelargonium × asperum*): Tender perennial, 24 inches tall, with silver-gray dissected leaves edged with white; rose-scented lavender-pink blooms in summer.

9. **Silver tansy 'Jackpot'** (*Tanacetum niveum*): 18-inch-tall perennial with white, daisylike blooms all summer; finely cut silver-gray foliage.

10. **Mexican bush sage 'Purple Velvet'** (*Salvia leucantha*): 2- to 3-foot-tall tender perennial with lance-shaped, gray-green, aromatic leaves; showy purple bloom spikes midsummer to late summer.

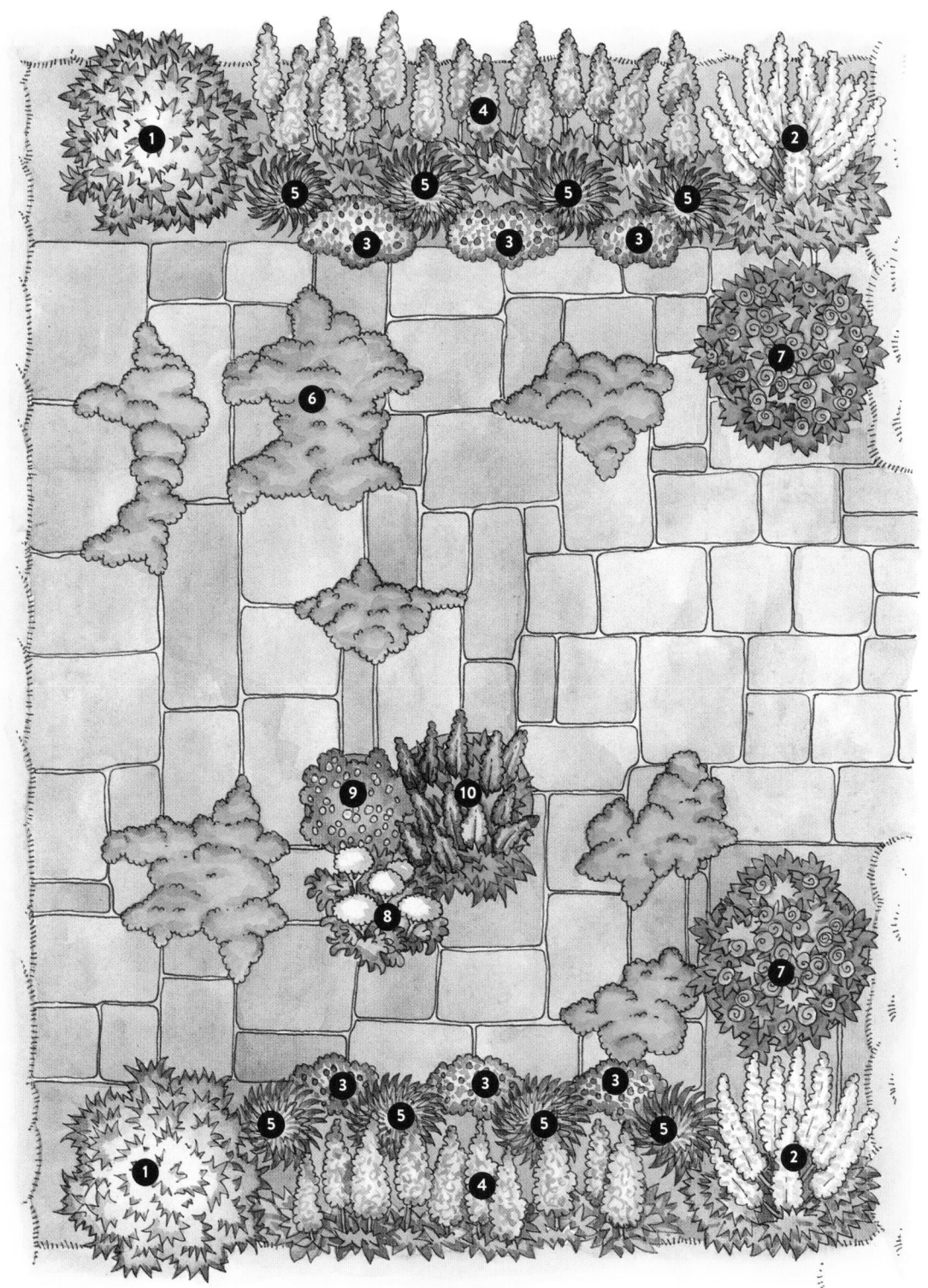

Spiritual Retreat Garden

Modeled loosely on a cloistered medieval monastery garden, this herbal oasis includes a bench for sitting and meditating among raised garden beds. Enclosed by a clipped hawthorn or bayberry hedge, the garden feels secluded and separated from the often-hectic outside world—even if it happens to be located on a rooftop in center city.

Pink-flowered soapwort naturalizes along the base of the hedge and offers a continuous view of soothing color.

Although this garden includes herbs commonly grown during the Middle Ages, separated by their uses (household, kitchen, medicinal, and mystical), you could substitute your own favorites.

Hedge and Groundcover

1. **English hawthorn** (*Crataegus laevigata*): Deciduous, thorny shrub up to 15 feet tall; clusters of aromatic white flowers followed by dark red fruits.

2. **Soapwort** (*Saponaria officinalis*): Single-stemmed perennial up to 2 feet tall; clusters of pink blooms in midsummer to late summer; roots used to make soap.

Household Herbs

3. **English lavender** (*Lavandula angustifolia*): Branching, aromatic shrub up to 3 feet tall; flowers used in bath and laundry.

4. **Madder** (*Rubia tinctorum*): 4-foot stems; panicles of tiny, greenish white flowers in midsummer; reddish brown roots used to make red dye.

5. **Woad** (*Isatis tinctoria*): Biennial or perennial, 3 to 5 feet tall; small yellow flowers appear in spring of second year; bluish green oblong leaves used to make blue dye.

6. **Agrimony** (*Agrimonia eupatoria*): Upright stems up to 5 feet tall; spikes of small yellow blooms in midsummer; aromatic leaves used to make yellow dye and potpourri.

Kitchen and Salad Herbs

7. **Chives** (*Allium schoenoprasum*): Dark green, hollow, cylindrical leaves up to 10 inches tall; small, pale purple blooms in late spring; leaves used as flavoring.

8. **Sage** (*Salvia officinalis*): Woody-stemmed perennial up to 30 inches tall; gray-green leaves; purple-blue flowers in early summer; leaves used as flavoring.

9. **Calendula** (*Calendula officinalis*): 2-foot-tall branching plant; orange or yellow ray blooms add flavor and color to soups and salads.

10. **Garden sorrel** (*Rumex acetosa*): 1- to 2-foot-tall perennial with lance-shaped leaves; spikes of yellow or reddish flowers in spring; lemony flavored leaves used in salads, soups, and sauces.

11. **Borage** (*Borago officinalis*): Succulent stems up to 18 inches tall, with fuzzy gray-green leaves; nodding clusters of small, bright blue star-shaped flowers; use cucumber-flavored leaves and flowers (sparingly) in salads.

Medicinal Herbs

12. **St. John's wort** (*Hypericum perforatum*): Erect perennial up to 2 feet tall; bright yellow blooms in midsummer.

13. **Feverfew** (*Tanacetum parthenium*): Biennial or perennial up to 3 feet tall; white, daisylike flowers in midsummer; strongly scented leaves.

14. **Lemon balm** (*Melissa officinalis*): Loosely branched perennial up to 2 feet tall; clusters of tiny white flowers throughout summer; lemon-scented leaves.

15. **Licorice** (*Glycyrrhiza glabra*): Erect, branching perennial up to 6 feet tall; spikes of blue flowers in midsummer.

16. **Valerian** (*Valeriana officinalis*): 3- to 6-foot-tall stems with dark green, lance-shaped leaves and clusters of small white or pink flowers in midsummer; large, pungent-smelling rhizomes.

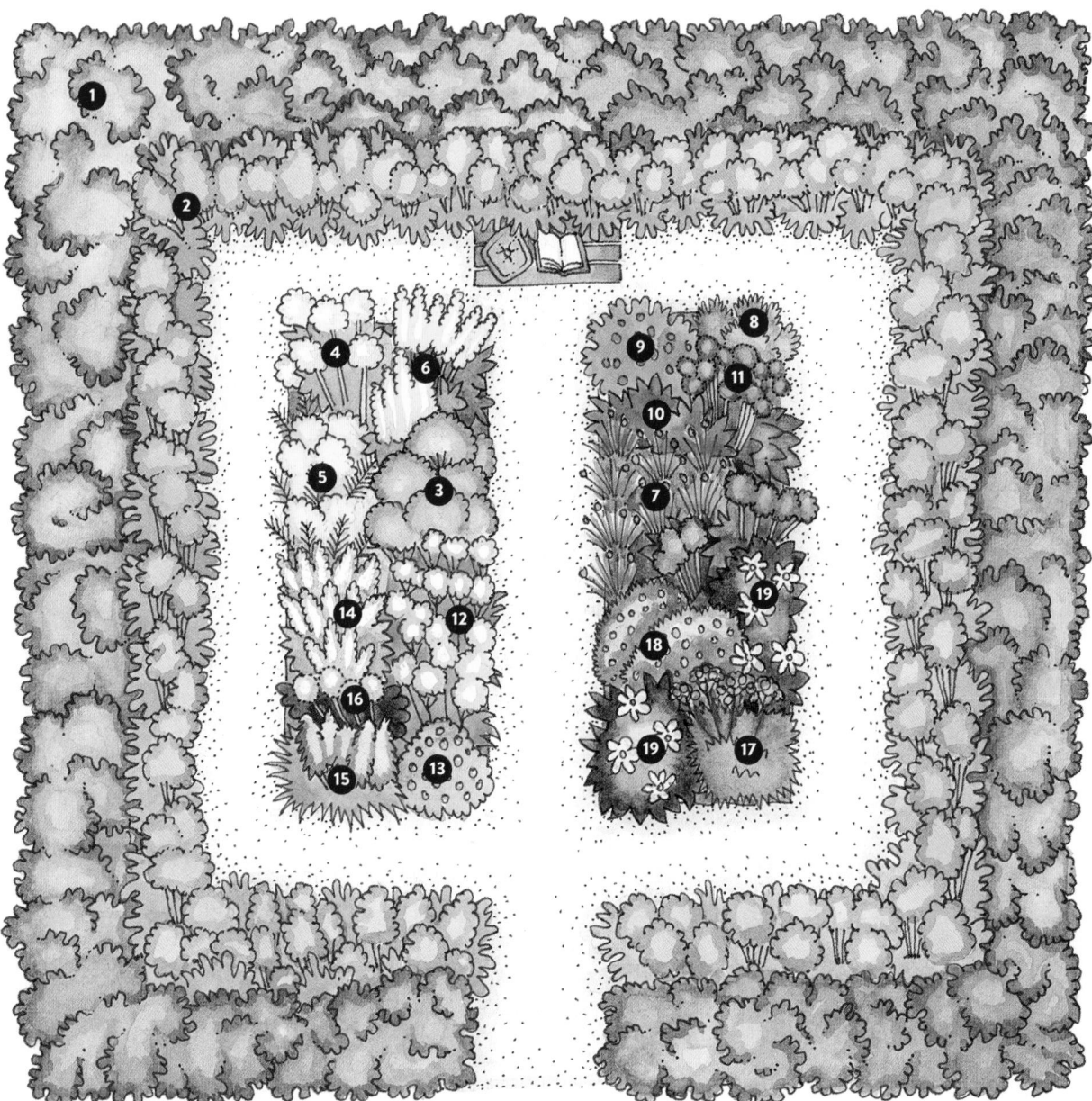

Sacred or Mystical Herbs

17 **Vervain** (*Verbena officinalis*): 2- to 3-foot-tall stems topped by slender spikes of small, tubular, pale purple flowers in midsummer.

18 **Rue** (*Ruta graveolens*): Semi-woody evergreen shrub up to 3 feet tall; grayish blue, spade-shaped leaves; bright yellow flowers throughout summer.

19 **Black hellebore** (*Helleborus niger*): Perennial up to 1 foot tall; deep green, evergreen leaves; white blooms in late winter.

A READER'S NOTES *on* HERBS

As mentioned in the Introduction, the favorite book in my library, *The Herball* by John Gerard, has a special sheaf of 18th-century notes bound into the book. These notes contain the therapeutic observations of one of the families who owned this priceless work during the past 400 years that have been passed down from generation to generation. I hope you will feel inspired to write your observations about herbs and their uses in these pages, making your copy of this book a one-of-a-kind reference.—M.J.B.

ACKNOWLEDGMENTS

At times our own light goes out and is rekindled by a spark from another person. Each of us has cause to think with deep gratitude of those who have lighted the flame within us.

—ALBERT SCHWEITZER

I HAVE BEEN VERY FORTUNATE to have so many people who were, and are, supportive of my lifelong interest in plants, people, and culture. My family has been a constant source of support and encouragement, from my first years of elementary school through graduate studies and into my professional life. When I was an undergraduate horticulture major at the University of Delaware, Professor Richard W. Lighty was an extraordinary and inspiring mentor who, during my first year at the University, invited me to prepare and deliver a public lecture on harvesting and processing herbs that was the beginning of my interest in this topic. This exceptional quality of mentorship continued through my graduate education at Harvard University, where I studied under Professor Richard Evans Schultes. The Botanical Museum of Harvard University, directed by Professor Schultes, was a remarkably inspiring place for a young graduate student to learn about ethnobotany and tropical plants because of its facilities, collections, and the multitude of world-class scholars who would visit the museum. Many of the graduate students who studied in the Biology Department with me during the 1970s are now considered leaders in their fields, and I am so fortunate to count a number of them as close friends.

My career at The New York Botanical Garden (NYBG) began in the fall of 1980, and I am grateful to the Board of Managers and Staff of the Botanical Garden for their support of the NYBG's International Plant Science Center, as well as my own studies, through all of these years and for their steadfast commitment to the institution's renaissance as one of the world's greatest botanical gardens. The comprehensive horticultural collections, groundbreaking public exhibitions, innovative educational programs, and unparalleled resources of The New York Botanical Garden's International Plant Science Center, including the Pfizer Plant Research Laboratory, Lewis B. and Dorothy Cullman Program for Molecular Systematics, Genomics Program, William and Lynda Steere Herbarium, C.V. Starr Virtual Herbarium, LuEsther T. Mertz Library, Institute of Economic Botany, Institute of Systematic Botany, Graduate Studies Program, NYBG Press, and international field studies programs, along with the dedicated staff and graduate students, have made this institution an ideal place for me to continue to learn about ethnobotany—particularly how traditional cultures have used plants for healing and to promote wellness.

My research and scholarly contributions to our understanding of tropical floras, ethnobotany, and ethnomedicine have built upon the work of others, as Isaac Newton wrote, " . . . by standing on the shoulders of giants." These giants have included my colleagues here at the Botanical Garden as well as the people I have worked with in remote field sites around the world who have helped guide my studies of plants and their uses. In addition, this group includes the remarkable collection of dedicated individuals at the Botanical Garden who support its daily operations, from upkeep of the landscape and buildings, to managing its resources, to raising awareness of its programs and administering the institution. And when my "light" (as Schweitzer called it) dims, I often find my "spark" by taking a walk through The New York Botanical Garden, enjoying the beauty of its historic landscape, its exquisite gardens, and reconnecting with nature.

A book that covers so many different topics, most of which are in a state of constant updating and evolution, can never be the work of a single individual. This book has been a community effort, building on the contributions of a previous group of authors to produce what you see in these pages. In addition, a number of people took time to review sections relevant to their specialties, kindly contributed directly to the chapters, or helped in some other way. I offer my heartfelt thanks to the following who graciously responded to my requests for guidance, wisdom, and inspiration: Mark Blumenthal and the staff of the American Botanical Council; Peggy Brevoort; Francisca Coelho; Paul Alan Cox, PhD; Mia D'Avanza; Linda S. Einbond, PhD; Margaret Falk; Fabiana N. Fonseca, PhD; Todd Forrest; Susan Fraser; Ashley Glenn; Katherine Herrera; Sara Katz; Steven R. King, PhD; Fredi Kronenberg, PhD; Daniel Kulakowski, PhD; Sally A. Leone; Gregory Long; Marie Long; Tieraona Low Dog, MD; Robert F. C. Naczi, PhD; Thomas Newmark; Emily Lewis Penn; Nancy Rutman; Stephen Sinon; Ina Vandebroek, PhD; and Andrew Weil, MD. I am deeply indebted to my family and dearest friends, who patiently understood my commitment to writing and rewriting during evenings, weekends, and vacation breaks and who offered their suggestions, answered questions, and vetted ideas for stories I wanted to tell.

The idea for this book was the result of a conversation I had in the Costa Rican rainforest with *Organic Gardening* editor-in-chief Ethne Clarke, during a Sacred Seeds meeting warmly hosted by Tom Newmark and Steven Farrell at Finca Luna Nueva. Sometimes it seems that our best ideas come during a break from normal routine, when novel thoughts can be fully explored without the limitations of busy schedules and, in this case, in a very special part of the world. A weekend brainstorming session, hosted by the book's editor, Karen Bolesta, at Rodale, outlined the shape of this book. Many thanks to Ethne and Karen for their ideas, support, and contributions, which made this project possible. And my gratitude to art director Christina Gaugler whose inspirational design and meticulous approach to photography and art make the story of herbs come alive in this volume, and to botanical illustrator Lizzie Harper for her beautiful renderings. Sincere thanks, as well, to many others who contributed their time and talent to photography and styling, nomenclature research, copyediting, layout, and indexing, including Nancy Ondra, Tom MacDonald, Paige Hicks, Hope Clarke, Erana Bumbardatore, Andrea Chesman, Keith Biery, Elizabeth Krenos, Wendy Gable, and Lina Burton.

I am particularly grateful to Vicki Mattern, who began this journey as my editor. Early on in our work together she became my coauthor as well, carefully preparing and updating significant portions of the text. This book would not be the comprehensive, rich, and joyful volume it has become without her wisdom, guidance, thoughtfulness, skilled writing, and encouragement all along the way. For those contributions I offer my most sincere gratitude and can only hope that, sometime in the future, I have the great fortune to work with her again.

Finally, my thanks to you, the reader, for your interest in nature's green treasures.

Michael J. Balick, PhD

RESOURCES

BOOKS

Burgess, Rebecca. *Harvesting Color*. New York, NY: Artisan, 2011.

Castleman, Michael. *The New Healing Herbs*. Emmaus, PA: Rodale Inc, 2009.

Hobbs, Christopher, and Leslie Gardner. *Grow It, Heal It*. Emmaus, PA: Rodale Inc, 2013.

Pitcairn, Richard H., and Susan Hubble Pitcairn. *Dr. Pitcairn's Complete Guide to Natural Health for Dogs and Cats*. Emmaus, PA: Rodale Inc, 2009.

Schlosser, Katherine K. *The Herb Society of America's Essential Guide to Growing and Cooking with Herbs*. Baton Rouge, LA: Louisiana State University Press, 2007.

Schnaubelt, Kurt. *The Healing Intelligence of Essential Oils: The Science of Advanced Aromatherapy*. Rochester, VT: Healing Arts Press, 2011.

White, Gregory Lee. *Making Soap from Scratch*. Woodstock, MD: White Willow Books, 2012.

Wulff, Mary L., and Greg Tilford. *Herbs for Pets*. Irvine, CA: Bow Tie Press, 2009.

BOTANICAL GARDENS AND ARBORETA

One of the most delightful ways to learn about herbs is to see them growing in gardens and nurseries. Many botanical gardens and arboreta have herb gardens designed to educate and inspire the public. For a list of public horticultural institutions, go to

http://en.wikipedia.org/wiki/List_of_botanical_gardens_and_arboretums_in_the_United_States.

Many botanical gardens and arboreta have Web sites rich in information of interest to herb gardeners and plant enthusiasts. For example, The New York Botanical Garden Web site is an excellent source of information on bibliographic, horticultural, and botanical research topics. Go to www.NYBG.org.

EDUCATION PROGRAMS

The organizations below offer specialized education programs about herbs, although this represents only a small fraction of the resources available to those who wish to learn more about herbs and their uses. Many universities, adult education programs, and local nurseries also offer courses on herbs.

Arizona Center for Integrative Medicine
The University of Arizona
PO Box 245153
Tucson, AZ 85724
http://integrativemedicine.arizona.edu
Founded by Andrew Weil, MD, the center focuses on education, clinical care, and research related to healing-oriented medicine, addressing mind, body, and spirit. Directory of integrative medicine practitioners.

Bastyr University
14500 Juanita Drive
Kenmore, WA 98028
(425) 602-3000 / www.bastyr.edu
This institution, devoted to natural health arts and sciences, has a certificate program in Holistic Landscape Design focused on the cultivation, aesthetic, ecological, and therapeutic attributes of medicinal and edible plants.

Maryland University of Integrative Health/Tai Sophia Institute
7750 Montpelier Road
Laurel, MD 20723
(410) 888-9048 / http://muih.edu
This institution has an academic and clinical focus on health and wellness, with programs that draw from contemporary science and traditional wisdom and includes an on-site Natural Care Center. Students can earn graduate degrees and certificates.

The New York Botanical Garden
2900 Southern Blvd
Bronx, NY 10458
(800) 322-6924 / www.NYBG.org
The NYBG Adult Education Program offers a variety of courses on herbs—from growing, to preparing, to their use in fostering wellness.

INFORMATION

American Botanical Council
PO Box 144345
Austin, TX 78714-4345
(512) 926-4900
http://abc.herbalgram.org
This organization provides accurate and reliable information on the use of medicinal plants for consumers, health-care providers, researchers, educators, industry, and the media.

American Herbalists Guild
www.americanherbalistsguild.com
The AHG Web site can help guide you to a professional herbalist and has many other resources, as well.

American Holistic Veterinary Medical Association
PO Box 630
Abingdon, MD 21009-0630
(410) 569-0795
http://ahvma.org
This association explores and supports alternative and complementary approaches to veterinary healthcare; a member directory is available at http://ahvma.org/Widgets/FindVet.html.

Dr. Duke's Phytochemical and Ethnobotanical Databases
www.ars-grin.gov/duke
This search engine compiled by James Duke, PhD, allows users to find chemical compounds, activities, and ethnobotanical uses of specific plants or to identify plants with a chosen chemical or activity. It includes links to other databases, including nutritional information.

Native American Ethnobotany Database
http://herb.umd.umich.edu
Based on the research of Daniel Moerman, PhD, this online database contains information on plants used by native peoples of North America for medicines, foods, fibers, dyes, and many other purposes.

The Herb Society of America
9019 Kirtland Chardon Road
Kirtland, OH 44094
(440) 256-0514
herbsociety.org
This group is dedicated to promoting the knowledge, use, and delight of herbs through educational programs and research, and by sharing the experience of its members with the community.

United Plant Savers
PO Box 776
Athens, OH 45701
740-742-3455
www.unitedplantsavers.org
This group seeks to protect native medicinal plants of the United States and Canada and their native habitats while ensuring a renewable supply of medicinal plants for the future.

USDA Plants Database
http://plants.usda.gov
This database compiled by the USDA Natural Resources Conservation Service provides information on North American plants, including taxonomy, growth habit, distribution, and photos.

MAIL-ORDER HERB SUPPLIERS

Horizon Herbs, LLC
PO Box 69
Williams, OR 97544
(541) 846-6704
www.horizonherbs.com

Johnny's Selected Seeds
PO Box 299
Waterville, ME 04903
(877) 564-6697
www.johnnyseeds.com/default.aspx

Mountain Rose Herbs
PO Box 50220
Eugene, OR 97405
(800) 879-3337
www.mountainroseherbs.com

Mountain Valley Growers
38325 Pepperweed Road
Squaw Valley, CA 93675
(559) 338-2775
www.mountainvalleygrowers.com

Pacific Botanicals
4840 Fish Hatchery Road
Grants Pass, OR 97527
(541) 479-7777
www.pacificbotanicals.com

San Francisco Herb Co.
250 14th Street
San Francisco, CA 94103
(800) 227-4530
www.sfherb.com

Sandy Mush Herb Nursery
316 Surrett Cove Road
Leicester, North Carolina 28748
(828) 683-2014
www.sandymushherbs.com

Well-Sweep Herb Farm
205 Mount Bethel Road
Port Murray, NJ 07865-4147
(908) 852-5390
www.wellsweep.com

Richters
357 Highway 47
Goodwood, ON
L0C 1A0
Canada
(905) 640-6677
www.richters.com

PHOTOGRAPHY CREDITS

All photography by Steven Foster, except the following:

Tom MacDonald/Rodale Images: pages ii, vi, 1, 3, 70, 74, 78, 310, 313, 316, 319, 320, 322–24, 326, 327, 329, 331, 334, 335, 337, 339, 366, 367, 370, 376, 377, 379, 382, 384, 386, 388, 392, 398, 403, 406, 411, and 428

Michael Balick: pages xiii, 10, 41, 73, 127, 141, 158 (bottom), 163, 186, 187, 209 (left), 223, 235, 238, 292, 298, and 430

Courtesy of Weil Lifestyle: page ix

Katherine Herrera/NYBG: page xi

Shutterstock/C Sa: page 7

Courtesy of National Library of Medicine: page 8

Getty Images: pages 11, 27, 315, and 341

Shutterstock/Rolf_52: page 15

Colourbox/Rostislav Ageev: page 17

The LuEsther T. Mertz Library of The New York Botanical Garden, Bronx, New York: pages 21 and 24

University Library, Leipzig, Germany /Archives Charmet/ The Bridgeman Art Library: page 26

123RF Stock Photo: page 94

Rooibos Ltd.: page 111

Shutterstock: pages 131 (left), 132, and 244

istock: page 155 (left)

Max Licher: page 197

Imageflora: page 252

Vicki Mattern: page 300

Rolv Hjelmstad: page 301

Shutterstock/gorillaimages: page 318

Mitch Mandel/Rodale Images: page 330

Getty Images/Emilie Duchesne: page 336 (right)

Getty Images/Asri' rie: page 336 (left)

Reed Rahn: page 342

Photodisc: page 361

Shutterstock/itakefotos4u: page 403

Shutterstock/Mat Hayward: page 405

Christa Neu: page 412

Sara Katz: page 413

Getty Images/Dan Moore: page 414

Patrick Montero: page 423

Rodale Images: page 424

Shutterstock/Nadia Borisevich: page 425

Robert Cardillo: pages 427 and 432

Shutterstock/Maria Gaellman: page 435

Matthew Benson: page 439

INDEX

Boldface page numbers indicate photographs or illustrations. <u>Underscored</u> references indicate boxed text, charts, and graphs.

Sage (*cont.*)

garden (*cont.*)

using for skin and hair care, 373

Mexican bush (*S. leucantha*)

in Silver Terrace Garden, 462, **463**

purple (*S. officinalis* 'Purpurascens')

in "Grand Opening" Entryway Garden, **456**, 457

in Kitchen Herb Garden, 446, **447**

silver (*S. argentea*)

in Silver Terrace Garden, 462, **463**

Sakau (*Piper methysticum*), 232–33, **232**, **233**

Salad burnet (burnet) (*Sanguisorba minor*), 262, **262**

Salix alba (willow, white willow), 256, **256**

Salves, 367, **367**, 369

Salvia argentea (silver sage)

in Silver Terrace Garden, 462, **463**

Salvia leucantha (Mexican bush sage)

in Silver Terrace Garden, 462, **463**

Salvia officinalis (sage, garden sage), **48**, 257–58, **258**

as healing herb, 348–49

in Healing Herb Garden, 448, **449**

purple (*S. officinalis* 'Purpurascens')

in "Grand Opening" Entryway Garden, **456**, 457

in Kitchen Herb Garden, 446, **447**

in Spiritual Retreat Garden, 464, **465**

using for skin and hair care, 373

Salvia sclarea (clary, clary sage, muscatel sage), **48**, 259, **259**

essential oil from, 358

in Garden for Fragrance and Beauty, 450, **451**

Sambucus canadensis (elder, black elder, elderberry, North American elder, elder flower), 260, **260**

as healing herb, 346–47

Sambucus nigra (elder, black elder, European elder, elderberry, elder flower), 260, **260**

in Four-Season Woodland Border, 458, 458–59

as healing herb, 346–47

in Healing Herb Garden, 448, **449**

Sambucus spp. (elder, black elder, elderberry, elder flower)

as dyeing herb, 399

using for skin and hair care, 372

Sanguinaria canadensis (bloodroot, red paint root, red puccoon), 261, **261**

as dyeing herb, 399

in Four-Season Woodland Border, 458, **458**

Sanguisorba minor (burnet, salad burnet), 262, **262**

Santolina, green (*Santolina virens*)

in A Formal Knot Garden, 442, **443**

Santolina chamaecyparissus (lavender cotton)

in A Formal Knot Garden, 442, **443**

Saponaria officinalis (soapwort, bouncing bet), 263, **263**

in Garden for Birds and Butterflies, 454, **455**

in Spiritual Retreat Garden, 464, **465**

Sassafras (*Sassafras albidum*), 264, **264**

in Four-Season Woodland Border, 458, **459**

Satureja hortensis (summer savory), 265, **265**

Satureja montana (winter savory)

creeping winter savory (*S. montana* ssp. *illyrica*)

in Rock Wall Herb Garden, 460, **461**

Savory (*Satureja*)

creeping winter (*S. montana* spp. *illyrica*)

in Rock Wall Herb Garden, 460, **461**

summer (*Satureja hortensis*), 265, **265**

Saw palmetto (*Serenoa repens*), 267, 267, **267**

Scabwort (*Inula helenium*), 189, **189**

Scale, 436

Scarification, 416, 418

"Science of Life." *See* Ayurveda

Scouring rush (*Equisetum arvense*), 164, **164**

Scrubs

household, 386

from nature, 389

for skin, 376

Seafood

herbs and spices and, 330–31

pairings with herbs and spices, 333

Seasonal tasks, 438

Season extension, 426

Sedge, cinnamon (*Acorus calamus*), 84, **84**

Sedum 'Dragon's Blood' (*Sedum spurium*)

in Rock Wall Herb Garden, 460, **461**

Seedlings

growing healthy, 416

hardening off, 416

transplanting, 416, **416**, 421–22

Seeds

harvesting, 433–34

morphology and, 56–58, **57**

propagation by, 414–16, 415, **415**, 418

indoors, 415, **415**, 415–16

outdoors, 414–15

special sowing techniques for, 416, 418

Self-heal (*Prunella vulgaris*), 242, **242**

Self-medication, cautions about, 81